AIDS
The Crime Beyond Belief

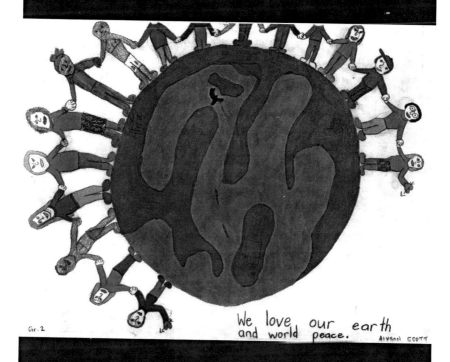

We love our earth and world peace.

William L. C. Scott & Donald W. Scott

Box 133, Station B,
Sudbury, Canada P3E 4N5
705-673-0726

Canadian Cataloguing - in - Publication Data:
Scott, William L.C.1955 -
Scott, Donald W. 1924 -

AIDS

1. Epidemiology - Popular works 2. Communicable diseases - Popular works 3. Kennedy, John F. (Fitzgerald), 1917 - 1963 - Assassination 4. United States - Politics and Government 5. AIDS 6. CIA - (Central Intelligence Agency)

l. TITLE

Copyright © William L.C. Scott and Donald W. Scott

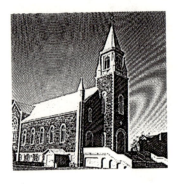

The Chelmsford Publishers
Box 133, Station B
Sudbury, Ontario
P3E 4N5

Marketing and Distribution:

Executive Services Limited
30 Brodie Avenue,
Sudbury, Ontario P3C 3M8
Canada
705-673-0726
wlcscott@yahoo.ca

All rights reserved. No parts of this book may be reproduced in any form or by any electronic or mechanical means, including information storage and retrieval systems, without permission in writing from the authors, except by a reviewer who may quote brief passages in a review.

Books

by William L. C. Scott and Donald W. Scott

Medical/Scientific/Historical

The Extremely Unfortunate Skull Valley Incident

The Brucellosis Triangle

Life: From Plants to Animals to Us

Amyotrophic Lateral Sclerosis

By Donald W. Scott

Medical/Scientific/Historical

Steve's Dream Catcher

Literary

Gertrude: Queene of Denmark

Hamlet: A Guide to Study

Paradise Lost: A Guide to Study

Celebrating Sudbury

The Twist (A play in three acts)

Order this book online at www.trafford.com/07-2675
or email orders@trafford.com

Most Trafford titles are also available at major online book retailers.

© Copyright 2007 William L. C. Scott & Donald W. Scott.
All rights reserved. No part of this publication may be reproduced, stored in a retrieval system, or transmitted, in any form or by any means, electronic, mechanical, photocopying, recording, or otherwise, without the written prior permission of the author.

Note for Librarians: A cataloguing record for this book is available from Library and Archives Canada at www.collectionscanada.ca/amicus/index-e.html

ISBN: 978-1-4251-4157-8

We at Trafford believe that it is the responsibility of us all, as both individuals and corporations, to make choices that are environmentally and socially sound. You, in turn, are supporting this responsible conduct each time you purchase a Trafford book, or make use of our publishing services. To find out how you are helping, please visit www.trafford.com/responsiblepublishing.html

Our mission is to efficiently provide the world's finest, most comprehensive book publishing service, enabling every author to experience success. To find out how to publish your book, your way, and have it available worldwide, visit us online at www.trafford.com/10510

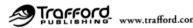 www.trafford.com

North America & international
toll-free: 1 888 232 4444 (USA & Canada)
phone: 250 383 6864 ♦ fax: 250 383 6804 ♦ email: info@trafford.com

The United Kingdom & Europe
phone: +44 (0)1865 722 113 ♦ local rate: 0845 230 9601
facsimile: +44 (0)1865 722 868 ♦ email: info.uk@trafford.com

10 9 8 7 6 5 4 3 2 1

AIDS
Acquired Immune Deficiency Syndrome

The Crime Beyond Belief

DEEP POLITICS OF THE UNITED STATES OF AMERICA

> "Thus I now refer to parapolitics as only one manifestation of *deep politics*, all those political practices and arrangements, deliberate or not, which are usually *repressed* rather than acknowledged."
>
> Peter Dale Scott; **Deep Politics and the Death of JFK** (Page 7)

One cannot study any major aspect of North American medicine of this age without concurrently studying economics and politics.

The Chelmsford Publishers in co-operation with Trafford Publishers

In Memoriam

The authors are grateful to the investors who have helped us publish *AIDS: The Crime Beyond Belief*. As an expression of our thanks, we list those investors and honour the memories of the following special people that they have nominated:

Armi Laine
April 1932 - December 2001

"A quiet, gentle man who loved and was loved by many"

Marlene A. Johnson & W. "Gus" Mazzuchin

Robert D. Popp
1919 - 2005

"A long career in high school teaching and preparing young people for a good future."

Mr. and Mrs. Harold W. Clark

Thomas McPherson Brown
1906 - 1989

"Author of *The Road Back - Rheumatoid Arthritis - Its Cause and its Treatment,* Professor of Medicine, Department Chairman, Developer of the antibiotic (tetracycline) treatment of rheumatoid diseases."

Mr. and Mrs. Harold W. Clark

John Gerard Laurian
April 1919 - December 1996

"The Golden Rule was his motto, for those he loved and respected. His goal was first things first - God, Family and Country. He gave himself completely to his beloved family, his Church and his nation. We thank God for him and his guidance during the perilous journey in seeking answers to our devastating local, national and world problems."

Peggy (Margaret) Laurian, Peggy, Linda, Jack and Vickie Lou

Garnett Carson
January 1968 - July 2006

"I would like to dedicate the publishing of this book to the authors who have diligently uncovered the truth. And also to the memory of my son Garnett and all others who struggle with health issues."

Victoria L. Dobson

Antonio Maiello
March 1907 - April 1982

"Until the day I die I will never forget the tears that came down from the eyes of your immobilized and speechless body as I as a very little boy made facial expressions of you."

Michael Pengue

DEDICATION

Dedicated to the late **Harold W. Clark**, Ph.D.,
Professor Emeritus George Washington University (Retired),
with profound respect and sincere affection.

First Edition

This first edition is limited to 2,000 copies,

of which this is number _____.

_____   _____
William L.C. Scott   Donald W. Scott

Contents

Books	iii
In Memoriam	vi
PREFACE	xvii
PRINCIPAL THESIS	xix
Contributing Theses	xix
The Mycoplasma Species	xx
A brief note on style and organization	xx
FOREWORD	xxiii
How We Began	xxiv
THE BACKGROUND	xxix
Part One: Holding A Patent On Death	xxix
PART ONE—The Discovery	1
Chapter One	3
The Profit Paradigm: From OIL to AIDS	3
AIDS: The Crime Beyond Belief	4
Section 1: Parsing our title: "AIDS - The Crime Beyond Belief"	4
Section 2: Nocard and Roux	8
Section 3: The Pathogenic Mycoplasma	8
Section 4: Hidden in Plain Sight: Holding a Patent on Death	9
Koch's Postulates; Pity the Poor Chimpanzee; Perhaps Dr. Lo's cited References Will Help; Dr. Lo Admits to an Error; Enough Already!	
Section 5: The Confluence of AIDS, CFS/ME and the murder of a President	18
Section 6: U.S. Military Medicine and the Uniformed Services University of Health Sciences	26
Section 7: The Concept of Co-Factors	28
Section 8. Dr. Ishii Shiro	29
Section 9: Dr. D. Carleton Gajdusek	35
Section 10: The Central Intelligence Agency (Part One)	47
Section 11: Luc Montagnier	49
Section 12: Monkey Kidneys	52
Section 13: Baylor College of Medicine	53
Chapter Two	57
The CIA plus Monkey Kidneys equals MKULTRA, MKDELTA and MKNAOMI	57

The Unelected Elite	62
The Central Intelligence Agency from 1952 until 1960	66
Iran	67
Guatemala	68
Vietnam	69
Belgian Congo	70
Cuba	72
Back to MKULTRA and its Subprojects	74
The Other Side of the AIDS Coin	76
Socio-Political	82

PART TWO—The Development and Testing of Pathogenic Co-Factors — 85

Chapter Three — 87
Robert Huebner and the Coughing Recruits — 87
Summary — 92

Chapter Four — 93
Bjorn Sigurdsson…Scrapie and Retroviral Diseases — 93
Summary — 97

Chapter Five — 99
Hilary Koprowski — 99
The Moribund Wistar… — 99
Solving the Polio Problem as a Cover for Co-factor Testing — 99
Summary — 105

Chapter Six — 107
The Henles — 107
Just Love Those Kids to Death — 107
Summary — 112

Chapter Seven — 115
The Belgians and the Portuguese — 115
Those Pesky Black Nationalists — 115
Belgium, the Congo and HIV-1 — 117
Portugal, Guinea-Bissau, Goa, Brazil and HIV-2 — 119
Summary — 120

Chapter Eight — 123
Testing bioweapons — 123
Postscript — 128

PART THREE—Deep Politics and the Murder of JFK — 129

Chapter Nine — 131
Shadow Government and Deep Politics — 131
November 22, 1963—Darkness at High Noon in Dallas: — 134

The murder of John F. Kennedy	134
The Central Intelligence Agency (Part Two)	135
The U.S. Military/Joint Chiefs of Staff	136
Israel and Ben Gurion	136
The French Military Algerian Faction	137
The Establishment	138
The Mafia	139
J. Edgar Hoover and the FBI	140
Richard Case Nagell	140
Some geographic sites you should know about	141
Cold Spring Harbor Laboratory; Plum Island	
Summary	143

Chapter Ten — 145
The Murder of JFK	145
Postscript	198

Chapter Eleven — 207
David Ferrie	207
The Nexus of the Assassination of JFK	
and the Development of AIDS; Tracy Barnes; E. Howard Hunt	207
The Canadian Connections:	
Pershing Gervais and James Earl Ray come to Canada	207

Chapter Twelve — 217
Lyndon Johnson 1963 - 1968	217
Johnson, Population Control	217
and the murder of President Kennedy (and AIDS)	217
Johnson, Population Control and AIDS	220
Martin Luther King	223
Robert Francis Kennedy	223

PART FOUR—The Deployment — 225

Chapter Thirteen — 227
1966: WHO is working on Smallpox?	227
Trade Your Old Diseases for New	227
Summary	229

Chapter Fourteen — 233
VO to SVLP to SVCP to VCP to HTLV	233
From Cancer to Lymphadenopathy and back to Cancer	233
Now that we've beaten Polio, let's tackle Cancer	233
The Special Virus Cancer Program	233
Gajdusek and Gallo…and Litton Industries	238
From VO to SVLP to SVCP to VCP by way of HTLV	244
From Cancer to Leukemia/Lymphadenopathy and back to Cancer	244

Chapter Fifteen — 249

- November 1968: Enter Nixon and Agnew…Stage Right — 249
- Henry Kissinger — 251
- AIDS: And the Deep Politics of the United States of America — 260
- The Nixon Presidency — 262
- The Election of 1968 — Richard Nixon and AIDS — 264
- June 9, 1969 — 264
- North Atlantic Treaty Organization (NATO)— — 275
- The CIA's Overseas Arm — 275
- National Security Study Memorandum - 200 (NSSM-200) — 276
- E. Howard Hunt: Foot Soldier in the Hidden War — 278
- The Election of 1972 — Watergate — 287
- 1975: Exit Agnew and Nixon…Stage Right — 294

Chapter Sixteen — 297

- Gerald Ford — 297
- Pardon? — 297
- Nelson Rockefeller — 298
- From the CIA basement to the Oval Office by Proxy — 298
  - Revealing CIA Mis-deeds
- Jimmy Carter — 299
- Back to MKULTRA — 301
- Ronald Reagan in the White House; William Casey in the CIA — 306
  - AIDS: Officially on the Record; Assassination Attempt
- George H. W. Bush and the First Gulf War — 308
- Let's start with the First Gulf War — 309
  - Saddam Gets Suckered In
- The First Gulf War — 313
- Gulf War Illnesses and the Riegle Report — 314
  - Captain Louise Richard; Defeat of the U.S.-led Coalition in the First Gulf War; Major Timothy Cook
- President William (Bill) Clinton — 340
  - Back to the Paradigm: Get Control of the Gulf OIL; Gulf War Mark Two; Special Flights to Saudi Arabia
- The Krever Commission — 347
  - The Whole Truth — Up to a Point
- Financing the CIA: Bre-X — 354
  - Bre-X: Do you wonder where the money went?; The CIA Tries Free Enterprise, and Finds that it Works!; Kissinger the Venal; First to the Freeport Story; The Précis; Days of Living Dangerously; Fast Forward to 1975; When Shall We Three Meet Again?; 1988; Unthinkable Thoughts; Another 1994 Item; Enter an Australian Spook; Good Corporate Citizenship; Back to Bre-X Basics; Enter J. P. Morgan; Sorting Out Who's On First The Phone Cal; Hypothesis; Bre-X: A Postscript

PART FIVE—World Health — 375

Chapter Seventeen — 377
AIDS, CFS, and Collateral Damage: — 377
The Common Cause — 377
Part One: AIDS and CFS — 377
   Robert Gallo and AIDS; Brian Mahy and CFS/ME
Collateral Damage — 389
   An overview of the pathogenic effects of the mycoplasma as a factor or co-factor in various diseases; the potential for damage to the human body by certain species of mycoplasma: a summary review; The Common Cause Hypothesis; Fritz Haber (1868 -1934)

PART SIX—The Media — 405

Chapter Eighteen — 407
The Media: Introduction — 407
The Dana-Farber Cancer Institute — 413
Media and Science Magazine — 417
   Enter Jean W. Pape, *et al.*; The Dog and Pony Show
A Special Report to The Journal of Degenerative Diseases — 429
A brief burst of reality almost spoils 'feel good' parade — 429
Denis St. Pierre Reports the News — 432

PART SEVEN—The Dawning Of Awareness — 437
Introduction — 439

Chapter Nineteen — 443
Hillary Johnson: A Prose of Reportorial Calm — 443
Tahoe-Truckee High School — 445
Lyndonville, New York — 446
Doctors Daniel Peterson and Paul Cheney — 446
Doctors David and Karen Bell — 450
Dr. Elaine DeFreitas — 451
The Kingston to St. Lawrence Valley 'Mystery Disease' of 1984 — 453

Chapter Twenty — 455
Edward Hooper: Enthusiasm and Good Counsel In Equal Measure — 455

Chapter Twenty-One — 459
Engage the Enemy — 459
Donald Gibson — 459
The Links to Watergate — 462
   The Johnson Shambles and the Presidential Elections of 1968

Chapter Twenty-Two — 467
Avian Flu…A Cautionary Tale — 467
An Analogy — 503

PART EIGHT — 507
The Scientific Paper Trail to AIDS — 507

Chapter Twenty-Three — 509
From Rosebury and Kabat to Eternity — 509
The Chemical and Research Paper Trail of AIDS — 509
The Concept of a Paper Trail - Part One — 511
  Ms. Shirley Bentley
The Concept of a Paper Trail - Part Two — 517
  Robert E. Lee
The Concept of a Paper Trail - Part Three — 519
  Ms. Candace Brown
The Concept of a Paper Trail - Part Four — 520
  Ms. Sue Oleksyn
Pre- and Post-1953 Research — 523
  Pre-1953 Research
  Post-1953 Research

PART NINE—As It Might Be: On Telling the Truth — 583
The Eternal Struggle: — 583
Authority versus Reason — 583

Chapter Twenty-Four — 585
The 9/11 Fraud — 585
 Mohamed Atta's movements on — 587
September 10 and September 11 — 587
President George W. Bush — 591
and $30 Billion for AIDS — 591
To control Health is to control Death...And make Money — 591
There are Many Battles, but only One War — 593
Authority versus Reason — 595
Christopher Hitchins — 595
Al Gore — 599
The Internet — 600
Dichloroacetate - DCA Two Cancers;Two Protocols; Two Outcomes — 602
Two Cancers; Two Protocols; Two Outcomes — 602
Two cancers; Two protocols; Two outcomes continued — 604
Medicine, Money and Health — 605
The Cancer Industry — 605
The AIDS Industry — 607
The Nexus of the Cancer Industry and the AIDS Industry — 610
SOUTH AFRICA — 613
AIDS: The Crime Beyond Belief — 614
Re-Birth of Democracy — 616
AIDS:The Limits of Belief/Disbelief — 617

EPILOGUE
619
    The Complete Paradigm of Life:
    623

APPENDICES
625
    Exhibit ONE
    627
    Exhibit TWO
    628
    Exhibit THREE
    629
    Exhibit FOUR
    630
    Exhibit FIVE
    631

BIBLIOGRAPHY
633
    Secondary Sources
    635
    Primary Sources A
    644
        Articles reporting critical research
    Primary Sources B
    646
        United States Government Documents; Isaiah 40; 1 Timothy 6

INDEX
649

PREFACE

The late J. S. McLean, founder of Canada Packers Limited, had a recipe for mince meat. This was not the sort of recipe one can find in monthly homemaking magazines, but was the recipe for the large-scale manufacture of mince meat. At a certain point in each year, tons of apples, currents, molasses, suet and other ingredients had to be combined and cooked, then canned, labeled and packed in boxes for shipment to food outlets in time for Thanksgiving and Christmas Holiday meals.

Only one man of record had the full recipe, J. S. McLean himself.

The recipe for the annual manufacturing operation was divided into something like five or six parts. Each part was entrusted to a Superintendent who was pledged to secrecy and who was charged with the responsibility for bringing together the required elements in the required sequence, form and amount and to supervise the blending of these elements until his part of the recipe was complete. At that point the superintendent would leave the cooking area and he would be followed by the next of the chosen few, each of whom would, in turn, do his part of the job. It is claimed that none of the five or six superintendents knew each other and each had only his particular part of the total recipe.

When each superintendent had completed his part of the enterprise, he returned his portion of the recipe to the safe in J. S. McLean's office until it was required the following year.

This analogy bears some resemblance to the history of the bringing together of all the elements involved in the discovery, development and deployment of the pathogenic co-factors which together result in the world-wide scourge of acquired immunodeficiency syndrome.

Thousands of people world-wide, but principally in the United States of America, contributed their talents to produce the pathogenic agents by which the terrible disease was communicated initially to selected victims for the purpose of limiting the rate at which the world's population was growing. Only a very small and self-selecting core knew what was going on and for what reason. Others may have had some inkling, but their knowledge was sufficiently amorphous and the risks to their well being sufficiently suspect as to limit any possible inclination to make public their suspicions.

This book presents in a clear and simplified form the process by which the pathogenic co-factors which present as acquired immunodeficiency syndrome have come into the human family. It involves the historical, scientific, political, medical, industrial, sociological, economic, financial, philosophical, military and, *overriding all else*, the *ethical* elements that enter into the mix.

Now, as with J. S. McLean and his mince meat recipe, you will have the full recipe for AIDS.

PRINCIPAL THESIS

The authors propose that, based upon the facts presented herein, the syndrome of disease symptoms which present as a consequence of an acquired deficiency of the human immune system, is principally caused by the action of a species of cholesterol-dependent mycoplasma in concurrence with the retroviral action of the zoonotic visna-derived lentivirus and/or other 'opportunistic' pathogens which present as Kaposi's sarcoma, *Pneumocystis carinii* pneumonia, diarrhea, dementia, lymphadenopathy, wasting, and various other endocrine-based disorders.

Contributing Theses

1. The up-take of pre-formed sterols, including cholesterol, by certain species of mycoplasma reduces cellular membrane integrity, and alters most endocrine-based metabolic activity, such as hormone production.
2. The reduction of cellular membrane integrity leads to cell death and hence reduces the production of essential neurotransmitters such as glutamate and other enzymes and may present as Parkinson's disease, diabetes type one etc.
3. The immune-suppressing mycoplasma without the visna-derived retrovirus or other opportunistic infections may present as chronic fatigue syndrome (CFS) or 'HIV'-negative AIDS.
4. The immune-suppressing mycoplasma together with the visna derived retroviral co-factor presents as an acquired deficiency of immunity. AIDS
5. Reduced human immunity opens the way for various opportunistic diseases such as Kaposi's sarcoma, Pneumoniae carinii pneumonia (PCP), dementia, etc. to present in victims.
6. Cellular damage also causes various collateral diseases such as cancer.

The Mycoplasma Species

It is critical to the understanding of the Principal Thesis of this study that the reader is aware of the *Mycoplasmas* and the role they play in human disease.

Mycoplasmas are the smallest and simplest self-replicating microorganisms lacking a cell wall, which appear to have originated from walled bacteria by degenerative evolution. Mycoplasmas have been discovered in plants, insects, and animals including humans. Rottem, *et al.* have demonstrated that certain species of mycoplasmas have an absolute growth requirement for the up-take of pre-formed sterols, including cholesterol. The impact upon cholesterol supply affects hormone generation, external and internal cell-wall integrity, cellular and humeral immune function, cellular metabolism, and hematopoiesis. These effects in turn present as factors or co-factors in health challenges such as AIDS, ALS, Crohn's, diabetes type one, Gulf War illnesses, Huntington's, lymphadenopathy, lupus, Lyme disease, multiple sclerosis, Parkinson's, rheumatoid arthritis, sarcoidosis, schizophrenia and Wegener's disease. Mycoplasmas thus represent extremely dangerous human health challenges that have been under-reported by the United States public health agencies to the end that their role in such diseases is essentially unknown to the average health professional and to the public at large. The natural etiological consequences of mycoplasmal infections have been augmented by U.S. Government biological research and testing dating especially from 1952 and by various national and international vaccination programs in the same period.

Refer to Appendices, Exhibit One. Popular medical dicta have it that the mycoplasmas are relatively minor factors in disease etiology. This exhibit suggests the falsity of such a claim.

A brief note on style and organization

To the extent possible, given the mix of so many elements that enter into the story of how AIDS came into the human family and how that family responded (politically, philosophically, ethically, financially, historically, scientifically, biologically, medically, and legally) we have attempted to present the evidence in chronological order. However, at times we have departed from that order with a clearly designated **'Interlude'** wherein we elaborate on some critical factor for the benefit of those readers who may not previously have associated that factor with AIDS. Also, at certain points we have inserted **'Exhibits'** along with a commentary, which deals with the scientific paper trail involved, placed against a background of the above list of factors. Finally, at various points we have used a simplistic **'Analogy'** also clearly designated, because we want to reach as wide an audience as is possible and not limit that audience to those who have a knowledge of the obscure jargon often utilized by professionals. We employ analogies that communicate the essence of an idea without using the usual obscure technical terminology.

FOREWORD

The acronym AIDS is made up of the first letters of the words in the phrase 'acquired immune deficiency syndrome' or sometimes 'acquired immunodeficiency syndrome.'

According to many medical history reference books AIDS was identified as a specific disease entity in **1981**. And therein lies our first anomaly. There was an earlier phrase that was strikingly similar to the one now in use to label the horrible epidemic that is killing over 8000 people a day. The earlier phrase appeared in **1971** when it was used by two medical researchers who were working at the Stanford University School of Medicine in California! The two researchers were Thomas C. Merigan and David A. Stevens. They had used the phrase in the title of an article published in the November-December issue of *Federation Proceedings* "Viral infections in man associated with *acquired immunological deficiency states.*" Note the acronym formed from the italicized phrase: AIDS. How does it happen that ten years before there was such an entity as **AIDS**, Drs. Merigan and Stevens were able to write about AIDS? Was it just a co-incidence, or is there more here than meets the eye?

To answer this question we will have to take a look at who the people were that coined the acronym and what they were involved in. And, we'll have to look at the institutions that were involved. What were they up to? Who was paying them and with whom were they working and for what reason? However, before we answer these and other questions, here is another strange thing about AIDS that the reader needs to know at the outset.

On **June 9, 1969**, Dr. Donald MacArthur of the Pentagon met in secret with a small group of Congressmen who were on a deep secret committee that monitored the work being done by the United States *in the field of biological and chemical weapons development.* They were gathered to approve the Congressional Black Budget items for the coming fiscal year: 1970. It is important to note this meeting because it means that the development of biowar agents was an official U.S. Government activity. It wasn't just a group of rogue lunatics abusing positions of power. *The Government of the United States as represented by the elected Congressmen of the American people was and still is heavily involved in finding ways to kill and maim human beings in order to advance Government policies and objectives.* As a consequence, the American people themselves are culpable in mass murder, for it was and is their agents who were then and are now doing the dirty work.

On June 9, 1969, Pentagon representative Dr. MacArthur told the peoples' representatives the following: "There are two things about the biological agent field I would like to mention. One is the possibility of technological surprise. Molecular biology is a field that is advancing very rapidly, and eminent biologists believe that within a period of 5 to 10 years it would be possible to produce a synthetic biological agent, an agent that does not naturally exist and for which **no natural immunity could have been acquired!** That's an 'acquired immune deficiency state'… AIDS!

We'll develop this critical June 9, 1969 meeting in Chapter Fifteen.

How We Began

In 1996 one of the authors [DWS] had the great good fortune to find Hillary Johnson's magnificent study of chronic fatigue syndrome, *Osler's Web*, in our local bookstore. I was just beginning my study of this terrible disease and a glance through the book made it apparent that it was an essential resource in my research. I bought it and read it over three times; each time finding new insights initially over-looked.

In a tone of reportorial calm, Ms. Johnson, herself a victim of CFS, traced the evolution of the disease from early 1983 through to July 19, 1995, when she reported:

> "…[Stephen] Straus responded in writing to a question posed to him through a public affairs officer at the National Institute of Allergy and Infectious Diseases. (He had refused all interview requests since 1987.) "I remain committed to helping resolve the numerous complex problems that chronic fatigue syndrome presents to its many sufferers," Straus wrote, "and foresee active involvement in the field for years to come."

The significance and irony of this statement will only be apparent to those who have read the preceding 684 pages of *Osler's Web* where the insidious intransigence of Stephen Straus and many of his colleagues in the National Institutes of Health and the Centers for Disease Control is developed. Hillary Johnson doesn't say it in so many words, but it is obvious that Straus and a whole range of others such as Robert Gallo, Robert Huebner, and Hilary Koprowski had something to hide. As Johnson's sub-title makes clear ['Inside of the Labyrinth of the Chronic Fatigue Syndrome Epidemic'] the N.I.H., the C.D.C., the United States Military and elements of the United States Government, have a need to obscure the truth about chronic fatigue syndrome.

In the course of my continuing research into myalgic encephalomyelitis, and after I had recruited the research talents of my son, William L.C. Scott, to help me in this endeavor, I had the further good fortune to discover Edward Hooper's equally magnificent book, *The River*.

In *The River*, Hooper does for AIDS what Johnson had done for ME: he traces the course of the disease from the trickling source of its earliest victims to the tragic epidemic sea of death, which it has become. He has tracked down and interviewed as many of those persons who were involved in treating and reporting upon AIDS as he could locate. And something strange has become apparent: most of Hooper's major players in the AIDS epidemic are the same players that we met earlier in Johnson's chronicle of ME!

Suddenly Johnson's statement about ME on page 95 of her book took on new meaning. Johnson had reported the findings of biochemist Susan Wormsley's 1985 research, which showed that "M/E [CFS] was the mirror image of AIDS."

Was there a link between these two new diseases, both of which had appeared in growing numbers in the late 1970's and early 1980's; both of which had 'no known cause'; both of which presented with an immune system dysfunction; and, both of which had no known cure?

The tragic answer that we have found over our twelve years of research is the same for all of these questions and that answer is "Yes". In *AIDS: The Crime Beyond Belief* we present our evidence. And, in presenting that evidence we want to express our profound respect for the wonderful work of Hillary Johnson and Edward Hooper. We and the whole world owe them our gratitude.

William L.C. Scott and Donald W. Scott, September 3, 2007

We began our research with a study of chronic fatigue syndrome [CFS], which began to appear in North America, Europe and Australia/New Zealand in epidemic proportions in the early 1980s. This study led us almost immediately into the labyrinth of acquired immunodeficiency syndrome [AIDS], the mirror-image of CFS, which began to appear principally in Africa (following an initial program begun in the 1950s and continued by a huge smallpox vaccination project by the World Health Organization [WHO] in 1968 and among the gay male population of the United States (following a free hepatitis vaccination program by the U.S. Government) in 1976. The advent of the AIDS epidemic was formally placed in the peer-reviewed medical literature with an article written by Dr. Michael Gottlieb, et al. and published in December 1981, by *The New England Journal of Medicine*.

Our continuing research into AIDS/CFS led us to a Patent of a '*Pathogenic Mycoplasma*' held by the American Institute of Pathology. This Patent whose principal investigator was Dr. Shyh-Ching Lo, asserted that "Patients infected with the *Mycoplasma fermentans* will be patients who have been diagnosed with AIDS or ARC, chronic fatigue syndrome..." and directed our attention to the species of micro-organism known as the 'Mycoplasmas'.

The mycoplasma soon became the key to our further study of AIDS and CFS and the list of diagnoses in Dr. Lo's Patent. To the latter list we were able from our search of the literature to add other diseases including but not limited to fibromyalgia, diabetes type one, amyotrophic lateral sclerosis, Parkinson's disease and cancer as diseases wherein the mycoplasma played a major part.

This latter reality brought us to the realization that the newly-patented 'mycoplasma' had been recognized as a potential population growth-rate control agent as early as 1953 and used in preliminary programs operated by the CIA. It was brought into mainstream U.S. Government research when the NIH established a Mycoplasma Laboratory under the direction of Dr. Leonard Hayflick, and revealed on June 9, 1969, when Dr. Donald MacArthur of the Pentagon secretly briefed several 'black-budget' Congressmen about research being done by the United States military into a '*new micro-organism that might be refractory to the human immune system.*' This description fitted the description of the mycoplasma, and made it dramatically clear that the pathogens responsible for AIDS and CFS were biologically engineered products of American laboratories and that these laboratories were working under the direction of certain factions of the United States Government. This latter realization tied our research into the politics of the U.S. and especially to the U.S. Government document known as NSSM 200 by Henry Kissinger on the need to limit the rate of world population growth. *AIDS and CFS would help achieve that objective if the pathogens responsible for them were widely disseminated among target populations in vaccines such as smallpox and hepatitis.* The evidence demonstrates that the contaminated vaccination programs began in the 1950s on a random test basis, were taken from CIA covert programs to a larger expanded program under the U.S. Agency for International Development in the early 1960s under Lyndon Johnson. The major 'smallpox' vaccination programs were undertaken in 1968 and the seeds of the AIDS epidemics were loosed into the human family. The crime beyond belief!

This book is a summary of our research. Don't 'believe it' and don't 'disbelieve it'. Just read the evidence, and then let your reason, further reading and conscience guide you.

THE BACKGROUND

PART ONE: HOLDING A PATENT ON DEATH

AIDS: Acquired Immune Deficiency Syndrome: A pattern of symptoms, which follow upon an induced compromise of a living organism's ability to resist disease. Popular mythology, promoted by certain social, political, defense and health interests primarily in the United States of America, but aided and abetted by factions in Great Britain, Canada, Australia, and Israel contend that the major compromise of human immunity which appeared in the 1970s principally among the native population of Africa and concurrently among homosexual men in New York, San Francisco and Los Angeles, was a natural transmission of an immune deficiency virus from certain non-human primate species to humans by accidental infection. The cited interests further contend that this deficiency was rapidly communicated by the migration of peoples from rural to urban centers, by increased ease of international travel, by a reduction of sexual mores, and by intravenous drug use.

A study of the evidence available but very hard to access in U.S. government documents, peer-reviewed medical and scientific articles, and historical records demonstrates that the compromise of the human immune system in the 1970s had its origins in scientific research rooted initially in the eugenics philosophy of a few wealthy American and British families and given a critical boost in 1952 when the election of Dwight D. Eisenhower brought elements of these factions into powerful positions within the new administration. These factions essentially co-opted population control as an official challenge to America.

The research of the eugenics advocates became a major concern of the C.I.A. and the defense Department. Initially conducted as a covert program under the umbrella program known by the cryptonym MKULTRA, with sub-programs known as MKDELTA and MKNAOMI, the covert efforts became more public when witting eugenist Lyndon B. Johnson succeeded anti-population control advocate, John F. Kennedy. Johnson established under U.S. government auspices, a Special Virus Leukemia/Lymphoma Program to advance the research.

The science of immune suppression was launched with the work of Dr. Robert Huebner who, in the 1940s had re-discovered the disease microorganism originally discovered by French scientists, Nocard and Roux of the Pasteur Institute in 1898 and labeled by them as a *Mycoplasma*. The *mycoplasma*, of which there are now several known species, as a particle of bacterial nucleic acid causes a severe reduction of human immunity by promoting the degeneration of certain immune system cells (principally lymph cells). When united as a co-factor with a zoonotic retrovirus of sheep popularly known as scrapie but more technically as visna, maedi or rida viruses, and the subject of Icelandic researcher Bjorn Sigurdsson working for the Rockefeller Medical apparat in the 1940s and later with the Rockefeller-financed Icelandic Institute of Experimental Pathology, the mycoplasmal/retroviral laboratory-engineered biological entity presents as the etiological foundation of AIDS.

The mycoplasma sans the retrovirus but likely co-factored with other viral entities such as human herpes viruses or Epstein-Barr virus can present as chronic fatigue syndrome or as collateral damage diseases such as Alzheimer's, sarcoidosis, Wegener's disease, rheumatoid arthritis and more.

PART ONE

THE DISCOVERY

Chapter One

THE PROFIT PARADIGM: FROM OIL TO AIDS

"It was about this time that a startled bystander watched one day as (John) Rockefeller, thinking himself alone in his office, jumped in the air, clicked his heels together, and repeated to himself, 'I'm bound to be rich! Bound to be rich! Bound to be rich!'"From: Collier and Horowitz (1977), Page 19

"Behind the visible government there is an invisible government upon the throne that owes the people no loyalty and recognizes no responsibility. To destroy this invisible government, to undo the ungodly union between corrupt business and corrupt politics is the task of a statesman."

President Teddy Roosevelt, 1912

Prevue: Being a collection of verbal snap shots (sections) which will enter more fully into our narrative as we present our evidence that one co-factor of AIDS (the mycoplasma) was accidentally discovered by Dr. Robert Huebner and that immune suppressing microorganism opened infected victims to a protean range of disease pathogens, including the retroviral disease of sheep (visna) researched by Dr. Bjorn Sigurdsson. The accidental discovery of the mycoplasma was followed by private (principally Cold Spring Harbor Laboratories) and U.S. government research (principally at Fort Detrick, MD) to determine whether it would be useful in enhancing the biowar weapons then being researched. When it was realized that it was, great effort was put into its development and later its deployment.

"The only thing necessary for the triumph of evil is for good men to do nothing."

Acquired Immunodeficiency Syndrome (AIDS) was officially entered into the record of medical history in 1981 when Michael Gottlieb, a Los Angeles medical doctor, coauthored a report on some gay male patients he had treated, who presented with an unusual cluster of signs and symptoms. The report was published in the Centers for Disease Control's (CDC) *Morbidity and Mortality Weekly Report* (MMWR). Although this date and article are now generally presented as the 'official' launch of AIDS, it was anything but!

AIDS: The Crime Beyond Belief

> "The date is June 5, 1981; the AIDS epidemic - or pandemic - has officially begun. In reality, of course, the AIDS epidemic started some years earlier, but June 5, 1981, is when information about the newly recognized condition was first released to the medical profession and general public."
>
> (Hooper, *The River*, Page 7)

Section 1: Parsing our title: "AIDS - The Crime Beyond Belief"

'AIDS': Drs. J. C. Samuels and G.H. Friedland in Conn's Current Diagnosis #8, state that Acquired Immunodeficiency Syndrome (AIDS) presents primarily as a defect in cell-mediated immunity which opens the way for opportunistic infections and certain malignancies in infected patients. Defects also occur in humoral immunity leading to pulmonary and sinus infections with bacterial pathogens. The effects are specifically tropic for T-helper Cells (CD4) Central Nervous System effects include dementia, myelopathy, and peripheral neuropathy. Infants can be infected in utero, perinatally or during breast-feeding. Blacks and Puerto Ricans, the authors note, '… have disproportionately high rates of the disease.' (Page 208) We have further comment upon the latter apparent ethnic discrimination by the syndrome in Chapter 23, where we present a discussion of a 1953 article by Dr. Maurice C. Shepard. There is a very real scientific basis for this characteristic.

AIDS: Presenting Signs and Symptoms:
1. Weight loss
2. Fevers or night sweats
3. Diarrhea
4. Lymphadenopathy
5. Oral Candidiasis
6. Oral hairy leucopenia
7. Chronic weakness or fatigue
8. Recurrent pneumonias
9. Uni- or multidermatomal herpes zoster infections

(Adapted from Conn (1991), Page 209)

Since the evidence we are about to present in this book demonstrates that HIV does not cause AIDS but is only one of many candidate co-factors, the diagnosis of AIDS is dependent upon the presence of certain disease states not otherwise ascribable to the so-called retrovirus. As Celia Farber writes in an article published in *Harper's Magazine* in March 2006, (See Ch. 23)

> "The clinical definition of AIDS in Africa...is stunningly broad and generic, and was seemingly designed to be little more than a signal for funding. It is in no way comparable to Western definitions. (See below: 'Case definition for AIDS in adults') The definition requires neither a positive HIV test nor a low T-cell count, as in the West, but only the presence of chronic diarrhea, fever, significant weight loss, and asthenia, as well as other minor symptoms. These happen to be the symptoms of chronic malnutrition, malaria, parasitic infections, and other common African illnesses...even when HIV tests are performed many diseases that are endemic to Africa, such as malaria and TB, are known to cause false positives." (Page 40)

The claim that a human retrovirus (HIV) similar to that in sheep (the visna virus) which causes the sheep diseases of visna, maedi and rida causes a human disease called 'AIDS' is a fiction created by certain United States scientists to hide the fact that what actually happens is that some disease pathogen lowers the human immune defence system and opens the way for several other diseases. And, so the story goes, if one possesses some of the latter diseases, even if one is HIV negative, one is diagnosed as having AIDS.

The jargon is hocus-pocus and is based upon the fact that several people who you will meet in the following pages and who hold various powerful positions are anxious to keep the truth from being known. Because the truth is, a crime beyond belief has been committed by these people and they (naturally) don't want to be called to account. Before we say more about the crime itself, we will finish this sketch of AIDS with the Samuels-Friedland case definition.

Case Definition for AIDS in Adults:
1. Candidiasis of the esophagus, trachea, bronchi or lungs
2. Coccidioidomycosis
3. Cryptococcus
4. Cryptosporidiosis
5. Cryptomegalovirus disease other than liver, spleen, or lymph nodes
6. Herpes simplex virus infection
7. HIV encephalopathy based upon so-called viral load*
8. Histoplasmosis at a site other than lungs, cervical, or Hilar lymph nodes
9. Isosporiasis
10. Kaposi's sarcoma
11. Lymphoma of B-cell or other specified type
12. Lymphoma of brain
13. *Mycobacterium avium-intracellulare* or *M. kansasii* disease
14. *M. tuberculosis* disease
15. *Pneumocystis carinii* pneumonia
16. Multi focal encephalopathy
17. *Salmonella* septicemia recurrent
18. Toxoplasmosis of the brain

* 'HIV tests detect footprints, never the animal itself.' (Farber, supra) Since there is no actual Human Immunodeficiency Virus that has ever been detected by scientists, but various tests demonstrate various levels of viral debris in the blood. Such debris can be the consequence of a variety of virus-destructive forces.

Farber also notes that in various health jurisdictions, the incidence of signs and symptoms required to establish an AIDS infection is of greater or lesser stringency. As Ms. Farber reports:

"The most stringent criteria (four bands) are upheld in Australia and France; the least stringent (two bands) in

Africa…It has been pointed out that a person can revert to being HIV negative simply by buying a plane ticket from Uganda to Australia."

(Note 1, Page 39)

There is no actual human immune deficiency virus, but something is killing millions of people annually by opening them to the diseases named. What is it? We will develop our answer to that question as we proceed. In the meantime, we must deal with the fact that the whole fiction of a retrovirus as *the sole cause* of a syndrome of illnesses was invented to cover what was actually at work in the human family. And what was at work was a micro-organism which was engineered in U.S. Government owned or controlled laboratories to kill or disable certain targeted people.

'THE CRIME'

To be convicted of a 'crime' it must be established by due process that someone acted or purposefully failed to act in such a way as to deprive another person of inherent rights by illegal means. To distinguish a crime from an accident or mistake, the perpetrator must have a motive, the means, and an opportunity to do the act or to fail to act.

Since the evidence that we have located over the past twelve years and which we summarize in this book demonstrates that the acquired immunodeficiency syndrome is the product of scientific laboratories owned or controlled by agencies of the United States Government, a study of AIDS is as much a political study as it is a medical study.

'BEYOND BELIEF'

An act sufficiently outside normal experience or reasonable or logical limits as to induce skepticism or doubt as to the likelihood of its existence is likely to be and in the case of AIDS already is an act beyond belief to the average citizen.

Section 2: Nocard and Roux

Drs. Edmund-Isidore Nocard and Pierre Roux worked with the Pasteur Institute in Paris during the turn of the 19th century where in 1898 they successfully cultivated the mycoplasma, bovine pleuropneumonia. They discovered that the microorganism was small enough to pass through an ultra filter, and that it combined some characteristics of a bacterium and some characteristics of a virus. However, unlike the virus that has a protein protective coat and cannot reproduce itself without taking over the nucleic acid of a host cell, the mycoplasma has its own metabolism and reproduction capacity outside of host cells. It lacks a rigid cell wall and is contained within a membranous envelope.

Because the mycoplasma lacks a cell wall and is so small, it tended to be ignored after its initial identification, and was not generally regarded as particularly dangerous to animals, including humans. It was the literal re-discovery of the mycoplasma some fifty years later by Dr. Robert Huebner that led to its identification as a very dangerous microorganism and to its becoming the subject of an intense, but largely secret study by the United States Government, especially the bioweapons military researchers and the Central Intelligence Agency. This intense study was to lead to the development of a retroviral/mycoplasmal combination (co-factors), which together constitutes the pathogenic instigator of AIDS, although the mycoplasma together with certain other pathogenic influences can present as an HIV-less AIDS.

Section 3: The Pathogenic Mycoplasma

A bacterium (plural: bacteria) is any of a group of minute single celled organisms that carry on activities of life including the capacity to reproduce their species. The latter capability requires nucleic acids. In the late 1800s two French Scientists, Nocard and Roux (See below number 7) discovered that there was a species of organism even smaller than bacteria without a cell wall, but able to self-replicate. They labeled the species 'mycoplasma', but because it was so small as to limit ease of study by scientists, it did not enter into medical studies for many years. In the early 1900s an American microbiologist,

Monroe Davis Eaton, realized that there was some type of pathogenic microorganism, which was at work in people ill with primary atypical pneumonia. Eaton was not familiar with the work of Nocard and Roux and he named it an 'Eaton Agent', which was replaced by some researchers with the name 'pleural-pneumonia organism'. An associated organism which was associated with degenerating adenoids was called a 'pleural pneumonia-like organism' (PPLO) by American researcher, Dr. Robert Huebner. (See Ch.3)

Later scientists agreed to standardize reference to the Eaton Agent/PPLO as a 'mycoplasma. As you will learn in this study, the mycoplasma is a critical agent in the on-set of many diseases, including AIDS, CFS and Alzheimer's. Of equal significance to our study is the fact that in 1993 the U.S. government patented the 'Pathogenic mycoplasma!'(See below: Hidden in Plain Sight)

Section 4: Hidden in Plain Sight: Holding a Patent on Death

There is a certain irony in the fact that when Dr. Shyh-Ching Lo of the United States Armed Forces Institute of Pathology in Washington, D.C. made application under the 'Patent Cooperation Treaty' to patent a "Novel Adherent and Invasive Mycoplasma" on December 1, 1992, he gave his address as '8700 Hidden Hill Lane, Potomac, MD, 20854, U.S.' Somehow, when one learns more about Dr. Lo, his living on a 'hidden hill' seems appropriate. Both the man and his work have contradictory qualities of being both public and obscure at the same time, as typified by this and other patents that the elusive doctor has applied for and received.

A hidden hill! Hidden…to prevent from being seen or discovered. Hill…a natural elevation of the earth's surface. It's hard to imagine being both hidden and on a hill…but Shyh-Ching Lo manages it; In fact, he lives there.

The subject patent was not Dr. Lo's first foray into the legal realm based on International Agreements and upon Article 1, Section 8 of the United States Constitution which states "Congress shall have power…to promote the progress of science and useful arts, by securing for limited times to authors and inventors the exclusive rights to their respective writings and discoveries." On June 6, 1991,

Dr. Lo had filed an application for a "Pathogenic Mycoplasma." For a year and three months his application had been examined by Primary Examiner, Christine M. Nucker, and her Assistant Examiner, D.R. Preston. Then, on September 7, 1993, Nucker and Preston accepted Dr. Lo's claim, and assigned his invention Patent Number 5,242,820 and so bestowed upon him the right to 'make, use or sell' the pathogenic mycoplasma.

Dr. Lo and the associate researchers with whom he had worked since their initial Application of June 18, 1986, immediately assigned his rights to their employer: The American Registry of Pathology of the Armed Forces Institute of Pathology, Washington, DC. Thus, the President of the United States, through the Joint Chiefs of Staff had an exclusive patent on death.

And it was hidden in plain sight. On a hidden hill, as it were.

If inventor Dr. Shyh-Ching Lo is something of a mystery or an enigma, then the subject of his science is even more so. According to the Patent document duly approved by Nucker and Preston, the 'new and useful process, machine, manufacture, or composition of matter, or any new and useful improvements thereof [to quote the Constitution], the 'Pathogenic Mycoplasma' is now the exclusive intellectual property of Dr. Lo and his assignees for 17 years. Almost as if one had patented a "Dangerous Weapon"!

The title does not make sense. 'Pathogenic' means 'disease causing'. A 'Mycoplasma' is defined as a *naturally occurring microorganism without a cell wall*. Just what has Dr. Lo claimed as his exclusive intellectual property?

Before we examine Patent Number 5,242,820 in more detail, we need to answer an anticipated question: What does a pathogenic mycoplasma have to do with AIDS and ME and with a crime that is beyond belief? Part of the answer is found on page 20 of the document where Dr. Lo tells us that of the patients who have mycoplasma infection:

> "Some of these patients who have been diagnosed as having AIDS or ARC, Cchronic [sic] Fatigue Syndrome, Wegener's Disease, Sarcoidosis, respiratory distress syndrome, Kikuchi's disease, autoimmune diseases such as Collagen Vascular Disease and Lupus and chronic debilitating diseases such as Alzheimer's disease."

Thus Dr. Lo's Patent is linked to AIDS and 'CFS' as well as several other of the neuro/systemic degenerative diseases. The link to a crime beyond belief will be developed over the course of this book.

He who pays the piper, calls the tune. On page one of his Patent Dr. Lo reveals an important fact:

> "The invention described herein was made in the course of work under a grant or award from the United States Department of the Army."

In this curt statement Dr. Lo tells anyone who wants to know that the development of this disease-causing microorganism is an undertaking of the military. The Pathogenic Mycoplasma is a weapon, not made of iron or steel, but of living matter. It is a biological warfare weapon. It is something that the United States Military had been working on for some time and it has the ring of a microorganism referred to on June 9, 1969 when Dr. Donald MacArthur of the Pentagon told a group of Congressmen in a secret meeting:

> "Molecular biology is a field that is advancing very rapidly, and eminent biologists believe that within a period of 5 to 10 years it would be possible to produce a synthetic biological agent, an agent which does not naturally exist and for which no natural immunity could have been acquired."

'For which no immunity could have been acquired.' That is a disease agent against which the body would have an acquired immune deficiency! The disease agent, MacArthur continued, '...would be refractory to the immunological and therapeutic processes upon which we depend to maintain our relative freedom from infectious disease.'

Was he talking about AIDS?

We'll discuss this fully in Chapter Fifteen, Section Two.

Back to Dr. Lo's Patent

On page three of his Patent, Dr. Lo makes the statement:

> "HTLV-III/LAV is believed to be the causative agent of AIDS."

Again, Dr. Lo is misleading his readers. "HTLV-III" is the

initialization of 'human T- [for 'thymus'] cell leukemia virus.' LAV is the initialization of 'lymphadenopathy virus.' Both are now seen as being a so-called 'human immunodeficiency virus' [HIV]. In the early 1980's when scientists in America, led by Robert Gallo, and scientists in France, led by Luc Montagnier, were trying to isolate a possible AIDS-causing virus, terminology was naturally imprecise. Then, on July 18, 1983, Montagnier described to an AIDS Task Force Meeting, with Gallo in attendance, a strange particle that his laboratory had isolated from the blood of an AIDS victim. According to Mathew Gonda, an NIH Microscopist who was also in attendance, the new isolate appeared to be the 'equine infectious anemia virus.' It is passing strange that the first look at a possible AIDS-causing organism seemed to have come into the blood of its human victim from a horse! But more of that later. At this point we need only note that Montagnier's isolate was labeled by him as a 'lymphadenopathy virus.'...LAV.

Later, Gallo purported to have found the same isolate on his own, and he labeled his version HTLV lll. Montagnier decided that Gallo had stolen his intellectual property and sued for damages. But again, this is not the critical element in the story. We are concerned with Dr. Lo using both Gallo's isolate which he called HTLV lll and Montagnier's isolate which he called LAV in the same sentence and then claiming that 'HTLV-lll/LAV' jointly 'is believed to be the causative agent of AIDS'. Such a linkage suggests that both Gallo and Montagnier see the peculiar isolate as the cause of AIDS and that is just not true.

Although initially Montagnier felt that since the isolate was a viral particle, and was found in the blood of an AIDS victim, and obviously had no logical reason to be there, that it might be the sought-for AIDS virus...if such actually existed. However, as his research continued, Montagnier soon came to the opinion that LAV was **not** the causative agent in AIDS.

By 1993, when Lo received his Patent for the Pathogenic Mycoplasma he surely had to have known of Montagnier's more considered and decidedly more logical view that LAV was a co-factor to the mycoplasma in the etiology of AIDS!

Furthermore, Dr. Lo must surely have been aware of the fact that both the term "HTLV- lll" and "LAV" had been replaced by a label which reflects another Gallo flight of fancy: "HIV"...'human immunodeficiency virus.' Suddenly, on lines 69 of page 3 and 1 to 5, page 4, of his Patent, Dr. Lo confirms the reasonable supposition that he was indeed aware of this semantic switch by writing without any explanation for the switch that:

> "Furthermore, HIV infected patients often show a wide variation in times of disease incubation and speed of disease progression. It is not known whether any specific infectious agent other than HIV can be responsible for the complex pathogenesis often seen in this disease."

Thus, after introducing the misleading statement that "HTLV-lll/LAV is believed to be the causative agent of AIDS", Lo is suddenly on to "HIV" as the cause and even more subtly confusing, he employs the Montagnier theory of co-factors in the etiology of AIDS.

Why would a supposedly precise scientist such as Dr. Lo mislead his readers so insidiously? We will not attempt an answer to that question at this point, but we will suggest that the pattern of obfuscation is there, and that it appears to be intentional.

Koch's Postulates

Robert Koch (1843-1910) was a German physician who suggested that a set of four conditions would establish that a particular organism was the etiological agent of a disease. Koch's postulates have been a touchstone for medical professionals ever since.

These postulates are:
1. The same organism must be found in all cases of a given disease.
2. The organism must be isolated and grown in pure culture.
3. Organisms from the pure culture must reproduce the disease when inoculated into a healthy, susceptible animal.
4. The organism must then again be isolated from the experimentally infected animal.

To his credit, given his senior research post with the United States Military, Dr. Lo appears to be aware of Koch's postulates for he tells us "...[T]he human retroviruses have not fulfilled Koch's postulates." [Page 3, ll 61-2] That is, HTLV-lll/LAV does not cause AIDS!

This significant scientific position goes a long way towards explaining the incidence of people with HIV who do not present with AIDS, and of others without HIV who have died of AIDS.

Pity the Poor Chimpanzee

Suddenly Dr. Lo makes a critical statement:

> "The chimpanzee is the only primate other than man found to be susceptible to infection by HTLV-lll/LAV. However, overt AIDS manifested by the development of opportunistic infections and/or unusual malignancies has not yet been seen, despite evidence for persistent infection and/or viremia in experiments on this species."
> Gajdusek, D.C., et al. *Lancet I, 55* (1985) [Page 3; ll 53-9]

In other words, one can put the HTLV-lll/LAV *cum* HIV into the target chimpanzee or human body, but AIDS does not present. In the course of this study we will have occasion to refer to other U.S. Government documents that make this same point: *HIV does not cause AIDS* [See Ch. 14, "SVLP to SVCP..."]; however, we again want to point out how ambiguous Dr. Lo is in making his case that he and his laboratory have evidence that merits a Patent on a Pathogenic Mycoplasma.

The reference to the fact that only chimpanzees and humans among the primates are susceptible to infection by HTLV-lll/LAV is partly attributable to the cited work of Dr. Gajdusek, but something important is left unsaid. Who established as a scientific fact this shared susceptibility of chimps and men? Was it Drs. Koprowski and Huebner? And were they working in the Lindi Chimpanzee Colony in the then Belgium Congo back in the early 1950's? We'll consider this possibility later.

However that may be, the fact that only the chimpanzee among primates would allow scientists to test their engineered HTLV-lll/LAV pathogens exposed these poor creatures to great hazard.

In other places Dr. Lo writes totally meaningless sentences, such as:

> "Furthermore, *M. fermentans incognitus* can be grown in a variety of commonly used mycoplasma media, whereas *M. fermentans incognitus* cannot." [Page11; ll. 49-52]

Perhaps Dr. Lo's cited References Will Help

A careful reading of Dr. Lo's Patent is a most unsatisfying experience for a reasonably informed reader. It is characterized by imprecision, confusing references, misspelt words, and ambiguity.

When one turns to his References [Item 56 of his Patent] in search of greater clarity, one is not enlightened to any great extent. Of the eight References he lists, five are to his own work, two are to 'Marquart, *et al.*', and one is to 'Hu, *et al.*'. All dated on or after 1985. Wasn't there anything to be learned in the literature after his brief allusion to 'B. Frank in 1889' [Page 2, l 43] and C.J. Krass in 1973 [Page 2, l 44] that would be relevant to his 'discovery'?

Further along in the Patent, under the heading: 'Description of the Background Art', Dr. Lo does add some more sources, but the earliest of these is dated 1981, (1) then he skips to 1983 (2), 1984 (5), 1985 (2), 1986 (3), 1988 (1). The cluster in this group can be understood by examining the titles: all deal with the increasing volume of studies into AIDS, but few have any specific reference to the 'mycoplasma.'

Actually, there was much significant reporting upon the nature and importance of the mycoplasma, especially in the period of the late 1940's and into the 1970's, which would be extremely relevant to any claim to have discovered a new species...even one with so vague an assigned title as 'incognitus.' But one would never know that from reading Dr. Lo's Patent.

We undertake to fill in the blanks in Dr. Lo's 'history' in **Part II** of this work, and to present evidence of what he was really trying to patent in Chapter 14. In the meantime we offer further examples of carefully contrived ambiguity.

Dr. Lo Admits to an Error

The confusion in the first nine pages of U.S. Patent Number 5,242,820 is not cleared up when on page ten of that document; Dr. Lo admits that initially his laboratory thought they were dealing with a virus:

> "The presently identified mycoplasma like many other mycoplasmas has many of the characteristics of a virus, which resulted in its identification as such in the original

patent application (Ser. No. 875,535, filed Jun. 18, 1986). Further research then showed characteristics which were not typical of classic viruses, thus the characterization as a VLIA in Ser. No. 265,920, filed Nov. 2, 1988. Additional research has now revealed characteristics traits of a mycoplasma as fully explained below." [Page10, ll 49-58]

Dr. Lo's tantalizing suggestion in this quotation that characteristic traits of a mycoplasma will be "fully explained below" is just not realized. One of the glaring errors, to which we have already alluded, [see the final sentence in *Pity the Poor Chimpanzee*, above] states that the *M. fermentans incognitus* can and cannot be grown in a variety of media. We must put this contradiction down to poor proof reading, but equally egregious errors cannot be as readily excused, and one must wonder whether they are thrown in to confuse rather than enlighten the reader.

Let's consider two examples. On page 10, lines 60 to 66 Dr. Lo has this to say:

"A mycoplasma (*M. fermentans incognitus*) according to the invention, in persistently infected cells, is (sic) deposited with the American Type Culture Collection under Deposit No. CRL 9127, deposited on Jun 17, 1986 *M. fermentans incognitus*, itself is (sic) also deposited with the American Type Culture Collection under Deposit No, 53949, deposited on Sep. 29, 1989."

Again, just what does this paragraph mean?

If we accept the standards of normal English language syntax and ignore a couple of Dr. Lo's grammar errors, he is essentially saying: "*M. fermentans incognitus* was deposited with the ATCC on June 17, 1986 under Deposit No. CRL 9127. *M. fermentans incognitus* was also deposited with ATCC on September 29, 1989 under Deposit No. 53949."

All of the rest of his paragraph is meaningless verbiage. Why, for example, employ the word 'mycoplasma' in the first sentence together with the parenthetical '*M. fermentans incognitus*'? Why not cut to the quick with the apparent subject immediately?

Then, what does he mean by 'according to the invention'? Does he mean 'as specified in the invention application'?

Finally, consider his adjective phrase: 'in persistently infected cells.' Does it modify 'invention' or is it the 'M. fermentans incognitus' or perhaps it qualifies the bare subject 'mycoplasma'? Who can reasonably tell? And what are 'persistently infected cells'?

But enough of this effort. Not intended to be a nit picking exercise, it is, rather, an effort to pin down precisely what Dr. Lo and his laboratory claim to have 'invented.'

One last example will be considered. On page 11 the following paragraph occurs:

> "*M. fermentans incognitus* was also found to be distinct from any other known strain of Mycoplasma. One unique feature of *M. fermentans incognitus* is its ability to catabolize glucose both aerobically and anaerobically and also to hydrolyze arginine. *M. fermentans incognitus* cannot hydrolyze urea in a biochemical ssay (sic). When grown in culture, *M. fermentans incognitus* produces a prominent alkaline shift in pH after an initial brief acidic shift. The only other human mycoplasma which is known to metabolize both glucose and arginine is the rarely isolated *M. fermentans*." [Page 11; ll 33-43]

It is to be noted that in the first sentence Lo reports that the *M. fermentans incognitus* is 'distinct'. Then, in the second sentence it is 'unique'. Then he interjects with a fine lack of coherence, two unrelated ideas. Finally, in the last sentence of the paragraph he contradicts the first two sentences by reporting that the *M. fermentans* is neither distinct nor is it unique!

Dr. Lo confuses the issue further by using 'catabolize' in sentence two and 'metabolize' in sentence five. These words are essentially synonyms and precision should require that he use one or the other but not switch part way through his hypothesis.

Enough Already!

It would be possible to trace such confusing semantics throughout the whole document. However, that would be a waste of time. Sufficient evidence has been adduced to demonstrate that intentionally or unintentionally, Dr. Lo has presented the world with a document that defies understanding.

Why he has done so, only he and his cohorts know. It could be that Dr. Lo was being intentionally obtuse, and lacking a real invention worthy of a Patent, presented examiners Nucker and Preston with several pages of data tied together by meaningless rhetoric. The data and examples can be accepted as given, but there is no invention to be protected!

Why, then, did Dr. Lo apply for and ultimately receive, a Patent on the 'Pathogenic Mycoplasma'? For Control! *By having a Patent on the Pathogenic Mycoplasma, no matter how bogus, the U.S. Government has one more control on researchers who seek to study the agent in question.*

We will defer stating our final view until Chapter 17. It is sufficient at this point to suggest that if one is serious about understanding the pathogenic mycoplasma, one must not seek such understanding by studying Dr. Lo's Application, but one must get back to the basics by considering the history of the mycoplasma that Dr. Lo has left out. Only then will we learn what he and his colleagues were really trying to patent when they first entered their Application on June 18, 1986.

It is important to realize from the outset, that the mycoplasmas appear to be at a critical juncture between living organisms and non-living chemicals. Dependant upon level of concentration, pressure, temperature, and pH, mycoplasmas can move from a fluid state intimately involved in the metabolism of life forms and a crystalline state subject to all the laws of physics as they apply to crystals.

Section 5:
The Confluence of AIDS, CFS/ME and the murder of a President

"So we began to study the political 'terrain' upon which the Kennedy and King assassinations took place. By the end of this seemingly unrelated investigation, Jackie's proposed link between the politics of Camelot and the development of AIDS-like viruses seemed frighteningly plausible.
"It was during this bleak period of American history that biological weapons contractors began to realize the possibility of genetically engineered virus delivery systems for untraceable genocide."Leonard Horowitz (1996, Page138)

President John F. Kennedy was shot several times by unknown shooters at 12:30 P.M. Central Time on Friday, November 22, 1963, in Dallas, Texas and died shortly afterwards at Parkland Hospital. AIDS was officially entered into medical literature in 1981. Approximately eighteen years separate the two events, yet we title this section *AIDS and the Murder of a President*.

With an eighteen year interval between these two dates, how could there be a possible link between them? To most readers they are disparate entities, but over the past twelve years of research by the authors, it has become clear that the murder of President John F. Kennedy and the advent of an epidemic which today (September 2007) is claiming an estimated eight thousand (8,000) lives a day are critically and strongly linked. In fact, the murder of the President in 1963 was quite likely necessary if the planned and pending epidemic of AIDS were to come to pass.

As we shall demonstrate in Chapter Three, the AIDS epidemic began serendipitously in the late 1940's - early 1950's when Dr. Robert Huebner discovered that an unusual microorganism which was causing pleural pneumonia in U.S. naval recruits, was also causing the adenoids of some of them to 'spontaneously degenerate'. The adenoids spontaneously degenerated because, among other things, the recruits' immune system, upon which living organisms depend to protect them from disease, was being severely compromised by the mystery microorganism.

The microorganism, which Huebner called a 'pleural pneumonia-like organism' (PPLO) was actually a Mycoplasma, and one of its most important qualities was that it was refractory to that critical immune defence system. In other words, the mycoplasma could cause a deficiency of acquired immunity, and cause many affected victims to lose their ability to ward off such diseases as *Pneumocystis carinii*, lymphoid interstitial pneumonitis, respiratory syncytial virus disease, Kaposi's sarcoma, and others.

The mycoplasma as a critical disease pathogen had first been discovered by Drs. Nocard and Roux of the Pasteur Institute in Paris in 1898. (See below) However, because the mycoplasma lacks a cell wall and is very hard to identify, the medical profession essentially lost sight of it. Although its initial discovery did not attract much attention or follow-up, its re-discovery by Huebner caught the attention of several people who had a strong if not pathological interest in any disease agent that had such dangerous potential. Those people were the eugenicists largely led by the Rockefellers, who were dedicated to the idea that it was necessary to limit the rate at which the world's population was growing.

To the eugenicists and to those who sought ways to weaponize disease, something that was refractory to the human immune system and could cause cells to spontaneously fall apart was worthy of very serious study, and that study is just what it was given. AIDS was on the way.

At first, the study was privately undertaken by the various eugenicists, but it got a big boost when, in 1952 Dwight D. Eisenhower was elected President of the United States for it permitted the private sector searchers to covertly highjack the public sector health agencies and tie them to the search for ways to slow down the world's population growth rate.

Planning for the murder of John F. Kennedy began almost as soon as he took over as President in 1961. Although there were a number of factions, as we shall develop, who wanted him dead almost as soon as he was elected, the one faction with much to lose if he remained in power and was re-elected in 1964, was the population growth rate control faction. Eight years of planning and action during the Eisenhower administration were threatened by John F. Kennedy.

A clash of ideologies linked AIDS to the murder of President John F. Kennedy.

But, for the authors, the population control freaks and assassinations were the last things on our minds when we began the studies, which have led to this report. We started with just one thread and followed it through the labyrinth of disease and public health agencies and wealth and it has led us out of darkness and into the light of the truth about AIDS and about the murder of the President.

Although we did not realize it at the time, we had actually begun our study of acquired immuno-deficiency syndrome (AIDS) in June 1995, when one of us (DWS) was asked by a lady with chronic fatigue syndrome to help her with the many and tragic problems that accompanied her illness. Besides the terrible burden of symptoms such as extreme fatigue, severe headaches, nausea, disorientation, arrhythmia, mood swings and others, the disease had led to her being bullied by her employer, largely neglected by her union, cheated by her insurance carrier, given cursory care by her medical care professionals, victimized by the casual but expensive neglect by members of the legal profession, and subjected to passive and active discrimination by work place associates and the public at large.

DWS set out to help her with her heavy burden, and early on in that effort was greatly blessed to find a book in a local store titled *Osler's Web* by Hillary Johnson. This marvelous book by an author who was herself a victim of CFS promised in its sub-title to present an account of "the Labyrinth of the Chronic Fatigue Syndrome Epidemic." The author did that and more.

But right at the outset of his study there were two factors that Ms. Johnson presented in her 'Acknowledgments' that puzzled him and raised nagging questions that accompanied him through all his subsequent reading and research. First, there were these lines on page ix:

> "Attorney Quinlan J. Shea Jr., formerly of the National Security Archive in Washington, D.C., and an expert in the Freedom of Information Act, lent his considerable expertise to my efforts to acquire documents from the government through FOIA. On my behalf, he met for long hours with NIH staff to negotiate the release of documents, and vigilantly monitored the government's processing of records, without once abandoning his quick wit. Quinn also took an active role in advising me on other crucial First Amendment issues that erupted during the course of reporting this book."

What? Did a sick patient have to use high powered and informed attorneys to find out facts relating to her disease from the National Institutes of Health?

This question was raised again on page xi where, in her note on 'Methods', Ms. Johnson wrote:

> "The National Institutes of Health were minimally responsive, ignoring repeated entreaties for compliance and even, upon appeal, an order to comply by the assistant secretary of health, James Mason." What were they trying to hide? Why the secrecy about a tragic disease [CFS] that officially came onto the scene in 1981, the same year that AIDS had been recognized as an infection in the human family?

This question of secrecy was soon followed by another question, raised by Johnson's comment on page x:

> "In addition, their [Charles Ortleb and Neenyah Ostrom] commitment to investigating the nexus between AIDS and CFS in the face of antagonism from many sources is deserving of the greatest respect."

Again we had to ask why certain 'health' authorities would resist the investigation of anything, let alone the nexus between two terrible new diseases, one disabling and one lethal.

The author (DWS) set out upon his journey of discovery, guided by two quotations that Hillary Johnson presents early in her study. The quotations are both from a work by the great Canadian physician, Sir William Osler [1849 -1919]. They are: "The edifice of medicine reposes entirely upon facts…truth cannot be elicited but from those which have been well and completely observed." And, "Emulating the persistence and care of Darwin, we must collect facts with open-minded watchfulness, unbiased by crochets or notions; fact upon fact, instance upon instance, experiment upon experiment; facts which fitly joined together by some master who grasps the idea of their relationship, may establish a general principle."(Sir William Osler, *Counsels and Ideals*)

These quotes matched sentiments, long held by DWS, but given balance and perspective when he took a Master of Science degree at the University of Guelph. The essence of the program was the scientific method, frequently advanced by Dr. Harvey Caldwell: "When faced with any human or scientific problem, collect data, classify that data, formulate hypotheses about the relationship of the data, design ways to test those hypotheses, and alter the hypotheses as the test results require. If you do this, the nature, origin and solution to the problem will be apparent."

DWS re-read *Osler's Web*, and then prepared and circulated an eight-page questionnaire with some fifty questions for CFS victims to complete. Thus his study began with hard data, not with the sarcasm and smart-alec contempt shown by so many government doctors of the NIH and CDC and by media asset writers such as Dr. Edward Shorter in his rant *From Paralysis to Fatigue*.

With the data drawn from over fifty actual victims, DWS drew up a list of signs and symptoms of chronic fatigue syndrome and took it to the library of Laurentian Hospital, Sudbury, where the library staff was wonderfully helpful, and to the library of Laurentian University, which had inherited a broad range of rather dated medical texts from a former, but now closed, Sudbury hospital.

The data search paid off: it soon became evident that the signs and symptoms of CFS were almost exactly the signs and symptoms of an ancient bacterial disease called chronic brucellosis. The literature also revealed something very significant: human brucellosis had largely disappeared from those areas of the world where the pasteurization of milk and milk products had become almost universal. The disease persisted in countries where pasteurization was largely absent!

That was a critical clue: the evidence was compelling that *the disappearing brucellosis was coming back in the form of a new variant termed chronic fatigue syndrome.*

But brucellosis was not the only disease that the literature linked to CFS. One nagging hint of a question alluded to by Johnson was clearly enunciated on page 95 of her book where, discussing certain scientific experiments performed by Susan Wormsley of Cytometrics Laboratory of San Diego on blood from AIDS and CFS victims, Johnson made the observation that: *the results were the mirror image of each other!*

Thus, to the research into CFS and brucellosis was added a study of AIDS. At this point in the journey of discovery, there arose the startling possibility that not only were CFS and AIDS aspects of the damage done by the same pathogenic organism, but that the so-called 'opportunistic diseases' of AIDS such as *Pneumocystis carinii* pneumonia, and Kaposi's sarcoma have direct etiological links to the same organism.

It was soon to become evident that the failure of the medical profession to realize or at least in some cases to acknowledge the relationship between these apparently diverse diseases had its origin in the politics of health and the pursuit of power.

Part of the problem also derives from the fact, sometimes unwittingly but often intentional, that the same disease agents are given different labels by different scientists from different backgrounds...which was a 'technique of obfuscation' well-summarized by Serge Lang on page 392 of his important book,

Challenges. A case in point: as will be demonstrated later in this study, the so-called 'prion' conjured up by Stanley Prusiner, the 'amyloid' so critical to the work of Carleton Gajdusek, the 'lentivirus' of Bjorn Sigurdsson, and the 'mycoplasma' of Nocard and Roux are all slightly variant aspects of the same disease organism. All are derived from bacterial DNA/RNA (deoxyribonucleic acid or ribonucleic acid) and all stem from the essence of the *life force*.

At a point some five years into his research two important things happened for DWS. First, he was greatly encouraged by the interest taken in the work by his son, Bill. Although faced with the challenge of earning a living, a challenge DWS was spared because (at the age of 71) he was on a comfortable retirement pension, Bill began to devote more and more of his time as a volunteer research assistant for the Common Cause Medical Research Foundation. Thus, the one researcher became two. Besides editing *The Journal of Degenerative Diseases*, now in its seventh year of publication, we have written four periodic reports on our work in the form of books (See the Bibliography), and have together held seven Common Cause Conferences.

Second, DWS had the opportunity to read another magnificent study titled *The River*, by Edward Hooper. At his suggestion Bill also studied this history "…to the source of HIV and AIDS" and we have built upon it ever since. *The River* reflects Hooper's honesty, diligence, intelligence, sense of fair play and great humanity. Although we were to differ with Ed Hooper on certain details, his 1070 page report must rank among the greatest such works in history. *The River*, together with *Osler's Web*, should be the *beginning* for anyone interested in the truth about AIDS and CFS/ME.

However, these two studies are only the starting point for any honest researcher into the twin tragedies of AIDS and CFS. One must turn to the official documentation prepared largely by United States Government Agencies, and scientific researchers writing in peer-reviewed journals if one is to learn how AIDS and CFS came into the human family.

The latter advent of AIDS/CFS can, as a purposeful, scientific consequence, be seen to date from 1952 when Dwight D. Eisenhower was elected President of the United States.

However, this specific time and the specific and readily verifiable events that followed have a background which must be summarized briefly.

Before presenting such a précis we extend our great debt to Dr. Leonard Horowitz, author of *Emerging Viruses...AIDS and Ebola*. Where appropriate throughout this brief summary of AIDS, we will specifically acknowledge the three authors noted above. The others to whom we are indebted are listed in the Bibliography, but generally speaking, for ease of reading, are not specifically referenced in this study.

At the outset we want to make it clear that we do not extend the benefit of the doubt to many of the people who have been involved in these terrible crimes against humanity. We are well aware of and greatly respect the grand themes of English Common Law, including the principle that a person should be considered innocent of a crime unless proven to be guilty. However, bearing in mind the fact that, as we shall present, many of the major actors have been demonstrated to be liars, and/or thieves, and bearing in mind that the vast files of the CIA which recorded the discovery, development and deployment of the pathogenic agents giving rise to AIDS were ordered destroyed after the Watergate scandal became public, we assert that the accused criminals are guilty unless someone, somewhere, can come up with clear evidence to the contrary. *We are more concerned for the millions of innocent victims than we are with the few liars and thieves.*

Let us emphasize—CIA Director, Richard Helms, ordered Dr. Sidney Gottlieb of the CIA to destroy the paper trail of the covert CIA/Military programs:MKULTRA, MKNAOMI and MKDELTA. Only 171 pages of primary data, much of which is made up of commentary by certain U.S. Senators, survived and were only discovered after Jimmy Carter ordered an intensive search. Several hundred other pages of secondary U.S. Government documents were also ordered destroyed but by various accidents, they escaped the shredders. We have in our files the 171surviving pages of MKULTRA as well as many of the other documents noted. If you want to study these and other sources that we have employed, we will help you get copies. In the meantime, we treat the criminality of Richard Helms, Sidney Gottlieb, Robert Gallo, Brian Mahy, David Baltimore and others as assumed wherever the evidence has been purposefully destroyed by anyone 'in the loop.'

Let us also state at the outset: our goal is to place a short, readable, summary of the long dark road to AIDS in the hands of as many people as is humanly possible because we want the forces of light to triumph over the forces of darkness.

For the authors, the study of CFS/ME led inexorably and logically to the study of AIDS and the study of both led to the study of the politics. *There was a clear confluence of AIDS, CFS/ME, and the murder of the President!*

Section 6: U.S. Military Medicine and the Uniformed Services University of Health Sciences

As we have already seen, the U.S. Military working in some instances with the CIA has been deeply involved in biological warfare weapons development and testing. We develop this aspect of our study further in Chapter Fifteen, but at this point it is necessary to emphasize one important aspect of the military in medicine. That aspect is that in many respects, the military medicine is not the medicine of the mainstream. For our purposes this aspect is best demonstrated with reference to the Uniformed Services University of the Health Sciences (USUHS). This institution is a school for the training of military doctors, which, as the name makes clear, is run by the Department of Defence. The USUHS publishes an annual Calendar in which subjects of study are summarized. In the 1993-1994 academic year that Calendar had a six- page summary about 'Mycoplasma Infections.'

The latter section contrasts with the *lack* of serious attention given this topic in most other North American (especially U.S.) schools of medicine. Most general practice medical doctors receive little or no information about the mycoplasma. This lack of attention to the mycoplasma and its effects upon human health show up in many ways to the great disadvantage of the victims of the diseases listed by Dr. Shyh-Ching Lo (See Section 4 above, and Ch. 22) in the U.S. Patent cited. It is therefore appropriate at this point to share with you information about the mycoplasma that is given to doctors in the U.S. Military but generally speaking is not given to civilian doctors.

The course section titled "A. Mycoplasma infections" states:

> "Mycoplasmas belong to the class Mollicutes. Mollicutes are the smallest organisms capable of self-replication in cell free

media. Unlike viruses, Mollicutes have both DNA and RNA. They are tiny bacteria that stain gram-negative because they lack a ridged cell wall."

"*Mycoplasma fermentans*, *M. penetrans*, *M. genitallum* (sic), *M. hominis* and *Ureaplasma urealyticum* are the mycoplasma organisms that are known to be transmitted sexually."

"The incidence rate of genital mycoplasmas is significantly affected by the type of contraception, the number of sexual partners, socioeconomic states, degree of cultural tradition, as well as hormonal status."

"Results obtained in vitro suggest that mycoplasmas act as cofactors with the human immunodeficiency virus (HIV) in the development of AIDS and mycoplasmas, including *M. fermentans*, *M. pirum*, and *M. penetrans* have been isolated from HIV-infected individuals. These mycoplasmas have the capacity to invade cells and to be potent immunomodulators. They can produce systemic infections in HIV-infected individuals, but their pathogenic role in association with HIV remains to be determined."

Clinical and Pathological Changes:

"A. *Mycoplasma fermentans*

"The most serious presentation of *M. fermentans* infection is that of a fulminant systemic disease that begins with a flu-like illness. Patients rapidly deteriorate developing severe complications including adult respiratory distress syndrome, disseminated intravascular coagulation, and/or multiple organ failure."

"The organs of patients with fulminant *M. fermentans* infection exhibit extensive necroses. Necrosis is most pronounced in lung, liver, spleen, lymph nodes, adrenal glands, heart, and brain."

This passage is startling in many ways, but the most important thing to note is that, while the rest of North American medicine is preaching the "HIV as the sole source of AIDS" doctrine (See Chapter 23: *2000*…letter to *Harper's* from Drs. Marlink and Wilfert), U.S. Military doctors are taught otherwise!

Section 7: The Concept of Co-Factors

Reference was made in the previous Section to the belief that "…mycoplasmas act as cofactors with the human immunodeficiency virus (HIV) in the development of AIDS…" A definition of cofactors is appropriate at this point: "…a substance which acts with another substance to bring about certain effects…" from Webster's New Explorer Medical Dictionary. (1999, Page 127)

That is it in a nutshell: it takes at least two 'substances' to present as the 'effects' known as AIDS. One of the substances is a species of mycoplasma, and one (among many others) is the retrovirus visna adapted to humans from sheep.

In the conventional literature about AIDS, one usually encounters the claim that "Human Immunodeficiency Virus" - (HIV) - is the single or lone source of the disease. As you will learn in later pages of this study, there are many people in positions that count who repudiate any suggestion that there are at least two factors at work. One of the most vocal of the latter is Robert Gallo who expresses 'astonishment' (his exact words are: "Recently - and to me astonishingly - they [the mycoplasma—Ed] have been proposed as a primary co-factor…in AIDS by Montagnier" Gallo, 1991 Page 286) that people would pay any attention to such 'co-factor' theories.

It is apparently a part of a very deliberate campaign to remove the whole idea of the mycoplasma from serious consideration. However, in their unguarded moments, the mycoplasma deniers often let it slip that the microorganism does have a very significant role in AIDS.

Even Gallo has been caught off base in this matter. In an article in Discover Magazine, and quoted by Bruce Nussbaum, Gallo wrote:

> "…the AIDS retrovirus 'goes into hiding' once it invades the human body. 'It remains in the T cell until the cell is kicked into action by another infection. The virus comes out of hiding, reproduces and spreads.'"(Nussbaum, 1990 Page 324)

Note Gallo's reference to 'another infection'! That, by another name, is a co-factor.

Section 8: Dr. Ishii Shiro

Dr. Ishii Shiro was the head of biological weapons research for the Japanese military during World War Two. His notorious Unit 731 which was code-named a 'Water Purification Unit' (WPU), tested a wide range of biological agents on many Chinese cities, and upon Allied prisoners of war (Australian, British, American and Chinese, primarily) held by the Japanese. At War's end, Ishii Shiro first staged his own death and funeral, but was finally found out by the occupying American forces and taken to Tokyo where he worked out a deal to tell the Americans all that he and his co-workers had learned about a wide range of biological agents in return for amnesty and non-prosecution for war crimes.

Much of what he revealed has already been widely reported in the world press, *but there was one area where the information has been kept as a closely guarded American secret.* That information deals with what Ishii Shiro's unit did in the islands of New Guinea and New Britain after they invaded that area at the beginning of the war. All that is known is that the Japanese had established a bioweapons test site on the north coast of New Guinea. What they tested there and upon whom they tested have never been revealed by the Americans.

However, our research indicates that work was being done, possibly using the sheep visna virus as an inoculant. Work in this field had already been under way in Japan in 1942, and it is our hypothesis that Lt.-Gen. Ishii Shiro, M.D., through officers and units of the Japanese military under his control vaccinated several members of the New Guinea Fore Tribe with sheep-derived visna with the intention of monitoring the effects on a human population over an extended period of time. However, the Japanese had not counted on the fighting effectiveness of the Australian defenders of New Guinea, and were forced to retreat and to abandon the study the following year.

Evidence to support our thesis is scarce because as we reported above, *the Americans have kept their New Guinea secrets to themselves.* For example, Norman Covert devotes just half a page to what the Americans received from Ishii Shiro and all of that deals with Unit 731 in Manchuria (Covert, 1997 Page 21). *He says nothing about the Water Purification Unit in New Guinea, and we would know even less than we do if it were not for Yuki Tanaka, a visiting Japanese research fellow at the Australian National University. In his book, based upon Japanese sources and post-war Allied investigations of war crimes... limited and warped as such investigations turned out to be.*

From Tanaka we learn that Japan had established a 'Water Purification Unit' (WPU) (*i.e.* a biological weapons test site) on the north shore of New Guinea near what are now the ports of Jayapura/Aitape (location somewhat indeterminate) and about 500 kilometers from Madang. Madang in turn is about 150 kilometers north of the area of New Guinea where the Fore tribe lives. All of this area, together with the neighboring island of New Britain, during the 1942 Japanese occupation was under the supervision of Japanese medical doctor, Ishii Shiro deputy and biowar weapons researcher/experimenter, Captain Hirano Einosuke. Einosuke was head of the WPU stationed on Rabaul, and strangely enough he had brought some sheep with him from Japan for 'experimental purposes'! (Tanaka, Page 154)

What might be the significance of all of this, given the fact that the Americans who had secured the information from Ishii Shiro have never revealed what they learned to the rest of the world? Probably this: Sheep were the known major reservoir for the visna retrovirus (goats and mink being minor reservoirs), which presents as the sheep diseases visna, maedi, rida, and progressive pneumonia (and is very close genetically to the so-called HIV virus.) Biowar weapons researchers have had a long history of being interested in the visna retrovirus and it is entirely likely that Captain Hirano, as part of his research under Gen. Ishii Shiro, would know of the disease and would have an interest in finding out what he (and hence, Shiro) could about human susceptibility to it if it could be persuaded to jump species. To learn of this possibility would require testing, but, such testing would be very dangerous not just to the test subjects, but to those doing the testing and even all of humanity. No one could possibly guess what would happen if a group of humans were infected with the visna retrovirus. The consequences of turning a retrovirus loose in the human species might do damage in excess of that done in 1918 with the outbreak of a swine-based influenza that killed up to 20,000,000 people.

The latter danger would require that any testing be done in an area remote from any heavily populated area, such as in mainland China or Manchuria or even Japan itself. So what might Ishii Shiro, through his military underling, Captain Hirano, decide to do? Just this: travel overland in New Guinea south from Madang into some of the most remote and isolated areas in the world...into the area where the Fore peoples of New Guinea live. Once there, his forces could round up fifty or so healthy male test subjects and inoculate them with some fluid from visna-infected sheep. Then, over the following fifty years the Japanese researchers could monitor what happened to the isolated Fore peoples by annual or more frequent visits.

This fantastic scenario is not as weird as it might at first appear. Skipping ahead twenty years (to 1962), and referring to the *Special Virus Cancer Program*, Progress Report #8, one learns that in April 1964, blood from sheep carrying 'miscellaneous viruses' (?) was injected into twelve primates by Dr. P. Gerber to see how the primates would be affected. (Page 284) Working in the same program was none other than Dr. Carleton Gajdusek. (See Section 9 below) In April and May of 1966 Dr. Gajdusek injected eight primates with the mashed up human brain from a Fore victim of Kuru who had died of that disease in the remote mountains south of Madang! Kuru is a human disease caused by a slow virus which is related to the same virus which infects sheep with visna/maedi/rida!

Also reported in the same SVCP (*Progress Report #8*) are reported experiments wherein Drs. Rauscher, Davenport and Jensen injected a species of mycoplasma (unspecified) into 2 primates! The source was 'bovine.'

Of significance here is the fact that all three of the doctors named later turn up in Dr. Leonard Horowitz' book, *Emerging Viruses*. However peripheral their role might have been, it was at least sufficient for them to be identified by Dr. Horowitz as being involved.

As we have already noted, Ishii Shiro was protected from being tried as a war criminal when he worked out a deal with General Douglas MacArthur to spare his life in return for sharing all he knew about Japan's biological warfare research, including the tests in New Guinea, with the American military. Despite the fact that many hundreds, if not thousands of Allied prisoners of war had been slaughtered by Ishii Shiro, he was not tried by a War Crimes Court, but was instead essentially on the payroll of the American taxpayers until the end of his life.

To emphasize the betrayal of all of those Allied prisoner's of war who were murdered by the Japanese, and to make the point very clear that they were indeed murdered, that they hadn't died natural deaths from malaria or beriberi, we quote from Tanaka directly:

> "The War Crimes Section obtained information from Kiyama's juniors in the 81st Naval Garrison Unit. According to Kubo Saichiro, at the end of 1943, some men (prisoners of war-Ed) were ordered to dig two large holes. About 10 POWs were brought to the place by truck and divided into two groups. POWs in one group were decapitated by an officer, and the others were given lethal injections. The following is the testimony of another of Kiyama's juniors, Hosaka Katsumi: The executions were carried out by bringing one prisoner at a time to the front of the hole, making him lie flat on his back, opening his shirt and giving him an injection in the arm…I am not familiar with medical matters, but I think most of them took about 15 minutes to die. I remember one survived as long as 25 minutes. When one POW was dead, he was dropped in the hole and the next man was given an injection…"

Tanaka continues:

> "It seems that these POWs were injected with various poisons in order to test their effectiveness. Neither Kubo nor Hosaka knew who the doctors were or where they came from…It seems a strong possibility that the doctors were from the 24th Field Epidemic and Water Purification Department…(Shiro's command- Ed)
>
> (Tanaka, 1998 Pp. 156-7)

The perpetrators of these terrible crimes against humanity were given immunity from prosecution by General Douglas MacArthur. This is a blatant betrayal of trust. Just as commanders in battle are right to expect those under their command to do their duty…those who do the actual fighting have a right to expect in turn that their commanders will be loyal to them. Tanaka tells us that "the War Crimes Section apparently did not investigate further." (Page 157)

Were the criminals and their commanders (including Ishii Shiro) spared prosecution because they gave details as to how they had murdered prisoners of war? Of course not. The latter information was merely chaff from the mill. *Ishii Shiro and his deputies were spared prosecution because they gave much more important information to General MacArthur.* Just what was that critical information? Did it have something to do with sheep that had been brought all the way from Japan for 'experimental purposes'? After all, Shiro's deputy Captain Hirano admitted that he had such sheep in his Water Purification Unit.

And if the sparing of these criminals had anything to do with sheep, was it that sheep blood-borne visna disease was inoculated into members of the Fore tribe in the area, who were to be observed for several years to learn the consequences of such activities?

We don't know. We only know that General Ishii Shiro and his researchers (including Captain Hirano) were spared prosecution for war crimes.

We will return to this area of New Guinea and the Fore tribe in the next Section of this chapter when we consider the work of American Nobel Laureate, D. Carleton Gajdusek. In the meantime, we will take a moment to reflect upon General Douglas MacArthur.

— *An Interlude* —

General Douglas MacArthur is considered by millions of people, especially Americans, to be a great hero. His 'story' is dramatically presented in a movie titled *MacArthur*, with the lead role played by Gregory Peck. Who couldn't help but be impressed? The battle fatigues, the high peaked military hat, the jaunty corncob pipe? Dramatic lines such as "I shall return."

And then he returns, wading through knee deep water to a shore already secured by the 'grunts' who did the fighting and the dying and who bore the scars of shrapnel and bullet wounds. The 'grunts' like those whose murder was to be forgiven by the same MacArthur. In return for information about how those murders were committed or (possibly) how a sheep lenti virus had been planted into the blood of Stone Age Fore tribe natives of New Guinea.

General Douglas MacArthur who was later to establish his headquarters in Tokyo's Dai Ichi, as Supreme Commander, Allied

Powers (SCAP), had a Deputy...Major General Alonzo Fox, who in turn had a son-in-law named Alexander Haig; who in turn had been a Colonel in the Pentagon in the months leading up to the assassination of President John F. Kennedy. Colonel Haig's job in those days was to act as the bearer of 'voice only' messages among the Joint Chiefs of Staff. Messages so secret that under no circumstances could they be put into writing (even in code) and once received from whatever source could not be noted by a memo or any cryptic reminder. Colonel Haig who had been recommended for his job by Defense Secretary, Robert McNamara, a professed friend of John F. Kennedy!

But MacArthur also had a chief of Army Intelligence...General Willoughby, who would have received whatever 'intelligence' General Ishii Shiro delivered to the U.S. biowar researchers, and would have passed that intelligence on to the appropriate Army personnel for whatever action they deemed fit to take.

If, and at this point we acknowledge it as an 'if', subject to a more positive statement after we have presented some 300 pages of further evidence, the information would have gone to the head of research at the U.S. Army Walter Reed Hospital, Joseph Smadel. And Smadel would have passed the information on to someone who might follow up on whatever secret information they had received from Ishii Shiro.

However that may be, in 1954 Smadel directed Dr. D. Carleton Gajdusek to New Guinea via a stop over with Frank Burnet, a friend of an American named Henry Kissinger, of Australia. And it was in New Guinea where Gajdusek lets on he 'happened upon' the Fore tribe of Stone Age people *suffering from a sheep visna disease which they called Kuru*. (Dr. Gajdusek later experimented under direction of his friend and colleague, Robert Gallo with a Kuru- infected brain mashed up and injected into primates?)

Shortly before sending Gajdusek off to New Guinea, Smadel had also linked a Rockefeller-sponsored biological researcher named Hilary Koprowski to Karl Meyer of the University of California which in turn led to Koprowski's work in the Belgium Congo where he experimented by inoculating primates with a 'polio' vaccine. And later still, several researchers wondered whether by accident, that polio vaccine had been contaminated by primate kidneys and hence caused AIDS to jump species from primates to man.

We'll discuss all of these subjects and meet all of these people as we present the results of our research. We will also meet Alexander Haig and Generals Fox and Willoughby when we look at the assassination of John F. Kennedy and then the removal from office of Spiro Agnew and Richard Nixon. It may appear to those who have depended upon *The New York Times* or *Time* magazine as if there are no possible links. But, we'll see.

End of an Interlude

The rot of American expediency provides nutrient for the deep roots for AIDS.

In passing, and on behalf of human decency, we apologize to the slaughtered prisoners and the Chinese victims of Japanese biological weapons usage who were abandoned by the United States and the 'American Caesar', and we trust that to some extent, this study will make up for that betrayal of the murdered.

Now we will look at an American researcher who turned up in the New Guinea region of the Fore tribe, some ten years after Ishii Shiro and his gangsters left: Dr. D. Carleton Gajdusek.

Section 9: Dr. D. Carleton Gajdusek

In the Preface to his Nobel Lecture of December 13, 1976 D. Carleton Gajdusek stated:

> "In 1951 I was drafted to complete my military service from John Enders' laboratory at Harvard to Walter Reed Army Medical Service Graduate School as a young research virologist, to where I was called by Dr. Joseph Smadel."
>
> (Page 165)

Like so many other statements of 'fact' by the people whom we have identified as researchers in the laboratory-created AIDS co-factors, this simple passage by Gajdusek is laden with ambiguity and raises many questions for the researcher. For example, in 1951 Gajdusek was 28 years old, somewhat older than average to be 'completing' military service. Where was he earlier when he apparently did his initial service? Nowhere in this autobiography does he acknowledge that at some point during the Korean War he had been hastily thrown into a U.S. Army uniform and rushed out to Korea to help cope with an outbreak of hemorrhagic fever on the Hantaan River in Korea.

Although vigorously denied by the U.S. government at the time, later evidence makes it evident that the U.S. military was heavily engaged in biological warfare weapons development and deployment in Korea and that the outbreak of a hemorrhagic fever was an example of one of the dangers of bioweapons: the risk of disease agent 'blowback' upon the users.

Further collaboration of American use of biological weapons in Korea was later provided by E. Howard Hunt who was to gain notoriety in Dallas on November 22, 1963 when he was arrested while trying to ride a freight train from behind Dealey Plaza after the murder of President John F. Kennedy and still later when he was arrested in Washington, D.C. for his role in the Watergate break-in. Hunt was in Korea at the time of the Hantaan River outbreak of hemorrhagic fever. Although not involved in the latter event, he admitted to involvement in other biowar activities. (Endicott and Hagerman)

Further evidence of the American efforts to develop and deploy biological weapons around this same time comes from Ed Regis, *The Biology of Doom*. Regis reports:

> "But if the [U.S.-Ed] Air Force wanted an incapacitating biological device in its inventory, *Brucella* was what the Army Chemical Corps was offering to fill in with. In 1951, therefore, the Air Force formally standardized the *Brucella* suis biological bomb, which thus became the official American biological weapon." (Regis, 1999 Page 139)

The dispatch of Gajdusek to Korea is significant because it clearly links him to Dr. Joseph Smadel and biological warfare activities.

Several questions occur: had Gajdusek been given credit for service at Rochester University in lieu of military service? This, of course, was quite common during that period when several government agencies recruited young college students for (often) covert duties. Philip Agee is one example. (Agee, 1975) This possibility is rendered more likely when one learns that his degree work at the University of Rochester was paid for by the U.S. Navy.

Another question is, what would Gajdusek have known about hemorrhagic fever that made his presence in Korea so critical? Had he been involved in biological weapons research prior to his rush into uniform? After all, Rochester has emerged in our research as one of the major biowar research institutions of that time.

Furthermore, how would Joseph Smadel have known about Gajdusek in order to be able to 'draft' him for special service? This someone who knew Gajdusek and his prodigious talent must have passed a recommendation to the military. Was that someone John Enders at Harvard? After all, Enders was an early researcher into scientific subjects that later turned out to be very significant in the analysis of AIDS. For example; Gallo notes that it was Enders who first 'grew the polio virus in cell culture.' (Gallo, 1991) What link might polio have with biological weapons? As we shall see when we look at the work of Hilary Koprowski (Ch. 5) the development of polio vaccines was a possible cover for more insidious ends, and in passing (above) we noted that it was Smadel who in January 1952, recruited Koprowski to do his 'polio' vaccine work. (Hooper, 1999 Page 413) This likelihood is further advanced when Gallo states that he had worked extensively with both Enders and Koprowski. (Gallo, 1991 Page 315)

Enders is also the subject of speculation by Lee who has written:

> "...Enders and Peebles (1954) recovered simian (ape) 'foamy' virus from measles patients during the era. ...This historic finding, occurring in 1954, would appear to be a first recognition of simian/monkey viruses present in humans... Though AIDS is reported to be related to a primate virus (SIV-1) that has invaded humans through some apparently random process, investigation of historic medical literature shows substantial indication that many primate/monkey/simian viruses have invaded many species including humans and that many of these invasions appeared to begin in a Petrie dish in the laboratory." (Lee, 1989 Page 48)

Ed Hooper cites Enders' work nine times in the index of *The River*. Thus, when in 1954, Dr. Carleton Gajdusek was suddenly sent off to New Guinea, under the sponsorship of Dr. Joseph Smadel, Chief of Microbiology at the Walter Reed Army Institute of Research, Washington, D.C., and lets on that he just happened to stumble upon the Fore tribe, tragically infected with a variant of the sheep retroviral disease visna named Creutzfeldt-Jakob disease in humans, we are entitled to challenge his account about how it all came to pass.

It is our hypothesis, which we have discussed briefly with Gajdusek, that the Fore tribe of New Guinea had been vaccinated with a sheep-derived retrovirus in 1942 by Japanese General/Doctor Ishii Shiro's biowar researchers. (See Section 8 above) And that Gajdusek had been sent in 1954 to see how the tribe were thriving... or failing to thrive.

He found just what the Japanese had theorized: the Fore tribe was being decimated by visna *cum* 'kuru' (the Fore name for the disease) *cum* Creutzfeldt-Jakob disease. That Gajdusek was familiar with Sigurdsson's work is evident in the following extract from his diary entry of February 6, 1962:

> "This morning I was up before sunrise typing up the Slow Virus Infection abstract. I have submitted one paper on kuru in childhood and another on slow virus infections in which I shall develop the possibility of kuru-scrapie slow virus and temperate virus analogies and our current approach to the problem..."

Below, we will demonstrate how he and Huebner helped tie visna to kuru to Robert Gallo's work on AIDS. In the meantime, we have presented two of the five critical horsemen of the AIDS apocalypse: Ishii Shiro and Carleton Gajdusek. Three others of critical early significance, Bjorn Sigurdsson, Robert Huebner and Robert Gallo, we develop in separate chapters below. There were thousands of others involved in the creation of the AIDS plague...some witting, some unwitting. Some were dramatically important, such as Hilary Koprowski and Alton Ochsner, and some simply laboratory workers. There were also those who financed the research such as the Rockefellers and the Morgans, and those who paved the way politically, such as Nelson Rockefeller and Lyndon B. Johnson and Richard Nixon.

But, before we start the more specific and detailed study of AIDS with the appointment of Nelson Rockefeller as Assistant Secretary of Health, Education and Welfare (HEW) by President Eisenhower in April, 1953, we present a brief summary of the key scientific facts about the disease and its apparent links to visna/Creutzfeldt-Jakob disease and Carleton Gajdusek.

Early in our research, we had read some secondary sources before we learned that we must turn to the primary sources ourselves. (See Ch. 22: The Scientific Paper Trail to AIDS) In our early reading we came upon Arno Karlen's, *Man and Microbes*.

In Karlen's subtly dishonest book we read the following about Carleton Gajdusek:

> "In the late 1950s reports appeared of a strange new disease that was slaughtering the Fore tribe of Papua New Guinea. Virtually nothing was known of the disease, and little more of the Fore, who lived a Stone Age existence in New Guinea's isolated highlands. An adventurous young American virologist, D. Carleton Gajdusek traveled to Fore territory to study the epidemic."
>
> "Nothing like this outbreak had ever been seen. The disease struck mostly women and children, causing loss of coordination, tremors, paralysis, and dementia; wasting (by the way, the Icelandic term 'visna' means 'wasting' in that language! Ed) and death followed the first symptoms within a year. The Fore called it 'kuru, the trembling disease, and were convinced its cause was sorcery. Gajdusek had nothing to go on; the disease might be genetic, infectious, or the result of some environmental toxin. He began a one-man epidemiological study by walking from village to village for 2,000 miles, collecting data and samples."
>
> (Karlen, 1995 Page 197)

We puzzled over the apparent relationship between the sheep disease, visna, and the human disease Kuru (Creutzfeldt - Jakob disease) and decided to follow this gushing account of the intrepid selfless Gajdusek and his courageous 2,000 mile hike in a territory about 30 miles wide and sixty miles deep. He would have to have crisscrossed the territory some sixty-six times!

Among the documents that we dug up was the Volume 15, Number 2 issue of *Grand Street* magazine Fall: 1996. On page 15 of

Grand Street was the following account of Gajdusek's 'one-man' trip in New Guinea:

> "We arose at 5 A.M. and by 6:15 our entire patrol was on the trail. We number some seventy-two carriers, six boys, eleven police, and a contingent of a dozen or more Mobutasa men and boys who have come with us. A group of Agamusei people came along as well. Thus our line was about a hundred strong."

So much for a 'one-man' expedition. However, included in the same issue was a photo of Gajdusek at work in the jungle, with Dr. Vincent Zigas and an Australian government employee named Jack Baker. On the table are several books, a journal called *Clinical Methodology*, a large dish with what appears to be a human brain in it, a large microscope, some sort of lens, and even a bottle of Quick ink. On the wall behind there appears to be a heater or air conditioner and a radio. Karlen's account had at the least been a flight of fancy, so we decided to phone Gajdusek and talk with him personally to resolve some of the contradictions.

Besides, we wondered, why would Karlen feel obliged to promote the idea of a one-man expedition by a lone intrepid Gajdusek? Did Karlen want to obscure the fact that 'our line was about a hundred strong.' Also, we learned, Gajdusek soothed the sorrow of relatives of dead Fore whose brains were pickled and dissected, with many gifts. Who was paying for those? We phoned Dr. Gajdusek at the National Institutes of Health. We recount the conversation in our earlier book, *Life*, and will not repeat it here. But in response to our expressed skepticism about how he happened to turn up in Fore territory where he 'encountered' kuru and our expressed doubts that he had paid his own way, Gajdusek first asked "Who do you think paid my way?" We suggested that the U.S. Military had. A further discussion followed, but we kept no notes so we cannot be precise about it, but Gajdusek promised to send us a package of his research material. "If you can find any link to biowar research in the package," said Gajdusek, "You are welcome to it."

True to his word, a heavy parcel arrived from Gajdusek the next day by Fed-Ex®. The label showed that it had been shipped, not from NIH where we had talked with him, but from none other than Fort

Detrick, Maryland; the site of American biowar weapons research.

We will give more details about Gajdusek's gift to us later, but enough to say at this point that among the documents was his Nobel Lecture of 1976, and a chapter titled "Infectious Amyloids: Subacute Spongiform Encephalopathies as Transmissible Cerebral Amyloidosis" written by Gajdusek for the textbook *Field's Virology*, and a copy of a 1959 article titled simply "Kuru", by Gajdusek and Vincent Zigas in the aforementioned photograph in New Guinea. A brief comment upon each.

From the 1959 article "Kuru", we were interested to note that as early as 1958 Gajdusek had sent four Kuru-infected brains to Professor Oscar Vogt in Neustadt, West Germany for analysis. We also noted that in the infected brain of the Kuru victims there was a marked proliferation of astroglia and microglia. This, we realized, was also a characteristic of the brain of amyotrophic lateral sclerosis victims, and has a significance in cholesterol generation.(See below: Ch. 17; part 4) We also noted that the report stated: "...recent research has demonstrated abnormalities in serum ceruloplasmin and copper transport and associated abnormal depositions of copper in the body." This we were able to tie in with Andre Voisin's important book: *Soil, Grass, and Cancer*. We discuss the latter in more detail in Chapter 23.

From Gajdusek's chapter in *Field's Virology* we learned much of great significance to our study of AIDS and CFS and the collateral damage of other, related, diseases. For example, on page 2853 he describes the 'infectious amyloid' whose qualities resemble that of Prusiner's 'prion'. Gajdusek states that, "Since the unconventional and atypical viruses of SSVE (kuru, CJD, GSS, scrapie, BSE) have been identified as infectious amyloid molecules, our laboratory has slowly switched to designating them as *infectious amyloids* instead of *unconventional viruses*. Others have accepted the term prions for these agents." (Page 2862)

Is the mycoplasma really an amyloid or a prion? We look further at the answer to this possibility in Chapter 17 below.

But of equal importance to us was Gajdusek's observation that:

> "Hadlow, *et al.* have shown that the first appearance of scrapie virus in naturally infected young lambs occurs at 10 to 14 months in the tonsils, suprapharyngeal and mesenteric

lymph nodes, and intestine, suggesting infection by alimentary tract." (Page 2881)

Tonsils! We had started our research looking at infected *adenoids* in naval recruits! We will be returning to the amyloid but will cite one further paragraph at this point so that you may early on think about what Gajdusek wrote in 1996 and what Dr. Shyh-Ching Lo had written some three years earlier when he achieved his Patent of the Pathogenic Mycoplasma. Gajdusek writes:

> "The suspicion has been awakened that many other chronic diseases of man may be infectious amyloidosis. (Mycoplasmal infections? - Ed) Data from both the virus laboratory and from epidemiological studies have accumulated that suggest that multiple sclerosis and Parkinson's disease, disseminated lupus erythematosus, juvenile (type 1, insulin-dependent) diabetes, poliomyelitis, some forms of chronic arthritis, and even schizophrenia may be slow virus infections with a masked and possible defective virus as their cause." (Page 2888)

Compare the above list of possible disease consequences of an infectious amyloidosis with Dr. Lo's list:

> "Some of these patients who are infected with *M(ycoplasma) fermentans* incognitus will be patients who have been diagnosed as having AIDS or ARC, Cchronic (sic) Fatigue Syndrome, Wegener's Disease, Sarcoidosis, respiratory distress syndrome, Kibuchi's (sic) disease, autoimmune diseases such as Collagen Vascular Disease and Lupus and chronic debilitating diseases such as Alzheimer's disease" (Page 20)

As already mentioned, we will be returning to these and other disease lists but here we will only ask: is there a common cause for all of them, and is that cause an amyloid, a prion, or a mycoplasma? And was Ishii Shiro trying to answer this question in 1942 by infecting members of the Fore tribe with the sheep disease called visna? And did General MacArthur extend a freedom from prosecution for Ishii Shiro in order to find out? And was Carleton Gajdusek sent out to New Guinea in 1954 to see what had happened to the infected tribe members? And did what he found lead him to do the later work he did with Robert Huebner, Robert Gallo and Joseph Smadel? And did the work of all of these, incorporating what had been learned in New Guinea act as one of the factors in the creation of AIDS and CFS/ME and collateral damage such as the diseases listed by Gajdusek and Lo?

Before we answer any of these questions, we will present evidence of what transpired scientifically, medically, and politically following Gajdusek's return from New Guinea.

An Interlude on the Scientific - Biological - Medical Background

Human beings, like other living organisms, are built up of individual cells. Such organisms can range from one cell (the bacterium) to (a fully grown human) fifty trillion cells.

Relative to the total mass to earth's being, only a relatively small part plays a role in the make up of living organisms, whether the one cell or the 50 trillion cell variety. Those elements of the earth that make the greatest contribution to living organisms are only four in number: carbon, hydrogen, nitrogen and oxygen. These four elements (CHNO) constitute about ninety-eight percent of plant and animal (the latter category includes humans) matter. The other two percent is made up of trace elements such as sulphur, potassium, etc. Startling, but true. Check it out in the New York Public Library's *Science Desk Reference*...Page 101! Thus, as an absolute fact, the stuff of physical life is in very limited supply and those 'what have it seeks to keep it' and when they need more they seek to take it from other living beings.

The four elements in the ninety-eight percent part (CHNO) exist as atoms which, in varying composition, combine to form five nucleic acids: guanine, cytosine, adenine, thymine and uracil, which in turn present as either the fundamental blueprint for the carrying life form, deoxyribonucleic acid (DNA) using the thymine, or working drawings as it were for the manufacture of individual life form components, ribonucleic acid (RNA) using the uracil.

These nucleic acids combine in sixty-four groups of three (trinucleotides) some of which go together to form twenty amino acids which, when strung together and folded according to their inherent impulse, form the 60,000 + proteins of which the body is made.

The fundamental life form is the cell, and the fundamental features of the cell are:

1. It is bounded by a unique membrane of lipids. (Basically fats)

2. The membrane has a variety of protein doorways (David Goodsell's analogy; see Bibliography), which regulate what can get in and out of each cell.

3. The membrane has two layers of lipid with water repellant heads facing in and out to maintain the integrity of the cell's interior. What is in the cell stays in and what is outside the cell stays out.

4. **There are periodic molecules of cholesterol which lend the membrane flexibility or fluidity.**

5. The commonly accepted explanation of how the cell membrane is constructed and how it functions was postulated by Drs. Garth Nicolson and S. Jonathon Singer in 1972 and is called 'the fluid mosaic model'.

6. The basic cell model is maintained in all cells of the body, but a wide variety of specialized features make the cell fit into the body in the form needed to fulfill specific functions.

7. Inside each cell are several organelles (tiny organs) which are to the cell what specific organs (the heart, liver, etc.) are to the whole body - i.e. the mitochondria are the tiny organs which generate the energy needed by the cell to do its job.

8. No two cells are directly linked, but they communicate across gaps known as synapses, which are crossed by neurotransmitters such as glutamate or dopamine.

9. When the cell wall is destroyed, lesions are left behind and these form the basis of many of the neurosystemic diseases such as multiple sclerosis and Parkinson's disease.

We have placed point number four in bold type because the loss of cholesterol in the membrane wall is the starting point for most of the degenerative diseases, and cholesterol is lost to the actions of various mycoplasma species which up-take pre-formed sterols from host cells to meet its own growth requirements. A further disease factor originates in the fact that many of the essential hormones that the healthy body needs are built from cholesterol and if there is a reduction in cholesterol due to mycoplasmal up-take, there will be a potential loss of hormones.

The reduction of hormones, in turn, reduces the glandular regulation of bodily metabolism.

To trace the progress along the scientific path which developed sequentially as the political, military, covert forces made possible, we interleave as noted on the 'Contents' page at the appropriate chronological points the first page of the scientific articles which report that progress.

We want to emphasize that the sources selected are primary peer-reviewed articles and government documents which can be referred to by the readers who wish to do so. This is the hard evidence, hidden in plain sight! How that paradoxical condition came about begins with Nelson Rockefeller and ends with eight thousand people dying every day from AIDS.

However, before we turn to 1952 and Dwight D. Eisenhower's election as President of the United States, we need to make a clear statement about the human capacity for evil. We feel thus obliged because there is a view among an apparent majority of ordinary people, that "we" are good and "they" are bad. The "we" of course are those with whom we feel an affinity or kinship. The "they" are those who we are told are our "enemies."

We do good things; they do bad things.

Because of this psychological mindset, there is a resistance to believing anything bad about "us". Such a mindset keeps us from looking reality straight in the eye. In order to help the reader suspend his emotional resistance to what we are about to reveal in this study, we want to share the following well-supported truth with you. It has to do with "us" when we were engaged in fighting Germany, Italy and Japan from 1939 to 1945.

The Japanese, we now know, were engaged in horrendous biological weapons research and there is evidence that such were employed on a limited basis, including their test programs on Allied prisoners-of-war. There is also evidence that the Germans had evaluated the possibility of using chemical and/or biological weapons, but that they had decided against it.

The above we can read and accept because "they" do not have the same high moral qualities that "we" possess. To disabuse any readers who share this "we"/"they" dichotomy we ask you to consider carefully the following signal from Winston Churchill to his Chiefs of Staff on

July 6, 1944:

> "I want a cold-blooded calculation made as to how it would pay us to use poison gas, by which I mean principally mustard. We will want to gain more ground in Normandy so as not to be cooped up in a small area…
>
> "I quite agree it may be several weeks or even months before I shall ask you to drench Germany with poison gas, and if we do it, let's do it 100 per cent. In the meantime, I want the matter studied in cold blood by sensible people and not by that particular set of psalm-singing uniformed defeatists which one runs across now here now there." Churchill to COS, PRO, PREM 3/89.   Quoted from Bryden (1993)

There is no "we" and there is no "they": there is only us, and all are capable of any evil if given the necessary impetus and possessing the necessary lack of truly held moral standards.

End of an Interlude

Finally, before we leave Carleton Gajdusek, we should note the following:

> "To Joe Smadel I also owe the debt of further sponsorship and encouragement, and recognition of my scientific potential for productive research which led him to create for me several years later a then-unique position as an American visiting scientist at the National Institutes of Health."
> (Gajdusek, *Ibid*, Page 165)

In this acknowledgment, we see the tying together of the Department of Defense and the National Institutes of Health. And, we see a continuum from Enders to Gajdusek to Smadel to Koprowski to the Henles to Gallo and hence to AIDS.

But this continuum required an executive agency and that agency had been created in 1947 by President Harry Truman who thought that he was creating an agency which would gather together all intelligence being collected by several independent government departments and thus be able to present the President with a complete, coherent overview of world affairs. However, that Central

Intelligence Agency (CIA) was co-opted in 1952 by Allen Dulles and Nelson Rockefeller when they gained authority with the election of Dwight Eisenhower as President of the United States.

Section 10: The Central Intelligence Agency (Part One)

The Central Intelligence Agency (CIA) was created in 1947 by President Harry Truman to bring together intelligence gathered by numerous other intelligence agencies operated by the various branches of the military and other government departments and make such coordinated material available to the president. Its founding guidelines stipulated that the Agency was to operate in foreign intelligence gathering only and was not to participate in domestic politics. However, according to later comments by Truman after his retirement, and evidence gathered by a variety of political researchers, the CIA secretly extended its mandate by moving beyond foreign intelligence gathering to actual participation in all manner of foreign policy decisions and activities, including the waging of 'hidden wars' upon perceived enemies, and it illegally extended its activities onto the domestic front.

During the Eisenhower administration this activist role of the CIA was greatly expanded under the direction of Nelson Rockefeller who had been appointed by Eisenhower to run the Agency.

It was this extended and corrupted Agency that was largely beyond the supervision of Congress, which began the campaigns against nations with which the United States was technically at peace. Among their first covert sorties were those that destabilized Iran and returned the unpopular (even hated) Shah to the throne; destabilized and ultimately led to the overthrow of the legally elected government of Guatemala; planned and executed the abortive Bay of Pigs invasion of Cuba; and, began the US covert involvement in Vietnam.

In a review of a recent book on the history and role of the CIA by Tim Weiner, Legacy of Ashes, which we have not had the time to read and report upon, reviewer Wesley Wark rhetorically asks, after tracing Weiner's incomplete record of CIA trouble making in the world (including the observation that 'The U.S. Intervention in Iran in 1953 continues to reverberate in that country and throughout the

Middle East'):'Maybe it's time to draw the curtain on the CIA?'[The *Globe and Mail*, July 21, 2007] Wark then answers his own question by quoting Weiner:

> "The war in which we are now engaged may last as long as the Cold war, and we will win or lose by virtue of our intelligence."

Wark editorializes: "It's a sobering thought, and true." The inference is that the CIA, warts and all, will help 'us' win that 'war in which we are now engaged'!

A sobering thought indeed! Neither Weiner, if we can judge from a single review, nor Wark appear to be aware of the extent to which the CIA is the source of world problems and not part of the solution for those problems, including how the CIA, reflecting the will of the establishment, led the way in the development and deployment of biological weapons in Korea, China, Vietnam and as we detail herein, the development and deployment of the pathogenic co-factors that present in the victims as AIDS.

In essence, the CIA in 1952 became and still is, the armed wing or covert army of the shadowy entity variously known as the 'establishment' or the 'supragovernment' or the 'shadow government' of the United States, and this role will become apparent as we re-examine its history.

On this theme we cite Professor Carroll Quigley:

> "The Council on Foreign Relations (CFR) has come to be known as 'The Establishment,' 'the invisible government' and 'the Rockefeller foreign office.'"
>
> (Quoted by Barrie Zwicker; 2006 Page 240)

In summary: Behind the front of the apparent Government of the United States with its legislative, executive and judicial branches there is another 'government' made up of powerful people in finance, industry, law, media, and banking, who exercise power behind the scenes in the direction of public activities and foreign relations. Until 1947 this ill-defined but non-the-less real force exercised its power through the constitutionally established government, but with the establishment of the Central Intelligence Agency in the latter year by President Harry Truman, it secured in essence its own executive arm.

The baleful influence of this executive arm of the Establishment has demonstrated its power to the present authors in many ways since its inception. Although the average reader will have a great deal of difficulty accepting some, many or most of the consequences we list below, we cite them here to get our opinion clearly on the record. And we ask only that they be held in mind as we begin our study. In Chapter 24 we will return to them. Here is our initial list of CIA initiated actions which have significantly de-stabilized the world: destabilizing Iran in 1953; invading Cuba in 1961; executing a President in 1963; overtly involving the United States military in Vietnam in 1964 after the staged 'Gulf of Tonkin' incident; deposing Spiro Agnew and Richard Nixon in 1974; invading Iraq in 1991; staging the World Trade Center and Pentagon attacks on the United States in September, 2001; and the subsequent invasion of Afghanistan.

But, over-riding all else, as we attempt to establish in this study, is the development, testing and deployment of biological agents presenting as the epidemics of AIDS and CFS/ME, and the increasing incidence of other diseases linked to immune deficiency, endocrine disbalance and neuronal damage, such as Alzheimer's, amyotrophic lateral sclerosis, fibromyalgia, lupus, multiple sclerosis, Parkinson's, sarcoidosis, Wegener's, and others.

Beyond belief if your belief is casually held, but not beyond belief if you are able to take each incident and follow the evidence where that evidence leads, regardless of how much it challenges the most deeply held convictions.

Continued in Chapter Nine: See: 'The Central Intelligence Agency (Part Two)'

Section 11: Luc Montagnier

To introduce Luc Montagnier we will first quote from his nemesis, Dr. Robert Gallo:

> "Mycoplasmas are like viruses, rickettsiae, and chlamydia in that they are small enough to pass through an ultra-filter (450 nanometers). They differ from them in being able to have their own complete metabolism and reproduction outside of cells. In this sense they are more like the larger microbes,

such as bacteria, fungi, and parasites. Unlike bacteria, they do not have a rigid outer cell wall but only a membranous envelope. This is one reason for their particular characteristic of extreme variability of form - both size and shape. They were first isolated in 1898 by Edmond Nocard and Pierre Roux in association with a fatal pneumonia of cattle known in Europe since the seventeenth century. In humans, one type causes pneumonia. More often, mycoplasmas are a most unwanted but common accidental laboratory contaminant of cell culture systems. Recently - and to me astonishingly - they have been proposed as a primary co-factor not as an opportunistic infection, but a real co-factor in AIDS by Montagnier, who now further suggests that they are the chief cause of the death of the T4-cells, based mostly on his recent results detecting some in his cultures of the AIDS virus. Montagnier is also recommending treating AIDS with antibiotics - which do inhibit mycoplasma and which he finds also inhibit his T4-cell culture death when used with blood containing HIV and also apparently carrying mycoplasma. I do not agree with the recommendations, on the basis of our work or on what evidence I have seen; nor do I think it has logical merit. *Nonetheless, this surprising view, which has been chiefly presented in press conferences, has given, and may do so for a while, added longevity to confused and confusing (to others) arguments that HIV is not the primary cause of AIDS.*"

(Gallo, 1991 Page 286 footnote)

We have chosen to use Gallo's own words quoted exactly so that it is clear that we are not selectively warping the case he is trying to make. Gallo is saying that the so-called HIV causes AIDS. ('so-called'...please note that we have a problem using the HIV acronym because we just cannot locate any objective, scientific evidence that says such a single-factor immune-deficiency causing retrovirus exists. There is evidence of an adapted sheep retrovirus (visna) that in some cases of so-*called* AIDS acts as a co-factor, but not as a sole pathogenic agent. However, for the present we will use it until by clear scientific evidence we establish an alternative reality.)

Besides using Gallo's own words, we have used his critique of Luc Montagnier's thesis that the HIV is a co-factor able to have its way because of the immune system modulation by a species of mycoplasma. In passing it is to be noted that Gallo (in the italicized sentence at the end of the quotation) dismisses all the careful scientists who have taken much the same stand as that taken by Montagnier. We note, especially, Dr. Peter Duesberg who is discussed further at the end of Chapter 23 of this study.

We will be coming back to this dichotomy over the next several pages, but we want to be on record that Montagnier's thesis makes the most objective sense, and we refer again to the case against Gallo's stance by Professor Serge Lang who writes as follows:

> "**1. No scientific piece of evidence.** Some scientists (including Peter Duesberg and Kary Mullis, independently), have pointed out that there is no scientific piece of evidence showing that HIV causes any disease. For instance Kary Mullis is quoted in an interview (*California Monthly*, September 1994 Page 20):
> "What happened was simple I don't understand why it never happened to other people. In the late 1980s, I was working for several companies that were using PCR to detect HIV sequences. I would get into a little situation where I'd have to write a little report on what was going on at one of the companies. And I would find myself in a position of having to write a sentence that said, 'HIV is the probable cause of AIDS.'
> "I figured out there must be a standard reference or two I could use to back up that statement. So I yelled across the room, 'What's the reference for 'HIV is the cause of AIDS'"? Some guy said, 'Oh you don't need a reference for that. Everybody knows that.' And I said, 'I think it should be footnoted. When you make a direct statement like that, you give it a source. You say, 'Here's how I know that's true. I think its good form."
> "So he said, 'Why don't you cite this Centers for Communicable Diseases [CDC] report?' He gave it to me. It was a stupid little thing, without scientific merit; you might as well quote *The New York Times*. So I went to other people in the lab, and I started looking at the scientific literature, and I began to notice nobody ever quoted a scientific paper

to back up the notion that HIV causes AIDS."
(Quoted in Lang, 1998 Pp. 613-4)

It is important to know the author of this quote (Kary Mullis) won the Nobel Prize in Chemistry in 1993 for the discovery of the polymerase chain reaction [PCR].

The essence of the Robert Gallo versus Luc Montagnier difference thus boils down to a re-play of the Galileo Galilei (1564-1642) versus the Roman Catholic Church on the question is the earth or the sun the center of our galaxy? The Pope, the College of Cardinals and the Inquisition (authority) said that the earth was the center of the galaxy. Galileo (science) said that the sun was at the center. Galileo had his carefully drawn charts and models to demonstrate his interpretation of observed data. The Church had its authority and all the strength that comes from such.

This archetypal model is replayed in this present study.

Section 12: Monkey Kidneys

Edward Hooper (1999, Page 1059) devotes three inches of his index to the subject of 'monkey kidney tissue culture'; hence, it is appropriate that we comment upon the significance of 'monkey kidneys' at this point.

We first became interested in the role of the *monkey kidneys* when we read a 1961 article in the *Journal of Pathology* and written by R.M. Chanock, D. Rifkind, H.M. Kravetz, V. Knight, and K.M. Johnson of the National Institute of Allergy and Infectious Diseases. First, our interest was aroused by the title: "Respiratory Disease in Volunteers Infected with Eaton Agent; A Preliminary Report." The 'Eaton agent' referred to was (as we have already mentioned in Section 3 of this chapter) later identified as a species of mycoplasma. Further, we noted that the article had been 'communicated by Robert J. Huebner, April 19, 1961', who we discuss in chapter three below. The date was significant because it demonstrated that at that early point in time the mycoplasma was entering into the research being conducted. Far from it being a relatively innocuous agent as Gallo tried to let on in the quotation in Section 10, the mycoplasma was obviously important to these researchers. The date was also significant because it followed the

April 13, 1953 decision of Allen Dulles to establish the MKULTRA and the MKDELTA covert programs involving 'biological and chemical' materials. (Richelson, 2001 Page 10) The MK of these cryptonyms we interpret to refer to 'monkey kidneys' and we develop the evidence in Chapter Two.

However, our major interest derived from the statement that: "During the course of these studies 14 strains of the agent (*i.e.* the mycoplasma—Ed) were recovered in monkey kidney culture." (Page 887)

Section 13: Baylor College of Medicine

We draw attention to the College of Medicine of Baylor University in Houston Texas because Baylor has appeared many times in our research, and references will recur throughout this study in many different contexts.For example, on page 362 of the *Special Virus Cancer Program, Progress Report #8*, Baylor is listed as a Contractor to study the possible viral etiology of malignancies in primates. Also, Joseph Melnick who is referred to 16 times by Ed Hooper (1999) played a significant role in developing various pathogenic agents on monkey kidneys.Baylor University has also cropped up in our research as being an institution involved in biological testing on human subjects. See, for example, page 82 of the U.S. Senate Hearings on the subject (1977). In our Chapter 23 we refer to the Huntsville Mystery Illnesses, which involved Baylor.

Finally, in Chapter 15 we refer to the insidious role of Leon Jaworski of Baylor University Law School in respect to the Watergate scandal.

All in all, Baylor is one of the several American institutions doing much of the questionable activities to advance the agenda of certain powerful interests in the 'deep politics of America.'

An Interlude on Bacterium, Virus and Mycoplasma

A Rather Strained Analogy Between a bacterium, virus and mycoplasma breaching the immune system of a cell and a city under siege by a busload of terrorists

A bacterium carrying bacterial toxin seeking to enter a human cell can be likened to a bus loaded with terrorists who are intent on passing through the gates of a walled city to loot that part of the city's wealth as they may require. If the toxic terrorists succeed in breaching the cell wall they move from one molecule to the next, killing the cell and loading the parts onto the bus. (See Page 118, Goodsell 1996) The bus itself, as distinguished from its passengers the terrorists, will have certain fixed parts, or 'organelles' which are necessary for its functioning, but will require constantly replenished supplies of energy to operate. The terrorists on the 'bus' are living creatures who also need a constant supply of nutrient to survive.

If the toxin does not succeed in killing the cell, the organism of which it (*i.e.*: the human body) is just one part, may launch a counter offensive and destroy the bus. However, the terrorists who traveled on the bus may escape and still be alive, even though their bus is destroyed. Not all the escaping terrorists are the same. One part of their group is made up of masters called DNA. The other part is made up of followers with a more limited function called RNA. When their 'bacterial bus' is destroyed, some of the DNA and RNA are able to self-assemble protein flack jackets to protect themselves and flee the bus. When thus clad they are called DNA or RNA 'viruses'.

Other parts of the DNA or RNA only have the capacity to slip on a membrane coat before fleeing the wreckage of their bus and they are DNA or RNA mycoplasma.

The fleeing viruses and mycoplasmas look for other vehicles, either other bacteria or even cells of their erstwhile enemy, that they can get into and find shelter. If the virus or the mycoplasma can access a new host cell, the damage that they can do is what we call 'disease'.

Over the past couple of centuries the health professionals have largely tended to focus upon the disease-carrying bacterium (the 'bus') or the disease agent (the 'terrorist') called the virus. However, there has been a neglect of the nature and presence of that other terrorist called the 'mycoplasma'. The latter neglect was initially due to the fact that the mycoplasma, without a cell wall, was very hard to detect. Later, as we shall see, the neglect of the mycoplasma was studied and purposeful.

Stemming from the consolidation of great wealth in the hands of a relatively small number of families such as the Carnegies, the DuPont's, the Rockefellers and the Morgan's, there was *the development of a movement to limit population growth*. This 'eugenics' movement had its roots in the period from 1900 to the 1930's, and became manifest as official United States Government policy during the Eisenhower administration, and was advanced by the actions of Lyndon B. Johnson and his successor, Richard Nixon following the assassination of John F. Kennedy.

The establishment of the Federal Reserve banking system in 1913, the product of political juggling by Senator Nelson W. Aldrich of Rhode Island and a German banker named Paul M. Warburg, and signed into law by President Wilson on December 23, 1913, effectively surrendered an important constitutional power of the people at large to a small bevy of rich Americans. In this Act wealth was further consolidated into the hands of the few.

The effort by John F. Kennedy in 1962-63 to take back the constitutional right of government "To coin money, regulate the value thereof, and of foreign coin…" [The Constitution of the United States, 1787 Article I, Section 8] which had been surrendered by Congress under the direction of Senator Nelson Aldrich earned Mr. Kennedy the anger of people such as Nelson Aldrich Rockefeller, David Rockefeller and other representatives of wealth and banking institutions was just one of the factors that led to the murder of Mr. Kennedy on November 22, 1963.

The similarity of the names: Senator Nelson Aldrich and Governor (later Vice-President) Nelson Aldrich Rockefeller is more than a co-incidence as we shall establish further along.

In the early years of the twentieth century, the Rockefellers turned their attention and the tremendous power of great wealth to *the control of the nation's health*. This control would later be extended to the whole world through the agency of the World Health Organization. Although the control was purportedly sought so that the Rockefellers could help humanity protect its health, the evidence now is that it was designed as one more device for the few to dominate the many. When one controls another's health, he also controls another's death.

The Rockefeller apparat control of health, extended world wide through the World Health Organization, was to lead to the scourge of AIDS and is still engaged in such activities as the pending but carefully planned 'avian flu' pandemic. Although this statement may at this point sound completely nonsensical, we ask for your suspension of disbelief until we have had a chance to demonstrate the links between HIV (AIDS) and the so-called 'avian flu'. One source can be found, for example, in the article by Burroughs and Edelson (1991) "Medical Care of the HIV-Infected Child", with their discussion of the '*Mycobacterium avium* complex'. One can note in passing that Dr. Margaret Burroughs at the time she co-authored this critical article was a 'Postdoctoral Fellow, Department of Microbiology, *The Rockefeller University*, New York'.

The baleful Rockefeller wealth domination of the health of much of humanity had in its founding years, the input of Dr. William Welch of Johns Hopkins and of Simon Flexner who was to be appointed President of the Rockefellers' Medical Research Institute. The latter was largely responsible for placing the direction of medical research and practice under the direction of the power of wealth, rather than the medical and scientific realities of health and saw the number of medical schools pared down from 162 in 1906 to 131 four years later. The 'blessing' of the American Medical Association made sure that only 'approved' health care would be available to the people of the United States. Welch, at the same time, helped set a precedent of hiding certain medical realities which the power people deemed should be kept from the rest of the population.

The latter influence prevails to this day. Anyone with access to the Johns Hopkins Family Health Book (self-touted on the cover as 'America's #1 Medical Authority') will search in vain for any reference to the **mycoplasma** and to **Bang's disease or brucellosis**, both of which are critical if one is to know the true facts about AIDS. To allow information about brucellosis and the various mycoplasmal species to become widely known would threaten the grip that wealth has over health.

End of an Interlude

Chapter Two

The CIA plus Monkey Kidneys equals MKULTRA, MKDELTA and MKNAOMI

1952–1959…While Eisenhower golfed on the White House lawn and Nelson Aldrich Rockefeller labored in his war room

In April 1953, Nelson Aldrich Rockefeller was named Undersecretary to Oveta Culp Hobby, Eisenhower's Secretary of the newly amalgamated Department of Health, Education and Welfare.

Reports from the time indicate that Rockefeller didn't seem to take any significant degree of interest in any of the three major challenges of the Department. Routine matters of health, education and welfare were being looked after by the Rockefeller family's various charities and related institutions. To seasoned onlookers, Undersecretary Nelson Rockefeller seemed to have something else on his mind. As William Mitchell, a long time Social Securities Administration official expressed it:

> "'(Rockefeller) never impressed me as being either an effective or even particularly imaginative person…and he seemed to work through advisors that were hazy figures on the periphery of the internal administration. They were people who apparently were tied in with numerous Rockefeller outside interests, and I personally think he would have been a hell of a lot better off if he'd left them where they were.'" (Collier & Horowitz, Page 271)

If it was not health, education and welfare that were drawing Nelson Rockefeller's interest and efforts, what were?

Perhaps there is a clue in the fact that upon his arrival at HEW, he immediately set up what he called a 'war room'. The imagery is significant. Largely ignoring the regular staffers and allowing activity in the Department to unfold as it should, Nelson Rockefeller brought in several shadowy figures from the Rockefeller family apparat and worked diligently and secretly at something for eighteen months.

Then, apparently satisfied that he had accomplished all that he had set out to accomplish at HEW, he asked Eisenhower for a new job, and Eisenhower had one waiting for him: Special Assistant for Cold War Strategy.

Despite the unusual title and Rockefeller's claim that the post was meant to put him in a position to give "advice and assistance in the development of increased understanding and cooperation among all peoples," in fact, say Collier and Horowitz, the post made Nelson Rockefeller the President's coordinator of the Central Intelligence Agency. Eisenhower had wanted someone who would, in effect, stand between him and the public when it came to matters dealing with morally questionable activities. Not that Eisenhower objected to doing such deeds; he simply did not want to be questioned about them. 'Plausible deniability' was born during Eisenhower's watch.

An example of this way around being held morally responsible for his actions is seen in his order to assassinate Patrice Lumumba, the charismatic leader of the citizens of Belgium Congo as that colony was making its way towards self-government. Questioned about Eisenhower's role in the decision to murder a nationalist leader, a CIA official said that the President gave the order 'with a wink and a nod', but never said so in so many words. Everyone at the meeting knew what was to be done, however Eisenhower was later able to say to reporters that he had never given such direction to his staff.

However, before we examine Rockefeller's activities in the CIA, we must return briefly to his eighteen months in the war room of HEW. What was it that he and his team of outsiders, brought in from various 'Family' groups, were doing?

The answer to this question is difficult to find. Not only did the work going on in the war room proceed in absolute secrecy, but later official and semi-official writers and researchers have little or nothing to say publicly about it.

For example, Edward Shorter, a media asset in respect to the duplicitous role of the government and the medical hierarchy in hiding the truth about chronic fatigue syndrome, wrote a text about the National Institutes of Health titled *The Health Century*. Although nominally funded by The Blackwell Corporation, *The Health*

Century is a propaganda piece intended to take public attention off the politicalization of this government agency. Morton Blackwell was a New Right leader in the Reagan White House whose fellow Republicans like Jesse Helms and Pat Robertson were known for their neo-Nazi positions.

The Health Century makes a brief but gushing mention of the Rockefeller Institute for Medical Research...i.e. "In this sea of American scientific mediocrity an island of excellence—indeed brilliance—stood out: the Rockefeller Institute for Medical Research which opened in 1901..."

But it says absolutely nothing about Nelson Rockefeller and his eighteen months of secret activity. Although we have not been able to find any explanation of what Rockefeller was up to, we are satisfied from indirect evidence that he was busy splicing the hitherto largely apolitical National Institutes of Health into the largely secret health-related and very political activities of the U.S. Military and the newly emerging CIA.

To start at the beginning when Truman signed the Act to create the CIA, its budget was to come largely out of money originally spent by the Department of Defense. Fletcher Prouty tells us that:

> "As originally created, the OPC (Office of Policy Coordination) was totally separate from the CIA's intelligence collection (another function not specifically authorized by law) and analysis sections. The OPC's chief had been nominated by the secretary of state and approved by the secretary of defense. The funds for this office were concealed, as were much of the CIA funds, in the larger budget of the Department of Defense. Policy guidance and specific operational instructions for the OPC bypassed the director of central intelligence completely and came directly from State and Defense. In other words, the OPC was all but autonomous." (Page 27)

Nelson Rockefeller was to change that, and to go even further, but first, he had to work within HEW to establish the necessary channels of communication, control and finance. *HEW was to become an agency researching ways to kill rather than just an agency to research ways to protect life.*

With this re-structuring mission accomplished, Nelson Rockefeller was ready for his next assignment: to join Allen Dulles in the Central Intelligence Agency and to get on with the business of population control. President Eisenhower was willing to oblige and thus it was that in the fall of 1954, Rockefeller and Allen Dulles were united to begin whatever evil works they had dreamed of. The executive instrument of such works was to be the highly secret Planning Coordination Group, or as it was renamed, the Office of Policy Coordination. In place of the structure outlined above, the new OPC was to be made up of Rockefeller, along with the Deputy Secretary of Defense, and CIA Director, Allen Dulles. With whom, essentially, was the CIA to be 'coordinated'? Why none other than the U.S. Department of Defense and the Department of Health, Education, and Welfare.

What, exactly, had Nelson Rockefeller done?

He had first fractioned off a larger CIA budget from the Defense budget, and then he had incorporated a large part of the HEW budget into financing CIA research.

The latter move was not just insidious; it was ingenious for it gave CIA 'black ops' research a respectability from being done under the aegis of HEW, as well as a great cover. In addition, it gave CIA research a lot more money than it would otherwise have had. Finally, it effectively removed direction of the Office of Policy Coordination from HEW and Defense and put it under himself.

Rockefeller was ready to proceed with his 'family agenda', including population growth rate reduction. His next step was to bring on board several of his operatives from his pre-government role in Central and South America, such as E. Howard Hunt.

Most people who remember him at all, first learned of **E(vert) Howard Hunt** when he turned up in news reports as one of the 'masterminds' of the Bay of Pigs invasion in 1961 and later when he was photographed dressed as one of three 'tramps' who were riding out of town in a freight car from behind Dealey Plaza in Dallas, Texas on November 22, 1963. Then he is met while testifying before the Senate Select Committee on Presidential Campaign Activities (the 'Watergate Hearings') about a break-in of the office of a Dr. Fielding, the psychiatrist who had Daniel Ellsberg as a patient; and, later still when he was arrested for his role in the Watergate break-in. It is not that Hunt was a brilliant man who had much to offer his country but just had a streak of bad luck with everything he touched. The truth is that he was stupid and had a knack for fouling up whatever he turned his hand to. As Kenneth Galbraith has suggested about Whittaker Chambers, Hunt was not only a member of the extreme right wing cabal involved in all of these crimes, he was 'luminously insane.' But, stupid or otherwise, he was a loyal operative of the Rockefeller apparat.

Lunacy doesn't seem to be a handicap when working with this cabal. Indeed, it may well help ensure steady employment.

Thus, when Rockefeller joined Allen Dulles at the CIA in late 1954, he brought E. Howard Hunt with him. According to Hunt himself in his book, *I Came to Kill*, he had worked for Rockefeller in South and Central America where he had participated in assassinating politicians and others who opposed the baleful Rockefeller influence in those areas. He had also worked with Tracy Barnes, a Rockefeller relative by marriage who had been Hunt's Bay of Pigs co-worker.

In 1955 E. Howard Hunt was assigned to the North Asia Command of the CIA to participate in the joint CIA- Military attempt to cause disease epidemics in both North Korea and China. The use of biological weapons had begun earlier in that war, and in the course of carrying out secret raids, two U.S. intelligence operatives, John T. Downey and Richard Fecteau were captured. Hunt wrote of these two tragic victims of U.S. duplicity that the CIA assumed they had 'told their captors everything.' He was right; they had. (For more detail, see Endicott and Hagerman: *The United States and Biological Warfare*)

We draw special attention to E. Howard Hunt in order to demonstrate the Rockefeller link to the Bay of Pigs, the murder of John F. Kennedy, and the removal of Richard Nixon as President. We do this, not to join the other critics of the Rockefellers and their role in American history, but to prepare your psychological readiness to acknowledge the Rockefeller role in unleashing AIDS into the world, and the evidence which we present in this study.

For years the Rockefellers have employed professional public relations experts to convey a picture of a great family, wealthy because of their astute business acumen, but willing through their charitable works, to share their wealth with humanity. For much of humanity, especially for many American citizens who have been reared on a pliant media diet this image is hard to surrender, but the facts speak for themselves.

This 'Rockefeller' public persona is essentially fraudulent. From the massacre at Ludlow to the massacre at Attica certain members of the Rockefellers have demonstrated their capacity to be ruthless if need be to ensure that their wealth…the answer to all their problems…remains intact. And, as Ferdinand Lundberg has so brilliantly summarized in Chapter Five of *The Rockefeller Syndrome*, their 'charities' have served to preserve their hold on and control of their wealth, rather than serve as conduits to human betterment. The latter may, incidentally, be advanced to a degree, but only as a way to continue the Rockefeller hold upon it and the evil that it helps to obscure.

The Unelected Elite

Before we leave this subject, we must declare that not all the 'Family' who benefit from the wealth, were and still are culpable nor even witting of what is going on. We suggest that many have been largely put out to pasture by the self-perpetuating clique who have subtly but effectively seized control of this 'Rockefeller' power. If certain members do not demonstrate to the self-selecting core-perpetrators of the cabal, the necessary black qualities to carry on the *modus operandi* they are ignored in splendid isolation. We further want to make clear that although we use the 'Rockefellers' as the name for the apparat involved in the secret domination of American power, there are many others in the 'Establishment', including the DuPonts and the Morgans, who are linked in the shadows as the 'unelected elite'. To emphasize this point we feel that it is necessary to quote extensively from Collier and Horowitz, pages 275 and 276:

> "By the mid-1950s, the United States was locked into its global crusade and the Rockefeller family was established as an important resource in the life of the nation. If it was not quite the 'Rockefeller conspiracy' some charged, it did have the appearance of careful organization. Through its connections with the Chase Bank and the Standard Oil

companies, and its association with such great Wall Street investment and law firms as Kuhn, Loeb; Lazard Freres; Debevoise, Plimton; and Millbank, Tweed, the family had its fingers on the pulse of the country's industrial and financial heartlines. Through the Rockefeller Foundation, the Council on Foreign Relations, and the Republican Party, it was connected to the highest directorates of national policy. Whenever members of the power elite gathered to make the crucial decisions of the postwar period, one or two of the key individuals would inevitably be drawn from the executive levels of the institutions with which the family was deeply involved. Men like John J. McCloy, C. Douglas Dillon, James Forrestal, Robert Patterson, Robert A. Lovett, the Dulles brothers, and Winthrop Aldrich *were never elected to office*, but wielded a power that was in many ways greater and more sustained than that of the elected officials they served."

And, in support of the Collier & Horowitz thesis we quote Arthur M. Schlesinger, Jr., from page 128 of his book, *A Thousand Days*:

"(Kennedy) was little acquainted in the New York financial and legal community - that arsenal of talent which had so long furnished a steady supply of always orthodox and often able people to Democratic as well as Republican administrations. This community was the heart of the American Establishment. Its household deities were Henry L. Stimson and Elihu Root; its present leaders, Robert A. Lovett and John J. McCloy; its front organizations, the Rockefeller, Ford and Carnegie foundations and the Council on Foreign Relations; its organs, *The New York Times* and *Foreign Affairs*."

In 1955, Nelson Aldrich Rockefeller was the figure from this establishment in the key position to advance the Rockefeller 'interests' by virtue of his personal qualities of a pleasing public persona, which cloaked a well-contained contempt for ordinary humans. Included in their interests was that of controlling the rate of growth of the world's population.

Here is how it came about that he was able to indulge this compulsion.

On July 26, 1947, as we have mentioned above, President Harry Truman signed legislation which created the Central Intelligence Agency. There is now evidence that he did not know exactly what it was that he was creating, and he is quoted by Merle Miller in Plain Speaking:

> **(Miller)** "…you were responsible as President for setting up the CIA. How do you feel about it now?"
> **Truman:** "'I think it was a mistake…And if I'd known what was going to happen, I never would have done it.'"(Page 419)

Within the Truman-created CIA, on April 13, 1953, Allen Dulles, acting on a proposal from Richard Helms, his Deputy, launched a program to develop a capability in the covert use of biological and chemical materials. Research into biological and chemical weapons had actually been going on for years, dating back at least to 1942 when the United Sates joined with its allies, Canada and Great Britain, in work involving both. But, what was important about Richard Helms' proposal was that the plan included the verb "use" and designated that the activities were to be "covert".

The program was to be designated **MKULTRA**. Although not known at the time, the initials MK stood for 'monkey kidneys' and the 'ULTRA' was to indicate its umbrella-like nature which would allow it to go far beyond any known or stated limits. It was sold to President Eisenhower by telling him that what was going to be researched was the Chinese success in making American prisoners-of-war 'falsely confess' to war crimes such as the use of biological weapons in the Korea War. As we have seen, the confessions were actually true, but the United States Government and army apologists liked to let on to the world that they had been extracted from prisoners by 'brain-washing'. Eisenhower went along with the explanation for its need and it was soon up and running.

Shortly after the Watergate break-in and its links to the Nixon White House were discovered, Richard Helms directed Sidney Gottlieb to destroy all MKULTRA files. The efforts were largely successful and only a few pages escaped the shredders and were to be discovered later in an intensive search on orders from President Jimmy Carter. In those few pages published by the U.S. Government Printing Office, Carter's new CIA Director, Admiral Stansfield Turner reported:

> "MKULTRA was an 'umbrella project', under which certain sensitive subprojects were funded, involving among other things research on drugs and behavioral modification. During the Rockefeller Commission and Church Committee investigations in 1975, the cryptonym became publicly known when details of the drug-related death of Dr. Frank Olson were publicized…"

The red-herring was being drawn across the trail, and it had originally been provided by none other than Nelson Rockefeller! What was it that he was trying to draw attention away from? It was the major research that had been launched when he had become Eisenhower's man in the CIA, and that research involved the work of Dr. Robert Huebner who had discovered that a microorganism that he called a 'pleural pneumonia-like organism' could cause the 'spontaneous degeneration' of lymph tissue such as adenoids.

What? The lymph tissues, which provide the major human defense against opportunistic diseases such as Pneumocystis carinii pneumonia (PCP) and Kaposi's sarcoma (KS) even against certain cancers, could be caused to degenerate?

A victim whose lymph tissues had degenerated, or even reduced significantly in function, would be almost certain to die! The population control advocates' dream. Death would be even more certain if, along with this immune-system suppressor, a retrovirus such as the visna virus of sheep could be introduced at the same time or at some later point in time, to the target.

Fortunately, the Rockefeller Medical Institute had just such an expert on 'lenti-viruses' on hand in the person of Dr. Bjorn Sigurdsson. Dr. Bjorn Sigurdsson had spent two years with the Rockefeller Institute in New Jersey studying plant, animal and human viruses and he was now ensconced in Iceland as the head of an institution to do research into novel disease agents: The Institute of Experimental Pathology, financed in large part by Rockefeller wealth.

Sometime later, after Huebner had re-discovered the PPLO (it had earlier been identified as we noted in Chapter One, in 1898 by Drs. Nocard and Roux of the Pasteur Institute, but then largely ignored), other scientists (headed by Drs. R. M. Chanock and Leonard Hayflick) realized that the PPLO was actually a species of mycoplasma and they signed a letter to that effect which was published in Science, Volume 140, page 662, on May 10, 1963. (Ch. 22) We shall have much more to say about Hayflick and Chanock (a particular favorite of Gina Kolata and *The New York Times*) and their links to AIDS, later.

That PPLO *cum* mycoplasma correction was made in 1963, eight years after Nelson Rockefeller and his fellow CIA alumnus, Allen Dulles, had started to work on the mystery agent which promised to be refractory to the human immune system. Even though they had no knowledge of how deadly the microorganism that they were working with actually was, and even though they did not know its true nature, those who labored in the fields of MKULTRA research got immediately to work to follow up on the possibilities, including the possibility that they might unleash another Black Death plague in the world. (See Dr. MacArthur's testimony)

Getting to work meant finding research physicians who were amoral enough to use human beings as guinea pigs and such physicians were found. Among them were Dr. Alton Ochsner of Tulane University in New Orleans, LA, Drs. Robert Chanock, Robert Couch and Vernon Castle of Baylor College of Medicine in Houston, TX. And Dr. Herald Cox, of Lederle Laboratories in New York.

MKULTRA was under way.

To test the efficacy of such a theoretically perfect weapon component, it would be necessary to grow as much PPLO or mycoplasma on monkey kidneys as required for the growing demand of the researchers and to test these cultured agents on someone, somewhere, and if it worked, it would be important to get it into the blood of targeted victims. We will summarize the progress made in all of these areas after we first present an overview of other CIA activities of the times. Such activities laid the foundation for five decades of political corruption throughout the world.

The Central Intelligence Agency from 1952 until 1960

William Blum left the State Department of the United States Government in 1967 because of his opposition to what the United States was doing in Vietnam. In 2005, his book, the Third Edition of *Rogue State*, was published by Common Courage Press. The book gained notoriety when it was revealed that none other than Osama Bin Laden had read it and had urged readers throughout the world, but especially readers in the United States, to get the book and read it. *Rogue State* is a very readable account of the many crimes against humanity that have been committed by certain forces within the United States against several foreign nations since the CIA was created in 1947 and then given its head by Dwight Eisenhower in 1952.

We took Osama Bin Laden's advice and bought and read *Rogue State*, and we are pleased to urge you to do the same. It presents a well-researched and humane account of world history from c.1945 to the present, and the baleful role of the United States in that history. Furthermore, it presents that U.S. record in more detail than we can do here. Our major study is how the co-factors that present as what is now called AIDS were discovered, developed and deployed. In order to present that story, we first had to present in outline the story of the CIA and all of the evil that has grown from that Agency as a counter to the glib and self-serving picture depicted by much of the major media, and to present the background from which the AIDS mentality sprang. We chose the following five examples of that background, but to read a fuller account we recommend William Blum's *Rogue State*.

We will save what Mr. Blum says about AIDS until Chapter 16.

Iran

Allen Dulles had a long and devious history in activities of the Middle East, but Iran began to receive more of his attention when, in April 1949, as a private lawyer for the New York law firm of Sullivan and Cromwell, he arrived in Tehran as an adviser to the Shah, twenty-nine year old Mohammad Reza Pahlavi. The Shah was engaged in an intense struggle with his subjects who seemed to put more trust in their populist, somewhat eccentric, leader, Mohammad Mossadegh. Dulles' links with the Shah paid off for both after Eisenhower was elected President and essentially sheltered himself from the covert activities of the CIA which followed by appointing Nelson Rockefeller as his special assistant in CIA matters.

After Dulles' appointment as Director of the CIA, and with the later support of Nelson Rockefeller as the Chair of the nebulous Planning Coordination Group, Dulles led the United States' efforts to depose Mossadegh and keep the Shah on the throne. The illegal and indeed criminal actions of the Dulles/Rockefeller alliance were apparently successful. Largely against the will of the people of Iran, the Shah remained upon the throne and the United States took control of its oil production. However, we qualify this success with our reference to 'apparently successful'. The promising dawn of a democratic movement was quashed by a repressive Iranian secret police and opposition to the Shah went underground until the resistance burst its bonds and the country fell into the hands of the Ayatollah Khomeini and all that followed.

It is important to note that the turmoil and challenge that exists today grew from U.S. covert crimes against another nation…the War of Terror…U.S. terror against the world had started.

Guatemala

The apparent success of the Dulles/Rockefeller CIA efforts in Iran emboldened them to continue, and they found their next target in Guatemala.

In 1951 Jacobo Arbenz was elected President of that country. He was a left-leaning, somewhat cautious advocate of social reform. But he was first and foremost, a democrat and one of his first acts was to legalize the Communist Party…the first nation in Central/South America to do so. Despite the fact that the total number of communists in Guatemala was less than the number of communists in San Francisco, Arbenz' actions excited a near frenzy in the Council on Foreign Relations and in the Eisenhower administration.

A Council on Foreign Relations spokesman went on record as declaring that the election of Arbenz was "…quite simply put the penetration of Central America by a Russian-dominated communist group."

When Arbenz legally and with full due process enacted legislation to expropriate several large estates and turn title of the land to Guatemalan peasants, the CIA, in January 1954, began its campaign to depose Arbenz and to replace him with a U.S. military-dominated dictatorship. The campaign was successful and a long, dark night of U.S.- trained murder squads killing thousands to teachers, clerics, nuns, left-wing lawyers and other 'communists' was launched.

Year's later one of the CIA operatives confessed that those murdered actually were not ranting communists who were taking their orders from Moscow. He said, "They were very honest, very committed. This was the tragedy - the only people who were committed to hard work were those who were, by definition, our worst enemies." American state-sponsored terror continued on its path of evil.

Vietnam

When the French Army was finally defeated in Vietnam on May 7, 1954, Eisenhower turned to Allen Dulles and the CIA to keep all of what had once been called "French Indochina" from becoming another 'communist's state.' Dulles was more than willing to tackle the job and with the support of Nelson Rockefeller, Vice-President Richard Nixon and Admiral Arthur Radford (another 'hawk' who could well be described like Whittaker Chambers in John Kenneth Galbraith's words as 'luminously insane' and who, as chairman of the U.S. Joint chiefs of staff, had assured a congressional committee on the eve of France's defeat…that France had arrived at 'a favorable turn in the war') he and Nelson Rockefeller went to work to replace the French in Vietnam.

Eisenhower accepted the view of these criminals and he allowed the gradual involvement of the U.S. in that country. (For more of the story of Vietnam see the following in our Bibliography: Stanley Karnow: Vietnam; John Newman: JFK and Vietnam; and Neil Sheehan: A Bright and Shining Lie)

However, *Eisenhower's acceptance of the U.S.'s growing role was more by default than by intention. Actually, he was opposed to getting involved in Vietnam, but since he had largely abdicated from his proper role as the leader of the United States Government, that involvement developed under Dulles and Nelson Rockefeller. Here, as summarized from Fletcher Prouty's account. (Bibliography: Pages 51 -56)*

"It was January 8, 1954…Eisenhower…was presiding over a meeting of the National Security Council when the subject turned to U.S. objectives and courses of action with respect to Southeast Asia, the President said…'with vehemence': 'There is just no sense in even talking about the United States forces replacing the French in Indochina…I cannot tell you how bitterly opposed I am to such a course of action. This war in Indochina would absorb our troops by divisions!'

"President Eisenhower could not have expressed his views on the subject of a 'Vietnam War' more forcefully. He knew that we did not belong there. Yet less than a month later, on January 29, 1954, many of the officials who were at that meeting, including the vice-president, the secretary of state, the secretary of defense, and the director of central intelligence, ignored the President and made plans to get on with the business of making war in Indochina."

Thus, by default of active, involved leadership, Eisenhower allowed the United States to get involved in Vietnam.

Note the pattern: the President just didn't know what was going on.

Belgian Congo

From 1885 until 1908 this large equatorial country in central Africa became a Belgian colony and was known as the Congo Free State, and from 1908 until 1960 when it became independent, it was known as the Belgian Congo (pop. approximately 35 million - 1991). Today it is variously called Zaire or The Democratic People's Republic of the Congo. Essentially, it is the basin of land drained by the Congo or Zaire River, which rises near Uganda and flows south and west to the Atlantic as the White Nile flows north to the Mediterranean.

A smaller country, known simply as Congo (pop. approximately 2.5 million - 1991), flanks the north and westerly shore of the Zaire River. Occupied by France in the early 1800's, it gained independence in 1960, and like its neighbour, Zaire, was wracked by civil wars.

For purposes of this study, we will focus solely upon Zaire, as an example of the tragedy of the local inhabitants engaged in a century-long struggle to be rid of foreign masters and the subtle imperialistic ambitions of the United States to acquire an empire in fact, but not in name.

But, there is another and more pertinent reason to focus upon the former Belgian Congo. That reason is found in the fact that the Belgians for ten years prior to Zairian Independence, had fought a very cruel fight to retain command of its resources and, when the Americans offered them assistance in the period following the election of Dwight Eisenhower, they jumped at the chance.

The assistance in question was not the traditional armed help that America often offered right wing colonial or dictatorial rulers, but was a new type of assistance: a plan to reduce the population significantly and, to facilitate that plan, help in murdering national leaders such as Patrice Lumumba.

As we have seen, the population reduction plan required on-site laboratory facilities for an American 'polio' researcher named Hilary Koprowski of the Wistar Institute in Philadelphia, and also required several hundred chimpanzees and some other primate species. The primates would provide monkey kidneys to be harvested and shipped to the Wistar Institute or sent to Belgium or, in some cases, retained and used in the Belgium Congo.

In passing we must note that working alongside Koprowski was a German researcher named Fritz Deinhardt who had received some special training at Wistar, and had then traveled to the chimpanzee facility in the Congo to experiment on chimpanzees with a hepatitis B vaccine that he was attempting to develop. Hepatitis will figure in this study later on in three American cities: New York, San Francisco, and Los Angeles, and involving homosexual men in those communities. The same population was to present with the earliest North American cases of AIDS.

As suggested, Camp Lindi was a combination chimpanzee farm and research laboratory in the Belgian Congo near the City of Stanleyville. It was situated on the north shore of the River Congo, near the junction of the Lindi River.

The Camp had its inception in 1955 when Dr. Hilary Koprowski, an employee at that time of the Rockefeller-controlled Lederle

Laboratory, met with an ex-patriot Polish veterinarian named Dr. T. J. Wiktor in Muguga, Kenya at a WHO-sponsored conference.

Notice the concurrence of the date (1955), Rockefeller, and WHO.

Wiktor referred Koprowski to Ghislain Courtois of Belgium who was currently Director of the *Laboratoire Medical* in Stanleyville, the Belgian Congo. Koprowski shared an expensive plan with Courtois: the Belgium Government would establish the Camp Lindi complex, and would allow and indeed work with Koprowski and Deinhardt in developing vaccines on **monkey kidneys**, with an emphasis on chimpanzee kidneys.

Now notice the monkey kidneys and the MKULTRA-MKDELTA CIA programs were just getting nicely under way in the United States.

Strangely enough, the Belgium Government was enthusiastic about expending large sums of money in a monkey colony in a country which they knew that they were about to lose to rebel nationalists! Besides building the camp and paying hunters to capture and deliver hundreds of chimpanzees to Camp Lindi, the Belgium Government assigned Courtois, and two other Belgian doctors, Gaston Ninane and Paul Osterrieth to the undertaking.

Why were the Belgians willing to expend this money and effort?

They said that it was done in the hopes of finding a polio vaccine, grown on monkey kidneys, which would *save the lives of the citizens of the Congo with whom, paradoxically; they were engaged in a nationalist civil war.*

As the use of 'monkey kidney' implies, they were actually working with the Rockefeller - American eugenics fanatics in the CIA programs: MKULTRA and MKDELTA. The war against the nationalists was to continue, but it would be a one-sided, secret war using syringes rather than guns.(We are greatly indebted to author/researcher, Ed Hooper and his book *The River*, for the wonderfully detailed accounts of Camp Lindi.)

Cuba

The Cuban conspiracy of Allen Dulles, Richard Bissell, Richard Nixon, E. Howard Hunt and Tracey Barnes (a Rockefeller family member by marriage) was different than the covert wars waged against Iran, Vietnam, Guatemala, and the Belgian Congo. The Cuban crime was planned and put together during the Eisenhower administration, then was to be carried out in a form much in excess to anything Eisenhower thought that he was approving. The plans would be put in motion when Vice-President Nixon succeeded Eisenhower as President.

Eisenhower had approved a relatively low key plan to train some forty to sixty Cuban exiles as guerillas and to land them in Cuba where, it was claimed by the Dulles brain trust, they would soon be joined by thousands of disaffected Cubans who wanted to get rid of Fidel Castro. During the election hiatus between the Eisenhower administration and the anticipated Nixon administration, the plans changed dramatically and secretly and instead of a band of fifty guerillas, the invasion force of Cubans was expanded to the size of a Brigade.

And Eisenhower didn't know how the original plans as described to him had been changed!

The Brigade was to be landed from three ships supplied by CIA operative (later President) George H. W. Bush working under the cover of an oil drilling supply firm, and was to be supported by American air cover. Some of the American planes were to be painted with Cuban logos to make it appear that they were actually being flown by rebellious Cuban Air Force pilots. Then, President Nixon was to order the American military to join the fray in support of the 'democratic' invaders, and the rebelling Cuban Air Force.

Or so it was thought; but, a funny thing (in fact, several funny things) went wrong on the way to the American invasion of Cuba. First, Richard Nixon was defeated by John F. Kennedy in the election of November 1959. Second, the Cuban people rushed to the invasion site, known as the Bay of Pigs, to repel, not to support the Brigade. The latter was soon being decimated. Third, President Kennedy, who had gone ahead reluctantly with the Dulles plan, would not be suckered into sending U.S. air support nor ground and navy forces.

The Bay of Pigs failed; President Kennedy publicly took the blame; Allen Dulles and Richard Bissell were fired after a decent, face-saving interlude, and John F. Kennedy vowed to break up the CIA and throw it to the wind. This was the transition point between the dark era of

1952-1960 and the era of dawning light of the Kennedy thousand days. The crimes of America in Iran and Guatemala were done, but the agony lingered on and festers until this day. The crime against Vietnam was still in progress and John F. Kennedy was working towards withdrawing the U.S. from that betrayed nation. But the terrible crime against the Belgian Congo and the world crept along in the sewers of American life, hidden even from John Kennedy, himself, until November 22, 1963, and Lyndon B. Johnson was enabled to come out of the traitor's closet where he had sheltered for three years as Vice-President.

But, the seeds of AIDS were well and deeply planted with the work of scientists from Fort Detrick to Johns Hopkins and the "44 colleges or universities, 15 research foundations…12 hospitals or clinics, and 3 penal institutions" referred to by Admiral Stansfield Turner who were working in the MKULTRA/MKDELTA programs.

We will trace those plantings as reported in the peer-reviewed medical and scientific journals and in government documents, as we follow the political record from 1952 until the present in Chapter 23: The Scientific Paper Trail to AIDS. Many readers will express incredulity at the idea that such a heinous crime would be placed in the media for all to see, but this was a major part of the plan to hide the reality. Hide the record in plain sight!

By the CIA/Pentagon links to the NIH and CDC established by Nelson Rockefeller from 1953 to 1955, money could be spent, eminent scientists hired, and research could be conducted as if it were growing naturally out of the search for health. Hide the use of chimpanzee kidneys under the search for a polio vaccine. Hide the infection of millions of Black citizens of Africa under the gift of a smallpox vaccine program. Pay for it with American taxpayers' money except for that portion paid under the 'Black Budget' necessary for the financing of the most blatant activities.

However, John F. Kennedy stood in the way.

Back to MKULTRA and its Subprojects

These are just five of several instances where, while President Eisenhower golfed on the White House lawn, Nelson A. Rockefeller and Allen Dulles, on behalf of what Professor Donald Gibson refers to as "...the Establishment, East Coast Establishment, Higher Circles, financial establishment, Wall Street, or upper-class elite" plotted to spread American terror throughout the world. We cite these examples to make the secondary point that the operative words in describing all of them are 'bullying, inhumane, and selfish.'

However, the primary point that such instances serve to make is that the climate was sufficiently immoral to allow the makers of MKULTRA to embark on a plan to use Dr. Robert Huebner's medical science to kill off millions of human beings in an effort to slow the rate at which the world's population was growing. If a disease agent could lower the human immune system sufficiently by causing the 'spontaneous degeneration' of lymphoid tissues, then those infected would be exposed to opportunistic diseases including those caused by retroviruses, heretofore only a health threat to sheep, then death was sure to follow.

Only gangsters whose daily work included Iran, Guatemala, Vietnam, the Congo and Cuba could seek to advance such an evil enterprise, and just such gangsters were in place to do so, but as we have noted, John F. Kennedy stood in their way.

They began by growing the mycoplasma on the kidneys of monkeys, so that this relatively unknown pathogen could be available to selected scientists to work out the necessary details of how to develop the ideal weapon of an undeclared biological war against unsuspecting and defenseless people, especially those of Africa and the Third World.

Because they had no idea what they would need nor where their necessary research would lead, their evil project had to start as an 'umbrella' project, and specialized subprojects must be capable of being followed up on as experience demonstrated to be necessary. Project 'monkey kidney umbrella', code named **MKULTRA** was launched.

We will review what remains of the MKULTRA records in Chapter 16, but note at the outset the comment of a 'Mr. Brody' who was, as Admiral Stansfield Turner described him to the Senate Hearings, "...a long-time member of the CIA...To my knowledge, there was no Presidential knowledge of this project at the time."

As Eisenhower golfed on the White House lawn, the Rockefeller agenda of population growth rate control got under way.

The Other Side of the AIDS Coin

To this point, we have been examining the evidence that Nelson Rockefeller, first as an Undersecretary of HEW and later as Eisenhower's point man in the CIA, had been able to tie the Rockefeller Family interest in population control into a covert program of the CIA under Allen Dulles. This program under the umbrella of MKULTRA, and the latter's subprojects, MKDELTA and MKNAOMI, took the work of Robert Huebner and the latter's re-discovery of the mycoplasma and began the search for ways to utilize the mycoplasma as a strategic weapon. Thus there was a continuum from Rockefeller to Allen Dulles to the CIA to HEW to the National Institutes of Health and to the National Cancer Institute (NCI) under Robert Gallo to AIDS.

That was one side of the AIDS coin.

There was another side, even though in the final analysis, both sides were aspects of the same coin. The other side of the AIDS coin consisted of Vice-President Richard Nixon, businessman Roy L. Ash, American Cyanamid, Litton Industries and Dr. Robert Ting to Robert Gallo and hence again to AIDS.

We will develop more about Richard Nixon in Chapter Fifteen, however at this point we must introduce him, since, while the President was golfing on the White House lawn, Vice-President Nixon was engaged in other things. Those other things included the cultivation of certain wealthy friends such as the above-mentioned Roy L. Ash.

Roy Ash is probably a far more important person in the development and deployment of AIDS than he has ever been given credit (or blame) for, and we must summarize him at this point.

Ash began his working career at eighteen, working for the Bank of America from 1936 until 1942. At this point, although with no undergraduate degree, he was able to enroll in the MBA program at Harvard where he was a classmate of Robert McNamara and a member of a group of ambitious young men who were classed as 'whiz kids'. It is important to note that both he and McNamara held strong 'population growth rate control' ideas, although until John Kennedy's death, McNamara was reticent to publicize these views.

Ash returned to the Bank of America until 1949 when he

moved to Hughes Aircraft where he remained until 1953. At Hughes Aircraft, Ash became familiar with Nixon who was first a Congressman, 1947, and after 1950 a Senator, until elected Vice President in November 1952, and assuming office in 1953. Ash had been one of the contributors to Nixon's infamous private fund used to complement his Congressional pay, which when it was revealed to the public almost caused Eisenhower to drop him as his running mate. However, Nixon out-maneuvered Eisenhower on this one by making his famous televised speech about his wife's 'Republican cloth coat', and stayed on the ticket.

Ash and Nixon had known each other over the previous six years…Ash as a high finance officer with Howard Hughes Aircraft and Nixon as a Congressman and Senator with an interest in military contracts. When Nixon assumed his duties as Vice President in 1953, Ash suddenly resigned from Hughes and participated as a founder of a new corporation called Litton Industries, Ltd.

As Vice-President, Nixon continued his interest in defence contracts and by 1956 had become Chairman of President Eisenhower's Committee on Government Contracts, and in this role was instrumental in directing hundreds of defence contracts to the new Litton Industries, Ltd., as well as continuing contracts directed to Hughes Aircraft.

Thus, Litton was off to a good start under Roy Ash and his fellow whiz kids who were participating in a very sophisticated fraud scheme designed to bilk investors out of billions of dollars.

It worked this way…and here we will quote from Robert Monks and Nell Minow's book *Power and Accountability*:

> "Some of the cleverest people in America - Ford Motor Company's 'best and brightest', Roy Ash and Tex Thornton - with their 'whiz kid' credentials, brought forth to a hungry public the new phenomenon in the form of Litton Industries."

"Litton was as close to glamorous as a business can get. With its former movie headquarters in Los Angeles, with Crosby Kelly, the inventor of 'financial public relations,' and with a record of increasing quarterly earnings for over ten years, Litton seemed able to do anything, despite the fact that no one could single out any particular value that was added…"

"The story ended badly. Litton's radiance ultimately became tarnished. The stock 'tanked' in 1968. That is, the stock fell 18 points in one week. It did not merely fall in an orderly manner; it disintegrated."(Pages 38–9) With parts of heavily compartmentalized Litton Industries, Ltd., falling apart in 1968, Roy Ash took on another job for Richard Nixon. In April, 1969, Nixon was just assuming his new office as President of the United States, and Ash became Nixon's chairman of the President's Advisory Council on Executive Organization."

Now, with Litton Industries 'disintegrated' in 1968, one could not be blamed for assuming that Litton was out of action. This was not the situation. Over the years from 1953 to 1969, Litton had emerged in a variety of forms, including Litton Bionetics, Inc., and Litton Systems, Inc., and Bionetics Research Laboratories, Inc., and Litton Data Systems Division…and many more. So, when Litton Industries, Ltd. 'tanked' in 1968, the body of corporations assembled by the whiz kids, continued to fly blindly around like a decapitated chicken, and by 1972 it was a holding company listed among the 50 largest corporations in the United States!

How could a huge corporation built upon fraud survive and even thrive as its crimes were revealed? There are probably several aspects to the answer to this question, but one of the important reasons for its survival was simply this: Richard Nixon was able to channel billions of dollars in defence contracts to his old friend, Roy Ash. Taxpayers' money flowed into Litton in all the latter's corporate manifestations and, in return, the covert evil of the CIA was able to acquire a corporate partner in its schemes. And one of those schemes involved the development and deployment of disease pathogens that finally led to AIDS.

And where did the covert and the corporate meet? What was the nexus of biological evil?

The meeting of the covert and the corporate was the MKULTRA, MKDELTA efforts of the CIA working with Litton Industries, Ltd. The nexus or linkage was supplied by the United States Government and Nixon's 'war on cancer' program.

And who were the key people at the actual meeting point of the covert and the corporate under the aegis of the U.S. Government besides those in the shadows that we have been examining to this point?

The two key people in the actual science of developing a new microorganism, one which does not naturally exist and which is refractory to the human immune system were Robert Gallo for the CIA-covert and Robert Ting for the corporate with Henry Kissinger directing on behalf of his sponsors, the Rockefellers and their cohorts.

An Interlude

Acknowledgment: We are greatly indebted to Edward Hooper, author of *The River*, for many of the details recounted in this 'Interlude'. However, the speculative elements are our own.

In November **1955**, David Carr of Manchester, England, joined the Royal Navy. Upon his enlistment, he was given the full range of vaccinations that all British servicemen were required to accept.

In January **1956**, on H.M.S. Ceres he was given two further vaccinations. His medical record states that one vaccine was a "pretreatment" while the other was listed as "ATT". The ATT may have been a booster of antitetanus toxoid, but the other was then and is still a mystery. What was David Carr being "pretreated" for? Ed Hooper interviewed the senior officer of the Institute of Naval Medicine in Gosport, England, looking for answers. That officer said "*it sounds like he was being pretreated for something he was going to be exposed to*," such as malaria. I pointed out that members of the armed forces had also been used as guinea pigs in germ warfare experiments during this period, and the officer agreed that such trials took place. He promised to investigate discreetly, but he never got back to me with any results."

Three years later, in late summer **1959**, David Carr died of what appears to have been AIDS, but with one exceptional and vitally important difference, he does not appear to have been infected with the so-called human immunodeficiency virus or HIV! **AIDS without HIV!**

Here is what we believe happened.

In the 1940s and 1950s and probably longer than that, the United States Navy co-operated with the British Navy and the Royal Canadian Navy in testing various biological, chemical and radiological weapons.

For example, our research has provided us with sketchy but genuine details about a Canadian warship, which, in the early 1950's, joined with several American warships at sea south of Newfoundland. At a particular point an American bomber flew over them, spreading a plume of mist. All the ships were drenched with whatever it was being thus disseminated. Years later we were approached by a young man in Ottawa, Canada, who told us that his father had been on the Canadian warship and that some ten years later had begun to present with symptoms of amyotrophic lateral sclerosis. Not only that, but four other crewmen who had served with him in the same ship at that same time, had also developed symptoms of ALS. In all five cases the symptoms worsened until all five were crippled and ultimately died of the disease. Given the fact that the crew of the Canadian warship was approximately six hundred, the incidence of ALS is extremely high, and the only thing that any of the five men could identify that might have triggered the disease in them was the American spraying in the 1950s.

We are continuing our research into this tragedy, but we are finding it hard to get any answers at this late point in time. However, we are satisfied that the United States Navy was heavily engaged in biological weapons testing and that they were able to recruit the co-operation of the British and the Canadian forces in their efforts.

In support of this hypothesis is our experience with another testing program that was conducted in Canada within the same time frame.

We have learned that the Canadian Government directed the Dominion Parasite Laboratory in Belleville, Ontario, Canada, to breed one hundred million mosquitoes a month and to deliver these to Dr. Guilford B. Reed, Head of Biology at Queen's University in Kingston, Canada. In his laboratory, Dr. Reed contaminated the mosquitoes with unknown pathogens supplied to him by the United States Military. The disease-contaminated mosquitoes were then delivered to the Canadian Military in Kingston, Ontario. The Canadian Military shared the contaminated mosquitoes with the United States, and both the Canadian forces and the American forces carried out a series of tests in various geographic areas and then monitored the health of that area to determine how many people presented with what signs and symptoms over the days and weeks ahead.

When we learned of this program, we contacted Queen's University, the Canadian Military, the Department of Veterans Affairs, the Prime Minister of Canada, and other politicians, including

The Hon. Diane Marleau, Member of Parliament for the Federal Riding of Sudbury and who is our local M.P.

Queen's University was very rude and unco-operative. Initially, they had threatened to sue us if we persisted in presenting our findings to the public. We encouraged them to sue, and they immediately dropped that threat. Now, they simply do not reply to our letters. The Canadian Military has not replied to any of our queries. The Prime Minister, The Rt. Hon. Jean Chrétien, also never replied, nor did the Minister of Veterans Affairs.

On our last encounter with The Hon. Diane Marleau, she asked, "Has the Military ever replied to you about their use of mosquitoes in testing programs?" We replied that they had not. At that Ms. Marleau said something very revealing: "They haven't replied to my letter, either. You know, the Military is a power unto itself. It doesn't tell us anything that it doesn't want us to know."

This episode demonstrates that the Military of both the United States and Canada have participated in programs which test the efficacy of new biological weapons. It further demonstrates that certain institutions such as Queen's University co-operate in such programs while posturing as law abiding upright models of social responsibility. It is also evident that someone, other than the politicians who are nominally in charge of such things, are really directing things from the shadows.

What does this all have to do with David Carr who died a way back in 1959? Just this: it is altogether likely that at some level of the Royal Navy there was someone in a position to order the RN Medical Institute to participate with their American allies in testing a new biological weapon. The weapon would be the PPLO or mycoplasma, re-discovered by Dr. Robert Huebner and known to reduce the capacity of the human immune system and so expose the victim to opportunistic diseases which ordinarily he would be able to resist. This would be a 'pre-treatment' with another pathogen (probably one linked to the visna virus of sheep) to follow, which, in David Carr's case was never delivered. Despite that fact, Carr developed a range of illnesses based upon his immune deficiency, and he died. AIDS without the HIV!

In other words HIV (if it even exists) does not cause AIDS…it is just one of many pathogens which can take advantage of an immune system which is rendered refractory to such insults.

We will return to this subject in Chapter Sixteen where we present details about Gulf War Syndrome and Major Timothy Cook of the Canadian Military and Captain 'Craig" Hyams of the United States Navy.

End of an Interlude

By November 1959, the shadow government of the United States, with its covert CIA army ready and willing to wage war anywhere in the world, including a secret strategic biological war against the growing population of the Third World, was suddenly faced with an unexpected crisis: the anticipated successor to Eisenhower, Richard Nixon, was defeated in the election of that year by John F. Kennedy.

Socio-Political

Although we identify the election of Dwight D. Eisenhower as the specific date of activities that have led to the development and deployment of the co-factors (actually, as we shall develop, the 'co-factors' are biologically, probably aspects of one principal factor) which together present as acquired immunodeficiency syndrome, we must summarize *the critical elements which constitute the background* of the post 1952 political events. *Among these elements are the concentrations of great wealth in the hands of a few families.* That concentration of wealth has in many instances, passed from the actual families to a self-perpetuating power structure operating on its own momentum. The families, although still nominally controllers of the wealth and power, are largely put out to a comfortable pasture.

The initial corruption of American society, now a corruption extending world-wide, which has taken place as a consequence of this consolidation of wealth is evident in many crimes ranging from the 1963 murder of John F. Kennedy to the current invasion of Iraq but most tragically, it is evident in the 8,000 AIDS - related deaths a day and the disablement of many thousands of other human beings, world-wide, from diseases such as chronic fatigue syndrome, and (quoting from a Patent of a '**Pathogenic Mycoplasma**' held by the

United States Government and dated January 6, 1991) "Wegener's Disease, Sarcoidosis, respiratory distress syndrome, Kibuchi's (sic) disease, autoimmune diseases such as Collagen Vascular Disease and Lupus and chronic debilitating diseases such as Alzheimer's disease."

To the above official acknowledgment of pathogenic mycoplasma illnesses we, with assurance, can now add diabetes type one, many forms of cancer, Crohn's-colitis, Lyme disease, multiple sclerosis, Parkinson's disease, Rheumatoid Arthritis, and others. All can be traced to a disease microorganism called the 'mycoplasma', which can in turn be linked to the bacterium *Brucella* that we referred to above.

PART TWO

*THE DEVELOPMENT AND TESTING
OF PATHOGENIC CO-FACTORS*

Chapter Three

ROBERT HUEBNER AND THE COUGHING RECRUITS

When Robert Huebner was asked in the early 1950's by the United States Navy to help solve the recurring problem of a chronic but relatively mild form on pneumonia in Naval recruits, he agreed and set to work. Later, he reported his findings in a 1953 article in the *Proceedings of the Society of Experimental Biology and Medicine*. But, the article didn't focus upon the pneumonia. It dealt with a secondary phenomenon: the isolation of a disease agent from the adenoids of his naval recruits. The adenoids in the cases of chronic pneumonia presenting in the recruits were undergoing **spontaneous degeneration** in tissue culture!

This phenomenon of spontaneous degeneration of living tissue was to set the course for the remaining life and research of Robert Huebner, for it was to lead to the isolation and engineering of one of the critical co-factors of AIDS, and, as you shall learn, it also set Huebner on the path to his own death.

Robert J. Huebner can be pointed to as the father of AIDS.

Huebner followed his 1953 article with a series of further research reports spanning the years to 1971 when in the latter year he is credited with a total of 61 citations in *Progress Report #8* of the *Special Virus Cancer Program*, and by 1978 he appears in *Progress Report #15* as a member of one of the SVCP Committees. Among his SVCP committee colleagues are three others worthy of note: Dr. Robert Manaker who as we shall see in Chapter 14, contributed his initial "M" to the strange antecedent program titled MK-SVLP; also listed is none other than Dr. Robert Gallo who was to later 'co-discover' HIV with Luc Montagnier; and, another key figure in the creation of the AIDS co-factors, George Todaro.

Thus, Huebner started with an atypical pneumonia [which is a characteristic of AIDS], moves into the degenerating adenoids [which are **lymph** tissues] and then he becomes an important researcher in a program mysteriously labeled with a code name: **MK-SVLP** [where the 'L' stands for 'leukemia/lymphoid'] and in 1965 [right after Lyndon B. Johnson had won the election in his own right as President of the USA] the 'MK' is dropped from the original code name, and SVLP comes out of the covert shadows into the relative light of day, as a mainstream US Government research enterprise, Huebner is still right there. As we have already mentioned, the Program known as MK-SVLP is an apparent attempt at obfuscation which we will develop further in Chapter Fourteen.

Then, when Nixon declared his war on cancer in 1971, Huebner made a career change. His friend, Robert Gallo, tells it this way:

> "When Huebner announced his virogene-oncogene hypothesis, he had already worked for many years and with much success in the Infectious Disease Institute of the National Institutes of Health. His decision to move at this time to the National Cancer Institute, also at NIH, coincided with President Nixon's declaration of his 'great war on cancer' in 1971."

We shall see why it was that Huebner made this 'move' at this time, but first let's continue with his pneumonia to adenoids research. When we do that you will see how the spontaneously degenerating adenoids were to lead to his work in cancer and finally, how it came together as a co-factor in AIDS. (We realize that there is no such thing as 'spontaneous degeneration', that there is *something* that is causing the adenoids to degenerate. However, the terminology is Huebner's so we will go along with it for the time being.)

At this point we refer you to Exhibit Two in the Appendices. There you will note the adenoids at the top and back of the nasal cavity. And note in passing that they are just behind the receptor neuron olfactory node which allows certain air-borne molecules breathed into the nose to enter the brain and register as odors. Later we will demonstrate how this fact figured in the death of Dr. Huebner, but first we must continue with the adenoids.

The adenoids are one of the first lines of defence in the immunological processes in the body (and keep this in mind when you read Dr. MacArthur's statement to the Congressmen that we report in chapter fifteen, that a new lethal biowar agent the Pentagon's eminent biologists were working on would be "…refractory to the immunological and therapeutic processes upon which we depend to maintain our relative freedom from infectious disease.")

In the immunological processes upon which we depend to maintain our health, the adenoids play a guardian role. They capture samples of the air that is being drawn into the lungs.

If that air has some pathogenic agent (such as a species of airborne mycoplasma, the adenoids will not stop it, but will react to it, warning the immune system of the affected individual that something is wrong with the air that he is breathing. The re-action to one of the pathogens - various mycoplasmal species- which humans can breathe (*i.e.* that are transmitted by 'aerosol') is 'spontaneous degeneration', which was just what Huebner had noted in his study of pleural pneumonia! That's why Huebner devoted further attention to the degenerating adenoids than to the pneumonia itself. He wanted to find out what it was that was causing the pneumonia, but he was more concerned about the concurrent adenoidal disease.

At first, he could do no better than label the pathogen as a 'pleural pneumonia-*like* organism' or PPLO. He chose this name because the pathogenic agent found in the infected lungs that was causing the chronic pneumonia in the naval recruits was the same pathogenic agent he had found in the degenerating adenoids and which was called a 'pleural pneumonia organism' (PPO).

It is worth noting in passing that Huebner had adopted a new name for the lung disease that was interfering with the Navy's training programs. He called the disease "acute respiratory disease" or ARD. This acronym is startlingly close to another 'acute respiratory' illness, the *severe acute respiratory syndrome* or SARS, which we will look at in chapter seventeen.

After Huebner, *et al.* had published their findings, several other biologists corrected him. It is not, properly speaking, a PPLO that is causing the ARD and the concurrent spontaneous degeneration of the adenoids they told Huebner. The PPLO, they pointed out, is really a micro-organism identified in the late 1800's by two French scientists [at the Pasteur Institute, Nocard and Roux]. The PPLO is actually a **'mycoplasma'.**

A Brief Anticipatory Interlude

At this point we want to draw your attention to something that you need to know as early as it can logically be introduced. This is just such a logical point.

It needs to be noted that the mycoplasma which Huebner stumbled upon in the late 1940's and early 1950's became a subject of much covert research. After all, if the Military is looking for a bioweapon what would be better than one which causes human tissues to spontaneously degenerate? The resultant research, much of which we have now succeeded in tracking down and which we recount in the coming pages, led to the Patenting of a **pathogenic mycoplasma** by the United States Department of Defence. The nominal 'inventor' of this disease-causing mycoplasma as we have reported in chapter one, was Dr. Shyh-Ching Lo of the American Registry of Pathology and the Patent was granted on September 7, 1993.

The critical details that you need to know are on page 22 of that Patent. On that page it is asserted that persons infected with the mycoplasma will be those who have been diagnosed as having either AIDS or CFS or other disease entities such as those we summarize in chapter seventeen. All have to do with some mysterious disease agent that affects the respiratory system…including the one that got Huebner his job with the Navy in the first place.

End of an Interlude

Three micro-biological researchers [Rottem, Pfendt, and Hayflick] were able to demonstrate in 1971 how the mycoplasmal damage is done. It seems that certain species of mycoplasma, because they are only *particles* of a complete DNA/RNA have no capacity to manufacture their own growth requirements. To make up for this short-coming, while still possessing the essential urge to live, these species can up-take pre-formed sterols from their host and incorporate these sterols into their own being. Ultimately the loss of such sterols by the host cell, within which the mycoplasma has taken shelter, especially from their membranes, both external and internal, leads to the death of the host, and further damage is then done. The damage that is done is broadly categorized as 'degenerative' and there's where we came in…studying Huebner's work with the *spontaneously degenerating adenoid tissues* in Naval recruits.

Here, apparently, is what was happening, and how this led in turn to AIDS.

The naval recruits, sharing cramped sleeping and living quarters were exposed to and inhaled air breathed many times over by all of them. In such an environment any pathogenic microorganism was not received and then exchanged for fresh and non-contaminated air, but was constantly being re-introduced into the lungs to challenge the immune defence processes provided by the body. In time those recruits with the least immune defence, would begin to present with the lung infection and in some cases with degenerating adenoids. And it is at the latter point that we began our study of Huebner with his naval recruits; acute respiratory disease; degenerating adenoids; PPLO and finally the mycoplasma.

The same principle appears to be at work today in certain work situations and the incidence of disease. For example, the largest employee groups presenting with chronic fatigue syndrome are schoolteachers, hospital workers and airline flight crews. All are exposed in their work to closed space and re-circulated air for lengthy periods of time.

Huebner followed up his initial work with the help of Drs. Manaker, Todaro and Aaronson and as we shall demonstrate, all figure significantly in the so-called *Special Virus Cancer Program*. For example, on page 327 of Progress Report #8 of the SVCP, Todaro is credited with an article titled, "Rapid detection mycoplasma-infected cell cultures", while on page 282 of the same document, Manaker is reported to have experimented with primates by inoculating 33 chimpanzees with the mashed up tissue of diseased human lymph glands. Finally, on page 303 of the document we find that two of these researchers, Todaro and Aaronson, were busy with Huebner himself working with a mouse sarcoma virus. (You will recall that Kaposi's sarcoma is an important symptom of AIDS.)

Summary

In the late 1940's and early 1950's Robert Huebner went to work with the U.S. Naval Medical Research Unit No. 4 to study chronic and recurring respiratory diseases. In the process of doing his research, he realized that the organism which gave rise to one such disease also infected the adenoids of the recruits. Further research showed that the microorganism involved in the adenoidal degeneration, which he had first labeled as a pleural pneumonia-like organism, was actually a bacterial DNA/RNA particle called a mycoplasma. Huebner and his Navy employers quickly realized that the mycoplasma had great potential in a field of research that greatly interested them all: biowar weapons development. Other researchers such as Todaro, Aaronson and Hayflick were recruited to covertly pursue the latter prospect. One of the co-factors of AIDS, the mycoplasma, was well on its way to being put to work to reduce the rate of world population growth.

Chapter Four

BJORN SIGURDSSON…SCRAPIE AND RETROVIRAL DISEASES

In 1946 the United States' chief of biological weapons development reported to the Secretary of Defence that the research scientists had managed to *isolate the disease active principal of bacteria in a crystalline form*. This accomplishment held great significance for the creation of effective biowar weapons. One of the major problems encountered in biowar research prior to this was the fact that bacteria were very hard to keep alive and dangerous until they could be used against an enemy. Further, methods of dispersing bacteria, such as putting them into bombs, often killed the payload before a disease epidemic got started. Finally, it was hard to target an enemy without exposing one's own forces to the disease agents being used. There was always the great danger of 'blow-back' as happened in Korea when the U.S. tried to use the Hantavirus against the North Korean forces. (Chapter One; Section Nine)

Now, if one could take only that part of a disease-carrying bacterium, and remove just the part that specifically caused the disease from its source in the form of crystals which would be easy to carry and easy to target on a foe, one would obviate many of the problems. This is just what George Merck and his researchers had learned how to do by 1946.

Reports as to just which bacteria were used in developing this crystalline and highly portable disease agent are still hidden in the Pentagon archives; however, circumstantial evidence suggests that one of them was based on the *Brucella* bacteria. This highly contagious capsulated bacteria causes disease in both animals and humans. The disease that presents was named after Sir David Bruce [1855-1931], a British bacteriologist who was studying the disease on the island of Malta. The symptoms of brucellosis are dramatically similar to the symptoms of chronic fatigue syndrome…just what Merigan and

Stevens and others in the biowar weapons program were working on in the 1960-70's: weakness, extreme fatigue, night sweats, generalized aches and pains.

Whichever bacteria it was that Merck was talking about, the potential was clear. The disease active principal could be removed from its living source as inert crystals, and then could be communicated to the target with more precision by way of various vectors: aerosol, insect bites, or food chain. And, furthermore, regardless of which bacteria it was derived from, the new bioweapon had to be tested.

Biological weapons testing pose great hazards to all of humanity, including the testers and their families. One way to limit such danger is to do the testing in a remote, hard to access place such as an island…preferably a foreign island, such as Iceland.

That's where Dr. Bjorn Sigurdsson of Iceland enters into the history of AIDS.

Bjorn Sigurdsson was born in Iceland in 1913 and died from kidney cancer 49 years later (1959). At the age of 24 he had graduated in medicine from the University at Reykjavik, and did further studies in Denmark. In 1941 he made another career move: he entered the **Rockefeller Institute** in New Jersey to study plant virology and animal virology to complement his existing expertise in human virology. From plants to animals to humans! You'll learn the significance of this continuum later, and we'll learn that Robert Gallo had been an early student of the science. However, at this point we need only note the entry onto the scene of the Rockefeller Institute.

Sigurdsson apparently made quite an impression upon the powers that be in the Rockefeller Empire, for, after completing his plants to animals to human's virology, he returned to Iceland with a $200,000 grant from the **Rockefeller Foundation** to establish an Institute of Experimental Pathology. Get that name: 'experimental pathology'. Everyone understands 'experimental' meaning to test ideas about something, and when it is coupled with 'pathology', the origin and nature of diseases, the name of Sigurdsson's new Institute is at least highly suggestive.

Sigurdsson was on his way to discovering the other factor in the AIDS co-factors: the retrovirus. Let's trace his progress.

As luck would have it, and just after Sigurdsson's return to Iceland, a rather remote Island in the North Atlantic which at that time was under the control of the United States' Government, a 'mystery' disease broke out in the northern part of the country. But Sigurdsson was on hand to rush to the main town affected, Akureyri, and give the victims the benefit of his education in virology.

In Akureyri, Sigurdsson found that some 1,116 school children and young adults had become ill with a disease that looked for all of the world like brucellosis, but with a strange presence in a few cases of paralysis. Furthermore, something even stranger presented. In five of the children Parkinson's disease developed, and rapidly progressed, killing the victims.

One must keep constantly in mind that this outbreak of what appeared to be a bacterial disease (brucellosis) *without the presence of the bacteria* itself developed at almost the same time that George Merck was reporting that his researchers had managed to isolate the disease active principal from bacteria such as *brucella*.

Then something else occurred that merits reporting. After the outbreak of what came to be called 'chronic fatigue syndrome' a contingent of scientists, doctors, and other researchers arrived in Akureyri from none other than the Rockefeller Institute to measure the extent of the epidemic, and the continuing consequences. Sigurdsson was, of course, on hand to make his patrons at home.

After the Rockefeller contingent had completed their survey, Sigurdsson went on with his work in an area largely unexplored up until then: **retroviruses**.

Before going further let's recapitulate what we have noted thus far. In the United States Robert Huebner was working towards the discovery of the nature of the various mycoplasma species, which is essentially a virus without a protein coat. Because certain species of the mycoplasma have an absolute growth requirement for the up-take of pre-formed sterols (including cholesterol...and keep this in mind when we get to that portion of this study that focuses upon Dr. Robert Gallo) they can cause the 'spontaneous degeneration' of the cells that they invade. If they do not cause sufficient damage to kill the cell, they at least compromise its capacity to defend itself from other disease agents, such as those which present as Kaposi's sarcoma, pneumoniae carinii pneumonia, lymphadenopathy, and so on.

In Iceland Bjorn Sigurdsson was busy searching for the secrets of the retroviruses. After all, one of the better-known retroviruses was one that infected sheep, [with sheep raising a major industry in Iceland] and was called 'Visna', which means 'wasting' in Danish. As a matter of fact there are three variants of the visna virus: Visna, itself, plus Maedi [name derived from the Danish for 'shortness of breath'] and a third referred to as PPS...because it causes a 'progressive pneumonia of the sheep', and is sometimes referred to as OPP or 'Ovine Progressive Pneumonia.'

There are two factors worthy of note here. One is the fact that the diseases in the sheep have so much in common with AIDS and CFS in humans. The wasting quality is characteristic of both, and the significant linkage to respiratory illnesses is another. In fact, in one tribute to Sigurdsson published in 1991, the late doctor was credited with laying "the base upon which AIDS research was later built." This despite the fact that AIDS was not officially known until 1981 and Sigurdsson had died 22 years before!

The principal symptom of visna is that derived from the extreme itch, which accompanies the disease. This leads infected sheep to rub themselves against trees or posts until their wool is 'scraped' off and hence is called scrapie. The latter word has now entered into the lexicon of western medicine where it is defined as a usually fatal disease of the nervous system characterized by emaciation, weakness and paralysis and caused by a slow virus. On autopsy the distinguishing feature of an infected brain and to a limited extent certain other organs such as the heart, is the presence of intracellular fibrillary tangles.

It was to this group of retroviruses that Sigurdsson largely devoted his research after he had finished up his 1946 to 1948 work on the mystery outbreak of CFS among school children and had acted as escort for the visiting Rockefeller investigative team.

Thus, while Huebner was appearing in the literature with articles such as "Isolation of a cytopathogenic agent [the mycoplasma] from human adenoids undergoing spontaneous degeneration in tissue culture" based upon military financed research, Sigurdsson was appearing with articles such as "Visna, a demyelinating transmissible disease of sheep" based upon Rockefeller financed research.

Here you have the co-factors of AIDS: the mycoplasma and the retrovirus.

Concurrent with the work of Huebner and Sigurdsson was related work by several other scientists most of whom were to appear in the

Special Virus Leukemia/Lymphoma/Cancer Reports a few years later. Among those who will turn up later in this study are J. B. Moloney, a great friend of Robert Gallo. Moloney even misappropriated money to help Gallo according to Gallo's own admission. Another interesting researcher whose work is reported in the literature of the period is Dr. Brian Mahy. [Chapter seventeen, below] Like Moloney, Mahy was not only someone whose work is tied in closely with AIDS/CFS/ME research, but also like Moloney, Mahy misappropriated over four million dollars given to him by Congress to study CFS. Then there is Dr. Maurice Hilleman who later turns up as the Chief Virologist for George Merck Pharmaceuticals. [You may recall that Merck was once the Head of the Biological and Chemical Weapons research for the U.S. Government.] Finally, in this time frame there was another Rockefeller protégé: Dr. Hilary Koprowski, whose research deserves a separate chapter (below), for he took the science of Huebner and Sigurdsson and turned their results into the crime beyond belief: AIDS.

Summary

Bjorn Sigurdsson's whole career is colored by the fact that in the early 1940s he attended the Rockefeller Institute to study plant and animal virology. Since he was already an accomplished and well-regarded medical doctor, the focus upon plant and animal diseases is very suggestive. Also, the fact that the microorganism known as the mycoplasma infects plants, animals and humans can provide a reason for extending his scientific foundation beyond that which he already possessed. In addition, the wartime efforts to adapt certain animal diseases to affect humans as biological weapons [brucellosis for example] suggest that his links with the eugenics-minded Rockefeller Institute and his broadened studies were not based simply upon a professional desire to be better informed.

It is evident that Sigurdsson was an early recruit to the Rockefeller stable and that his long-term goal was to master zoonotic diseases such as the retroviral sheep disease, Visna. The Rockefeller Foundation advanced such work by funding Sigurdsson's Reykjavik-based Institute of Experimental Pathology. Sigurdsson was also on hand in Iceland to monitor the evident trial of a disabling disease, which possessed many of the same symptoms as Chronic Fatigue Syndrome.

Chapter Five

HILARY KOPROWSKI

The Moribund Wistar...
Solving the Polio Problem as a Cover for Co-factor Testing

By 1952 two important scientific factors for the ultimate development of the co-factors of AIDS were in place, albeit in a rudimentary and poorly understood way. There was the immune suppressing mycoplasma re-discovered by Dr. Robert Huebner and there was the retrovirus based upon the research of the visna virus by Dr. Sigurdsson. It was enough to require some sort of testing to determine whether the promise that the co-factors combined in a vaccine carrier seemed to hold, could in fact be realized. This state of knowing some things but not knowing others was not enough to prevent further efforts to put what was known to work as soon as possible. Robert Gallo himself admitted as much when he wrote in another context:

> "Some commentators on the history of science have noted that scientists did not need to understand any fundamentals or mechanisms to come up with antibiotic cures for some bacterial diseases, nor did Sabin, Salk and *Koprowski* need to know how the polio virus worked to develop their vaccines."

So it was with the powerful and hidden patrons of those scientists whose scientific research could be put to work to develop a deadly pathogen based upon the co-factors being developed.

The PPLO of Huebner, which he soon learned, was a species of mycoplasma, did not have to be understood in order to see that its great capacity to compromise the immune system and to cause the degeneration of cells could be an important component of a new microorganism in the search for biological weapon agents. A microorganism composed of co-factors, which did not naturally exist, as Dr. MacArthur was later to tell certain Congressmen on June 9,

1969, but one, which would be refractory to the human immune system. At the same time these patrons saw that the mycoplasma if united with the visna retrovirus of Sigurdsson could open the way for the latter disease agent and other opportunistic diseases to have their way within the body of a targeted victim. The mycoplasma would lower the immune defence system and the retroviral RNA of visna could then access selected cells and direct those cells' DNA to reproduce copies of its mutated self.

And this is just what happened.

If we skip ahead to July 1972, and if we study the *Special Virus Cancer Program, Progress Report #9* we find on page 39 the following statement:

> "We have for the first time demonstrated that the…RNA directed DNA polymerase, **can be activated** by alteration of the physiological endocrine balance."

The RNA directed DNA polymerase is the retrovirus at work. It can be put to work if the endocrine balance of the body is altered… and that is just what happens when the mycoplasma up-takes pre-formed cholesterol to meet its own absolute growth requirements. When the cholesterol is up-taken, the production of hormones in the endocrine system is **altered** because it is cholesterol from which the secretory glands manufacture hormones. The altered endocrine system in turn adds to the already compromised immune system.

However, the researchers of 1952 did not understand the mechanics of the pathogenic co-factors. All that they and their patrons knew was that the mycoplasma altered the cellular immune defence and that this compromised defence permitted retroviruses, such as visna of sheep, to do something they couldn't do before: invade the cell's DNA and create in humans the scrapie already seen in infected sheep.

Huebner's and Sigurdsson's work could be united. What was needed was some scientist of sufficient skill to do the science and to combine them in a suitable vaccine and of sufficient moral deficiency to permit him to undertake such a task. Also, there had to be a place to do the work…one, which was totally and completely under the control of the patrons. There also had to be a cover story so that when the world saw the skilled scientist in the new physical facility doing all manner of biological research, there would be no suspicion that the goal of the whole enterprise was to slow the rate of growth of the world's population. Finally, there had to be a way to get the new co-factors into the blood of the targeted victims without them knowing that they were being doomed to a terrible death.

And this is where one of the Rockefellers enters the scene as an active participant, rather than simply as the source of direction and funding.

In November 1951, war hero General Dwight Eisenhower was elected President of the United States. Between the date of his election and the day that he took office, he had to put together a Cabinet to run the vast machines of the bureaucracy. One person that he had to recruit was obviously one of the most political of the powerful Rockefeller family: Nelson Rockefeller.

To most peoples' surprise, Nelson Rockefeller chose the job of Undersecretary of Health Education, and Welfare [HEW]. At last one of the scions of one of the world's most ardent eugenics-driven families had a toe-hold in government. And when:

> "…he became an administrator in charge of the new agency's $2 billion budget and 35,000-member staff; he began immediately setting up a **war room**…(H)e seemed to work through advisors that were hazy figures on the periphery of the internal administration. They were people who apparently were tied in with the numerous Rockefeller outside interests."

And Nelson Rockefeller's major outside interest was eugenics, and to advance this passion his new assignment would allow him to co-op the public health agencies into the biowar weapons research of the military.

After these agencies of health and defence had been melded and the Department of Health was effectively a Department of Death, Rockefeller was appointed as Eisenhower's 'Special Assistant for Cold War Strategy.' Effectively, Rockefeller was in command of the Central Intelligence Agency, and was ready to declare a covert war against a major enemy: humanity. He began by taking direction of the CIA program known as MKULTRA that had been launched in 1953. Ostensibly, the program was to be a secret study of 'brain-washing' in response to the work of the Chinese on prisoners of war from the Korean conflict. Under Rockefeller the MKULTRA expanded from one secret program to one program that held within itself several other secret programs, including MKNAOMI and MKDELTA, and quite possibly the MK-SVLP we have already encountered.

But, we are getting ahead of ourselves. We must first go back to 1952 and the research of Huebner and Sigurdsson. The eugenicists, led by the Rockefellers, needed someone to bring Huebner's mycoplasma and Sigurdsson's retrovirus together, and their man to do this was right there. Ready willing and able: Hilary Koprowski.

Hilary Koprowski had been born in Poland, educated as a microbiologist, and fled to Italy ahead of the German invaders. He immigrated to Brazil where he was employed by none other than the Rockefeller Foundation. Following the war he moved to the United States where he found employment with Lederle Laboratories, the pharmaceutical arm of American Cyanamid. He worked with Dr. Herald Cox from 1946 to 1950 developing a polio vaccine. American Cyanamid and Herald Cox were secretly engaged in biological weapons research as a photo in the official history of Fort Detrick was later to reveal, for there, right in the front row was Dr. Herald Cox.

The man, Hilary Koprowski, a Rockefeller alumnus, was available to follow up on the Huebner/Sigurdsson research. Now, to find a place.

The place had to be somewhere that did not have a solid, informed Board of Directors already in place. Further, there could not be pre-existing staff already doing professional research. The answer was found when the Wistar Institute in Philadelphia was suddenly activated to be more than a biological museum as it had been. Then, in 1957 Hilary Koprowski was named its director. Koprowski moved rapidly to convert it into a beehive of biological research activity. The frontispiece of such activity was to be a search for an effective and safe polio vaccine. The suggestion came from Dr. Joseph Smadel of the U.S. Army Walter Reed Hospital. That was to be the cover, and like many covers devised by those working on covert programs, it had to have a level of legitimate activity in its professed field. Koprowski gave it this quality by doing extensive work in polio vaccine research. However, all the evidence points to other work going on beneath the surface that had to do with Huebner's mycoplasma and Sigurdsson's visna retrovirus.

The evidence for this conclusion lies in the fact that one of Koprowski's early colleagues in his extended and re-furbished research laboratory was one named Leonard Hayflick. Dr. Hayflick turns up later in the history of AIDS development when it is reported in the SVCP, Progress Report #8, that when the public health agencies/department of defence partners in biowar research decided to establish a Mycoplasma Research Institute, they appointed Hayflick to run it.

With the man and the place established, and with MKULTRA help in financing the activities, thanks to Nelson Rockefellers' role in the Eisenhower administration, the answer to the question of a suitable cover was already at hand. On his transfer from Lederle it was decided that Koprowski would simply bring with him his Lederle research on polio vaccines, together with another Rockefeller alumnus, Tom Norton, to the Wistar.

The role of the CIA in financing the acquisition and re-modeling of Wistar is now hard to determine since, when the Watergate scandal broke, all known MKULTRA documents were collected and destroyed. However, a few pages managed to escape the destruction and these are now available to us. From these pages there are several references for the need of secure research and testing facilities, including a new wing for a hospital that was to play a part in the on-going efforts. We develop these facts in Chapter Sixteen, Section Three under MKULTRA.

Thus, during the time frame, 1950-1960, Koprowski did his cover work on developing a polio vaccine while engaged in some mystery work for which he lost all record during a move! Unfortunately his dates on all of this are hopelessly inconsistent and suggest that the records were not lost but were destroyed. For example, he stated at one point that the records of his work from 1956 to 1970 had been lost when he moved to the Wistar in 1956! In other words, he 'lost' his records *before* they were made!

However that may be, while engaged in whatever he was engaged in, Koprowski was also busy establishing a chimpanzee camp in the Belgian Congo. Ostensibly, the chimps were to be used to test his evolving polio vaccine, but therein lays another problem for him. It seems that the number of chimps used for polio research were reasonably well accounted for, and according to AIDS-historian,

Edward Hooper, this figure falls well short of the number of chimps actually sacrificed during the period. Something other than polio vaccine was being tested at Camp Lindi in the Congo.

The missing chimps were not those used concurrently by Friedrich ("Fritz") Deinhardt when he was testing a hepatitis vaccine upon which he was working. Plain and simply…several chimps were used to test something that Koprowski and his colleagues wanted kept off the record.

We think that the evidence we now have is sufficient to warrant us declaring that Koprowski and certain others were working at Wistar to create a co-factor pathogen based upon Huebner's mycoplasma and Sigurdsson's retrovirus and that this pathogen was then tested on chimps at Camp Lindi.

Furthermore, given the fact that the mycoplasma has a very serious adverse effect upon the liver due to the up-take of liver-produced cholesterol, Fritz Deinhardt's hepatitis vaccine was a correlative program which would find a role in the hepatitis program in New York, Los Angeles and San Francisco in the mid-seventies, when gay men were offered a free hepatitis vaccine.

Koprowski and Deinhardt had something else in common besides testing mystery vaccines on chimps in the Belgian Congo. Back in Philadelphia both worked very closely during this period with Drs. Werner and Gertrude Henle at the Children's Hospital of Philadelphia. We shall learn more about the fate of children in the care of the Henle's in chapters six and nineteen.

However, at this point we need to consider the use of children by Koprowski as human guinea pigs for his research products. In this area, Koprowski had an interesting agreement with the Clinton State Farms (Prison for Women). Under this agreement and with the consent called in all cases 'informed volunteer consent' pregnant inmates who delivered their children in prison were 'requested' to have their babies vaccinated by Dr. Koprowski with his 'polio' vaccine. And here we have a very suggestive and intriguing development. The evidence is that in late 1957 or early 1958, a newborn baby of an inmate received Koprowski's 'polio' protection. Then, sixteen years later this vaccinated child born in Clinton and used as a test object by Koprowski had, by 1973, become a promiscuous drug addict in New Jersey, and had a baby of her own. And here is where the suggestive and intriguing development occurs: *five years later, in 1979, the baby died of AIDS! That was two years before AIDS was first reported in the medical literature!*

Obviously too young to be a drug user or promiscuous, it seems evident that she had caught the disease at birth from an AIDS-infected mother. Where else, in 1979, could a 16 year old have contracted the disease? The reasonable explanation is that Koprowski's neonatal vaccination was the source of the mother's disease. Then, as often happens, the mother, although a carrier, presented no signs of the disease herself, but passed on a more virulent disease agent to her child at birth. We will come back to Clinton State Farms and the use of children as unwitting guinea pigs.

However, before leaving Koprowski we need to note that many scientists observed during this period that Koprowski had a very special friend named Robert Gallo. It was, said one scientist who knew both men well, a 'father-son relationship'! The significance of this warm friendship will become evident in Chapters 13 and 17.

Summary

Hilary Koprowski was another scientist in the Rockefeller stable of scientific talent, joining Bjorn Sigurdsson, Edward Lennette and others. As the Director of the Wistar Institute, Koprowski worked to develop a polio vaccine as suggested by Joseph Smadel of the Walter Reed Research Institute, in January 1952. At the same time he was engaged in a number of mystery activities that required testing on children, prison inmates and chimpanzees in the Congo. All these activities can be linked to later manifestations of the AIDS- CFS/ME epidemics to officially hit the world in 1981.

All of these factors must be studied together especially as they are related to the work of Dr. Hilary Koprowski in the Congo. We expand upon this in Chapter Seven.

Chapter Six

THE HENLES

Just Love Those Kids to Death

The reader of Hillary Johnson's magnificent history of Chronic Fatigue Syndrome, *Osler's Web* meets Werner and Gertrude Henle, a husband and wife biological research team who emigrated from Germany to the United States in the 1930's, in the earliest pages of the book:

> "…the Henles were known reverentially as the 'mother and father' of Epstein-Barr virus; those who had the opportunity to study with the distinguished team universally referred to themselves as children of the Henles."

One such worshiper was biologist Dr. Evelyne Lennette who, according to Johnson, 'was a self-described child of the Henles.'

When the names of Werner and Gertrude Henle are couched in such gentle family analogies, it is hard to think of them in terms of biological warfare weapons development. Hard but necessary. Let's start looking at the Henles' presence in the literature of biowar research by referring to an early but valuable document: "*Bacterial Warfare. A Critical Analysis of the Available Agents, Their Possible Military Applications, and the Means for Protection Against Them*" by Theodor Rosebury and Elvin A. Kabat, asssisted by Martin H. Boldt. Originally written in 1942, and we take a closer look at this paper in Chapter 23.

A place to start in an analysis of Rosebury and Kabat's article, *Bacterial Warfare* is the References cited by the authors, and when one does that one can note in the 306 citations the following:

> 30. Burnet, F. M. 1940
> 31. Burnet, F. M. and Rountree, P. M.
> 46. Cox, H.R. 1940 (Koprowski's colleague and former boss)
> 47. Cox, 1941
> 296. Henle, W. 1941

These references are selected from the total list because, as we shall see in the pages ahead, Frank Burnet has ties to a **Dr. Carleton Gajdusek** and to **Henry Kissinger**; while Dr. Herald Cox has ties to Hilary Koprowski; and, **Werner Henle** casts a shadow of his presence over both AIDS and CFS/ME, and has ties with all the major people who appear in the literature of these plagues. In fact he and his wife, Gertrude, are cited several times in both Edward Hooper's seminal history of AIDS, *The River*, [eleven citations in the index] and in Hillary Johnson's seminal history of CFS/ME, *Osler's Web*, [six citations].

And it must be noted that the Henle's appear in the Progress Reports of the *Special Virus Cancer Program* with dramatic frequency:In 1977 in *Progress Report #14* alone, Werner Henle's current research is cited 27 times, with additional citations for Gertrude! Let's see what Werner and Gertrude were up to in the late 1950's...the time frame where the evidence strongly suggests that Hilary Koprowski was busily translating the mycoplasmal studies of Huebner and the retroviral studies of Sigurdsson into a viable biological co-factor pathogen, while Fritz Deinhardt (an employee of the Henles at the Children's Hospital of Philadelphia) was concurrently studying hepatitis and how the cholesterol-producing liver re-acts to cholesterol-consuming mycoplasma.

When one examines the work of the Henle's during this critical period one begins to feel that they were not just the loving godparents of all those sick children at the Children's Hospital of Philadelphia [CHOP]. In fact, Fritz Deinhardt as a fellow in the Henle's laboratory was actually reporting to the Henle's as his boss during his hepatitis research. Furthermore, it turns out that the expenses for all of this were being paid for by the *Armed Forces Epidemiological Board!* And talk about the Henle's love of children given their long service at CHOP, well, Fritz Deinhardt, their research Fellow, turned up at the Willowbrook Home for Handicapped Children where he experimentally exposed the children to hepatitis so that he could study the progress of the disease on a controlled (and totally defenseless) group of human guinea pigs.

It was shortly after his hepatitis experiments upon the Willowbrook children that Deinhardt flew off to the Belgian Congo with Hilary Koprowski. In the Congo, at the chimpanzee farm at Camp Lindi, the Henle's employee Deinhardt experimented on the chimps with hepatitis pathogens while Koprowski experimented more or less on the record with polio pathogens. That, at any rate, was the cover story and such work did, in fact, go on. However, as Edward Hooper has so astutely pointed out: when one adds together the chimps used for polio experiments and those used for hepatitis experiments, the total falls dramatically short of the number of chimpanzees that were used for admitted medical research at Camp Lindi! Something other than polio and hepatitis was being researched and that we declare with confidence was the co-factor pathogen of immunosuppressant mycoplasma and retroviral visna.

The Henle's who loved children are the godparents of AIDS.

But how about all of those researchers who said of the Henle's that the latter were their figurative father and mother? Evelyne Lennette, for example.

Well, it turns out that there was an Edwin Lennette working with none other than Robert Huebner and together they were studying such esoteric matters as the induction of lymphoma and xenotropic viruses. And later on, Edwin Lennette would work with a veterinarian named Dharam Ablashi who came to be regarded as an expert in chronic fatigue syndrome. Later still Dharam began to work closely with Evelyne Lennette in the same specialized field: both were 'experts' in CFS/ME. But there was more to Edwin Lennette than that. *During World War Two he had worked for the Rockefeller Institute in Rio de Janeiro in Brazil with none other than Hilary Koprowski.*

Furthermore, there is evidence that the pathogen labeled HIV-2 which, strangely enough is the dominant strain of HIV found in former Portuguese colonies, and in Brazil, which is culturally and linguistically linked to Portugal, has genetic links to two of Lennette's special fields of study: equine encephalitis and yellow fever.

So, just where are we? Well, Edwin Lennette and Hilary Koprowski had worked together for the Rockefellers in Brazil during World War 11. Then, Lennette turned up working with Robert Huebner who had discovered the role of the PPLO or mycoplasma in the 'spontaneous degeneration' of the adenoids and the suppression of the immune system.

Later, Koprowski began work at the Wistar Institute in Philadelphia where he co-operated with Werner and Gertrude

Henle who, in turn, had contracts with the United States Army to do research into hepatitis for which enterprise they recruited a research fellow named Fritz Deinhardt. About the same time they acted as the intellectual 'father and mother' to another Lennette engaged in microbiological research: Dr. Evelyne Lennette. Dr. Evelyne Lennette would later emerge as a dictatorial leader of research into an AIDS 'mirror image' called CFS/ME when the latter disease hit the world with dramatic virulence in 1981.(We refer to Dr. Evelyne Lennette as 'dictatorial' because, when we attempted to interview her by phone about her early work, she refused to discus it with us, and she rigorously controlled who could and could not attend any research conferences into the nature of CFS/ME.)

Oh what tangled webs we weave…But the question is: Was there a link between Evelyne Lennette and her figurative father-mother figures, the Henles, and the Edwin Lennette who had worked with both Koprowski and Huebner and other scientists who in turn had spawned AIDS and delivered it to humanity?

Hillary Johnson named her study of CFS/ME astutely when she titled it, *Osler's Web* for in this great book many of the same cast of characters who appear in Edward Hooper's equally magnificent history of AIDS [*The River*] are woven together in a complex web far too intricate to be simply coincidence. There's a master spider in the shadows.

We'll answer further questions of Lennette involvement later in Chapter Nineteen below. In the meantime, let's take a further look at the Henles.

In chapter four above, we noted that Hilary Koprowski, when he joined the Wistar Institute in 1957 had entered into an agreement with the Clinton State Farms (Prison for Women) wherein he could vaccinate newborns with some of his mystery vaccines. It turns out that Werner and Gertrude Henle also had their own agreement with that institution wherein they could vaccinate female 'volunteers' with a hepatitis vaccine being developed by their research fellow, Fritz Deinhardt. The Henle's then co-operated with Deinhardt to write a report to the Armed Forces Epidemiological Board titled 'Viral Hepatitis'.

An Interlude: David Carr: Pretreated! But for What?

As we have mentioned earlier, in 1959 a British sailor named David Carr from Manchester died of AIDS-related illnesses such as *Pneumocystis carinii* pneumonia [PCP] and cytomegalovirus [CMV]. How is it possible that a death can occur in 1959 that is tied to an acquired immune deficiency disease, when the disease now known as AIDS was not even existent in the world? And how can we suggest that Hilary Koprowski and others were responsible for the development of AIDS when, at the time of David Carr's death in 1959, the whole 'Koprowski Krowd' was still labouring in the fields of militarily-financed research in Philadelphia and the Congo?

The answers to these and other questions suggest that some three to six years before Carr's death, he had been infected with a precursor disease agent based upon the earliest application of Huebner's mycoplasmal research. Just where was Carr during that latter time frame? It turns out that four years before, in 1955, Carr had joined the Royal Navy. At that time, as we have seen, he had received the usual battery of vaccines given recruits into the military. However, in 1956 (three years before his death) in addition to the usual vaccines, Carr had been given an 'ATT' injection and, it was noted on his medical records, he was 'pretreated'! But, the records do not say what he had been **pretreated** for. According to Edward Hooper, to whom we are greatly indebted for this information, a senior British Navy medical officer commented when asked: "It sounds like he was being pretreated for **something he was going to be exposed to.**"

Is it possible that David Carr in 1956 had been pretreated with Huebner's immune suppressing mycoplasma with the view to subsequent treatment with a Sigurdsson retrovirus or other disease pathogen that would flourish when the victim's immune defence system had been compromised? We'll leave the answer to this question until later, but in the meantime we want to make it clear that there existed then and there continues to exist, a level of covert communication between certain factions within allied services that would have been at work in respect to such research at the time Carr received his 'pretreatment.'

As soon as the potential of Huebner's discoveries became evident, (*i.e.* the late 1940's to the early 1950's) certain officers in the Royal Navy, and possibly in the Royal Australian and the Royal Canadian

Navies, would have been briefed and their co-operation invited in exploring the phenomenon further. The present writers have in their files a confidential memo written by a Canadian military doctor, Major Tim Cook, to his Commander-in-Chief, General Baril. In the memo Major Cook advises Baril that the mycoplasma is not a factor in Gulf War Disease. If Cook really believes that, all well and good, but…we also learned that Major Cook then sent a copy of the memo that he had written for his commanding officer to an officer in a foreign military service! And just who was the recipient of this betrayal of military duty and trust? The memo was sent to Captain Kenneth Craig Hyams of the United States Navy's biological warfare research organization. The successor group to that for which Huebner had been working in the 1940-50's.

There is also evidence that certain ships (and crews) of the Royal Canadian Navy co-operated around this time with the U.S. Navy in testing various aerosol disease agents. Later, several exposed crewmembers developed amyotrophic lateral sclerosis. We develop this theme of collusion between the U.S. military and the Canadian military in Chapter 16.

End of an Interlude

Summary

By the latter half of the 1950's, Werner and Gertrude Henle were well tied in with two important research streams. One stream, being developed by Koprowski grew out of Huebner's earlier work with naval recruits and the mycoplasma-induced adenoid degeneration and immune suppression. The other stream, which also grew out of Huebner's work with the mycoplasma and the latter's deleterious effects upon the liver, dealt with hepatitis. Both the immune suppressive qualities of the mycoplasma and the damage to the liver had to be tested upon chimpanzees and both Koprowski and Deinhardt began vaccine-testing programs at Camp Lindi with the co-operation of the Belgian government of the Congo. Furthermore, tests upon women and children under state control in prisons and homes for mentally and physically handicapped children took place.

The Henle's provide an active and important link between Koprowski and Deinhardt and so figure as important contributors to the ultimate achievement of a new microorganism, one which does not naturally exist and which is refractory to the human immune system. Just what Dr. MacArthur knew was coming when he briefed select Congressmen on June 9, 1969. (Ch.15)

However, besides the fatal pathogen promised (that for AIDS) MacArthur had promised another pathogen, one, which would disable by altering the immune system (CFS/ME). The Henle's were well positioned to participate in this endeavor as well.

Chapter Seven

THE BELGIANS AND THE PORTUGUESE

Those Pesky Black Nationalists

At the end of World War Two, imperialistic nations such as France in West Africa, Algeria and Vietnam [the latter they fondly labeled '*French* Indo-China'], Great Britain in India and the Middle East, Holland in Indonesia, Belgium in Central Africa (The *Belgian* Congo), and Portugal in West Africa had a big problem. In many cases Black 'colonial' troops had served the imperial powers' interests well. Field Marshall Sir Archibald Wavell, for example, paid high tribute to his Black forces recruited from British East Africa, who had done such a tremendous job against the forces of Japan in the Battle of Burma. Now, many of these same battle-trained 'colonials' were aspiring to independence, and each imperialist power responded in its own way.

In general terms, the British benefited from having elected a post-war socialist government with Clement Attlee as Prime Minister. Attlee and his Labour Government set about to negotiate India's independence, and to a lesser extent independence for Kenya, Uganda, and Ghana. But France, Holland, Belgium, and Portugal tried to maintain the old order by brutal repression of nationalism in the colonies. Those pesky Black (and Brown) nationalists!

The situation was complicated by a dawning of a new imperialism for the old. Although mouthing anti colonial slogans, powerful forces in the United States embarked upon the creation of an American Empire to replace the crumbling empires of European nations. Blithely blind to the reality of what they were doing, the leaders of the U.S., while condemning colonialism, did all that they could (through the CIA) to support the anti-nationalist activities of France in Vietnam, Belgium in the Congo and Holland in Indonesia. As it became evident that such efforts were doomed to ultimate failure, and the European powers were forced to withdraw their flagging and defeated armies, the U.S. needed a new strategy...especially in Africa.

That strategy was provided by the Rockefellers and their Council on Foreign Relations allies and it consisted of a program of genocide in resource-rich Africa. First, kill off the nationalist leaders like Patrice Lumumba and replace them with puppets and well-armed warlords to fight among themselves. Then, introduce a lethal new biological weapon which is refractory to the human immune system and which is spread by fluid exchange [including vaccines, blood transfusions, sexual intercourse and illicit injected drug use] and the Black Continent with its wealth will fall easily into the hands of the U.S. military/industrial complex.

As we have already noted, this strategy received a big boost when the U.S. elected General Dwight Eisenhower as President in 1952. With Nelson Rockefeller militarizing the Public Health Agencies [Centers for Disease Control and the National Institutes of Health] while concurrently initiating the covert programs of MKULTRA, MKNAOMI, and MKDELTA (and possibly MK-SVLP) and, with the Dulles brothers, Allen and John Foster respectively, directing the new instrument of state terrorism called the CIA and the foreign policy establishment, **the secret American war of world conquest was launched.**

In the atmosphere of international discord that characterized the times and, with a cold war between two dominant ideologies, communism and capitalism, raging, America sought covert allies for their secret war. Such allies were readily found in Belgium and Portugal, and a little later, in the Apartheid regime of South Africa (Chapter 24). The French were pre-occupied with armed conflict in both Algeria and Indo-China, while the British were dis-engaging from their former colonies, and the Dutch were growing increasingly anxious to get out of their former colonies. But Belgium and Portugal maintained an obstinate urge to do what they could to hold onto the wealth they controlled in Africa.

As we noted in an Interlude above, ["David Carr: 'Pre-treated. But for What?"] there was a small clique in Great Britain privy to the genocide and co-operating in it, but this was not on the same level as the co-operation which was provided by Belgium and Portugal.

Belgium, the Congo and HIV-1

The evidence [scientific, historic and political] now available to the AIDS researcher demonstrates to a compelling degree that certain people in Belgium were determined in the 1950's to do all that they possibly could to destroy the national aspirations of Black leaders in the Belgian colonies and to replace these with puppets. These aspirations were supported by the United States in pursuit of its neo-colonial scheming. Historically and politically, Dwight Eisenhower by a 'wink and a nod' ordered the CIA to kill Lumumba, and to instigate a move to replace him with Moise Tshombe in copper-rich Katanga Province.

Although the actual murder of Lumumba took place a few weeks into John F. Kennedy's administration (after the latter's surprise defeat of Richard Nixon) utilizing an 'assassination capability' under MKULTRA, (Richelson, 2001 Pp.37-38) the Belgian/U.S. co-operation had been initiated early in the 1950's. However, our emphasis is upon the scientific evidence and we must précis that here.

In the 1950's a Belgian physician named Ghislain Courtois was placed in charge of a significant Belgian medical research laboratory in Stanleyville in the Congo. In this role, he presided over two important medical research activities. Despite the fact that the area was plunging towards independence and people like Courtois ran the very real risk of being turfed out of the country, a significant new and large addition to his laboratory was built. In addition, at a place close to but difficult to access from Stanleyville, the Belgian government financed the establishment of Camp Lindi where, it was announced; over one hundred chimpanzees (the primate species which, genetically, most closely resembles that of humans) would be assembled for medical scientific research.

Belgium was about to embark upon a biological warfare route to maintain its imperial possessions. It was not to be something new for them. As far back as 1928 Captain Graveline of the Belgian Army had written an important study titled: "The possibilities of Bacterial Warfare" which was published in the *Archives d' medicin belges*. (Cited in Rosebury and Kabat; Page 89 Ch. 24)

Soon after the establishment of Camp Lindi, in 1957, none other than Hilary Koprowski arrived for a visit to the medical laboratory and chimp farm. At the time of Koprowski's visit, he was still an employee at Lederle where he was working with biowar weapons researcher, Dr. Herald Cox. If one needs some clues as to how involved in biowar research Cox was, one can find such in the facts that (a) the microbe responsible for Q-fever, *Coxiella burnettii*, is jointly named after Herald Cox and Frank Burnet of Australia, and Q-fever is identified in the June 9, 1969 Hearings (Ch.15)) as a biowar agent being worked on by the Pentagon, and (b) Cox is also cited by Rosebury and Kabat. Thus, in one geographic location (Camp Lindi) one sees bacterial research, Frank Burnet, Herald Cox, Hilary Koprowski, the Belgium Government, the June 9, 1969 Pentagon Budget Meeting and 'monkey kidneys' all brought together.

At any rate, Koprowski saw fit to visit the Belgian research installations in 1957, shortly before he went to the Wistar Institute, and to re-new his association with several Belgian researchers. Two significant details emerge from such records as survive of the Congo laboratory, the chimpanzee camp, the Ghislain Courtois research, the Koprowski/Belgian co-operation in subjects such as rabies research and the development of oral polio vaccines. One significant detail is that both Koprowski *and* the Belgian scientists involved later 'lost' their records. The second significant detail is that while in the Congo, Koprowski co-operated with the Belgians in testing polio vaccines.

In respect to the latter vaccine test program several other details emerge which are disturbing. First, although the polio vaccine was to protect **children** from the ravages of polio, Koprowski also insisted on vaccinating all *adults* that he could, with the help of the Belgian Army, get his hands on. Furthermore, evidence now has come to light that Koprowski vaccinated hundreds of Blacks in the Congo and in Rwanda-Burundi, but, he failed to note this in his [already skimpy] records. *These geographic areas later became known for the early appearance of AIDS and later for the high incidence of AIDS.*

There are further areas for concern, and these revolve around the fact that although the first vaccines used had come from America, it wasn't long before a 'polio' vaccine was being manufactured under vague auspices in Belgium. Discussion of this aspect of the U.S./Belgian co-operation is vehemently denied by all parties, despite the preponderance of evidence that plain and simply, Belgium co-operated with the U.S. to concoct a vaccine for the Black citizens of Central Africa.

Finally, it is our duty to report that the areas whose citizens were first vaccinated by the U.S./Belgian efforts were the first areas from which HIV-1 emerged on a large-scale epidemic basis. And, we need to report; the species of pathogen is that which is now known as **HIV-1** as distinguished from another species known as **HIV-2**.

And therein lies another story…the story of Portugal and AIDS.

Portugal, Guinea-Bissau, Goa, Brazil and HIV-2

According to a strange story that is heard throughout the world, there was once a green monkey that bit a Black woman and transmitted a simian immune deficiency disease agent to her. Patient Zero one might call her. The said lady then had intercourse with someone to whom she passed the SIV, who had intercourse, etc. and before long an infected person had intercourse with a Canadian airline steward who, although celibate while in his home country and heterosexual when visiting Africa or wherever it was that he picked up the SIV (now known as HIV) turned homosexual whenever he visited the United States. In the U.S. travel-enabled as he was with his airline employee pass, he scooted around New York, San Francisco and Los Angeles having sex with some 2,500 gays. And that, according to the official story is how AIDS came to be in Africa and among homosexuals on the American east and west coasts.

Patient Zero plus One you might call him, but according to the U.S. Centers for Disease Control his real name was Gaetan Dugas.

Imagine anyone in his right mind believing this myth or any part of it to the effect that AIDS came out of monkeys in the jungle into the human family!

Such a myth makes it impossible to account for several anomalies.

First, there is the anomaly that there are two **major** HIV streams: HIV-1 and HIV-2.

Does the presence of a second strain suggest that perhaps a blue monkey (Yes, Virginia, there are blue monkeys known in formal company as *Cercopithecus mitis schoutedeni*) bit a Brown woman in Brazil?

Or does it suggest something more supportive of our research evidence: that AIDS was developed in American laboratories and that HIV-1 started off in the Lederle Lab and was the seed for HIV-1 presenting in Belgian-controlled Congo and other places, while HIV-2 came from some other laboratory? A laboratory in or associated with Brazil and Portugal- such as Brazilian Hospital laboratories greatly influenced by Dr. Alton Ochsner of Tulane University in New Orleans?

Let's consider the evidence about HIV-2.

The first, and indeed the absolute, fact about HIV-2 that one must face up to is this: the major areas of the world which are infected with HIV-2 are areas where the Portuguese language is spoken. These include the former African colonies of Portugal, the Goa enclave in India, and Brazil. How might one account for the strange fact that essentially, HIV-2 is the variety of immune deficiency disease that occurs primarily in Portuguese-speaking former colonies?

Our research suggests very strongly that a so-called smallpox vaccine was grown on Rhesus monkey kidneys (Hence, 'MK' and initially from the Yerkes Primate Farm in Atlanta and later from the Delta Primate Farm in Covington, LA. Hence, CIA program MKDELTA) at Tulane University under the direction of Dr. Alton Ochsner. Dr. Ochsner had very strong ties with Brazilian (as well as other South and Central American) medical institutions, which in turn, had strong scientific ties with the health establishment of Portugal itself. Ochsner was recruited in 1955 and 1957 to work with the U.S. Army and Air Force on some highly secret project, the details of which have still not been released by the U.S. Government. (Haslam, 1995 Page 182) We suggest that Ochsner, through his strong Brazilian medical contacts participated in early smallpox vaccination projects in Brazil, and then by way of a co-operating vaccine laboratory in Lisbon, in other Portuguese speaking colonies.

Thus, HIV-2 is largely limited to Brazil and the former Portuguese colonies.

Summary

There are two main streams of the so-called HIV current in the world. How can one possibly account for that fact? One can, of course, just ignore the problem. Or, one can accept the quaint official myth that HIV-1 came into being when a green monkey bit a Black woman and HIV-2 came into being, perhaps when about the same time a blue monkey bit a Brown woman. Easy myths to memorize and quote, but not nearly as likely as the science that traces from PPLO in naval recruits to a visna co-factor from sheep, engineered by U.S. government owned or co-operating agencies.

One can accept the myths or face the fact that HIV-1 and HIV-2 were developed in such American military controlled laboratories, and that changes occurred when Belgian and Portuguese controlled labs took over some of the vaccine production.

Chapter Eight

TESTING BIOWEAPONS

On September 29, 1994, the *Delaware State News* ran a story with the heading: "GAO lists government experiments on 500,000, 1940 - 1974" written by Karen MacPherson and distributed by Scripps Howard News Service.

The GAO is the General Accounting Office of the United States Government and the 500,000 is the *known* number of citizens of the United States who were used as guinea pigs to test various radiation, biological and chemical experiments sponsored by the federal government. As the report goes on to say, "...the numbers of experiments and people involved may rise as more information is made public by the Pentagon."

There is no indication in the report as to whether the 500,000 includes tests on citizens outside of the United States (probably not) such as Black citizens of South Africa offered for testing by the apartheid government of the day. Nor is there any indication whether the number includes tests on Canadian, British or other allied countries' armed forces (probably not) in places such as Suffield, Alberta, Canada, or on the high seas when various aerobic disease agents were tested on the crews of American and Allied navies.

In other words, about one out of every 600 Americans were tagged (many or even most), secretly to be gassed, irradiated, poisoned or otherwise assaulted by their government to find out whether they would die, catch a disabling disease, lose their minds. And all of that in the 'land of the free'! Can you imagine the carnage if the U.S. were a dictatorship?

There are several things in the news story that should be commented upon. First, the numbers only apply to people used as test objects up until 1974. Our research has suggested that tests were continued and probably greatly increased from 1975 to the present. Our evidence, presented elsewhere in this study, establishes that the school children who became ill in Lyndonville, New York in 1984 were fed goats' milk contaminated by a mycoplasmal species. The teachers in the auxiliary staff room of Tahoe-Truckee High School in Incline Village, Nevada, were undoubtedly exposed for long hours to air that carried a mycoplasmal species. The homosexual males of New York, Los Angeles and San Francisco who accepted a 'free' vaccine to protect themselves from hepatitis were more than likely seeded with the AIDS co-factors at that time.

But not only were these people the direct test objects, their family members and fellow workers and neighbors were just as much test objects, and many were seriously sickened or even killed as happened in the community of Huntsville, Texas, and reported by three courageous, determined and well-informed ladies. (Chapter 23)

There is also much evidence that either purposefully or accidentally, hundreds of thousands of people living in an area radiating out from a point on Long Island Sound across from Plum Island, were victims of two laboratory pathogens which present as Lyme disease and as West Nile Fever.

Readers must also note that, subsequent to the release of this already limited information, the Congressional Committee receiving it was directed by President Clinton to limit their further research to those involved in radiation experiments! *They were to ask no questions about tests involving chemical or biological disease agents!*

Our conservative estimate would be that, if one figures in all of those left out of the 500,000 count, *at least one million American citizens have been assaulted by their own government.*

When, on June 9, 1969, Dr. Donald MacArthur of the Pentagon told the black budget Congressional sub-committee members that he was assured of the feasibility of an AIDS pathogen by certain 'eminent microbiologists' you can be sure that the latter knew of what they were promising because they had already seen enough early test results, and even more test subjects would be similarly victimized in the coming years.

The tests were bad enough, but the deployment of the confirmed research product AIDS co-factors would be even worse. That would constitute the crime beyond belief.

An Interlude on Nelson Rockefeller and the Rockefeller Apparat

The wars that the American people have allowed themselves to wage on behalf of the wealthy power core, including that in Vietnam for oil, tin and tungsten; that in the Middle East for oil; and finally, that secret war in Africa for that continent's great untapped resource base, and employing the de-population strategic weapon of AIDS, have all been contrived by the forces and power of great wealth, and in 1973 Nixon was being double-crossed while himself double-crossing others.

The major actor in the Rockefeller stable of talent was Henry Kissinger (see below) but, before we get to him, let's start back in 1943 in Brazil where the Rockefellers ruled supreme. Who was in the stable then?

Edward Lennette worked at the Yellow Fever Research Service in Rio de Janeiro, Brazil, for, nominally, the Brazilian Ministry of Health and the Rockefeller Foundation. One of his areas of research was an investigation of encephalitis. One of the experiments he participated in involved the Venezuelan equine encephalomyelitis virus [VEEV]. Thus, Lennette was right in on the ground floor of biowar weapons research for, when Dr. MacArthur of the Pentagon was briefing the Congressmen about Pentagon research in that field, on June 9, 1969, (see above) he was asked what pathogens were being worked on. MacArthur replied:"…Incapacitating agent (among others): Venezuelan equine encephalomyelitis virus [VEEV] (and) Lethal: Yellow fever virus"!

Hilary Koprowski (Ch.5) also turned up in Brazil in 1940, where he, too, worked for the Rockefeller Foundation! One of his fellow researchers was Edward Lennette, and consequently, one of his areas of expertise was VEEV, which, as one author points out was later put to use in the development of a vaccine by Koprowski and the U.S. Army and whose potential as a 'biological warfare agent was swiftly recognized.' In 1944, Koprowski used his Rockefeller links to immigrate to the U.S. where he first worked for the Rockefeller Institute. Then, he went to Lederle Laboratories and association with Herald Cox, whom we have already met. [We have noted elsewhere that the disease pathogen *Coxiella burnettii* had been named in honour of Herald Cox and Frank Burnet. *C. burnettii*, in turn, is the causative factor in Queensland fever (Q-fever) and the latter was also identified by MacArthur in his report to Congress, as a 'disabling' bioagent being worked on by the Pentagon.]

From Lederle and some early and mysterious trips to Belgium and the Congo, Koprowski arrived at the Wistar Institute and was a part of much that followed.

Meanwhile, in another part of the stable, Dr. Bjorn Sigurdsson (Ch. 4) was also working for the Rockefellers. In the early 1940's Sigurdsson was working at the Rockefeller Institute in New Jersey. Later, with hundreds of thousands of Rockefeller dollars he returned to his native Iceland, to study 'experimental pathology'. He was just in time to experience the first major outbreak of a mysterious 'incapacitating' disease agent that hit over 1,000 Icelandic students, five of whom developed Parkinson's disease and later died. From there he went on to study the nature of the sheep retroviruses, which co-incidentally, are a major component of the 'lethal' disease pattern called HIV-1, and which by being able to take over the reproductive mechanism of its host cell [RNA-directed DNA polymerase], can perpetuate itself in its victim.

In the 1970's Fritz Deinhardt looms very large in the *Special Virus Cancer Program*. In *Progress Report #8* alone, he is cited 19 times. An expert, it would seem, in cancer. But, it wasn't always so. In fact, back in 1958 the record shows that he was a great colleague of Hilary Koprowski, and, when Hilary was in the Congo testing something on chimpanzees at Camp Lindi, there also was Fritz Deinhardt plying the poor chimps with a hepatitis vaccine that he was researching. Of special interest to us in this book about AIDS, was that part of Deinhardt's work focused upon the role of hormones in contagious liver diseases. This research becomes even more pertinent when one has a chance to study the SVCP, *Progress Report #9*, for in the latter document the following, as we noted earlier, is reported as an important discovery:

> "We have for the first time demonstrated that the virogenic markers, group specific antigens (g.s.) and RNA directed DNA polymerase; can be activated by alteration of the physiological endocrine balance."

What is so relevant about this discovery (made for the first time!)? To begin with, the 'endocrine balance' has to do with the role of the hormones, and the role of the hormones has everything to do with the ability of certain mycoplasmal species to alter that endocrine balance. Here is how it works: When roused to action by some trauma, certain mycoplasmas will up-take pre-formed cholesterol from its host cell. Cholesterol, in turn, is antecedent to the production of hormones in certain secretory glands. If the cholesterol supply is limited due to mycoplasmal up-take, then the supply of certain hormones is ipso facto also limited. Hence, the significance of Deinhardt's hormone research vis a vis hormone balance, hepatitis, and chimps in the Congo.

However, of significance to us at this point is the fact that Deinhardt's work was to a large part financed by the Rockefeller Foundation.

Put Fritz Deinhardt in to the Rockefeller stable of talent.

We have noted the role of certain Belgian scientists in a variety of Koprowski-related activities. However, we should take particular note of Dr. Ghislain Courtois. It turns out that in 1955, before embarking upon a vaccination program in Central Africa where the records of just what was being vaccinated against had been lost, Dr. Courtois was brought to America for a three-month study session. *He started this tour at the Rockefeller Institute in New York, and then he continued his studies at Rockefeller-sponsored labs in Trinidad and Rio de Janeiro.*

Then in 1958, a very critical year in the history of AIDS, Dr. Courtois visited the Wistar Institute for a training course. After this course, he traveled to Tulane University in New Orleans for further 'study'. Tulane was a significant Rockefeller-dominated research center for biowar weapons development. However, at this time it is enough to note the large role played in the education of Dr. Courtois by the Rockefeller apparat.

With the 1952 election of Dwight Eisenhower and the latter's appointment of Nelson Rockefeller to HEW, the Rockefeller apparat had its first official link to the Government of the United States. From 1952 until 1960 the apparat and the CIA were essentially one and the same. From the 1960 election of John F. Kennedy until the latter's assassination in 1963 by the CIA many of the Rockefeller apparat's programs were put on hold until 1963 when the assassination of Mr. Kennedy brought Lyndon Johnson to the Presidency. Johnson in turn brought the CIA hidden war agenda, including the development and deployment of the biological world population growth-rate reduction co-factors involved with AIDS and CFS/ME back to full, albeit covert, action.

But, by 1968 when the CIA hidden war in Vietnam had, also under Johnson, become a hot war involving the US Military and thousands of American casualties, the Democrats were replaced by the Republicans in the Legislative branch of government, and the Executive branch of government was headed by Richard Nixon.

During the Johnson administration, the Rockefellers had significantly more clout than under the Kennedy administration (See Ch. 21 below), but, with the election of Richard Nixon and the appointment of Rockefeller protégé Henry Kissinger to Nixon's Cabinet, the Rockefeller apparat once more had a greatly enhanced role in government. But, as it was to turn out, they did not have nearly as much clout as they thought they would. But that story lies ahead.

Postscript

June 28, 2007—As we complete this final draft of *AIDS: The Crime Beyond Belief* we have heard television news reports that startling evidence of Central Intelligence Agency misdeeds are being made public by the CIA's current chief, Michael Hayden. Reports in the June 27, 2007 Globe and Mail gives more details.

The action is deemed to be a coming clean of the 'agency's most egregious excesses over the previous quarter-century.'

The summary of these misdeeds reveals nothing not already known to scholars and researchers. Why Mr. Hayden has chosen this time to put this nonsense out can only be guessed at. To the present writers it is another example of what we term 'limited hang-out'. That is, put a bunch of details out which are already well known to those who are students of reality in CIA affairs, but which will seem to those citizens who largely confine their exposure to the pablum of New York Times journalism to be 'shocking' misdeeds. Thus pacified that they are still living in a 'good' society where the 'truth' finally gets told, the majority rests.

We ask one question: where are the thousands of pages of documents that detail the MKULTRA, MKNAOMI and MKDELTA programs?

PART THREE

DEEP POLITICS AND THE MURDER OF JFK

Chapter Nine

SHADOW GOVERNMENT AND DEEP POLITICS

"The real truth of the matter is, as you and I know, that a financial element in the large centers has owned the government ever since the days of Andrew Jackson."
President Franklin Delano Roosevelt, Feb. 23, 1945

Events do not just 'happen', they are 'performed'. As random and as spontaneous as events may appear, they all represent reactions to influences brought to bear over time. The influences may be subtle and generally overlooked by the majority of those affected or participating or they may be blatantly promoted and obvious. However that may be, the events of history are in reaction to the influences at work.

Events may be immediate, clear cut and obvious, or they may extend over a long period of time, insidious and hard to discern, but they are events none-the-less.

The murder of John F. Kennedy was an immediate, clear cut and obvious event which took place in Dallas, Texas at 12:30 Central Time on November 22, 1963. The infection and death of millions of citizen's world wide, but especially in Africa among the Black population, has drifted insidiously onto the world scene, hardly perceptible at the outset, but occurring with the same finality as that of the death of Mr. Kennedy.

For each event, there is a cause, and following each cause there is an effect.

In this study we are searching for the cause of a murder and the cause of an epidemic.

There are those who suggest that the cause of the murder was that a young man (Lee Harvey Oswald) with serious mental challenges, sought emotional satisfaction in bringing down from the heights of public acclaim another young man (John F. Kennedy) who had achieved much in his short life.

There are those who suggest that the cause of the epidemic (AIDS) was that a green monkey being slaughtered for food by a Black woman, bit its butcher and so infected her with a simian virus that destroyed her immunity to many diseases. She subsequently passed her immune deficiency to male sexual partners.

Two events; two causes; two effects. But were the events random, and the causes spontaneous, and the effects without cautionary lessons for mankind? In other words, was each event the outcome of planning or of chance?

If you believe the easy popular story that each event…the murder by a 'lone nut' and the epidemic by the 'bite of a green monkey', you are a co-incidence buff. Or, if you believe as we do, based upon hours of research and interviews, that each event is a consequence of planning by someone somewhere with the power to initiate the action, then you are a 'conspiracy buff'.

A conspiracy buff is someone who believes that significant events, especially those tragic in outcome, must be rigorously examined in order to determine true causes with a view to preventing a recurrence of similar tragedies. A coincidence buff is someone who believes that chance rules the world and no lessons can be learned from history.

We are conspiracy buffs and we believe that the murder of Mr. Kennedy and the millions of deaths of Africans from AIDS can be determined by the careful and honest collection of actual data about all aspects of these events.

We recognize that the term 'conspiracy buff' has been presented by those who deny the organized criminality of the murder and the epidemic as someone who is at least marginally nuts or at most, is completely and irrationally paranoid. We accept the conspiracy buff label despite the connotations conjured up by those who would have us believe that coincidence is the operative word. *We suggest that those who urge the acceptance of coincidence can be broadly divided into two camps: there are those people who benefit from the hiding of the reality, and those who are too lazy or intellectually unable to study and evaluate the evidence. Both of these groups resist change.* On the other hand, those who believe that the reasonable collection of facts leads to the truth are the people who would have history provide guidance for humanity in the years ahead, and who make an effort to effect positive change.

We believe that those who planned and carried out the murder of

Mr. Kennedy were members of the same group of powerful people who planned and carried out the development and deployment of the pathogenic co-factors that now present as AIDS. We have determined from the evidence, and we present much of that evidence in this study, who it was that had the motive (warped as such was) the *means*, and the *opportunity* to execute both crimes.

This latter affirmation brings us to the question of just what or who that 'group' was and is. It has been variously termed a 'shadow government' or an 'invisible government' or a 'secret team', or, as Peter Dale Scott calls it 'the deep politics of America.'

We don't want to get hung up on debating detail about the nomenclature used, we want simply to present the evidence that there is in reality, a power block that rough hews our political and social destiny and that has the capability of killing a president in broad daylight or of planting a population-reducing disease in a whole continent. To the extent possible this power block will operate through and co-opt to their own ends, the apparent political structure of society, but if they must go outside those accepted parameters and kill or otherwise remove its leaders, it will do so.

It will kill Mr. Kennedy or it will force Richard Nixon out of office, or it will develop and deploy a deadly disease pathogen, but that power block will have its way, which can only be stopped by an informed and aroused citizenry. In any event it is a power force to which we must respond.

To quote Professor Peter Dale Scott:

> "We shall see…that beneath the open surface of our society lie connections and relationships of long standing, virtually immune to disclosure, and capable of great crimes, including serial murder. To the stock objection that it would be virtually impossible to assemble a murder conspiracy without leakage, the response is that an existing conspiratorial network or systems of networks, already in place and capable of murder, would have much less difficulty in maintaining the discipline of secrecy."(Scott, 1993 Page 17)

We list some of those 'systems of networks' below.

November 22, 1963—Darkness at High Noon in Dallas: The murder of John F. Kennedy

Two persons are essential for a successful assassination where the true criminals want to avoid being identified as such: someone must do the actual killing and someone else must be assigned the blame. A 'patsy' in other words.

To achieve these two essentials generally requires someone to put the plot together, and he (or she) must have access to people who can put him in touch with known killers who will do the job and access to someone that can be controlled to such an extent that he will be in the right place at the right time and who will have a persona which will make his role as a killer seem believable.

In a clear dictatorship, where effective and unquestioned power lies in the hands of one or two people, putting these elements together can be achieved with varying degrees of ease. However, in a democracy, the organizers of a complicated plot such as that which led to the murder of President Kennedy in Dallas, Texas on November 22, 1963, much has to be done subtly and silently through intermediaries and in language which cloaks the meaning of necessary communications.

To prevent a vigorous and thorough investigation of the crime after it has been accomplished requires that the people at the base of the crime constitute a broad, powerful and strongly motivated coalition of forces.

Let us start our summary of Mr. Kennedy's murder with the people who made up the latter base.

Although the great grief of many persons, America- and worldwide, following the assassination shows the deep affection of many millions of people for Mr. Kennedy, a long and careful study of the evidence shows that the base in terms of *effective* power was indeed wide. The main elements of the base were the CIA itself; major elements of the Military; the Israeli Mossad; elements of the anti-Algerian independence officers' corps in the French Military; the 'Establishment', especially those that represented banking and oil interests and included persons from these interests within Mr. Kennedy's own inner circle, such as Robert McNamara and McGeorge Bundy; the Mafia, especially the Jewish Mafia families built around Meyer 'Little Man' Lanky and his 'soldier', Jack Ruby, but also certain Italian Mafia families such as those who were tied in with criminal labor union leaders such as Jimmy Hoffa and with Carlos Marcello of New Orleans; the leadership of the Federal Bureau of Investigation (FBI); fundamentalist Bible-belt politicians; the American Medical Association, especially parts of the executive who were engaged in biological weapons research involving 'immune suppressant agents'; the China Lobby; members, more or less fanatical, of the population control school; and finally, but significantly, large parts of the major media. Some of these elements of the base were in two or even three of the sub-groups. Henry Luce, for example, was a powerful media boss, and a devoted member of the China Lobby, while Meyer Lansky was both a member of the Jewish Mafia and also of the Israeli Mossad.

With such an extensive and powerful base, the grief of the people may be, as it was with the murder of the President, wide and sincere; but, their effective power to investigate the crime and to bring the criminals to justice must be limited by the official agencies which were then and are now part of the criminal conspiracy. We will make a brief allusion to each of these factors; however, we are not going to try to completely review all the essential flaws in the 'lone nut assassin' cover since that is not our purpose here. Our purpose is to draw the line between the forces of light as represented by Mr. Kennedy and the forces of darkness as represented by Allen Dulles and those who were parts of the base of the assassination plot as set out above.

The forces of light stood in the way of the dark goals of each part of that base, but most importantly for our study, they stood in the way of mass murder and international genocide.

The Central Intelligence Agency (Part Two)

The CIA had finally been brought down to earth when Mr. Kennedy was not bullied nor embarrassed into taking their Bay of Pigs Cuban invasion bait, by sending in the United States armed forces to get the Cuban Brigade off the hook. Not only were many members in high places embarrassed, but other key leaders such as Allen Dulles and Richard Bissell had been fired over the fiasco and Mr. Kennedy had expressed an intention to 'break the CIA into a thousand pieces and throw the pieces to the wind.' However, once a spook, always a spook and Allen Dulles who was the key instigator and plot-designer still held the loyalty of several CIA operatives such as E. Howard Hunt and Rockefeller family-member, Tracy Barnes. Both the latter were key people in putting together the actual parts of the murder plans in the first place.

Not only that, but the infamous CIA MKULTRA umbrella had an 'assassination sub-project' under it to handle "executive action-type assassinations." (Richelson, 2001 Pp. 37-38)

The U.S. Military/Joint Chiefs of Staff

The U.S. Military harbored a great disdain for Mr. Kennedy, and people such as Admiral Radford and General Lyman Lemnitzer were active allies of Nelson Rockefeller and Richard Nixon. The final straw for the Military came with the November, 1963 decision of Mr. Kennedy to start removing 1,000 U.S. servicemen a month from Vietnam. The President was murdered before he could put his signature to the National Security Action Memorandum, and it was drastically altered by Lyndon Johnson as one of the latter's first actions as President.

Israel and Ben Gurion

It is on record that by the spring of 1963 the relations between U.S. President, John F. Kennedy and Israeli President Ben-Gurion, had reached a very low point. Mr. Kennedy was pressuring Israel to (1) stop work immediately on their building of a nuclear weapon; and (2) pay compensation to all Palestinians who had been expelled from Israel and whose farms, homes and businesses were being used by new Israeli settlers. Ben-Gurion would agree to neither demand.

Then, someone in Mr. Kennedy's office leaked information to Ben-Gurion that the U.S. President was carrying on a friendly and open-minded correspondence with the Egyptian President, Gamel Abdel Nasser. Ben-Gurion, already increasingly paranoid, saw this as a terrible threat to Israel's very existence and he ordered the

Israeli Mossad to monitor the situation and to take such action as the security of Israel seemed to demand. Ben-Gurion was well aware that Meyer Lansky of the Jewish Mafia in the U.S. was an overseas member of the Mossad, and he was also well aware that Allen Dulles was a firm friend of Israel in its fight with its displaced Palestinians.

The French Military Algerian Faction

From a very early point in his political career, John F. Kennedy had opposed the French presence in Vietnam and their rule of a colonial Algeria. In July 1957 he rose in the Senate and bluntly criticized France's struggle against Algerian rebels. He concluded: "...the essential first step is the independence of Algeria."

This speech set the tone for his attitude towards French/Algerian stress after he became President. Such a stance earned him the anger of a strong right-wing faction of the French Army and was to play a role in his murder. Officers, who, like many of Kennedy's other enemies, viewed the rebels as 'communists' saw Kennedy as a communist sympathizer.

Against this background we can now look at the ordeal of Private First Class, Eugene Dinkin. Dinkin was a young cryptographer in the United States Army, stationed in Paris in October 1963. His job was to receive coded messages from the Pentagon and convert them into English and pass them to the top command.

In October 1963 he received a coded message which directed that certain officers of the anti-Algerian independence clique—the OAS or 'Secret Army Organization' a cadre of disaffected right-wing French military officers—be asked to assist in the location of an assassination hit team for a 'wet-job' in Texas in November, 1963. Dinkin knew two important things: first, 'wet-job' was a term used for 'murder'; second, Dinkin knew from friends in the United States that John F. Kennedy was going to visit Texas in November.

Taking sufficient documents to support his discovery, Dinkin went AWOL and visited several Embassies in Europe to alert them so that they in turn could get the message to Attorney-General Robert Kennedy in Washington. He was turned away at several before being betrayed to the U.S. Army police in West Germany. He was arrested, heavily sedated and surreptitiously flow back to the United States where he was confined to a very secure mental hospital in Chicago. He was in that hospital when the President was murdered. He was subsequently interviewed by the Secret Service, then transferred to the Walter Reed Military Hospital in Washington, D.C. where he was subjected to very brutal interrogation and electric shock 'therapy' until he was 'able to recall that he could not recall having seen the coded request for help in locating an assassination team.'

The Warren Commission refused all calls to subpoena Dinkins and hear his story. (For further details on PFC Dinkins refer to Dick Russell. See Bibliography)

The OAS, however, apparently was contacted and did, indeed, provide any help they could, to advance the Kennedy assassination. Evidence of continuing OAS - CIA cooperation can be supported by the fact that for some unknown reason, E. Howard Hunt was sent to Madrid in March - April of 1963 to meet with Jean Rene Souetre, a former OAS officer who was extremely anti- de Gaulle and anti-Kennedy. Besides meeting with Hunt in Madrid, Souetre was arrested in Dallas on November 22, 1963 and flown out of the United States to either Montreal or Mexico City on a U.S. Government aircraft.

The Establishment

Our files demonstrate that the Establishment (See above: Chapter Two: The Unelected Elite) had several of its top luminaries within the Kennedy cabinet. Kennedy had gone along with the recommendations of some of his advisors and had approved their appointment, and with the recommendation that he retain Allen Dulles in the CIA and J. Edgar Hoover in the FBI because, given the narrowness on his electoral margin against Nixon, he felt obliged not to rock the boat any more than necessary.

Now the evidence is very compelling that certain of these Establishment appointees were actually privy to the plans being made by Allen Dulles to murder Mr. Kennedy. These included Robert McNamara and McGeorge Bundy and others. When a reporter in Washington phoned the Pentagon contact station in Dallas shortly after the word of the assassination broke on November 22, 1963, to enquire who had the critical control box in case a nuclear attack were imminent, the communications officer in Dallas jauntily replied: "Robert McNamara and the Joint Chiefs are President now."

When this interesting and unusual comment was reported it was dismissed by the media and the Warren Commission without comment. However, to those who have studied the coup attempt against Hitler in April, 1945, as Allen Dulles had done (and well-reported in Anton Gill's book, *An Honourable Defeat*: see Bibliography) will understand that a critical element in the planning is the appointment of a witting communications officer. In this light, the comment is not an innocuous error; it demonstrates that the Officer was aware of the decision to murder the President and an intention to replace him by a junta if necessary to quell any uprising.

The Mafia

To the uninitiated, the Mafia in the United States is a group of criminal families far on the outskirts of real America. However, to those who have studied the great power of crime families in America or even those who have simply read such best-sellers as Ovid Demaris' *The Last Mafioso*, that power extends into every corner of American life. The role of the Mafia in the 'deep politics' of America is set out in a compelling and meticulous study by Professor Peter Dale Scott. The Mafia is as essential to the American Establishment as is Standard Oil.

Most people also know that in 1963 Attorney-General Robert Kennedy was heavily engaged in his efforts to eradicate this blight from America.

Add to this the fact that not only was Meyer Lansky a great power in the Jewish Mafia, but was also a great supporter of the state of Israel and was actually a member of the Israeli intelligence apparat, the Mossad, one can begin to see that Allen Dulles could readily recruit the Jewish Mafia into the plans to assassinate the President. Then, when one realizes that Jack Ruby was a member of Lansky's crime family, his need to assassinate Lee Harvey Oswald after Police Officer Marion Baker failed to get the job done, is clear. It is also clear that the CIA and Richard Nixon among others were privy to and participants in plans to recruit the Italian Mafia, especially Carlos Marcello of New Orleans, in an effort to murder Fidel Castro. It therefore became easy to place the blame for the murder on the Italian Mafia and their Teamster friends, led by Jimmy Hoffa. Actually, the evidence is compelling that the Italian Mafia was peripheral to the Kennedy assassination, but they are easy targets for blame.

J. Edgar Hoover and the FBI

There is some evidence that the Director of the FBI, J. Edgar Hoover, a Rockefeller 'wannabe', had strong suspicions, drawn from his well-known proclivity for wire tapping, about the Dulles/CIA planning and he took no steps to prevent it. However, since even his best friends didn't appear to trust him, the planners certainly were not going to make him aware of what was going on. It was enough that the leading law enforcement agency in the nation took no action to thwart the criminals.

Years later, the Watergate tapes reveal the Rockefeller/Hoover links. (Ch.15)

Richard Case Nagell

"Wouldn't it be funny if they gave an assassination and the patsy didn't come?"
We referred earlier to Dick Russell's important study of Richard Case Nagell in *The Man Who Knew Too Much*. In that book, Russell develops the idea that for an assassination to succeed, it is absolutely necessary that a 'patsy' be identified and killed before he or she can establish his or her innocence. The obvious patsy selected for the murder of Mr. Kennedy was Lee Harvey Oswald. There were other patsies available in case Oswald did not turn up for work on the morning of November 22, 1963. Oswald was obviously going to be murdered in the second floor employees' lunchroom by Officer Marion Baker right after the murder of the President, however, the arrival on the scene of Roy Truly spoiled that plan and Oswald had to be shot dead right in the Dallas police station a day and a half late, by a Meyer Lansky 'soldier', Jack Ruby.

At this point we want to make the point that Oswald was clearly a patsy, and that Mr. Kennedy was not murdered by a 'lone nut', but by a wide-spread, effective and very powerful coalition. We want to make this point as strongly as we can because it is necessary to the major thesis of this study: the forces that murdered Mr. Kennedy were the same forces that had engaged in internal terrorist activities in Iran; had over-thrown the legal government of Guatemala; had set up the disastrous Bay of Pigs invasion; had covertly committed the United States to replace the French in Vietnam; and, most of all, had put into place the machinery to develop and deploy pathogens which destroy the human immune system and so expose millions of people, especially in resource-rich Third World countries, to a new pandemic exceeding the horror of the Black Death, or the 1918-1919 influenza epidemic.

The 'lone nut' thesis is essential to the conspirators' cover.

Some geographic sites you should know about

Cold Spring Harbor Laboratory

We first learned of the role of the Cold Spring Harbor Laboratories early in our research when we read Leonard Horowitz' account of an interview with Dr. Robert Strecker. (Ch. 7; Horowitz; 1996) Dr. Strecker has this to say:

"Robert (Strecker): Frank Fenner talks about all the characteristics...Ahh...It's out of...Cold Springs (sic) Harbor, that's the other great biowarfare palace. It's the Eugenics Institute...Cold Springs is in upstate New York ...(Editor's note: not really, it's on the north shore of Long Island.) That was the place started by Margaret Thanger and others. Now they're, of course, the big biological warfare place under the guise of just research.

> "Anyway, Cold Springs Harbor put out a big thing on MMMV, that is, the 'maximally monstrous malignant virus,' and then they gave all the characteristics. And they talked about what it would take to produce this kind of virus. And, of course, all the characteristics are exactly those of the AIDS virus except for one thing, and that is, aerosolized transmission - which we believe is potentially feasible. (Horowitz; 1996 Page 106)

Cold Spring Harbor Laboratories were the site for early eugenics research financed by the American 'nouveau riche' families...(the Rockefellers, Morgans, the Du Ponts, etc.). In 1943 some of its personnel and research projects were transferred to Fort Detrick, Maryland, when the U.S. government authorized its military to establish a base for biological and chemical research in co-operation with its British and Canadian allies.

Despite the latter establishment of 'Camp' Detrick, (later elevated to the status of 'Fort' Detrick), Cold Spring Laboratories continued as a scientific base for biological weapons research, including the precursor research leading to AIDS, under various obfuscating fronts. The usefulness of Cold Spring Harbor lay in the fact that although many U.S. Government personnel and agencies participated in its public and 'shadowy' activities it was to the public mind a 'private' research facility and as such somewhat beyond direct government oversight. What was 'government' and what was 'private' helped limit official oversight and hence resembled the strange commingling of the National Cancer Institute activities with the activities of private corporations such as Litton Bionetics.

An example of this government-private research activity is seen in Robert Gallo's description of Cold Spring Harbor meetings in *Virus Hunting* (Gallo; 1991, Pp. 155-6; 164-66; 170-71). These descriptions suggest open scientific enquiry and reporting, but the reader is left with more questions than answers.

Plum Island

Situated at the northeast end of Long Island is another, much smaller island called Plum Island. The significance of Plum Island to biological weapons research can be gauged by the difficulty in learning anything about it!

Before going further with Plum Island, a comment about 'islands' in general as sites for biological weapons research and testing. Any work with biological agents is dangerous and in an attempt to limit any danger that may exist from the accidental escape of disease agents, scientists have favored the location of such sites on islands, since the water boundaries for such not only limit random wanderers from the site, including many animals and many bird species, as well as itinerant travelers, but also serve to a considerable degree as biological barriers. Hence in this study and many others islands such as Iceland, New Guinea, Plum Island, Anticosti Island, figure extensively.

Lack of common knowledge about Plum Island is an example of a variant of Professor Frank Scott's 'negative template' discussed elsewhere in this study. The more obvious the 'official' references to a site (by government of pliant media assets), the less likelihood that top secrets will be linked to it. Fort Detrick has a 64- year history in biological weapons research (it was founded in 1943). It figures in all manner of bioweapons' research literature such as Ed Regis, *The Biology of Doom* (Regis; 1999) where there are two inches of Index references. But there's not a hint of 'Plum Island.'

We will have more to say about Plum Island in chapter seventeen, but the evidence demonstrates that Lyme disease and West Nile Virus epidemics have significant links to it, as do many other biologically significant agents such as various mycoplasma species and dangerous bacteria. (See Ch.16; Sect. 6: The Riegle Report)

Summary

People make history and history in turn makes people.

For our purposes (tracing the discovery, development, and deployment of AIDS) history begins in 1839 with the birth of John Davison Rockefeller and his establishment in 1870 of the Standard Oil Company. From the latter date to the present we have been able, through our study of wealth, media control and political power to formulate the following nine word summary of that history: OIL > WEALTH > ROCKEFELLERS > ESTABLISHMENT > MEDIA > POLITICAL POWER > CIA > AIDS.

Chapter Ten

THE MURDER OF JFK

This chapter, which attempts to set out the events in and around Dealey Plaza in Dallas Texas from November 22nd to 24th, 1963, begins with a quotation from the December 6, 1963 issue of *Life* magazine. (see Exhibit #4 in Appendices) We introduce this quotation because it demonstrates more than any other single media act how the events of that place and date were misrepresented to the world. If the most significant magazine in the world was ready, willing and able to distort events, lie about facts and condemn a man guilty before a trial, then all the so-called evidence that served to render Lee Harvey Oswald guilty of murder in the minds of the world, must be re-examined objectively. It has been our experience that as each individual part of the day's events are studied afresh, Lee Harvey Oswald emerges more and more as a patsy…just as he said he was.

For example, one of the *Warren Report*'s star witnesses was Howard Brennan. He reported that he saw Oswald *standing* in a sixth floor window and firing the final shot at Mr. Kennedy. Then, says Brennan, Oswald drew the rifle back into the room and with the gun at his side, paused to assess the damage he had done to his target, and then sauntered away from the window.

This eye-witness account was published in a *Report* to the new President by his Commission of seven august gentlemen. But consider: the sill of the window was one foot from the floor, and the window was open one foot…a total of two feet. If Lee Harvey Oswald was to stand and fire through the open window, he would have to have been an 18 inch tall midget!

So step-by-step, let's take a new look at Dealey Plaza on November 22, 1963, and compare the consciously created myths with what actually happened.

At approximately 12:30 p.m., Friday, November 22, 1963, in Dealey Plaza, Dallas, Texas, President John F. Kennedy was shot to death.

For over forty years, from mere seconds after the shooting until the present, thousands of people have challenged the "official" accounts of the crime. They have studied the amateur movies, the Polaroid shots, the great variety of other pictures, the sound tapes of the police channels, the spoken and written recollections of people present, the scientific analyses of sounds, bullets and wounds. They have read reports by the US government, and critiques of those reports. They have tracked the lives of many persons, and have examined the actions of Mr. Kennedy in the months leading up to November 22, 1963, and the actions of Mr. Johnson and Mr. Nixon in the years following. They have succeeded in prying out FBI, CIA, ONI and other "secret" files…always heavily blacked-out for "reasons of national security." Many scholars such as Professors Josiah Thompson, Peter Dale Scott and Phillip H. Melanson have written careful, analytical studies of Dealey Plaza at 12:30 p.m. on November 22, 1963, and of the web of persons linked to Jack Ruby and the strange, short life of Lee Harvey Oswald. But the subject was not one left just to the scholars with distinguished academic credentials and careers. Many persons one might label as "just plain folks" such as Harold Weisberg, Mary Ferrell, Sylvia Meagher and Penn Jones spent thousands of hours reading, researching and writing about the murder. There have been people with "first hand knowledge" whose work often seemed to be a dollop of such knowledge mixed generously with other people's research and leavened by a fanciful role for themselves. In the latter category Hugh C. McDonald and Robert Morrow come to mind. There have been writers whose work is often characterized by selective editing, under-stated or omitted evidence, devious distortions and a snide style. Their work, in sum, appears to have been written to order in an attempt to shore up the "official" explanation of the crime: a lone, lunatic communist with a cheap mail-order rifle, shot Mr. Kennedy to give himself a "place in history." An example of such trash, released to a chorus of hallelujahs from the mainstream media, is Gerald Posner's *Case Closed*.

The variety of data and facts adduced in all of this effort was mainly directed to answering two key questions:

1) Was there a conspiracy to murder the President? And
2) Has there been a cover-up after the fact?

The most careful and devoted of researchers, such as that

magnificent devotee to truth and justice, the late, great Harold Weisberg, can be so close to the subject matter, they sometimes overlook the key facts. Mr. Weisberg was so intent in sifting through all of the reams of obfuscating (intentionally so) minutiae of the *Warren Report* to establish that Dean Andrews had, indeed, been phoned on November 3rd by a Clay Bertrand and that Clay Bertrand was really Clay Shaw and Clay Shaw really knew David Ferrie, and David Ferrie was working with the anti-Castro Cubans in New Orleans, and Lee Harvey Oswald had managed to insinuate himself into this cabal...and so on...that the *key* fact was over-looked. *No real conspirator in his right mind would come forward after the crime to hire an attorney for another of the conspirators!*

And it is the principal thesis of this chapter that *the key evidence needed to establish without a doubt* that there was a conspiracy to murder the President, and that the conspiracy went far beyond a few disaffected Cuban, mafia or rogue CIA agents, and that there was a conscious, blatant distortion of facts and cover-up of the plot, was printed and distributed to over 20,000,000 persons within 14 days of the crime. We refer to the article mentioned above in the December 6, 1963 issue of *Life* magazine, purportedly written by the late Paul Mandel. In particular, we refer to paragraphs eight and nine on page 52F, in the piece fancifully titled, *End to Nagging Rumours: The Six Critical Seconds.* (see Exhibit 4 in Appendices)

The "end" of the "rumours"! - And here it is, over forty years later and the deceitful spirit of Paul Mandel still stalks the halls of *Life*, and *Random House*, and *CBS* in the form of an equally dishonest writer - Gerald Posner mumbling "case...closed."

At this point we re-state the two key questions relating to the murder of John F. Kennedy:

Was there a conspiracy to murder the President?

Has there been a cover-up?

Before dealing with these questions we would like to urge four things of all readers. First, put aside *all* pre-conceptions you may have or conclusions you may have reached about the crime. Second, view if at all possible, the Zapruder film of the assassination. Third, re-read the accompanying paragraphs high-lighted from Mandel's article in Life; and fourth, consider Mandel's article in the context of *Life* magazines' immediate, insistent, dishonest character assassination of

Lee Harvey Oswald which began as soon as *Life* could get their first post-assassination issue to print. Where do these four steps lead us?

The *first* and most obvious truth these steps establish is that Paul Mandel, through *Life* publisher C. D. Jackson and through *Life* magazine itself, told over 20,000,000 readers within 14 days of the crime a direct, obvious and very significant lie. As your review of the Zapruder film will reveal, Mr. Kennedy does *not* turn "his body far around to the right as he waves to someone in the crowd" as the article states. His throat is *never* "exposed-toward the sniper's nest - just before he clutches it."

Please savour what Life magazine was doing here. To put it in context:

On November 22, 1963 Abraham Zapruder took his new Bell and Howell 8mm movie camera and, accompanied by his office receptionist, Marilyn Sitzman, walked to the monument on the north side of Dealey Plaza. He mounted a six foot promontory at the west end of the monument with Ms. Sitzman holding him to keep him steady. As the Presidential motorcade approached, he set the lens on 'telephoto' and focused on the lead motorcycle, and then pressed the shutter release. Thus was the murder of the President to be captured in colour over a 22 second, 8mm piece of celluloid.

And that short piece of celluloid *never* shows Mr. Kennedy at any time, "turning...far around to the right" as *Life* states.

Life magazine lied!

The liars - Mr. Mandel who wrote the piece and Mr. C. D. Jackson who published it - were confident that they could get away with their gross misrepresentation of reality because their employer Henry Luce had bought the rights to the film and had restricted its viewing to a select few - including various investigative agencies and the Warren Commission.

What is the next key conclusion one can draw from these paragraphs?

It is evident that Mr. Mandel was aware of the opinions expressed by doctors at Parkland Hospital, that there was an 'entry' wound in Mr. Kennedy's throat just at the neck-line. The United Press International had quoted Dr. Malcolm Perry, a Dallas physician who was with the President in the emergency room of Parkland: "there was an entrance wound below the Adam's apple." This opinion was later agreed to by Dr. Kemp Clark who said: (as reported by Tom Wicker of *The New York Times*) "Mr. Kennedy was hit by a bullet in the throat, just below the Adam's apple...This wound had the appearance of a bullet's entry." Another person who should have been able to tell an 'entry' wound from an 'exit' wound was Parkland's Emergency Room nurse Margaret Henchliffe (later Margaret Hood) who told the Warren Commission that the neck wound was "a little hole [that looked like] an *entrance* bullet hole." (Emphasis added)

By the next day, when all the police reports were declaring that a lone assassin in the Texas School Book Depository had fired all the shots, the Parkland doctors were forced to speculate. Dr. Perry suggested to the *Boston Globe* "It may have been that the President was looking up or sideways...when the bullet or bullets struck him," while Dr. Charles McClelland declared that the President..."would have to have been looking almost completely to the rear."

It is one thing to observe an entry wound and another thing to speculate from whence the bullets came. However, it is a criminal act to lie about such wounds as Paul Mandel, C. D. Jackson and *Life* magazine did. What are we to conclude?

We can only conclude that the cover-up had begun.

But let's go back to the wounds - an entry wound from the front by the first of the bullets to hit either Mr. Kennedy or Mr. Connally demonstrates to an objective examiner that there was a shooter to the front of the President. However, other bullet wounds in the President's back and to the back of his head demonstrate that there was a shooter or shooters to the *rear*.

To a normal, mentally healthy examiner, two shooters provide *prima facie* evidence of a *conspiracy*...(although one poor soul, Jeremiah O'Leary, offered the "hypothesis of two lone nuts in Dealey Plaza firing within the same half-second.")

Thus we have the evolution of a big lie which we shortly examine, growing from the initial truth...the first-hand observations of Parkland doctors and nurses that Mr. Kennedy was wounded in the front and back, through to speculation as to how a shooter behind could hit his target in the front, to the lie by *Life* magazine that the Zapruder film shows the speculation to have been accurate.

But wait!

Wait!

The Zapruder film can be viewed by others...and as we have said, there is no sign of Mr. Kennedy turning around far to the right. A better story to *mask the conspiracy and continue the cover-up* was necessary. Enter Arlen Specter, Counsel to the Warren Commission assigned to the crucial "Area I" of the investigation: the 'Basic Facts of the Assassination'. Arlen Specter replaces Paul Mandel's first simple lie with one much more improbable, but also, one more difficult to disprove - a "Magic Bullet Theory" that will trace seven Kennedy/Connally wounds to one unusual bullet.

Mr. Specter, a protégé of John Mitchel, former Nixon Attorney-General, has since gone on to win election to the United States Senate.

Paul Mandel's attempt to mask any hint of a conspiracy by dismissing shots from the front and his recourse to a blatant lie are not the only items in these two paragraphs that should be noted.

Take a second look at line two of the second paragraph: "was 50 yards past Oswald and the..." Lee Harvey Oswald at the time the article appeared fourteen days after the assassination, was dead. He had been murdered right in the basement of the Dallas Police Headquarters while surrounded by over sixty police officers. He had been arrested in a movie theatre under very suspicious circumstances and had been "convicted" in the press by the comments of several police officers and government figures right from the moment he was arrested. William Alexander, the assistant district-attorney of Dallas County has stated, "We all knew the same man who killed the President had killed Tippit. *We had made up our minds* by the time we got [to the Texas Theatre]." Even if one accepts as somewhat possible his major premise that "the same man who killed the President had killed Tippit", one must puzzle over his initial logic—that a customer who doesn't buy a ticket to a theatre is probably the man who killed Tippit! During the struggle in that Theatre as Oswald was being arrested one police officer said, "Kill the President, will you." Shortly after, Police Captain Will Fritz said to the press, "This man killed President John F. Kennedy."

It is one thing for police officers who have been gathering evidence, talking to witnesses, studying "rap sheets", to develop an opinion about a suspect in a crime. However, proper police work requires that such opinions be privately held until a consensus is reached and the body of information warrants the formal laying of charges. But, for the assistant district-attorney on his way to a theatre where someone has been accused of entering without buying a ticket to say that "We had made up our minds by the time we got [to the Texas Theatre]" that the accused *gate-crasher* had killed a police officer and, therefore, had also killed the President is mind boggling. And when one of the arresting officers shouts, "Kill the President, will you", justice demands that how the association between gate-crashing and double murder was arrived at, must be revealed.

One can only conclude that well before the time of the President's murder and Oswald's arrest, someone, somewhere, had determined that Lee Harvey Oswald was going to be guilty of that murder and that select members of the Dallas police were privy to this fact.

At this point we must continue our study of the events in Dealey Plaza on November 22, 1963.

By writing that the President's limousine was 50 yards past "Oswald" *Life* re-enforces the theme that Lee Harvey Oswald was the assassin. Thus *Life* magazine, besides masking the evidence of a conspiracy and lying about the evidence, was to become the major factor in making Oswald the murderer in the minds of the world. And this mind set was to prove crucial for it made it easier to deny Oswald his legal rights. After all, he was the killer of John F. Kennedy...

But was he?

Ponder this: Ninety seconds after the final shot rang out in Dealey Plaza on November 22, Officer Marion Baker of the Dallas Police Motorcycle squad "encountered" Lee Harvey Oswald in the second floor employee lunchroom of the Texas School Book Depository. (At this point we would like to remark upon the *Warren Commission Report*'s choice of words. As we shall see, Marion Baker's meeting with Oswald on this occasion was less of an 'encounter' and more of a chilling 'confrontation'. But it served the purposes of the *Warren Report* to downgrade the meeting for reasons that will become obvious later in this study.)

Let's review Officer Baker's "encounter" by first reading the critical details from the *Warren Report*, then let's analyze certain words and phrases which we have underlined to determine just what these details tell us.

According to the *Warren Report*, parts of which are quoted below, Officer Baker was on one of the last motorcycles in the President's motorcade. As he turned right from Main Street onto Houston Street heading north towards the Texas School Book Depository, he heard shots that "sounded high…and I had a feeling that it came from the building…in front of me…or *to the right of it.*"

Officer Baker drove right to the front door of the School Book Depository building, leapt off his motorcycle and ran into the lobby of the building …and "asked *where the stairs or elevator was*…and this man, Mr. Truly…says…follow me." In their rush towards the North West corner of the first floor Baker was in such a hurry that he "bumped into Truly's back."

The elevator that they ran to was immobilized on the fifth floor because someone had not closed its door, so Truly led Baker up *eighteen stairs* to their left. Roy Truly circled left from the top of the first flight of stairs and started up the second flight. When he was almost at the third floor, *he realized that Officer Baker was not behind him!* So Truly turned around and ran back down the stairs to the second floor, where there was only one door through which Officer Baker could have disappeared. (Not the 20 doors he'd face had he taken the front door route!) That door led into a roughly triangular vestibule five feet across and eight feet wide. From the vestibule there were swinging double doors to the right and a single, windowless door straight ahead which led to one of the two employee lunchrooms. Truly opened the lunchroom door to see Lee Harvey Oswald near the middle of the room with a bottle of Coke in his hand and Officer Baker in front of him with his service revolver *pressed right up to Oswald's stomach.* When Baker heard Truly behind him he looked back and asked, "Do you know this man, does he work here?" Truly replied, "Yes." Baker then led the way out to continue up to the roof of the building.

What had led Baker to the lunchroom while Truly ran on ahead? Let's look at more of the *Warren Report* in detail. This is how the *Warren Report* recounts the incident! "As Baker reached the second floor…*he caught a fleeting glimpse of a man walking in the vestibule.* "Since" (the Report continues), "*the vestibule is only a few feet from the lunchroom door,* the man must have entered the vestibule only *a second or two before Baker arrived* at the top of the stairwell. Yet he must have entered the vestibule door before Truly reached the top of the stairwell, since *Truly did not see him.* If the man had passed from the vestibule *into the lunchroom, Baker could not have seen him…* With his revolver drawn; Baker opened the vestibule door and ran into the vestibule where he saw a man walking away from him in the *lunchroom.* Baker stopped at the door of the lunchroom and commanded, "Come here." The man turned and walked back *toward Baker. The man was holding nothing in his hands.*"…Truly thought that the officer's gun at that time appeared to be *almost touching the middle portion of Oswald's body."*

> "Within a minute after Baker and Truly left Oswald in the lunchroom, Mrs. R. A. Reid…saw Oswald…carrying a full bottle of Coca Cola."

That, in the fairest and most objective précis of the *Warren Report* pages that we are capable of, is the account of Lee Harvey Oswald on the second floor of the Texas School Book Depository *ninety seconds* after he supposedly murdered the President of the United States from the sixth floor!

Surely it merits a careful, phrase-by-phrase review, analysis and commentary, which we will now undertake. As we do so we want to make a personal observation. In the "Preface" to his valued and careful book, *Six Seconds in Dallas*, Professor Josiah Thompson pays tribute to Harold Weisberg's acute analyses, but he also notes Harold's "flaw" of "consistent shrillness." We know what Prof. Thompson has in mind. Mr. Weisberg's work is characterized by sentences like the following: "If 'sloppiness' were the acceptable apology, those who seek to defend this fraudulent [Warren] Report claim, there is nothing sacred or honourable or decent in our society. This is not sloppiness, not incompetence. It is a whitewash." Lines like these may indeed sound shrill, but we think it is vital that we never lose sight of the fact that we are not studying railroad timetables to determine the best schedule to get from New York to New Orleans. We are studying the murder of three (most likely four) men - Tippit, Oswald and Kennedy. All three were brutally shot dead within forty-eight hours and in the forty years since their deaths only one murderer has ever been tried and convicted in the deliberate, considered environment of a court of law with the proper evidentiary standards. Two of the murders are still unresolved - not because there is no evidence, but because the Justice Department of the United States, together with Presidents Johnson, Nixon, Ford,

Carter, Reagan, Bush, Clinton and Bush, Jr. have all failed miserably in discharging their obligation to the American people by refusing to study and act upon the evidence in the manner it warrants. Therefore, as we review details whose significance is so obvious, but which have been hidden or distorted or under-stated by the Warren Commission or the House Committee on Assassinations or the Rockefeller Commission, we struggle to contain our grief. Three husbands and fathers died in Dallas, Texas in November 1963 and justice should be done…but hasn't been. So please bear with us as we take you back to the preceding underlined phrases from the *Warren Report*.

Baker's reference to "it", when there had been at least three shots fired, suggests there may have been one shot from the Texas Book Depository ("it") and others from somewhere else. Not a strong point, but in a class with John Connally's cry after he had been hit, "My God, *they* are [not 'he is'] going to kill us all." (*Warren Report*, Page 63)

The reference to the building "to the right of it" is significant because that is the Dal-Tex Building and, as we shall see, strong evidence suggests that there were shots fired from there and that there was a criminal who was well-known to certain police forces, who was arrested as he exited the Dal-Tex Building. As well we learn later of another "boy" who was also an unauthorized trespasser in the building at the time of the shots, who was arrested, and then who simply disappeared from the police records. The Warren Commission's single-minded interest in and emphasis on only Lee Harvey Oswald must be borne in mind.

Officer Baker's request, while in the lobby of the Depository, for directions to "stairs or elevator" is a little troubling because there was an elevator six feet to his right and a flight of stairs three feet behind him. If, in his urgent rush, he had taken either, he could never have blundered his way into the lunchroom in the time he did, and since the building was (supposedly) new to him he needed someone to "lead" him so that he could avoid the labyrinth offered by the stairs and elevator to his right. If he had taken that route he would have had to choose between a total of 20 doors in making his way to the lunchroom. Also, it was a happy piece of good fortune that building superintendent, Roy Truly, was there to lead him. Again, as we shall see, there are problems of who Truly was initially with, and what he saw immediately after the shots were fired.

The fact that Officer Baker was so close upon Roy Truly's heels that he bumped into him has significance when we review what happened next...consider...point (v).

Although Truly starts up *18* stairs with Baker so close behind he bumps into him, by the time they get up those 18 stairs (10 feet, 6 inches), Truly is about *20 feet* ahead of Baker. You see, Truly is supposed to have reached the second floor landing ten feet up, and then circled to his left about 15 feet, and then to have been well on his way to the third floor, as Officer Baker was arriving on the second floor. So, in about six seconds Truly covers 35 feet and Baker only makes ten feet while Oswald, as we shall see, has covered only *two* feet - if the *Warren Report* re-construction is correct. It sounds almost as if Officer Baker, after his burst of speed to get into the lobby of the Book Depository and after he had, in his haste, bumped into Roy Truly's back, that on the way to the second floor he had *purposely* lagged behind his escort to avoid a further collision!

Baker's "fleeting glance" of Oswald just doesn't make sense. Bear in mind that Roy Truly came up the stairs and was facing almost directly the door to the vestibule. *He* did *not* see Oswald or anyone else ...so if Oswald were on his way into the lunchroom through the vestibule, he must already be well into the former. Then, after Truly had gone another 15 to 20 feet around to his left, Officer Baker arrived at the top of the stairs. If Truly could get 15 to 20 feet, surely Oswald could get the last two to three feet into the lunchroom before Officer Baker arrived.

The next underlined detail, "walking in the vestibule" is equally amazing. The vestibule is five feet across at this point between the doors. If Oswald were at least four feet into the vestibule when Truly passed and Truly then covered another 15 to 20 feet, how much "walking" space would Oswald have in the vestibule before Baker supposedly saw him? About one foot! Some walk!

As noted in (vii) above, the "few feet" from the vestibule door to the lunchroom was about five feet!

If Oswald entered the vestibule door a second or two before Baker came tagging along behind, where could Truly have been? To make it a "second or two" before he could get across the five feet of vestibule, *Oswald would have to have entered the vestibule as Truly passed by!* ("Hello Lee.", "Hello Mr. Truly.")

But Truly says he didn't *meet, pass* or even *see* Oswald on his way into the vestibule! One of the few statements in the whole account that sounds genuine.

This detail is one of the most critical in the whole account. If Oswald were in the lunchroom, rather than the vestibule, then as the Report observes, "Baker could *not* have seen him."

"Baker ran *into* the vestibule." Now, if Oswald is in the vestibule (where he must have been or Baker would not have been able to see him!) and Baker comes running in—then there would be a repeat of the earlier incident where Baker (running too fast behind Truly) had bumped into the latter! But no…

Oswald has miraculously evaporated from the vestibule and is now suddenly re-constituted in the lunchroom, where Baker commands him to "come here."

Note that in detail (xii) Baker had his revolver drawn and (as we shall note below—(xvi) the officer's revolver was touching the middle of Oswald's body suggesting that if it was Oswald who did the moving he was co-operative enough to press right up against Officer Baker's revolver!

Although to this point no mention has been made of a "bottle of Coke", the Commissioners want to have any reader ready for the fact that Oswald had not had time to buy a Coke!

Section (xiv) above.

Mrs. Reid remarked on the fact that at 12:32 (now just two minutes after Oswald had allegedly murdered the President) Oswald was four floors below his celebrated "sniper's nest" having an "encounter" in the lunchroom, and had then bought the Coke and continued his "flight" by sauntering off with his soft drink.

If one refers to the floor plans of the Texas School Book Depository, one finds that it is very unlikely that Lee Harvey Oswald could have murdered the President and then have leisurely "paused for another second as though to assure himself that he hit his mark" as Howard L. Brennan, one of the Commission's star witnesses, had claimed. After his "pause" to assess his handiwork (Brennan's claim) Oswald would have to run from the sixth floor south east window to the north west stairs, circling boxes of books along the way, then he would have had to pause, wipe his fingerprints off his rifle, hide it and cover it very effectively, then have taken off down the stairs where he would have to somehow *pass three workers on the fifth floor* at the south west corner who had hurried there after the shots and had then run down the same stairs that Oswald would have had to use. *None of the three saw him.* Neither did Victoria Adams see him descending and she claimed she was on the stairs moments after the shots were fired.

Furthermore, as he ran down the stairs approaching and then reaching the second floor landing he would be only ten feet above Roy Truly and Officer Baker on the ground floor who were starting up the flight from the first floor to the second, yet they did not hear Oswald coming down. *Then consider the ballet-like precision of the second-floor scenario:* Oswald rushes down four flights of stairs and, as he reaches the second floor he runs to the vestibule door 20 feet away. He then runs into the vestibule "a second or two" before Truly comes barreling up the stairs. But, Oswald is so far into the five-foot vestibule *that Truly cannot see him,* and Oswald then has only two more feet to go to pass through the lunchroom door. Truly circles swiftly to his left and covers 15 to 20 feet then starts up the next flight of stairs. As Truly disappears from the scene, Officer Baker comes puffing up to the second floor landing and then he is inspired to cross the landing to the 18" x 18" window of the vestibule door and lo and behold… there is Oswald *who has apparently been in an eight second "hold"* before entering the lunchroom…Bear in mind the Commission's critical observation—"*if Oswald had made the last two feet into the lunchroom, Baker would not have been able to see him*". However, Baker happily does see him in the vestibule so he, Baker, draws his revolver and "runs" in. Then the strange puzzle of the whole account…although Oswald was in the vestibule when seen, when Baker runs through the vestibule door Oswald has remarkably gone out of the vestibule and into the lunchroom. Officer Baker then has to open the door to the lunchroom and order Oswald to "come here." Oswald obeys and walks up so close to Baker that the latter's gun is right in the middle of his body! A person could get hurt that way.

At this critical point Roy Truly, having discovered that his follower had gone off track and, having re-traced his steps to the second floor, throws open the lunchroom door. There he is just in time to see Baker with his gun pressed to the stomach of a "startled" Oswald. When Officer Baker learns from Truly that "this man" worked at the Depository, he decides to continue his race to the roof—evidently on the assumption that no *employee* would shoot the President, only interlopers into the building would be worthy of questioning.

The Warren Commission, without a great deal of hesitation, reached the conclusion that Oswald was, indeed, in flight at the time he "encountered" Baker, and that he could have: accomplished the post-shooting "pause" as seen by Brennan; hidden the weapon; run down the stairs; engaged in the startling second floor landing ballet; and the unique vestibule sighting/lunchroom transplacement—all in ninety seconds!

At this point we must pause and consider what the Warren Commission was up to. The idea of a Commission was apparently broached by J. Edgar Hoover to President Lyndon B. Johnson by way of White House aide Walter Jenkins on *November 24, 1963*. Hoover stated, "The thing I am concerned about, and so is Katzenbach, is having something issued *so we can convince the public that Oswald is the real assassin.*"

In other words, don't *investigate*, don't consider the possibility of a conspiracy, and don't critically evaluate Oswald's "communist credentials"; just *"convince the public"* that *"Oswald is the real assassin!"* And *that* from the chief law enforcement officer in the United States!

It is necessary to reflect upon this gross statement before we consider the Commission's finding that Oswald was capable of such an action-packed ninety seconds.

Although it seems highly unlikely that the Oswald/Truly/Baker scenario unfolded as claimed by the Commission, let's look a little closer before we decide. First, there is the story of the bottle of Coke. Was Oswald actually holding a bottle of Coke when Officer Baker barged in upon him? If he were, then Oswald was definitely *not* the assassin.

The story that Oswald was holding a bottle of Coke when confronted by Baker in the lunchroom 90 seconds after the shooting was first reported by Chief Jesse Curry on November 23. The story recurred several times over the next few months until September, 1964, when Officer Baker was *finally* asked by the Warren Commission to write out his best memory of the incident. Baker wrote, "I saw a man standing in the lunchroom drinking a Coke." Here a very questionable change was made in his handwritten account—the words "drinking a Coke" had a line drawn through them and the deletion was initied by Officer Baker! The corrected version was then typed and it was that version that was entered into the record.

One must also consider the very credible evidence offered by Mrs. Reid. When she saw Oswald come from the lunchroom after Baker and Truly had re-newed their run for the roof, Oswald *was* carrying a Coke.

Let's examine one more item of clear evidence in respect to the 'Coke'. When Lee Harvey Oswald was arrested in the Texas Theatre at 1:55 p.m. he was taken downtown to police headquarters. There he was questioned by Captain Will Fritz of the homicide squad. Early in the interrogation Fritz asked Oswald if he had encountered a police officer as he was exiting the Book Depository. Oswald said that he had. Fritz then asked him where the encounter took place and Oswald replied that he had been in the second floor lunchroom *"drinking a Coke"* when Officer Baker rushed in.

It is evident that when someone was firing at President Kennedy, Lee Harvey Oswald was in the second floor lunchroom having a Coke.

Had Oswald lived and gone to trial, the alleged 90-second flight would never have been able to bear full and careful scrutiny.

> "…so we can convince the public that Oswald is the real assassin"   J. Edgar Hoover, November 24, 1963

But there would have been other evidence to convict him, would there not? For example, wasn't he seen in the window on the sixth floor of the Book Depository by witnesses below? Let's go back to the *Warren Report*. On page 75, the Warren Commission's star witness Howard Brennan, had this to say:"…he was *standing up and resting against the left window sill*, with gun shouldered to his right shoulder, holding the gun with his left hand and taking positive aim and fired his last shot."

How an objective, reasonable person can read this statement and not be totally disillusioned with the people who wrote the *Warren Report* and those who signed it, and those who accepted it, and those who still believe it, and worst of all, those who continue to defend it, is hard to comprehend. Let's examine the statement and consider it in relation to objective, determinable facts. "He was standing up," says Howard L. Brennan.

If you have access to the *Warren Commission Report*, take a look at Dillard Exhibits C & D following page 344. You will note that the southeast, sixth floor window in question is open about 12". Now take a look at Commission Exhibit No. 887, just two pages further on. Here you will note two details: first, the bottom of the window is about 12" above the floor; second, the window *for the re-enactment of Oswald's supposed shooting is not the 12" Oswald needed, but is closer to 16 or 18 inches…*

What do these details show us? They show that, if as Brennan says, "He was standing up" to shoot, that Oswald would have had to be approximately *two feet tall!* Furthermore, an examination of these three photos shows how blatantly the Warren Commissioners were prepared to adjust the evidence so it would help them in their primary goal: "… so we can convince the public that Oswald was the real assassin."

Imagine—a two foot midget with a four foot rifle standing at a window which is open only two feet from the floor!

What else does the Warren Commission tell us about Oswald's remarkable shots from the sixth floor? Well, let's flip over to page 127 where the Commissioners, apparently forgetting that they had earlier accepted Howard Brennan's eyewitness report that Oswald was *"standing in the window"*, now treat us to some further details of Oswald's "sniper's nest": "Three cartons had been placed at the window apparently to act as a gun rest." When one examines the pictures of the boxes on the sixth floor, one sees that on average they stand about 18" high. Two of them in a pile would give our 24" midget a gun rest three feet high. (Two were in a pile and one was on the floor) Either our short assassin would have to spring back up to Oswald's normal size, or with three boxes as a Warren gun rest he, as a midget, would have to stand on one other box and then shoot *through* the glass, or, Mr. Brennan would have to be in grave error. And, as a more detailed study reveals, Mr. Brennan was, indeed, a terrible witness to depend upon in the identification of Lee Harvey Oswald as the assassin.

Because Mr. Brennan was such a weak witness, the Warren Commissioners found it necessary, as had *Life* magazine some months before, *to simply invent a lie* and pass it off to the public. On page 78, with reference to the southeast window on the sixth floor of the Book Depository, the Report states that this window was "the only open window on that floor." *This is another direct, blatant lie.*

Actually, the Dillard Exhibits C and D as they appear in the *Warren Report* and as referred to above are cropped severely with five sets of windows removed from view. *The full picture shows two more windows open and other pictures by Charles and Howard Hughes show the same thing!*

Gerald R. Ford, who was later to be hand-picked as President by Richard M. Nixon, was to say in *Life* magazine of October 2, 1964, Howard Brennan "was the most important of the witnesses."

Indeed. When one is inventing an explanation for the murder of a President, it helps to have liars on your side.

Besides discrediting the testimony of Howard Brennan, the above gross incongruities (Oswald standing to shoot/Oswald behind three boxes to shoot/Oswald, as re-enacted in Exhibit 887, kneeling to shoot) point up another very important characteristic to note: The *Warren Report* is very fluid in citing "evidence". In one place it declares with certainty, what a few pages further on, is *replaced* by another certainty.

In the latter category is the famous police alert for: "an unknown white male approximately 30, 165 pounds, slender build…" Although the source of this "description" was never established, the *Warren Report* tries to make out that it came from Howard Brennan, by stating on page 146…"An *eyewitness* to the shooting *immediately* provided a description of the man in the window which was similar to Oswald's actual appearance." Since they had earlier said that there was only *one* eyewitness, then they must be alluding to Brennan, but this cannot be asserted with confidence because Brennan turned out to be a very unreliable witness—despite Gerald Ford's faith in him.

The fact seems to be that, like the situation noted earlier in the Texas Theatre arrest of Oswald, certain police officers knew before the President was even murdered, who they would be looking for after the crime had been committed.

    A chronological summary to this point:
    12:30 — Shots fired at Mr. Kennedy.
    12:30 — Howard Brennan sees the last shot fired from the southeast corner window on the sixth floor of the Book Depository.
    12:30:20 — Officer Baker roars up to front door of Book Depository—joined by Roy Truly.
    12:31 — Baker and Truly try to get elevator to go to the roof—use stairs.

12:31:30 — Up just 18 stairs, with Truly getting about 20 feet ahead of Baker in only a ten foot run, Baker has a confused impulse to enter lunchroom. Truly, as he nears third floor, notes Baker absence so heads back to second floor.

12:31:40 — Oswald met in lunchroom, holding a Coke. Truly catches up just as Baker thrusts gun up to Oswald's stomach. Truly identifies Oswald. Baker and Truly continue to the roof.

12:32 — Brennan tells some police officer (never really identified) what he had seen and points out sniper's nest.
Mrs. Reid meets Oswald on second floor, and he is holding a Coke!

12:34 — Oswald met at front door of Book Depository by NBC newsman, Robert MacNeil.

12:34:15 — Oswald leaves the Book Depository where he would pass Brennan and the mysterious police officer - but neither seems to have noted the murderer fleeing!

12:44 — After an *unexplained ten minute delay*, the description of Oswald broadcast over police radio channel.

12:45 — Buell Wesley Frazier leaves work just ten minutes after Oswald had left.

The events and *the accounts* of such events from 12:30 to 12:44 just reek with confusion, inconsistency, incompetence and cover-up. The confusion, a large part of which is understandable under the circumstances, was greatly compounded by several factors. First, Chief Curry of the Dallas Police, and Forrest V. Sorrels, Secret Service Chief-in-charge in Dallas, were in the lead car of the presidential motorcade. As they proceeded in the limousine and as they were entering the under-pass, they heard the shots. *"Get someone up in the railroad yard and check those people."* Then he and Sorrels, the two men who should have taken immediate charge of Dealey Plaza, roared off to Parkland Hospital with the wounded President.

Three factors are absolutely critical here. First, the absence of Curry and Sorrels left a huge vacuum at the crime scene where all manner of officers ran in all directions. Second, despite Curry's *obvious* conclusion that the shots had come from "up there" in the "railroad yard" (*i.e.* the grassy knoll) his absence permitted attention to be shifted to the Texas School Book Depository. Third, with Forrest Sorrels gone for about twenty minutes (on his round trip run to Parkland) unidentified "secret service agents" were able to head off any pursuit of persons apparently fleeing into the railroad yard.

Other serious consequences of a command vacuum: some buildings overlooking Dealey Plaza were never properly sealed; the "sniper's nest" in the southeast corner of the sixth floor *supposedly pointed out immediately by Brennan* was not "discovered" for forty-two minutes; a variety of agencies related directly or indirectly to law enforcement were functioning in various roles—(for example, ten minutes after the assassination seven Alcohol, Tobacco and Firearms agents were searching the Book Depository and the railroad yard); three "tramps" spotted in the railroad yard were able to evade apprehension on a first search and were almost able to leave town in a departing train before a second search discovered them; evidence of various kinds was seized from by-standers or otherwise removed—never to be seen again.

The total chaos that reigned in Dealey Plaza because of a leadership vacuum permitted anyone who so chose to walk out of the Texas School Book Depository or flee from the grassy knoll. Many employees, believing there would be no more work that day, left the building. Among them was Wesley Frazier, who had driven Oswald to work that morning. But Frazier was to figure in Oswald's destiny in other ways as well. His sister, Linnie Mae Randall had helped place Oswald in the Book Depository by telling him of a job opening. On November 22, 1963, she was to play a further role as we shall see.

Let's pick up our chronology where we left off. As we have seen, Howard Brennan supposedly saw Oswald *standing* in the southeast corner window of the sixth floor. He told a secret service man, who he later insisted was Forrest Sorrels (who didn't arrive back at the Texas School Book Depository until about 20 minutes later) what he had seen. Yet, it was to be over 12 minutes later before the "Brennan" description was broadcast and it was to be a mind-boggling *forty minutes* later that the Dallas Police made it to the "Brennan" sixth floor sniper's nest. In the meantime, Officer Baker and building Superintendent Roy Truly had made it down from the roof to welcome Sorrels back to the scene of the crime. Sorrels finds that although the front door of the Texas School Book Depository was well-guarded, the back door was wide open!

Let's go on from there:

12:50 — Sorrels asks Truly for a list of missing employees.

12:54 — A Dallas Police patrolman, J. D. Tippit contacts his dispatcher from Oak Cliff area where Oswald lives—is advised to "be at large for any emergency."

1:04 — Truly reports Oswald missing from the assembled work force. He was *one* of about *seven* missing employees—yet his name was at the top of the list, which also contained the name of Buell Wesley Frazier. Although Oswald had been in the lunchroom at 12:32 and Truly had said he was "O.K." Sorrels decides to dispatch police to Ruth Paine's home where Oswald had spent the previous night in Irving - but not to Frazier's home!

1:12 — Deputy Sheriff Luke Mooney discovers sniper's nest. Leans out window to call down to officers below that he had located "the location of the sniper"...just about *thirty minutes after Howard Brennan* had already supposedly reported the location to the police.
At about the same time, Lt. J. C. Day arrived at the Texas School Book Depository—*before* Truly reports to Captain Fritz that Oswald was missing.
Day goes to sniper's nest with Detective R. L. Studebaker to photograph the "nest" and look for fingerprints. Locates a box upon which he writes "from top of box *Oswald apparently sat on to fire gun.* Lieut. J. C. Day."

1:16 — Call from citizen in Oak Cliff - Officer Tippit has been murdered.

1:50 — Oswald arrested in Texas Theatre.

2:00 — (?) Sheriff Bill Decker calls Capt. Will Fritz from the Texas School Book Depository for a confidential discussion which he did not want to trust to a "phone or police radio."

2:15 —	Captain Fritz returns from the Texas School Book Depository and orders arrest of Oswald (?) He learns he's already in custody. Sends Serg. Rose to seize Oswald's belongings.
3:30 —	Police arrive at Ruth Paine's home in Irving. Find rifle missing! By a streak of good fortune Linnie Mae Randle arrives on the scene to report that she had seen Oswald arrive for a ride with her brother Buell that morning and Oswald had been carrying a wrapped package!
5:00 —	Captain Fritz decides to pick up Buell Wesley Frazier.

A review of this chronology reveals that out of the chaos created by the absence of Chief Curry and Secret Service Chief Sorrels, a pattern was emerging. It is not a pattern of evidence being discovered and fitted together, but rather a pattern of closing in on Lee Harvey Oswald *despite* the evidence, *not because of it*. Of seven names on a list, the emphasis on Oswald by Captain Fritz is to be noted. And when the police rush off to Irving, the presence of Linnie Mae Randle serves as a link between the supposed hiding place of Oswald's gun and Buell Wesley Frazier's car.

These and other factors tend to re-enforce the earlier evidence, that certain police knew who they were looking to arrest (as a second resort!) before the evidence had been discovered and analyzed. And nowhere is this impression more dramatically demonstrated than it is in Bishop's book, *The Day Kennedy Was Shot*. On page 348 of this insidious book where Bishop describes as we have noted the actions of Lieut. J. C. Day on the sixth floor of the Texas School Book Depository:

> "Then Day wrote on the box: 'From top of box **Oswald apparently sat on to fire gun.** Lieut. J. C. Day'. He tore the top off and took it back to headquarters." Emphasis added.

Lieut. Day had located the box in the south east corner of the sixth floor of the Texas School Book Depository shortly after 1:12 p. m. Pause long and deliberate on just how significant this passage is. Lieut. Day knows that it is Oswald's hand print on the box *before he knows what Oswald's hand print looks like!* He knows before he learns Oswald had a gun that the gun was not just owned by Oswald, it had been fired by him! But, far more puzzling is the fact that he knew Oswald's name *ten minutes before such an employee was reported* by Roy Truly to Captain Fritz as *missing!*

William Manchester in his equally insidious book, *The Death of a President* was to remark, "On November 22 [Oswald's] speedy arrest had been considered an achievement."

The achievement was Oswald's…that he had gotten away from his designated assassin, Officer Marion Baker, and had made it to his rooming house, and then that he survived his arrest in the Texas Theatre. On his own, he was safe. His greatest risk came when he was under the protection of the Dallas Police.

The so-called "flight" of Oswald is as confused and contradictory as his "encounter" with Baker; his standing in the window as witnessed by Brennan; and the rush by the police to his wife's Irving residence where Linnie Mae Randle happened by to bridge the garage-to-car gap of Oswald's rifle.

Let's start by seeing what the *Warren Report* has to say about Oswald's flight from the Texas School Book Depository. According to the *Warren Report,* Oswald left the Depository by the front door at the corner of Elm and Houston at approximately 12:34. Although he lived south and somewhat west, he walked seven blocks east on Elm, then caught a bus going west towards the point he had just left. The bus driver, Cecil J. McWatters, and a former landlady, Mary Bledsoe, recalled him being on the bus and McWatters gave him a transfer when he got off a couple of stops west. The Commission speculates that he walked south where he caught a cab driven by William Whaley at Commerce and Lamarr. He left the cab at Beckley and Neeley Streets, some distance south of his 1026 North Beckley rooming house, and backtracked to it on foot where he arrived at about 1:00 p.m.

Given the chaos and traffic congestion around Dealey Plaza, this scenario is not unusual. To go west, one could well walk east to escape the crowd, and then ride back to the west. The bus that McWatters and Bledsoe say Oswald was on did not go to North Beckley and a request for a transfer was reasonable. When arrested Oswald has such a transfer in his possession.

However, problems began to develop almost as soon as the police had established Oswald's movements. The main problem was posed when Roger D. Craig, a deputy sheriff of Dallas County, claimed that at about 12:45 (fifteen minutes after the shooting) he had seen a man that he later identified as Lee Harvey Oswald come down an embankment from the Depository on Elm Street and enter a light-coloured Nash Rambler station wagon which then drove towards the railroad underpass.

So now we have two "escape" scenarios—the McWatters/Bledsoe/Whaley route and the Roger Craig route. The Commission accepted the McWatters' version, although there were lies, distortions and time differences to complicate it.

For example, bus driver Cecil McWatters had first told the police that he remembered Oswald on the bus because Oswald had had an argument with a women passenger. However, when he was placed under oath to testify to the Warren Commission, McWatters admitted that it was a 19-year-old youth named Milton Jones who had had the argument in question.

Taxi driver William Whaley wasn't much better as a witness before the Commission. He had reported a wrong time on his manifest that acted as a log for his trips, and he also had three different points where he believed Oswald had left his taxi. In addition, he had Oswald wearing a zippered gray or blue jacket, rather than the rust-brown shirt he had actually worn. Finally, William Whaley got everyone confused about his identification of Oswald in a police line-up. First, he claimed that the police had him sign a statement about whom he had identified *before* he saw the line-up. Then he testified that "Oswald" (who was number two in the line-up) was actually number three.

Ordinarily, in a proper Court of Law, testimony such as that by William Whaley would have been thoroughly discredited. Only the Warren Commission could accept inconsistencies and pick and choose amongst the details for the ones they needed for their case... They had to get Oswald to 1026 North Beckley Avenue by 1:00 p.m. so that they could have him leave in time to murder a second victim, Officer J. D. Tippit at 1:15 p.m. Harold Weisberg's review of Whaley's "evidence" in *Whitewash* is still, after 44 years, the most incisive review yet pondered.

However, if the Commission did not accept the McWatters, *et al.* scenario, it would have been stuck with the testimony of Deputy

Sheriff Roger Craig that he had seen a light-coloured Nash Rambler station wagon pick Oswald up on Elm Street near the Depository fifteen minutes after the assassination. If they had accepted this story they would have inherited a much bigger problem than the one that they already had, for Craig's description of the station wagon and the dark-skinned Latin driver had already cropped up around Dealey Plaza on that November day in other suspicious circumstances. For example, a construction worker named Richard Randolph Carr had seen a heavy-set man with horn-rimmed glasses and a tan sport jacket *at a sixth floor window* of the Texas School Book Depository shortly before the assassination. After the assassination, Carr saw the same man walk a block and get into a light-coloured Nash Rambler, driven by a "real dark-complected" Latin. The Commission dealt with the testimony of Craig and Carr by simply suggesting they were mistaken. To admit to a get away car, the Commission would be admitting to a conspiracy.

So, by whatever route, Oswald did arrive at his 1026 North Beckley rooming house somewhere around 1:00 p.m. He went to his room where he apparently changed his shirt and put on a zippered jacket.

If he did arrive at 1026 North Beckley by 1:00 p.m. as the Warren Commission speculates, then he would have fifteen minutes to change his shirt, pick up his revolver, leave the house and walk several blocks to the corner of 10th Street and Patton Avenue where he is purported to have slain Officer J. D. Tippit at the Commission's stated time of "approximately 1:15 p.m. Not an impossible task…although he would have had to walk at a rate three times as fast *getting* to the scene of the murder as the rate he walked fleeing from the scene! One would expect the opposite.

But that isn't the only problem with Oswald's return to 1026 North Beckley at 1:00 p.m. and his departure at 1:03. Other strange things happened that suggest Lee Harvey Oswald was not just heading to a movie on an unexpected afternoon off.

First, there was the strange episode of a Dallas police car which, about one or two minutes after Oswald arrived at his boarding house, pulled up in front of his residence and sounded its horn. At the sound of the horn, Mrs. Roberts went to the window and put aside the curtain and watched as the police car paused, then pulled slowly away. Although she had seen a number on the vehicle, she could not recall the number with any certainty. The Commission dealt with this very unusual event by saying there were no police cars known to be in the area at the time therefore, Mrs. Roberts could not have seen one in front of her home. Then they went on to other things in keeping with their usual approach of ignoring anything that did not contribute to the establishment of Oswald's guilt.

There was another problem…when Oswald left the rooming house shortly after the police car sounded its horn and then drove off, Mrs. Roberts looked out the front window and saw Oswald standing at a bus stop which was for *north-bound* buses. The Commission, of course, needed to have Oswald walking quickly south—*not standing* at a north-bound bus stop. To deal with this anomaly, the Commission again just ignored it.

Their challenge to get Oswald to 10th Street and Patton while on his way to the Texas Theatre west of the Jefferson/Zangs intersection was made greater by the fact that to get *south and west*, their hypothetical route had him heading at a *very brisk walk south and east* to commit the murder of Officer Tippit then *taking a casual stroll to the movie house.*

Finally, with $14.00 cash in his pocket, why Oswald would attract attention and sneak into the Texas Theatre without buying a ticket and so give the man who had followed him (Johnny Calvin Brewer) an excuse to report him to the theatre manager raises interesting possibilities; but again, the Commission did not appear to be interested. As J. Edgar Hoover had suggested, their goal was still to "convince the public that Oswald is the real assassin" and contradictory claims were solved by picking the one that best fitted their need—to get Oswald at 10th Street and Patton Avenue by *1:15 so he could be fingered* as the killer of Officer J. D. Tippit.

Did Lee Harvey Oswald shoot Dallas Police Officer J. D. Tippit at the corner of 10th Street and Patton Avenue at approximately 1:16 p.m. on November 22, 1963? The Warren Commission has decreed that he did. Although it had taken some juggling with taxi-driver William Wayne Whaley's shifting testimony, and with the need to have Oswald walk swiftly south-*east* to get south-*west*, and although they had to ignore him standing at a north-bound bus stop, the Commissioner's got Oswald to the murder scene on time. At least to their satisfaction.

But, as asked above, did he commit the murder? Mrs. Helen Markham said he did. However, as we shall see, Mrs. Markham as a witness was in a class with Gerald Ford's favourite witnesses, Howard Brennan and William Whaley. Very little of what any of the three had to say was logical, consistent, or believable but the Commission accepted their testimony.

Let's start with Mrs. Markham's description of the man she saw shooting Officer Tippit. The *Warren Report* states: "Her description and that of other eyewitnesses led to the police broadcast at 1:22 p.m. describing the slayer as 'about 30, 5'8", black hair, slender.'"

Fine. Short. Straight-forward. Could apply to about 300,000 males in a ten-mile radius.

However, the Commissioners are again less than forthcoming about the description broadcast by Patrolman J. M. Poe. Actually the officer had also said that the suspect was wearing a "white jacket." Typical of their obfuscating writing habits, the *Warren Report* does not mention this fact until six pages later. One would almost think by the way the writers of the *Warren Report* let out dribs and drabs of contradictory details that they were counting upon their readers having short memories. To make matters worse, Officer Poe learned of the jacket's colour from Mrs. Markham and a Mrs. Barbara Davis. As we shall see, Mrs. Davis had seen a man leaving the scene; she had not seen the crime committed so she didn't necessarily see the man who had shot Officer Tippit. Thus, although both Markham and Davis said that the fleeing man had worn a "white" jacket, only Mrs. Markham had seen the shooting.

Another witness, Domingo Benavides, had also seen the shooting from about 25 feet away. However, *Benavides refused to identify Oswald as the shooter.* So, as with Howard Brennan, the Commission was stuck with Helen Markham…and her very confused and confusing testimony was to prove a boone to the Commission because it could pick and choose what they wanted from what she said and then invent things for her where needed.

Thanks to this latitude, the Commission was able *to ignore* the fact that Mrs. Markham had said Oswald wore a *white* jacket, when in fact the jacket found by the police and claimed to be the one Oswald had worn was a darkish green colour tending to blue!

Here we enter another chapter of Alice in Wonderland—just what colour was Oswald's jacket and what colour was the jacket of the man who shot Officer Tippit?

Here is a range of colours you can select between:

	Witness	Page & Source	Colour
1.	Markham	163 - *Warren Report*	"white"
2.	Westbrook	163 - *Warren Report*	"light-coloured"
3.	Roberts	163 - *Warren Report*	"gray"
4.	Callaway	164 - *Warren Report*	"tan"
5.	B. Davis	3H347	"black"

Actual colour in Groden's colour photo: green.

How did the Commission resolve the problem? They decided that *whatever colour it was*, the jacket belonged to Oswald.

But then, more problems with this chameleon jacket: it had laundry identification marks and dry cleaning marks that could not be traced and, investigation revealed that all of Oswald's other clothing had been hand-washed or cleaned.

At this point it is enough to try to put together a coherent picture, sustainable by reasonable evidence, of what happened in Dallas on November 22, 1963.

The Warren Commission would have us believe that:

At 12:30 p.m. Lee Harvey Oswald had fired three shots at President John F. Kennedy, hitting him and Texas Governor John Connally, killing the President. Oswald fired from a "sniper's nest" on the sixth floor of the Texas School Book Depository located at the north-west corner of Houston and Elm over-looking Dealey Plaza. After shooting the President, Oswald hid his rifle on the sixth floor, and then fled down four flights where he paused in the lunchroom for a Coke; there he "encountered" Officer Marion Baker and superintendent Roy Truly. After a chat, he continued his "flight" while they proceeded to the roof of the Depository. At 1:00 p.m. he arrived at his 1026 North Beckley boarding house where he changed his shirt, put on a green zippered jacket and, at 1:03 p.m. hurried over to the corner of 10th Street and Patton Avenue where he shot Dallas police officer J. D. Tippit to death and fled (at a rather casual pace) to the Texas Theatre some blocks away, discarding his jacket as he fled and saving money by sneaking into the Texas Theatre instead of paying.

What has our re-examination of events suggested to this point?

It is evident that no one saw Lee Harvey Oswald at the sixth floor window of the Depository. Howard Brennan's testimony is totally impossible. It is also evident that Oswald was holding a Coke ninety seconds after the shooting, and Officer Marion Baker lied about seeing him enter the lunchroom. It is also evident that the Dallas police began looking for Oswald long before they knew from their collected evidence that (a) he worked in the Depository, (b) he was missing from the Depository after the crime and (c) he had once purchased a rifle.

So far, from what we have seen of Oswald's movements and the quality of the "witnesses", the evidence is heavily weighted to the conclusion that Oswald did not shoot the President and that he was being pursued as a "patsy".

This being so, we must set aside the simplistic, highly unreliable scenario set forth in the *Warren Report* and go back to Dealey Plaza at 12:30 p.m. if we are to determine what had, indeed, happened.

As we have seen, as the shots rang out in Dealey Plaza, Officer Marion Baker concluded "it" came from either the Texas School Book Depository or the Dal-Tex building, and he opted to speed up to the former and rush in.

Officer Baker's actions must be compared with those of Officer Clyde Haygood, and the actions of both of them in respect to the whole question of the President's security in Dallas. The House Select Committee on Assassinations heard testimony from Captain Winston Lawrence about the motorcycle escort. In that testimony, Lawrence referred to both Baker and Haygood as "straggling". That is, they were off their proper stations in respect to the President's limousine and were further back than Captain Lawrence would have preferred.

Now, the fact that they were straggling is bad enough, but that will be examined later. At this point it is what each did when the shots rang out that we should examine. As we have seen, Baker rushed to the Depository, but Haygood sped down Elm Street to a point near the underpass. *Here, he dropped his motorcycle and ran up the grassy knoll. He, unlike Baker, thought the shots had come from the front and right of the President!*

What does the *Warren Report* have to say? Well, as we have seen, they spent a great deal of time on Officer Baker's actions - referring to him on several pages (10) but they dismiss Haygood's run in two sentences:

> "Bowers and others saw a motorcycle officer dismount hurriedly and come running up the incline on the north side of Elm Street. The motorcycle officer, Clyde A. Haygood, saw no one running from the railroad yards."

If one were to judge from the *Warren Report* only Clyde Haygood had made this egregious error...but their representation is seriously flawed. Let's consider the actions of Deputy Sheriff Luke Mooney who was standing near the corner of Main Street and Houston as the shots rang out. Rather than follow Baker towards the Depository, Mooney ran across the grass of Dealey Plaza, crossed Elm Street, and ran up the embankment, which came to be known as the "grassy knoll." The *Warren Report* doesn't seem to have been interested in this aspect of Mooney's day...although they do mention him in another context.

However, before we get to that, let's follow Mooney a little further. He had vaulted over the picket fence and was trying to decide just how to proceed in the railyard. Several other Dealey Plaza witnesses had begun to join him when an officer who was never identified, began telling the police that "Sheriff Bill Decker had wanted his men to go inspect the Depository Building." As a "Deputy", Mooney had no choice but to head over to that building.

But wait. Before he goes...let's review what was happening.

When the firing began, many people in a position to judge, were under the clear impression that at least some of the shots came from a "grassy knoll" to the front and right of the presidential limousine. Others had an equally clear impression that the shots came from the Texas School Book Depository. A few others identified places such as the Courthouse on the northeast corner of Main and Houston, or the Records building on the southeast corner of Houston and Elm, or "buildings" (plural) at the corner of Houston and Elm.

One of the first and best efforts to study the evidence on the question was Prof. Josiah Thompson who, in 1967, published his remarkable book, *Six Seconds in Dallas*. In his Appendix "A", Prof. Thompson published a map of Dealey Plaza and a list of all the witnesses he could locate and where possible, interview. He came up with 268 names and, of this number, 76 reported their impression of the direction of the shots. The majority said "the grassy knoll" (47%); the balance said either the Texas School Book Depository (38%) or "other" (15%).

So Clyde Haygood was not alone in his first impression and his run up the embankment …in fact, in terms of numbers, he was with the majority who believed that the shots came from the grassy knoll.

However, let's begin our review of this part of the study of Dealey Plaza, November 22, 1963 with what the *Warren Report* concluded. Here is their statement:

Speculation   There are witnesses who alleged that the shots came *from the overpass*.

Commission finding   The Commission does not have knowledge of any witness who saw shots fired *from the overpass*. Statements or depositions from the two policemen and 13 railroad employees who were on *the overpass* all affirm that no shots were fired *from the overpass*.
Most of the witnesses who discussed the source of the shots stated that they came from the direction of Elm and Houston Streets.
[Emphasis added.]

First, notice how the writers refer to the "testimony" that shots came from in front of the President as "speculation". Such a label reduces the specific testimony to a type of fanciful mental exercise.

Second, notice how the reference is to shots *"from the overpass"*. In all of our reading and studying of the events in Dealey Plaza on November 22, 1963, we never came upon any witness who suggested that shots came "from the overpass". The devious minds who wrote this let on that the "grassy knoll" and "the railroad yards" and "behind the picket fence" could all be lumped together as "the overpass", and then they could dismiss any shots from "the overpass."

No one ever said "from the overpass", but the writers of the *Warren Report* were careful to repeat "the overpass" four times, thus shutting out the evidence of the 47% of the witnesses who said shots came from in front of the President.

One more (out of many) devious tricks will be referred to here simply to alert you early on not only to *what* the *Warren Report* says but to *how* they say it. In this regard take a second look at the final sentence quoted. Here they refer to "most of the witnesses who discussed the source of the shots stated that they came from the *direction* of Elm and Houston Streets". The "witnesses" they refer to only discussed the source of the shots if they were asked by their questioner, and the questioners did not ask those whose answers might not fit their needs to "convince the public that Oswald is the real assassin". Then, when the majority of the witnesses on and around the overpass who *were asked* from what *direction* the shots seemed to come they indicated "the direction of Elm and Houston Streets"—which "direction" *included* the grassy knoll, the railroad yards, the monument and the embankment!

Where **did** the shots come from?

Let's look at some of the testimony of a representative selection of witnesses closest to the action.

Mr. Abraham Zapruder was standing on a portion of a monument about 30 feet from the street down which the motorcade was passing. What he *saw* was enhanced by the telescopic sight on his movie camera. But it was what he heard that we must consider, and Zapruder says he heard the critical shot that blew open the President's head "behind him and to the right."

The grassy knoll!

As we have seen, Chief Jesse Curry of the Dallas Police was in the lead car of the motorcade. The car was going under the overpass when the shots rang out and Currie grabbed his police car microphone and ordered: "Get someone up in the railroad yard and check those people."

The grassy knoll!

S. M. (Sam) Holland was a railroad employee who had one of the best viewing points in Dealey Plaza - he was on the "overpass" which, as we have noted, the Commission used to obfuscate the testimony of him and several others. Mr. Holland signed affidavit only hours after the shooting which reads in part:

> "I heard what I thought for the moment was a firecracker and [the President] slumped over and I looked over towards the arcade [upon which Zapruder was standing] and trees and saw a puff of smoke come from the trees."

The grassy knoll!

Roy Truly, the building superintendent of the Texas School Book Depository was out on the sidewalk near the front door when the shots were fired. Within sixty seconds, he was to lead Officer Marion Baker up to the roof of the building, but his first impression was that the shots came from the "vicinity of the RA or WPA project" [where Zapruder was standing].

The grassy knoll!

And so it was for 37 other witnesses on record.

There were also a significant number of witnesses (30) of record who believed the shots came from the Texas School Book Depository. For example, Secret Service driver of the presidential limousine, William Greer, claimed that the shots came from the Depository. However, an analysis of the Zapruder film shows that from the time the vehicle turned down Elm Street until the shots began; Mr. Greer kept his eyes on the grassy knoll ahead and to his right. Almost as if he was waiting for something. Then, when the shots began, he put his foot on the brake, instead of speeding up and held it there until the President's head was blown off.

In other words - it's probable that certain witnesses might have had a reason for identifying the Depository, if they were part of a plot to have the President hit from the front.

The evidence from bona fide witnesses is clear: there were shots from both the front and rear of the President when he was murdered. The attempt of the Warren Commissioners to pretend otherwise cannot be sustained in the face of open-minded, critical review.

The next question is—who fired the shots from back and front? There are some clues.

Lee Bowers, Jr. was a railroad towerman for the Union Terminal Company. His workplace was a fourteen-foot tower slightly to the west and north of the Depository. From this location he could look out over several lines of railroad tracks that ran roughly north and south, with a Texas and Pacific line running from the north end of the Depository to the west. He also had a good view of a large parking lot that filled in the space between many of the rail lines, and he could see part of Houston Street to his south and east. Most important of all, Lee Bowers had a very good view of the area behind the Dealey Plaza north monument upon which Abraham Zapruder stood and the picket fence to the west from whence Sam Holland and others had heard gun shots and had seen a puff of smoke.

Mr. Bowers' job required him to be alert and observant and in the hour before the murder of President Kennedy he noted some vehicles moving about and, at the time of the shooting his attention was caught out of the corner of his eye by a "flash" or something different from usual. It came from near two men standing behind the picket fence. A few minutes later, having learned of the shooting, he saw three men dressed somewhat as tramps, seeking to place themselves on freight cars of a train about to depart. Mr. Bowers reported the three men to the police, who with the aid of some Alcohol, Tobacco and Firearms Agents of the Treasury Branch, searched the train and found nothing. Then, as the train began to leave the rail yard heading south over the overpass, Lee Bowers spotted them again. Bowers, using the signal controls in his tower, stopped the train and reported the tramps. Again the train was searched and this time the three tramps were discovered, arrested and escorted up to Elm Street across Houston and along Houston Street to the police station. There, it is claimed, they were finger-printed and had mug shots taken, but these were "lost" soon after. Twenty-seven years later the Dallas Police Department let on that the records had come to light, but as we shall see, the records are inconsistent and contrived. The tramps were then allowed to leave by direction of Captain Will Fritz and some unidentified FBI agents.

These three tramps will, as we shall see, provide a link to the CIA and to the "Watergate" break-in, but that all comes later.

What does the *Warren Report* have to say about the three tramps? Nothing!

In a classic example of Prof. Scott's "negative template" the Commissioners, the Dallas Police, the FBI, and the Secret Service all omit reference to them. And little wonder - one of them is E. Howard Hunt, a long-time OSS-CIA spook and former Rockefeller employee who was recruited into the CIA by Frank Wisner at about the time the latter was handling the ex-Nazi Gestapo agents recruited into the CIA by John J. McCloy and Allan Dulles. Whether Hunt was shooting from the grassy knoll or was present in Dealey Plaza to witness the execution of his President can only be surmised as we will do later. At this point all the evidence suggests that the CIA was involved.

But, there was another building on Houston Street staring right down on the limousine as it crawled down Elm Street at Wm. Greer's shooting gallery speed...and that was the Dal-Tex Building of oil millionaire H. L. Hunt.

Almost immediately after the shooting of the President, a man unknown to a building security person came out of the Dal-Tex building and headed east on Elm Street. The security person reported him to police and the man was taken to the Police Station for questioning and identification. He gave an alias to the police, supported by a California driver's license - "Jim Braden."

It turns out that Jim Braden was really Eugene Hale Brading - a man with a "long arrest record, a long history of association with organized crime with links to Jim Hoffa's Teamsters Union and to Meyer Lansky's 'front man', Moe Dalitz."

So besides the CIA, elements of the Mafia were apparently involved in the Dealey Plaza shooting.

There is, however, evidence that a third group was linked to the shooting.

Joseph Adams Milteer was also in Dealey Plaza on November 22, 1963. He was standing on Houston Street, about sixty feet from the corner of Elm Street. Next to him were Pearl Springer and Carolyn Walther. Mr. Milteer was a right wing nut. He was a member of the Ku Klux Klan and the Congress of Freedom, Inc. The latter group met in New Orleans in April, 1963 when they discussed "the overthrow of the present government of the United States", including "the setting up of a criminal activity to assassinate particular persons." According to Prof. Peter Dale Scott, the report added that membership within the Congress of Freedom, Inc. included "*high ranking members of the armed forces.*" Thus, with the CIA-Mafia components, it is evident that the Congress of Freedom and other right wing factions participated in the murder of President Kennedy.

The important thing to note about Joseph Milteer is that the FBI was warned of a planned attempt on Mr. Kennedy's life on November 10, 1963 - eleven days before the assassination - and the FBI did nothing! Such a failure to take resolute action to prevent the assassination is prima facie evidence that J. Edgar Hoover and other senior officers in the Bureau were participants in the crime. Either directly, by heading off action on information that came from their vast network of informants (of whom, ironically, Oswald may have been one) or indirectly by simply doing nothing as evidence of the plot grew.

As well, the Secret Service was advised of the planned attack and if anything, they reduced their efforts to protect the President.

Finally, there is convincing evidence that the US Military Intelligence apparatus played an active role in planning and carrying out the execution. The presence of Military Intelligence Officer, James Powell in Dallas in contact with the H. L. Hunt family and Eugene Hale Brading help to establish this. It was probably through Military Intelligence that Generals Willoughby, Walker, Cabell and Wedemeyer were involved.

So—who fired the shots from both the front and rear of the President's limousine—at least four professional gunmen representing elements of the CIA, the Mafia, the Congress of Freedom, the FBI and Military Intelligence!

When one considers that in one place in the nation (Dealey Plaza) on November 22, 1963, there were assembled E. Howard Hunt (CIA) and Eugene H. Brading (Mafia) and Joseph Milteer (Congress of Freedom) and James Powell (Military Intelligence) it is ludicrous to suggest that co-incidentally there was a lone nut who shot the President.

The involvement of these various levels of the black espionage, terrorist, criminal and intelligence communities provided the assurance that once the President was dead; the nation would be kept well under control.

When Oswald was confronted in the second floor lunchroom ninety seconds after the last shot was fired at the President, Officer Marion Baker was to shoot him dead, trying to "prevent" his escape. When this part of the plan failed because of the timely return of Roy Truly to the lunchroom and to the fact that while awaiting a communication from his handlers, Lee Harvey Oswald had bought a Coke.

Baker had no choice but to let the designated, and now alerted, "patsy" leave the building.

Although further examination of the murder of Officer Tippit is required, there is as much evidence that Oswald did not murder him, as there is evidence that he did. However, with a corrupt Dallas Police force and a compromised, if not participating, FBI and Secret Service conducting the investigation, Oswald had little chance of escaping.

It is quite possible that the experience of having Officer Baker rush into the lunchroom and shove a gun into his stomach was enough to alert Oswald to the fact that he had come within two seconds of being killed at that point as a patsy for a crime he may or may not have known was going to take place.

Spared by the timely return of Roy Truly, Oswald may well have fled—*not* from the scene of a crime he had committed as the *Warren Report* would have us believe, but fleeing from those who would kill him. Hence his rush home to pick up his revolver.

This latter action raises the question that if he had indeed planned to murder President Kennedy, why would he not have taken the precaution to carry his revolver with him to work? Why wait until after the fact to pick it up? Furthermore, it is quite possible that Officer Tippit was a back-up hit man to murder the "fleeing" killer of President Kennedy and that Oswald simply beat him to the draw. Possible, but doubtful as we shall see.

The realization that he was being set up as a patsy would also account for Oswald's shouts in the Texas Theatre: "I am not resisting arrest! I am not resisting arrest!" He needed as many witnesses as he could attract in order to prevent his execution in the Theatre. The realization that he was being set-up probably accounts for the fact that, even though Johnny Calvin Brewer had pointed Oswald out to police in the Texas Theatre, the police began their search several rows away - possibly to give Oswald a chance to jump up and attempt to flee. Then, the police could shoot him dead. Oswald declined the opportunity and sat impassively until they reached his seat.

It was 1:50 p.m. when Lee Harvey Oswald was arrested in the Texas Theatre, and at 2:00 Sheriff Bill Decker called the Captain of Homicide, Will Fritz, to a private, and to this date, confidential discussion. It was only after this puzzling *tête-à-tête* that Capt. Fritz began his interrogation of Lee Harvey Oswald, the suspected assassin of President John F. Kennedy.

What was it that Sheriff Bill Decker communicated to Capt. Will Fritz that was so confidential that it could not be trusted to the telephone or the police radio channel? Did it have something to do with the fact that the intended patsy for the murder of the President had not been shot dead by Officer Marion Baker or Officer J. D. Tippit or by the Dallas Police in the Texas Theatre and that Capt. Will Fritz would have the unexpected challenge of interrogating a suspect? In fact, a suspect who might (alive) be able to successfully prove his innocence? Or, did Decker's highly confidential message to Capt. Fritz deal with the murder of a Secret Service agent behind the Texas School Book Depository? After all, it was only 18 minutes later that an A.P. wire story out of Washington (?) reported such an event.

At this point, we will suspend surmise and try to identify what transpired between 2:30 p.m. when Capt. Fritz began his "interrogation" of Lee Harvey Oswald on Friday, November 22, 1963 and the death of Mr. Oswald at approximately 1:07 p.m. on November 24, 1963 at Parkland Hospital.

The first and most important factor to note is that over the period that he was held, Lee Harvey Oswald was consistently denied access to legal council. As we shall see, various Dallas police personnel and other law enforcement officers tried to mask the fact that Lee Harvey Oswald was used in a totally criminal way during his so-called "interrogation". When we have examined the record of this terrible abuse of Mr. Oswald, we will advance an answer to the question asked by Harold Weisberg: "Cui bono?" That is, who benefited from this denial of legal rights to the accused assassin?

The second most important thing to be noted about what happened to Mr. Oswald during his approximately twelve hours of interrogation is the startling "fact" that the questions asked and answers given were not tape recorded or otherwise preserved!

Insidious apologists for the corrupt abuse of Lee Harvey Oswald, such as William Manchester, express wonder at this deficiency in proper police methodology. *"For some reason, which has never been satisfactorily explained, the [police] department's secretaries had been sent home. Thus the historian is deprived of even a shorthand transcript of these vital sessions."*

A third important factor that we will examine is the fact that, without advice of legal council, Lee Harvey Oswald did not want to discuss certain subjects that were raised. As we shall see, he was not being "sullen" or "un-cooperative" as the image painted by the police and the Press would have us believe - he was just being logical as any informed and intelligent person in his situation should have been.

Finally, we must note how the august gentlemen of the President's Commission, presided over by the Chief Justice of the United States Supreme Court glossed over the abuse of Mr. Oswald and what this cost the world in understanding who murdered President John F. Kennedy. When Lee Harvey Oswald came off the elevator on the third floor of police headquarters, flanked by detectives and arresting officers shortly after 2:00 p.m. on Friday, November 22, 1963, he looked straight at several news reporters and photographers and said, "I want a lawyer." The police hustled him down the hall to the office of Will Fritz, Captain of the Homicide Division.

"Fritz decided that he did not want a stenographer…nor did he desire a tape recorder."

Capt. Will Fritz asked a number of innocuous questions, which Oswald apparently answered in a calm, polite fashion. After several minutes of the exchange, Oswald asked, "Can I get a lawyer?" At this point Capt. Will Fritz began his exercise in duplicity that he was to maintain until Lee Harvey Oswald was safely dead.

"You can call one anytime you want." he said.

Taking this to mean that all he needed to do was say who he wanted, Oswald said, "I want John Abt. He's in New York."

"You can have anyone you want." repeated Fritz.

"I don't know him personally," continued Oswald, "but that's the attorney I want. If I can't get him, then I may get the American Civil Liberties Union to get me an attorney."

Any reasonable person would take this exchange to mean that Oswald wanted a lawyer, as he was entitled to have, before the interrogation continued. Capt. Fritz brushed it aside by saying: "You'll find a phone on the fifth floor. You can make the call yourself at your expense."

Then, with this superficial nod in the direction of the prisoner's rights, Fritz *went on with his questioning* until most legal offices were closed for the weekend! Again Oswald answered a series of questions that had nothing to do with any crime. These he responded to with candour and intelligence. Then he again drew the line …"I don't have to answer any questions until I speak to my attorney."

"Oswald, you can have one any time you want." said Fritz.

"I don't have the money to call Mr. Abt."

"Call him collect or you can have another lawyer if you want.

You can arrange it upstairs." But again, Fritz made no move to stop his questioning to permit Oswald to go "upstairs" or to secure legal council. After another hour or so, Capt. Fritz left his office and Oswald remained behind with Secret Service agent, Forrest V. Sorrels, an FBI agent and two Dallas detectives. Oswald refused to answer any of Sorrel's questions, but asked instead, "What am I going to be charged with? Why am I being held here? Isn't someone supposed to tell me what my rights are?"

"I will tell you what your rights are." Sorrels said. "Your rights are the same as any other American. You do not have to make a statement unless you want to. You have the right to get an attorney...You can have the telephone book and you can call anybody you want..." But, as with Capt. Fritz, this agent of the US Government ignored the reality of what was happening - that Oswald was *not free to call* whoever he wanted - and went on with his questioning.

Sometime after 5:00 p.m. Oswald was taken back to the fifth floor jail. At that point (which was after 6:00 pm New York time!) jail guard Jim Poppelwell came in and said, "All right, he can make his phone call." Poppelwell led Oswald to a glass booth that contained two pay phones and handed the prisoner a dime. Oswald asked: "How can I phone New York with this?"

"That's not my department," replied Poppelwell.

It is necessary to emphasize the reality of Oswald's situation. He has one dime. His $14.00 cash had been taken from him and the police would not return it to him. It was after 6:00 p.m. on a Friday and anyone who knows anything about the legal profession in New York would be aware that the offices of the major law firms would be shut down tight...not just for the evening (Friday), but for the weekend.

With his dime, Oswald called information New York, and asked for the telephone number of "John Abt." He was given the number "212-AC2-4611" of a "John J. Abt." He then called this number collect, but charges at the other end were declined.

Oswald had made his one entitled call!

He asked Poppelwell if he could try again. Poppelwell told him he'd ask Captain Fritz. Oswald then said he'd call his wife and ask her to try.

Downstairs, reporters were asking if Oswald had been permitted to call an attorney. They were told: "He's phoning one now!"

The dissembling and equivocating were to continue.

After being served a dinner, Oswald was again brought down to the office of Capt. Will Fritz. Again he answered some questions in a straight-forward way, but at others he balked - stating that he declined to answer certain questions until he had consulted with an attorney.

Thus, the Dallas Police, by their own contriving, were able to keep certain answers off such record as was being maintained by the simple expedient of effectively denying Oswald legal council.

At about 7:00 p.m. Capt. Fritz signed a complaint charging Oswald with the murder of Patrolman J. D. Tippit. As Jim Bishop was later to write:

> "Considering the magnitude of the case and the weaknesses of motive, Captain Will Fritz and his men had achieved remarkable results within six hours."

Indeed!

The fact is, with the rambling interrogation that was not recorded by either a machine or a competent stenographer; nothing Oswald has said provided anything that would have stood up in a Court of Law. Furthermore, with the evidence that he had been effectively denied legal counsel and had never been advised of the crimes he was supposed to have committed, any pretence of a case would have evaporated under informed scrutiny.

Capt. Fritz signed a complaint simply to have grounds for continuing to hold Lee Harvey Oswald incommunicado.

Not only was Lee Harvey Oswald denied legal counsel, and not only was his interrogation an unrecorded, totally useless star chamber, but every time he was moved, Oswald was subjected to shouted questions from reporters to which he tried to respond with deliberate replies. In addition he was subjected to a heavy tirade of insults! "Bastard!" "Son of a bitch!" "Why'd you kill the President?"

And through it all, Oswald held to a steady course: He would only co-operate in the unimportant things…when it came to significant legal points, he insisted on an attorney. He refused to sign a fingerprint card or take a polygraph test "without the advice of counsel."

On each of these occasions, Oswald expressed a need for legal representation, and his requests ultimately reached a handful of concerned civil rights people. One such person was Gregory Lee Olds, President of the Dallas Civil Liberties Union. At about 10:00 p.m., Olds phoned the Dallas Police Station and insisted on speaking with Captain Fritz. After being stalled for several minutes, Olds was finally put through to Capt. Fritz. He told the Captain of Homicide that the Civil Liberties Union "was anxious to see that Oswald had whatever legal representation he desired." The Captain replied that the "police department had been at pains to detail Oswald's rights, *but Oswald had declined all assistance.*"

This of course, was an outright lie. Oswald had been questioned without the aid of counsel for more than four hours. Then he had been given one single dime and the right to one phone call—well after New York law offices were closed.

Captain Fritz was a willing participant in making sure that Lee Harvey Oswald was denied legal counsel. We shall soon see why.

Gregory Olds did not give up. He phoned several ACLU Board members and called them to a special meeting at the Plaza Hotel. At about 11:00 p.m., after discussing the puzzle of Oswald expressing a wish for legal counsel in the media while Captain Fritz was claiming that he had "declined assistance," they determined to call Mayor Earle Cabell—brother of General Charles Cabell who had participated with Allan Dulles in the Bay of Pigs fiasco. Mayor Cabell refused to take the call from the ACLU on the grounds that he was "too busy."

At this point, the ACLU board members decided to go personally to the Dallas police station and, if possible, speak directly with Oswald. At the station they were shunted around until finally referred to Justice of the Peace, David Johnston. The judge assured them that Oswald's legal rights had already been explained to him and that he had "*declined counsel.*"

Another direct lie!

But the ACLU officers accepted the word of the Justice of the Peace for Dallas County and all except Gregory Olds left the police station.

Lee Harvey Oswald was left enmeshed in a web of Dallas police intrigue.

At this point we should note the strange role of Police Chief Jesse Curry. We saw earlier how, when the shots rang out in Dealey Plaza, marking the commission of the "crime of the century", Chief Curry, after ordering police up to the railroad yards, had sped off to Parkland Hospital. While chaos and confusion reigned back at Dealey Plaza, Chief Curry busied himself helping Jackie Kennedy get a drink of water. He hurried over to Love Field to oversee the activities around Air Force One and Two. He helped get an ambulance to take the body of John F. Kennedy from the hospital to Air Force One.

In a word—Chief Jesse Curry hid from the eye of the storm. He essentially abdicated his role as Chief of Dallas Police and he allowed Captain Will Fritz and Assistant District Attorney William Alexander to run the show. And, as will become clear, William Alexander had played an important role in the execution of President John F. Kennedy and in the framing of Lee Harvey Oswald. It was no mere co-incidence that the day before the President was murdered, Wm. Alexander had a visit from a Dallas night-club owner, Mr. Jack Ruby, who will turn up in this narrative shortly. But at this point it is important to emphasize that Assistant DA Wm. Alexander, Captain Will Fritz and Justice of the Peace David Johnston blocked Oswald's access to legal counsel by various subterfuges and, as Jim Bishop says, "They ignored their own Chief of Police to a marked degree."

Lee Harvey Oswald, the designated patsy, was being set up for his execution…because the first three attempts: in the lunchroom of the Texas School Book Depository; at the corner of 10th Street and Patton Street and then at the Texas Theatre had all failed. Now Capt. Will Fritz and Assistant DA Wm. Alexander had to bully Chief Jesse Curry into standing Lee Harvey Oswald up in front of several newsmen and a Mafia thug Jack Ruby so the latter could make another try to end the life of the lone, communistic, ex-marine who wanted to go into the history books as the killer of a US President, but who steadfastly refused to take credit for the act. A paradox that only seven august gentlemen on a Presidential Commission could rationalize.

The fourth attempt on Oswald's life was scheduled for 11:26 p.m. on Friday, November 22 when he was taken to the basement assembly room in the Dallas Police Station. He was set up at the front of the room in *front* of a protective shield! Jack Ruby, who later admitted he was carrying a fully loaded revolver, was allowed into the room without being challenged and even allowed to climb up onto a table about 20 feet from where Oswald was standing, and from where Ruby could see over the heads of the crowd of reporters. However, the crush of people around Oswald made it impossible for Ruby to shoot at him without risking a hit on someone else. As we shall see later, Ruby didn't want anyone else to get hurt—including himself. He just wanted to kill Oswald on orders from his Mafia/CIA employers. If he were to shoot and miss or just wound Oswald, he would never have another opportunity.

The press conference had not served its purpose of setting Oswald up for execution...but it did have some positive effects. It gave Oswald a further chance to state that he was being denied legal counsel and in reply to a question from a reporter: "Did you kill the President?" he was able to reply in a surprised tone, "No, I didn't shoot anyone, no sir."

Fortunately, this and other replies by Oswald were captured on tape and were subjected to psychological stress evaluation by George O'Toole, a former computer specialist who served with the CIA as Chief of its Problem Analysis Branch. His findings: Oswald was telling the truth when he said, "No, I didn't shoot anyone, no sir."

But the goal of Will Fritz and William Alexander was not to find who murdered President Kennedy—their job was to hold Oswald long enough for Jack Ruby to kill him.

After the so-called "press conference", Oswald was returned to his jail cell for an hour and then, at 1:30 a.m. on Saturday, November 23, he was again brought before Justice of the Peace Johnston where he was formally charged with the murder of *President Kennedy*. When Lee Harvey Oswald heard this charge he made a dramatically revealing comment: "Oh, this is the deal, is it?"

Again you must pause a moment to savour just what was happening to this victim of the powerful forces which had earlier executed the President of the American Republic. He was being railroaded. Even Jim Bishop, whose insidious style constitutes one of many sick chapters in the media character assassination of Lee Harvey Oswald acknowledges what Fritz, Alexander and Johnston were up to when he was arraigned in a hidden room, at 1:30 a.m., with no witnesses other than Dallas Police, FBI agents and Secret Service men, and then denied representation by legal counsel. "There could be but one reason for this," writes Bishop, "*to keep Oswald's mouth shut.*"

"I don't know what you are talking about." concluded Oswald as he was led back to his jail cell.

They had him in their web.

Ironically, his guards were to remark upon the fact that Oswald slept soundly—almost as if he were innocent of two murders in one day.

The next day was relatively easy for Oswald. He was "interrogated" for about two hours and fifty-five minutes in three different sessions. Each time he said there were certain things he would only discuss if he had an attorney! Thus, if Fritz, Alexander, Sorrels, etc. had really wanted to hear Oswald's answers to certain questions, they would have expedited the process of securing him legal counsel. But they did no such thing. *There was a strong need felt by his interrogators to keep answers off the record, not to get answers on the record.* In the meantime, the newspapers and radio reports, which were kept from Oswald, reported that John Abt had said Oswald had not been in touch with him, and even if he were, Abt believed his present client load would not permit him to accept the case.

No one told Oswald.

He also saw his wife, daughters ("Buy June some new shoes."), his mother Marguerite Claverie Oswald, and his terribly embarrassed brother, Robert Oswald, to whom he said, "Do not form any opinion on this so-called evidence." Advice which, tragically, Robert Oswald was to later ignore.

By 5:30 p.m. it was time for Fritz and Alexander to make another meaningless gesture towards Oswald's legal rights. Fritz okayed a visit to Oswald by Dallas Bar Association President, H. Louis Nichols. In a five-minute meeting, Nichols told Oswald that the Bar Association was obligated to provide legal counsel after his indictment. Oswald thanked him, but said he preferred John Abt or failing him, a lawyer from the American Civil Liberties Union. Nichols told Oswald it was his call and he did not have to respond to interrogation until represented to his satisfaction.

Nichols did not undertake to communicate Oswald's wishes to either John Abt of to the ACLU, and then left for home.

Oswald believed that sooner or later he would have an attorney with whom he could share his side of the story. He did not know that Fritz, *et al.* had to prevent this at all costs.

Again that night Oswald slept like an innocent man.

By late Saturday night, the participating elements of the Dallas Police Department had done their share of damage control. When

Officer Marion Baker had been unsuccessful in his assignment to kill Oswald in the second floor lunchroom immediately after the President had been assassinated, and when Oswald succeeded in getting back to his rooming house and then on to the Texas Theatre, the police had to engage in a holding pattern. If Jack Ruby had been able to get off a clean shot at the 11:30 p.m. "press conference", the task would have been completed. But that, too, failed. In the meantime, by keeping no notes or record of the "interrogation" and by keeping Oswald away from legal counsel, the police had kept certain facts *off the record*. Furthermore, by charging Oswald with two murders in the middle of the night way from all non-co-operating witnesses, the police had legal grounds to hold him. Finally, after being formally charged, Oswald was entitled to an immediate transfer to the Dallas County Jail. However, in that setting any chance to silence him without blatant police co-operation would be remote. Again Oswald's rights had to be completely ignored and Oswald had to be set up for his designated executioner: Jack Ruby.

And in that task, Ruby was ready, but not necessarily willing.

Late on Saturday evening, while Oswald slept for the second night, "as if he were innocent", the telephones in the Dallas Police Communication's Centre were ringing constantly. Callers from around the country asked for information tips and threatened Lee Harvey Oswald. One of the latter calls was taken by Lt. Billy R. Grammer, who paid particular attention to it because the caller had specific information about the planned transfer of Oswald to the Dallas County Prison the next day. Grammer beckoned his supervisor to listen in on another phone so *both, Lt. Grammer and Lt. Henry Putnam heard the caller say, "You're going to have to make some other plans, or we're going to kill Oswald right there in the basement."*

Grammer was sure he had heard the caller's voice before, but couldn't put a face to it. It was only after Jack Ruby was arrested that it suddenly came to Grammer who his caller had been. Grammer was convinced it was Jack Ruby who had phoned him a warning!

The telephone warning was passed on to Chief Curry, Captain Fritz and Lt. Decker. But they went ahead as planned and Lee Harvey Oswald was executed in the basement of the Dallas Police Station.

Finally the "patsy" was executed and out of the way…leaving certain peoples an open path to assert that a lone, lunatic communist had killed President John F. Kennedy. The path was open because *after several hours of interrogation there were no records of what was asked and what was answered.* As well, there were no lawyer notes of what the accused assassin had to say about who he was, who he worked for, why he was in the lunchroom with a bottle of Coke 90 seconds after the shots were fired in Dealey Plaza. All the data about his study of Russian language, his "defection", his mystery flight from London to Helsinki, his strange journey home, his rifle purchase, his New Orleans street fracas…all and much more was forever stilled by Mafia thug Jack Ruby and the Dallas Police.

Now all that remained was to get together seven august gentlemen who would ratify an almost perfect plan to remove President John F. Kennedy from the White House.

But before we get to that, let's take a few more glances at Dealey Plaza from 12:30 p.m. on Friday, November 22, 1963.

From that critical time of 12:30 p.m. many stories surfaced. Some as "nagging rumours" that made it into the newspapers or on to the radio and TV. Others that just floated around taverns and kitchen tables. Some were sufficiently strong that certain people and certain elements of the media sought to counter them. This campaign began immediately and continues to this day. Initially, as we have seen, it was *Life* magazine that led the campaign. This journal with its strong covert links through owner Henry Luce, publisher C. D. Jackson and Luce's wife Clare Booth Luce held the denial fort until the *Warren Report* weighed in with a special Appendix: "Speculations and Rumours."

One "rumour" is under-pinned by an Associated Press news item dated, "Dallas, November 22, 1963, 2:18 p.m." - "to the effect that a Secret Service agent had been shot and killed in Dallas." The first strange detail about this report is that it had the dateline "Dallas", *but it originated from the Washington bureau of AP.* The next thing to be noted is that it was reported on the radio for nearly two and a half hours before it was countered by a wire stating the report was untrue.

Then a report cropped up that a large blood stain was discovered in an alley behind the Texas School Book Depository. Several people who had rushed to Dealey Plaza when they heard the news of the assassination were turned away from the area behind the Depository by representatives of various law enforcement agencies. There were rumours that members of the Secret Service were behind the Depository immediately after the assassination, but this was denied by the Secret Service Agency.

At 6:10 p.m. when Air Force One landed at Andrews Air Force Base, some civilian workers discussed a removal of something from the aft cargo compartment to a waiting helicopter behind the plane and then a quick take-off while the new President and the Kennedy casket were dis-embarking from the other side.

Medical technicians at Bethesda Naval Hospital talked amongst themselves about the arrival of a body in the autopsy area shortly before that of President Kennedy arrived. They were told not to "log" it in.

Each of these rumours, taken by itself, doesn't shed much light on the other events of November 22. However, taken together, they suggest a very ominous possibility—a crime and a cover-up within the main conspiracy. The following scenario is speculative—but merits a careful review.

Immediately following the assassination of the President, one of the assassins fled from the scene - either from the Texas School Book Depository or the grassy knoll - as he fled he was challenged by a Secret Service agent who was not privy to the plot - nor was he there officially as part of the Sorrels/Lawson guard unit. The fleeing assassin shot him dead and completed his escape. When located some minutes later the agent was already dead and Lt. Bill Decker who had just returned from Parkland Hospital was told that there was a dead Secret Service agent in the back area. Decker immediately realized that this was not part of the patsy scenario and called Captain Will Fritz to the scene - refusing to state what the emergency was either by phone or police radio. Fritz and Decker agreed that a dead Secret Service agent would totally blow the "lone assassin patsy" plan. *If, as was by then apparent, Officer Baker had not killed Oswald in the lunchroom and the designated patsy had strolled out the front door of the Depository, a death behind the Depository had to be covered up.*

Sorrels and Fritz okayed the immediate delivery of the body to Air Force One, (SAM 26,000), where it was placed in a body bag and stored in the aft compartment. Someone in the Secret Service contingent reported the death to the White House Secret Service headquarters. Unaware of the plot to murder the President, the news was passed to an AP reporter who phoned it to the AP Washington bureau, which, in turn, put it out on the wire at 2:18 p.m. (Dallas time), where it circulated for two and a half hours until denied by the Secret Service when the news reached them.

The unknown body was taken by helicopter to Walter Reid Hospital where it was placed in a coffin and re-shipped to Bethesda where the assassination control centre had been established. Here it lay until the body of President Kennedy arrived and while the top brass supervised the carefully controlled autopsy. Then, at that point, the body of the unknown Secret Service agent was quietly interred and whatever family he had was quietly advised that he had died under "unfortunate" circumstances such as "suicide" following the failure of the Service to protect their much loved President.

This speculative diversion ties together several disparate details of record. The final event of November 22 that will be noted here is all on the record. But the Warren Commissioners were to refuse to weigh what they said about the day's events.

Before summarizing the unusual events of that day in the life of Donald Wayne House, we would like to pose two questions for you. First, what if they gave an assassination and the patsy didn't come? Second, how many people named "Hunsaker" do you usually encounter in one day? We'll comment after we've told you about Mr. House in Dallas on November 22, 1963.

At approximately 2:00 p.m. on November 22, Donald Wayne House was driving west from Dallas towards Fort Worth. He was en route to his home in Ranger, Texas another 80 miles further west. Suddenly a Tarrent County police car overtook House's 1957 green and white Ford with the Texas license number DT-4857. House was arrested and taken to the city jail and held for questioning by two FBI agents who were called to the scene.

House was asked to account for his whereabouts over the past six hours. He replied that he had decided not to go to work that morning in his hometown of Ranger. Instead, he drove over to Dallas to visit an old army buddy, *Randall Hunsaker*, in the suburb of Mesquite. In Dallas, at 10:30 a.m. he parked on Commerce Street (one of the three streets that converge under the railroad overpass at Dealey Plaza) and phoned *Randall Hunsaker*. Randall was not home, so House decided to watch the Presidential motorcade. After the assassination, and when he could get clear of traffic, he says he set out for home and had gone about 25 miles west when he was stopped by the police at 2:00 p.m.

The police told Donald Wayne House that he was being held in relation to the assassination of President Kennedy. Apparently, shortly after the murder, a Mrs. Cunningham had called the Grand Prairie, Texas police and told them that she had reason to believe that House was involved in the crime. She said that he was driving a 1957 green and white Ford with the license DT-4857! She also said that he was on the highway heading west from Dallas towards Ranger! How much more specific could one be?

Then, at 2:19 p.m. Dallas Police were alerted by a phone call. A two-tone green car at 5818 Belmont had been spotted by a neighbor and someone in the car had been seen removing a rifle. The police rushed to the address where they discovered a different car, but this one was registered to a *George F. Hunsaker*, of Dallas. Then word was received by all concerned that a lone, lunatic by the name of Lee Harvey Oswald had been arrested in Dallas. The FBI agents let Donald Wayne House head off for home - without them visiting his friend *Randall Hunsaker* and the Dallas Police lost interest in *George Hunsaker* and the rifle at 5818 Belmont.

Apparently the FBI believed that if someone else had been arrested, whoever that someone was must be guiltier than the person they had arrested. Never mind any claims and details provided by a Mrs. Cunningham.

What do you do if you give an assassination and the preferred patsy doesn't come? **Answer:** You have another patsy on the shelf to be developed as "the" assassin.

This is one possible interpretation of the strange experience of Donald Wayne House on November 22, and the unusual fact that he was trying to visit a friend named Hunsaker and a Hunsaker was involved in some way with a rifle transfer on the very day several rifles are fired in Dealey Plaza.

How many Hunsakers do you usually encounter in one day? **Answer:** *Two—if you are investigating an assassination.*

But, whether House was a stand-by and equally unwitting patsy, should Oswald slip the net, we'll never know. For the FBI went no further (at least on the record) with House, Cunningham or either of the two Hunsaker's.

It is quite possible that a Mrs. Cunningham had hard evidence that did indeed link Donald Wayne House to the murder. But again, we'll never know—unless somehow we get a *real* and *honest* investigation… before it is too late.

There are *hundreds* of similar damning incidents that careful, conscientious researchers have uncovered. Incidents, which point to a powerful, high-level conspiracy to kill President Kennedy and then to cover the crime up while pretending to investigate it.

The case made by Chief Justice Warren and the gangsters who essentially drafted the fiction of the *Warren Report* for him, including Arlen Specter, David Belin, Gerald Ford and the rest, depends upon it being established that Lee Harvey Oswald, working alone, got off three shots in six seconds with one of those shots being the 'magic bullet' which caused all seven wounds in both Mr. Kennedy and Texas Governor, John Connally, and was then recovered in pristine condition on a gurney in Parkland Hospital.

Nothing in the actual evidence supports such a preposterous scenario, and any careful student must conclude that efforts to demonstrate the dishonesty of the *Warren Report* is frustrated at every step by the Report itself, by many layers of government bureaucracy and by the dishonesty of the public version which was then and is today, advanced by a corrupt media. Space limitations prevent us from putting forward all of the details which support such a conclusion, but we will provide three brief examples.

The *Warren Report* itself, is a very dishonest piece of work, and was carefully designed by those who drafted it to confuse and mislead the reader. An excellent example of this is seen in the fact that when the Report was issued, followed by twenty-six volumes of so-called supporting evidence, **there was no index and no table of contents.** Thus, if a reader of the Report wanted to check out in more detail some point of interest, he would have to sift through the 26 volumes of what is often pure, irrelevant junk to find what he was interested in.

Such idiocy aside, it is to be noted that one of the Commissioners, John J. McCloy, had used just such a technique of obfuscation in his early years as a lawyer for the Chicago, Milwaukee & St. Paul Railroad. Author Kai Bird describes it this way:

> "While McCloy was diligently drawing up the receivership papers and taking various affidavits, the major shareholders

of St. Paul stock and the men who had appointed the company's board of directors, William and Percy Rockefeller and Ogden Armour, were quietly selling out. In a short time, few of the railroad's directors had any stock at all in their own company…In anticipation of the receivership, Kuhn, Loeb needed a legal device whereby none of the forty thousand individual investors, scattered all over the country, could attempt to exercise collective control over the reorganized railroad. To this end, McCloy, Swatland, and Douglas drafted an enormously complicated and wordy document…**The document had no table of contents and no index.** The language was all but impenetrable; one sentence ran to 2,250 words. Buried throughout the proposed receivership document was this essential fact: in order for any shareholder to participate in the receivership, he must give an unqualified proxy to the bankers…In these circumstances, it was not long before the Cravath receivership committee controlled an absolute majority of all shares." (Pages 65-66)

The sabotage of honest researchers into the contents of the *Warren Report* is well illustrated by the actions of Johnson's attorney-general, Ramsey Clark. When Jim Garrison subpoenaed certain documents necessary for the case that Garrison was building against New Orleans businessman, *Clay Shaw, Clark had all the requested documents transferred to the Archives where they were beyond reach for seventy-five years.*

An even more egregious example of Ramsey Clark's efforts to stifle honest study of the so-called evidence is seen in his appointment of a panel of 'experts' to review the autopsy at Bethesda Naval Hospital upon Mr. Kennedy. Serious questions had been raised by many well-informed and respected reviewers of the autopsy evidence. Clark decided to appoint a panel of review, so he turned to the Presidents of the following universities for their recommendations: University of Utah, Johns Hopkins U., and Michigan State University. All were universities with a heavy involvement in United States biological warfare weapons research. After a very superficial 'study' the Clark panel supported the original warped autopsy findings.

It may be relevant that Ramsey Clark's uncle, attorney Hal Collins of Dallas, was a "close personal friend" of Jack Ruby.

It is also interesting to note that Ramsey Clark turned up in Baghdad to participate as a defence lawyer for the late Saddam Hussein, expressing his hope that the former dictator would get a fair trial. In the light of his lack of demonstrated concern for the rights, even in death, of John Kennedy and Lee Harvey Oswald to have a fair and unbiased study of their murders, it is doubtful that Mr. Clark's concern is really justice. It is more likely the fact that, since it was the United States that had largely supplied Iraq with biological weapons, there was as obvious need to monitor Hussein's defence for any incriminating evidence that had drawn Mr. Ramsey to Baghdad.

Finally, the continuing role of the major media in obfuscating the truth about Mr. Kennedy's murder requires comment. The most recent example of this distortion was well demonstrated on Sunday, March 26, 2006, at 10:00 p.m., EST. on the Canadian Broadcasting Corporation's television program called *The Passionate Eye*.

The title of the segment was: *Rendezvous with Death: JFK & the Cuban Connection*.

It was almost two hours long, and for anyone who has studied the evidence with care, it is a distressing mess of lies, slander, disinformation, innuendo, rumor presented as fact, unsubstantiated claims, and in a word: crap. Let us summarize the tragic ordeal of watching such warping of history, then we'll consider where such programs come from, what motivates their writers, producers and exhibitors We'll begin with the article announcing the show in the *Toronto Starweekly* of Saturday, March 25, 2006. The heading for the story read "Shedding new light on Dallas."

The article is by author Jim Bawden, and he creates the impression of someone who has not read very much if anything about the assassination…other than a report that the crime did occur. Bawden cites purported 'new evidence' that has actually been known and studied for about forty years. Yet to him it is "as damning an indictment against one state as could be assembled. The rogue nation is Cuba."

We can't go into either Bawden's superficial nonsense in any detail, so just one example will have to do. Bawden cites the myth that Oswald had attempted to murder right wing Dallas retired U.S. General, Edwin Walker. It is a claim that also makes its way into the CBC film. Bawden puts it this way:

> "Relocating to Dallas with a Russian wife, he [Oswald] carefully planned to kill Edwin Walker…a bullet grazed the general, and Oswald successfully fled from the scene of the crime."

All manner of contradictory evidence that has been known and studied over the years by careful and obviously very moral researchers of the assassination, such as Peter Dale Scott and Harold Weisberg, are not mentioned, and many of the details that are known to those who seek to be informed are advanced by Bawden as 'startling new evidence'. The whole story of General Walker's 'near brush with death' at the hands of Lee Harvey Oswald is so totally flawed that one scarcely knows where to start to repudiate it.

The first mention of Oswald's attempt on Walker, as summarized by Dick Russell in his *The Man Who Knew Too Much*, "…had appeared in the *Deutsche National-Zeitung und Soldaten-Zeitung*, a right-wing newspaper out of Munich, West Germany, on November 29, 1963." That was just seven full days after the murder of the President, and four days *before* Marina Oswald purported to recall the event! It seems altogether likely that only after the German paper had come up with the story did someone suggest to Marina that Lee had indeed been involved! When this was suggested to Marina, she immediately took it up in an apparent desire to say what was needed to convict her dead husband of the crime and so ingratiate herself with the investigators, who had implied to her that she was in danger of being deported to the USSR.

Once she started on this track, her memories came flooding back with details that just did not match the evidence recovered by the police. For example, she remembered that Lee had taken his Mannlicher-Carcano 6.5 mm. rifle to do the job. However, the bullet that was later dug out of General Walker's wall was from a different make and caliber of rifle. She recalled that Lee had operated alone, but a neighbour of Walker who heard the shot, looked up to see three men fleeing from the scene…two in one car and the third in another car.

The authors of *Rendezvous with Death* apparently did not know these details, or chose to leave them out because they would show the dishonesty of their presentation. *Their motive in writing the screen script was not to inform with honest facts, but to mislead with everything from innuendo to outright lies.*

There are other grotesque lies in both Bawden's article and in the film itself. For example, both claim that Oswald's bullet 'grazed' the general. There is absolutely nothing in any evidence that we can locate which suggests that Walker was hit in even a superficial way. Furthermore, although Oswald was supposed to have fired three shots in Dealey Plaza in 6.5 seconds, he didn't have enough sense to fire a second shot at Walker after his first shot missed. And, although Oswald was only twenty feet from Walker and was firing into a lighted room, he missed his target, but he had managed to hit Mr. Kennedy who was 150 feet away and moving in a car.

We are tempted to develop much more of the evidence which shows just how dishonest or stupid or misinformed or insidious both the Toronto Starweekly report and the film are, but again we recognize that is not the object of this study. What is relevant to our study are the questions: *why do people in a position to report the truth to the public choose to lie and why, after forty-three years is the truth about Mr. Kennedy's murder so badly distorted to the public?*

Only one answer seems to make sense: it is necessary to continue to hide the truth about the assassination of President Kennedy because that keeps the role of the shadow government secret and that, in turn, keeps the origin of AIDS secret and the deaths of millions of people to this day and far into the future will continue without an honest adequate response. Those who exercised the power, which extended even to the public execution of a popular young president in broad daylight in the middle of a great city, must remain hidden if they are to maintain those powers. And those same rulers in the shadows who can order the murder of the President of the United States can also develop and deploy pathogens which are killing over eight thousand people a day.

Postscript

June 24, 2007—As we were preparing the final draft copy of this study for the publisher, we received a news clipping from *The Brainerd Dispatch*, dated May 23, 2007, from Ms. Peg Laurian. The clipping was titled *"Closing the book on the Kennedy assassination"* and it was a review of a book titled *"Reclaiming History: The Assassination of*

President John F. Kennedy" by Vincent Bugliosi. The review was written by Jim Newton of *The Los Angeles Times*, and it identified Bugliosi as 'an American master of common sense, a punishing advocate and a curmudgeonly refreshing voice of reason'. Also, according to Newton, 'From this point forward, no reasonable person can argue that Lee Harvey Oswald was innocent; no sane person can take seriously assertions that Kennedy was killed by the CIA, Fidel Castro, the Mob, the Soviets, the Vietnamese, Texas oilmen or his vice president, Lyndon B. Johnson—all of whom exist as suspects in the vacuous world of conspiracy theorists.'

That sweeping claim by Newton certainly stimulated us to learn more, but, stressed as we are by the pressure of time, and after having spent several years reading many hundreds of books and articles, and personally interviewing several key persons such as Marina Oswald, District Attorney Jim Garrison, Lee Oswald Marine acquaintance Kerry Thornley, Dealey Plaza witnesses Jean Hill and Beverley Oliver, Warren Commission Counsel David Belin, *Warren Report* researcher Harold Weisberg, and many more, and still more and more solidly identifying ourselves as in that 'vacuous world of conspiracy theorists', we had to check out Mr. Bugliosi's 'probing review' of the evidence. We decided to take one piece of evidence in the many problems presented by the official account that the Warren Commission published and check out our position against that of Mr. Bugliosi.

The facts that we wanted to compare were those relating to Lee Harvey Oswald and motorcycle police officer Marion Baker in the ninety seconds after the last shot rang out in Dealey Plaza at 12:30 pm on November 22, 1963.

If Lee Harvey Oswald fired that shot (and two others) from a sixth floor window of the Book Depository he would have had to walk kitty-corner across the building to the stairs, hiding his rifle on the way, then he would have had to run down four flights of stairs, then crossed from the second floor stairs to a door to a vestibule outside the employee's lunchroom, then entered the lunch room, took money from his pocket and bought a 'coke' from a pop machine in the middle of the room, removed the top and taken a drink or more. At which point Officer Marion Baker entered the lunchroom.

To get to the lunchroom, Officer Baker would have had to 'gun' his motorcycle fifty feet to the front door of the Book Depository, drop his cycle on the side walk and run into the building, pausing to ask Manager Roy Truly to 'Take me to the roof.' Mr. Truly would have had to lead him across the building to the stairs. The same stairs that Oswald would have had to come down to get to the lunchroom… and have started up the stairs ahead of Baker. Reaching the second floor, Truly would have had to circle to his right and start for the third floor. Half way up to the third floor Roy Truly would have noted that Officer Baker was **not** following him, he had to run back down to the second floor, but Officer Baker was nowhere in sight! Truly entered the vestibule and then entered the lunchroom where he saw Truly with his gun drawn and shoved into Oswald's stomach. Hearing the door open, Officer Baker had to whirl around and ask Truly "Do you know this man?" Truly replied, "Yes, he works here." At that point Baker went back to the door, following Truly, and they continued to the roof.

For Baker to be in the lunchroom with Oswald without Truly having met Oswald on the latter's way down meant that Oswald must already have been in the lunchroom when Truly passed by the outer door. When Baker arrived on the second floor landing while Truly had already been there and left without seeing Oswald, Baker claims that Oswald had not yet entered the lunchroom. Completely impossible!

Vincent Bugliosi says nothing about this total improbability in his 1,600 page book.

To check out how Bugliosi handled this one flaw in the *Warren Report* we went to Chapters bookstore and checked the index of his book. We looked up the relevant pages and found that Bugliosi says nothing about this total improbability. He repeats the confusing claims from the Warren Commission!

We then downloaded the 46-page introduction and the 15-page 'Book Two' on the computer and read those twice. The first time we read them to get the overall ideas they contained and the second time to make notes of our response. We made eleven notes that follow, together with the relevant extracts from Bugliosi's text.

From page xi, lines 3 to 7 Bugliosi writes:

> "…three shots rang out from the south easternmost window on the sixth floor of the building. One of the bullets struck

the president in the upper right part of his back and exited the front of his throat, another entered the right rear of his head, exiting and shattering the right side of his head."

Bugliosi writes these details as if they were settled facts about the case, but they are not. For example, there is considerable evidence from several sources that the bullet hole in Mr. Kennedy's neck (which went through the knot of his tie) is an entrance wound, not an exit wound. Second, Mr. Bugliosi states quite definitively that there were 'three' shots. Several sources say differently. Some say four shots, some say five shots. A Congressional Committee determined there were at least four shots.

Conclusion: Mr. Bugliosi does not start by citing evidence and then examining any differences that various sources may offer. He starts with a verdict and then follows that verdict with sixteen hundred pages of print.

This is in keeping with the scenario advanced right from the beginning that Oswald is guilty. Now let's look at the evidence as expressed by J. Edgar Hoover.

> "On November 24, 1963, in a phone conversation with White House aide Walter Jenkins, Hoover stated, 'The thing I am concerned about, and so is [Deputy Attorney General] Katzenbach, is having something issued so we can convince the public that Oswald is the real assassin.'"
>
> Scott (1993), Pp. 46-7

Bugliosi puts forward a most egregious related claim on page 977, line 22. After several pages of tendentious and unproven claims he advances this:

> "This book thus far has conclusively established one point: that Oswald killed Kennedy, and inferentially established another, that he acted alone."

On page xiv, line 40 Bugliosi states:

> "…when the vast majority of these conspiracy authors are confronted with evidence that is incompatible with their fanciful theories, to one degree or another their *modus operandi* is to do one of two things - twist, warp, and

distort the evidence, or simply ignore it - both of which are designed to deceive their readers."

Conclusion: Those who disagree with Mr. Bugliosi are dishonest.
On the next page (xv, lines 2 to 7) Mr. Bugliosi suggests:

"These conspiracy 'buffs' (as they are frequently called) are obsessed with the assassination, have formed networks among their peers, and actually attend conspiracy-oriented conventions around the country. Though most of them are as kooky as a three-dollar bill in their beliefs and paranoia about the assassination, it is my sense that their motivations are and patriotic and they are sincere in their misguided and uninformed conclusions."

Conclusion: Condemn those who disagree with Mr. Bugliosi as borderline lunatics.
On page xix, lines 19 to 24, Bugliosi writes:

"Apparently, then, such distinguished Americans as Chief Justice Earl Warren, Senator John Sherman Cooper and Richard B. Russell, Representatives Gerald Ford and Hale Boggs, former CIA director Allen Dulles and former president of the World Bank John J. McCloy (the members of the Warren Commission), as well as the Commission's general counsel, J. Lee Rankin…etc."

Here Bugliosi does what he says that he won't do…he appeals to authority in support of his rhetorical position, rather than to reason. And at least three of those to whom he turns as people to be believed without one troubling oneself to study the evidence, are, upon careful consideration and a study of the background of each very suspicious characters. The three are: Allen Dulles, John J. McCloy and Gerald Ford.

Allen Dulles, for example, once authorized the testing of a new 'truth' drug upon a group of people in displaced persons camps in post war Europe. The rationalization for selecting these people was that if they died, no one would miss them. John J. McCloy, as Governor of occupied Germany right after the war, authorized the recruitment of several former Nazis, many wanted for war crimes, into the service of American biological weapons research. He had these people put into

American military uniforms and transported to the United States under Project Paperclip. Gerald Ford was the top man on a secret list of Congressmen that the CIA helped finance in his bid for re-election. The CIA's involvement in domestic American politics was strictly illegal, but that didn't bother the insidious Gerald Ford.

Conclusion: Bugliosi says don't go by the evidence, just trust authority.

On page xxv, Bugliosi tells how he embarrassed a group of lawyers at a professional development get together by asking how many of them had read the *Warren Report*...Only a few had, yet many believed that Lee Harvey Oswald was not a sole lone-nut conspirator. When only a few lawyers admitted to reading the report, Bugliosi declares:

> "I proved my point." (Line 11)

Conclusion: Bugliosi believes that reading the Warren Report is the most important thing a person can do before he takes any stand upon the Report's validity. In other words, he establishes irrelevant criteria for decision making.

On the preceding page Bugliosi had asked the assembly:

> "What if I could prove to you in one minute or less that although you are all intelligent people you are not thinking intelligently about the Kennedy case?"

It was at this point he asked his question about reading the *Warren Report*. The fact that his audience had not read the Report he interprets as evidence that they were not thinking intelligently. Actually, it proved no such thing. An intelligent person can reach reasonable conclusions by studying the original evidence, not the conclusions supposedly based upon that evidence.

Conclusion: Bugliosi mis-interprets an answer to one question as an answer to a different question.

> "Of one thing I am certain. The Commission's conclusions have held up remarkably well against all assaults on their validity", says Bugliosi on page xxxii, lines 39 and 40.

However, several pages prior to this 'certainty' he had written:

> "The most recent Gallup Poll...shows that a remarkable 75 percent of the American public reject the findings of the Warren Commission."

The latter statement is a flat out contradiction to the preceding statement!

Conclusion: Switch your position if that proves necessary.

On page xxxv Mr. Bugliosi quotes Pierre Salinger about the *Warren Report:* "It listened patiently to everyone."

It didn't. The Warren Commission shut out of the process very many significant witnesses such as Private First Class, Eugene B. Dinkins. Many others were shut out because their testimony challenged the 'lone-nut' theory that the Commission had set out to prove.

Conclusion: Lie if necessary.

On page xlii, line 23 Bugliosi writes:

> "…Oliver Stone's 'military-industrial complex'"

Actually it was President Eisenhower who had first warned against such a powerful alliance, not Oliver Stone.

Conclusion: Mis-attribute sources.

Then, Mr. Bugliosi gets quite insidious in his rhetoric. On page 977 of the second document that we downloaded he writes:

> "…no group of top-level conspirators would ever employ someone as unstable and unreliable as Oswald to commit the biggest murder in history, no such group would ever provide its hit man with, or allow him to use, a twelve dollar rifle to get the job done…"   (Lines 25 to 28)

You are right Mr. Bugliosi, no one would and no one did hire Lee Harvey Oswald with a $12 mail order rifle to kill the president. They would do what they did…put a professional hit team in place, and have a 'legend' created for the patsy: Lee Harvey Oswald. Then, they would have Officer Marion Baker arrive in the lunchroom ninety seconds after the last shot, and shoot Oswald as he was 'rushing at me to try to escape.' Baker was about to do his job when Roy Truly arrived in the lunchroom.

Finally, on page 977 Mr. Bugliosi writes:

> "This book thus far has conclusively established one point, that Oswald killed Kennedy."

My, oh my!

It is our opinion that since Oswald was in the lunchroom when Baker entered, and then he was there at the time he was supposed to be five floors up, hiding a rifle. He had been set up to be there, and Baker had been set up to go to the lunchroom, kill Oswald while the latter was 'rushing at Baker' after Baker had stopped him in his 'flight' from the sixth floor.

The headline across the world would then have read: "President Kennedy Assassinated; Assassin Killed While Fleeing!"

But Roy Truly's unexpected return to the lunchroom spoiled that scenario.

Chapter Eleven

DAVID FERRIE

The Nexus of the Assassination of JFK and the Development of AIDS; Tracy Barnes; E. Howard Hunt; The Canadian Connections: Pershing Gervais and James Earl Ray come to Canada

This chapter deals with two people. One, David Ferrie, apparently a buffoon in New Orleans at the time that John F. Kennedy was assassinated, and the other, Dr. Mary Sherman, also of New Orleans and heavily involved in cancer research at Tulane University. What is the link between them? Well, first of all this unlikely pair seems to have been friends and working colleagues. But, more to the point of our study of the origin of AIDS, both died under very mysterious circumstances and both were working with monkey viruses which had been inoculated into mice? Of both these circumstances, more later.

David Ferrie was a bald headed man who wore a homemade red wig cut from a mohair rug. Apparently some childhood illness had left him without body hair, but that didn't seem to make him overly self-conscious for his attempts to cover the deficit were rather obvious, or even slap-dash. In addition to his homemade mohair wig, he used a red body crayon to draw on a pair of eyebrows. Invariably, these were drawn on with a rather high arch so that he seemed to have a constant look of surprise.

We never saw him, but we received a first hand and rather sympathetic description of him when we met personally with his nemesis, District Attorney Jim Garrison of New Orleans, who at the time of our interview just before he died had been re-elected as an Appeals Court judge. As noted, Garrison, while recognizing Ferrie's criminal flaws, had a certain sympathy for him. "He was used by all who knew him" or words to that effect was how Garrison described him. And somewhere along the line Garrison labeled him "an important figure is history."

That he was used (and likely murdered) by those who knew him emerges from our study of his days in New Orleans where he had a number of 'high friends in low places.' He was, for example, a part time employee of Guy Banister, an FBI 153153 agent in New Orleans working under the cover of being a Private Investigator. He was also a working member of the Carlos Marcello mob, and was in the courtroom at New Orleans on the morning of November 22, 1963 where Marcello was on trial for immigration irregularities. Ferrie was one of Marcello's defence team. Three things happened in quick order that morning…Marcello was acquitted, word that Mr. Kennedy had died of gun shot wounds in Dallas was received, and Ferrie left for Galveston, Texas for some 'ice skating' and 'duck hunting'. Ferrie was also an accomplished pilot who had flown for Eastern Airlines, but had been fired for molesting children on his planes.

Ferrie had other claims to fame. He was purported to have been a friend of Lee Harvey Oswald when the latter was a teen and had joined the Civil Air Corps. Later, when Oswald returned from his short 'defection' to the Soviet Union, Ferrie and Oswald apparently re-established some level of contact through New Orleans businessman, Clay Shaw.

On the day that President Kennedy was assassinated, someone phoned the District Attorney's office and said that Ferrie was likely to have been involved in the murder. When investigators visited his rooming house, they learned that he was on his ice skating trip to Galveston. The investigators promised to return later to question him. There was an early report that Lee Harvey Oswald when arrested in Dallas had been carrying David Ferrie's library card!

On his way home to New Orleans, Ferrie phoned his landlady who told him that he was the object of police interest. On hearing that, Ferrie delayed his return to New Orleans for a few days.

It is a complicated and convoluted story, but to cut it all to the quick we will accept the view of Professor Peter Dale Scott, who after detailed and fair-minded study, reached the conclusion that "Ferrie, as much as Oswald, was a designated 'patsy' or fall guy for the assassination." (Scott, 1993 Page 329)

The question must rise to readers' minds as to why we would

feature a chapter on such a strange person as David Ferrie in a study of the origins of AIDS. Just this: Ferrie had an altogether mysterious link with Dr. Mary Sherman of Tulane University Medical School and with Dr. Alton Ochsner of the same institution. And, as we have already pointed out Ochsner and Tulane formed the center of the MKDELTA biological weapons research activities following the election of Eisenhower and the appointment of Nelson Rockefeller to the literal command of the CIA.

When police attended at Ferrie's apartment after reports of the latter's death, they found some evidence that linked him very firmly to the MKDELTA activities. First, there were several cages which contained mice. And on those cages there were record cards which showed that the mice had been injected with some type of monkey virus! Remember the "MK' of MKULTRA, MKDELTA and MKNAOMI? And, apparently, from notations on the cards, Ferrie had been monitoring the mice for signs of cancer.

But the evidence of interest in cancer doesn't end there. Also in the apartment there were the remnants of a typescript document that dealt with the *induction of cancer into both mice and hamsters and the treatment of the diseased mice*. Unfortunately, this document was largely destroyed when the apartment was 'cleaned out' and only a few pages remain which are filed in the National Archives of Washington, D.C. (Haslam, 1995 Page 239) These were later called 'David Ferrie's Cancer Treatise', but the evidence suggests strongly that the article of which they were a part was not Ferrie's work.

In the few salvaged pages there were two pages of a bibliography and *those two pages tie in very dramatically with the research we report in this book*. For example, the bibliography lists (among others) J.J. Bittner, L. Dmochowski, L. Gross and J. Melnick. Bittner and Gross are both reported upon by none other than Robert Gallo in his *Virus Hunting*. Apparently Gallo and Ferrie were on the same research track! Dmochowski in turn, is cited 39 times in the *SVCP, Progress Report #8*. The latter report is the one which features the sixteen page report from Gallo on behalf of Bionetics Research, a Division of Litton Industries, (yet Gallo was supposed to be working for the U.S. Government) and titled: *"Progress Report on Investigation of Carcinogenesis with Selected Virus Preparations in the Newborn Monkey."* (Page 273)

Monkey viruses being tested? Like the work being done by David Ferrie?

However, we cannot devote time and space to reporting all of the dramatic evidence that we have located, which demonstrates that David Ferrie was somehow tied in with the Special Virus Cancer (formerly Leukemia/Lymphoma) Program. We cite just enough to show that David Ferrie was obviously a foot soldier for someone, somewhere, who was calling the shots (no pun intended) in deep politics. And yet he is portrayed by the media as a buffoon. How does a buffoon have friends such as Dr. Mary Sherman, medical doctor, lecturer at Tulane University School of Medicine, researcher in cancer and an important social figure in New Orleans circles? There is obviously much more to David Ferrie, friend of Lee Harvey Oswald and heavily implicated (by apparently carefully contrived evidence) in the murder of President John F. Kennedy.

That is why we place this short chapter here in a study of the laboratory origin of AIDS. David Ferrie with his historic links to the murder of John F. Kennedy on the one hand and with his scientific research into monkey viruses inoculated into mice on the other has a role (albeit apparently small and much of it likely contrived by the powers in the shadows) in two of the greatest unsolved crimes of history: the origin, source and nature of the AIDS epidemic and the murder of the President of the United States at high noon in a major city of the United States.

But, what about Mary Sherman? How does she figure in all of this? And what might her links be with the scientific paper trail to AIDS?

There is strong evidence that Dr. Mary Sherman was murdered on the night of July 21, 1964. Apparently she was murdered somewhere other than her apartment in New Orleans, and was taken home, laid upon her bed, was stabbed several times even though she was already dead; was covered with bed clothes that were set on fire, and then those involved fled without leaving any significant evidence.

The burned bedclothes hardly scorched the bed or the rest of the apartment but (!) the heat was great enough to burn her right arm, shoulder and rib cage enough to consume them totally! How such intense heat could be focused upon such a precise area to the neglect of the rest of her body and bedding in the surrounding area remains a mystery. But that is where the story ends.

We are heavily dependent upon the research and written account of the Dr. Mary Sherman murder by Edward T. Haslam (*Mary, Ferrie and the Monkey Viruses*, 1995), and we cannot go into any further detail here, except to ask: was Dr. Sherman severely injured while working on a powerful particle accelerator at Tulane University? And, near death from that accident, and because the research that she was engaged in was top secret was she finished off with a knife wound to the heart and driven home late at night and her 'murder' there staged? Did the hypothetical accident with a powerful particle accelerator burn off her arm and shoulder, including the bones? Was the work she was doing so top secret that it warranted the masking of the accident?

Here are two people, Dr. Mary Sherman and David Ferrie, both of whom died under very suspicious circumstances, whose deaths have never been adequately researched and who provide a link between the murder of President Kennedy and the monkey virus research of Dr. Alton Ochsner and Tulane University. That can be linked to the people and subjects of study involved in research into immune suppressant viruses!

As difficult as it is to believe, the evidence clearly demonstrates that there is a link between the murder of John F. Kennedy and the development of a world-population growth rate limiting pathogen that presents as AIDS.

AIDS is linked to MKDELTA, which in turn is clearly linked to Dr. Alton Ochsner and Tulane University Medical School. Tulane is linked to the Delta Primate Farm in Covington, La., where rhesus monkeys were raised and butchered so that their kidneys (MK) could be used to culture the mycoplasma (PPLO) of Dr. Huebner. The mycoplasma had to be tested on humans in Huntington Penitentiary, Texas, by Drs. Chanock and Couch (great favorites of Gina Kolata of *The New York Times*) but it also had to be tested on mice, as David Ferrie was doing at the time of his death. David Ferrie, in turn, was a close friend of Dr. Mary Sherman, a cancer expert at Tulane and a colleague of Alton Ochsner, while at the same time Ferrie was linked to Carlos Marcello of the New Orleans Mafia family, and Clay Shaw of the World Trade Mart. In addition David Ferrie was at least known to and known by Lee Harvey Oswald. Oswald had a Marine acquaintance in New Orleans named Kerry Thornley whose evidence about Oswald to the Warren Commission was most incriminating and much of it obviously false. Kerry Thornley before his death claimed that he had been recruited into certain covert activities by CIA operative, E. Howard Hunt who was later to be apprehended behind Dealey Plaza in Dallas, riding out of town on a freight train, on November 22, 1963. Hunt in the CIA had been involved in the use of bacteriological weapons against China and was later a key person in the Bay of Pigs fiasco where Allan Dulles, on behalf of his patrons of the Rockefeller apparat had tried to snooker President John F. Kennedy into invading Cuba. Hunt was later involved with the assassination of President Allende of Chile and the break-in of the office of Dr. Fielding, Daniel Ellsberg's psychiatrist in search of evidence linked to the Pentagon Papers leak to *The New York Times*. Hunt ended (as far as we know) his record of public service by being caught in the Watergate break-in scandal that terminated the political career of Richard Nixon and the rise to the role of Vice-President by Nelson Rockefeller.

In other words, it is all of a piece. *The United States has not been hit by a series of great individual tragedies over the years*…biological weapons development and deployment (including the AIDS and CFS/ME epidemics); the Bay of Pigs; the assassination of Mr. Kennedy; the Vietnam War; the Watergate Break-in; the Iran-Contra scandal; the First Gulf War; the September 11 attacks; the Iraq War…from 1952 to the present. The United States has been engaged in a great unrealized war between wealth and humanity which can be summed up in a single sentence: oil to wealth to Rockefellers to Establishment to media control to political power to CIA to hidden wars to open wars. David Ferrie, Kerry Thornley and Lee Harvey Oswald have been foot soldiers in that war (pawns); E. Howard Hunt a knight (albeit, a luminously insane knight). The rooks are 'homeland security'; the bishops are the Christian right spokesmen such as Charles Colson; the all-powerful queen is the establishment and the (now) symbolic king is the Rockefeller apparat.

Tracy Barnes

Tracy Barnes was a relative by marriage to the Rockefellers. He creeps publicly in to very few of the accounts about the sordid events of the

1950s and 1960s, but we include him in our study because of that link to the Rockefellers and his secret ties to the 'Establishment' first of the north eastern United States, and then extending into Texas through the Hunt and Murchison families. He was a critical link between the mechanics or lower 'gophers' of the secret government...the E.

Howard Hunt's and the David Ferrie's and the upper reaches of that secret government, Nelson and David Rockefeller, Allen Dulles, Richard Bissell, etc.

Tracy Barnes is the type who doesn't get his name into history books (or at least not into many of them), but who is vital to the functioning of the latter power block.

To give you some idea of the role of Tracy Barnes we quote the following passage from Kerry Thornley's fictionalized diary, The Dreadlock Recollections:

> "E. Howard Hunt writes in Undercover that he once received a cable signed jointly by Richard Bissell and Tracy Barnes summoning him to headquarters."

> "Bissell had succeeded Frank Wisner as chief of the Clandestine Services, and after hospitalization brought on by overwork Wisner had been assigned to the relatively relaxed post of London chief of station. As a special aide to Allen Dulles, Bissell had created the concept of the U-2 aircraft, and then managed that successful program. I had held several perfunctory meetings with Bissell during consultation periods in Washington and a lengthier one during a Latin American chiefs of station conference in Lima, Peru."

> "As principal assistant to Bissell, Tracy Barnes told me, I was needed for a new project, much like the one on which I had worked for him in the overthrowing Jacobo Arbenz. My job, Tracy told me, would be essentially the same as my earlier one– chief of political action for a project recommended by the National Security Council and just approved by President Eisenhower: to assist Cuban exiles in overthrowing Castro…"
> (Thornley; 1988-89 Page 51)

Note how, in this single excerpt from the diary of Kerry Thornley, a U.S. Marine acquaintance of Lee Harvey Oswald, there is a direct line from Oswald, through Thornley, to E. Howard Hunt (a Bay of Pigs planner; and, one of the 'tramps' arrested in Dealey Plaza, Dallas on November 22, 1963, and Watergate burglar!) To Tracy Barnes, a member of the Rockefeller family and apparat and Richard Bissell, a prominent University Professor of McGeorge Bundy and deputy to Allen Dulles...all the way to the President of the United States: Dwight David Eisenhower!

The Canadian Connections:
Pershing Gervais and James Earl Ray Come to Canada

Pershing Gervais was a character who turned up at various points in the tales circulating about Carlos Marcello, Lee Harvey Oswald, David Ferrie, Jack Martin, Clay Shaw and others in the confused world of New Orleans politics, law enforcement and underworld in the pre- and post - Kennedy assassination years.

He was the State's principal witness against Jim Garrison when the latter was charged with fraud, and when that effort failed in court, Pershing Gervais and his family disappeared from the New Orleans scene.

Some months later a reporter for the New Orleans newspaper, The Times-Picayune, was in Vancouver, Canada when she suddenly encountered Gervais on the street. Gervais was agitated by the encounter and urged the reporter not to reveal that she had met him. When she asked why she should keep that fact confidential, Gervais told a very strange story.

He said that after his testimony against Jim Garrison, certain un-named sponsors had thought it wise for Gervais and his family to leave New Orleans. The whole family was moved to Vancouver on false passports, and was provided with false school and health records. All had British Columbia Health Insurance cards and birth certificates with their new names. Asked about how he paid his way in Canada, Gervais said that he regularly received a cheque from a General Motors Automobile dealership.

Despite Gervais' pleas for continuing anonymity, the reporter published the story of her encounter and of the Gervais family's new identity. Shortly thereafter, the Gervais' returned to New Orleans where they faded from public interest and view.

The authors of this study deem the story to be very important because it is solid evidence that there is a power in the shadows that has high level but covert links between the United States and Canada, and by inference, between the United States and certain other countries such as Great Britain, France, Israel, and so on.

Who, for example, could get false Canadian passports for the whole Gervais family? Who could get B.C. Health cards for the whole family? And who could arrange for General Motors to pay Gervais a weekly wage for doing nothing?

We believe that it is someone in the Royal Canadian Mounted Police (RCMP).

Further evidence of this high level but covert (indeed, criminal) linkage is to be seen in the case of James Earl Ray, the purported assassin of Martin Luther King.

After allegedly committing this crime, Ray fled the United States to Toronto, Canada. In his possession were complete sets of false documents for three different Scarborough, Ontario men who matched the physical description of Ray. Using one set of identification for some months, Ray lived in Toronto before moving to England, where he was later to be apprehended and deported to the United States.

The same questions arise about Ray's false passports and other identification. Who was in a position to provide such documents months before the murder of the Rev. King?

Again, it is the opinion of the present authors that there is a covert linkage between the shadow powers in the United States and counterparts to such powers in other countries.

Why should one be concerned about such details when one is studying the development, testing and deployment of a lethal pathogen or co-pathogens involved in AIDS and CFS/ME?

The answer goes back to our original questions: what was chronic fatigue syndrome? Why were victims used so abominably by the medical profession, the legal system, the warped media? How did it happen that CFS/ME and AIDS, both characterized by immune system damage, had begun at the same point in history?

And, as our study here has reported the evidence has led us to our present conclusion that there are powers in the shadows which have had the motivation, opportunity, and resources to do the necessary research. Powers that are not just national in scope, but international.

The false papers of the Gervais family and of James Earl Ray tell us that we are right. We will cite further evidence as we continue this study.

Chapter Twelve

LYNDON JOHNSON 1963 - 1968

Johnson, Population Control and the murder of President Kennedy (and AIDS)

Lyndon Johnson did everything he possibly could to keep the truth about Mr. Kennedy's murder from the public. We noted in the previous chapter how Lee Harvey Oswald was arrested, detained in custody, questioned without the benefit of any stenographic record being kept, and most egregiously, denied access to legal counsel until he could be set up by the Dallas Police Department for execution by Jack Ruby.

The purpose was clear and the necessity for Oswald's delayed execution fortuitous.

First off, Lee Harvey Oswald had to be kept silent so that no details about who he was actually working for could become public. If he had proper legal representation, he would have been able to share with a lawyer facts that he was prevented from sharing because no legal council was available to him. But, within forty-eight hours he was dead and his side of the story forever hidden.

Oswald's execution by Officer Marion Baker had been delayed because the Book Depository manager, Roy Truly, had unexpectedly turned around on his way to the third floor of the Depository and had returned to the second floor where he threw open the lunchroom door and saw Oswald in the middle of the room, holding a bottle of soda and Officer Baker with his revolver shoved into Oswald's stomach.

This was approximately ninety seconds after the last shot was heard in Dealey Plaza. To get to the lunchroom Oswald would have had to wipe his rifle clean of finger prints; hide the rifle; run down five flights of stairs; pass three men and one woman without them seeing him; pass Roy Truly heading from the second floor to the third floor without Truly seeing him; get well into the lunchroom and get out money to buy the soda; open the soda and then at that point be confronted by Officer Baker with a drawn revolver.

Absolutely impossible to do.

Oswald was obviously innocent of the murder of Mr. Kennedy, although he may well have been a part of some covert intelligence activity. Because of the latter possibility he could not be afforded any opportunity to place evidence of his innocence upon any kind of official record.

Captain Fritz did his part. Jack Ruby did his part. Oswald was dead and beyond any chance of defending himself.

Now it was up to Lyndon Johnson, a liar and a traitor as we shall develop further, to do his part, and he did that very well, thanks to the help he received from others, such as his attorney-general, Ramsey Clark. Clark's actions show that he was party to the insidious cabal that was running the United States from the shadows, and which later required Ramsey's presence in Baghdad to "ensure that Saddam Hussein gets a fair trial."

Johnson's first step was to have his aide, Walter Jenkins, consult with longtime Johnson friend, J. Edgar Hoover. Hoover wrote a memo dated November 24, 1963…Just thirty hours after President Kennedy was shot. The memo read:

> "The thing I am most concerned about, and so is Mr. Katzenbach, is having something issued so we can convince the public that Oswald is the real assassin."
>
> (Quoted from page 251 of Michael Ewing, 1977)

We urge you to consider this memo very carefully. In it there is no hint of a suggestion that Lee Harvey Oswald may be innocent. There is no hint that evidence should be carefully and deliberately gathered and placed before a jury of citizens. Instead, the leading law enforcement officer in the United States suggests that even without a trial, Lee Harvey Oswald is guilty and the public must to be convinced of that. But, there was a great potential danger in placing honest evidence before a panel of ordinary citizens: they just might determine that there was more evidence suggesting that Oswald was innocent than there was evidence that he was guilty!

And if the dead Oswald were innocent, the real killer or killers must still be out there!

Lyndon Johnson came up with a great way around that problem. He would appoint a 'blue ribbon' Commission to examine the evidence and several months down the line, reveal their findings to the world. By then much of the public passion would have been tempered by the pliant media controlled by people like Henry Luce.

However, there were several big problems in appointing such a Commission. It would have to be certain to confirm the already determined fact that Lee Harvey Oswald was a 'lone nut' killer and that there was no conspiracy by men in the shadows. The best way around this problem was to appoint the right people. First, it would have to have such luminaries as Allen Dulles, who had been fired from the CIA by Mr. Kennedy for his disastrous Bay of Pigs adventure. Second, it would have to have John J. McCloy, a former member of the OSS and the major designer of the latter's successor organization, the CIA. McCloy had been the U.S. High Commissioner to occupied Germany after the Second World War, and in that position he had presided over an administration which engaged in several neo-Nazi activities. For example, he was High Commissioner when several war criminals were given false U.S. credentials and who, under Operation Paperclip, had been secretly transported to the United States for infiltration into certain American government agencies such as health and intelligence. Third, it had to have Gerald Ford. Ford was a Member of Congress who had a reputation of 'knowing where the bodies were buried' in Washington, D.C. He was also a great friend of J. Edgar Hoover and Richard Nixon.

Also on the Commission were Senator Richard Russell, Senator John Sherman, and Representative Hale Boggs. Each of these is worthy of careful review, but the essential thing about Russell and Boggs are the two facts that neither agreed with the 'single bullet' myth of Arlen Specter, and that both later expressed doubts about Oswald's guilt.

The Chairman of the Commission was Chief Justice Earl Warren. Warren, when he had heard that he was to be asked to take the job, had said that, for unknown reasons he would not. His opinion was delivered to Johnson, who invited him to the White House and asked him this way:

> "I said I didn't care who brought me a message about how opposed he was to this assignment. When the country is

> confronted with threatening divisions and suspicions, I said, and its foundation is being rocked, and the President of the United States says that you are the only man who can handle the matter, you won't say 'no', will you?"
> "He swallowed hard and said, "No, sir."
> "The Warren Commission brought us through a very critical time in our history. I believe it fair to say that the commission was dispassionate and just." (Johnson, 1971 Page 27)

By his appointment of the Warren Commission, and by the choice especially of Dulles, McCloy and Ford as Commissioners, Johnson successfully headed off a proper legal examination of one of history's great crimes. Simply put: The *Warren Commission Report* is totally beyond credibility and not only does it mask the truth of who killed Mr. Kennedy and why, but it most dramatically demonstrates the presence of and the power of a guiding force variously referred to as the 'shadow government', 'unelected elite', or the 'Establishment.'

Johnson, Population Control and AIDS

In his book, *The Vantage Point*, Lyndon Johnson writes this about population control:

> "When I pledged in my State of the Union message of January 1965 to 'seek new ways to use our knowledge *to help deal with the explosion in world population*' I was breaking sharply with Presidential tradition…When I entered office we were investing less than $6 million annually for population control. During my last year in the White House that investment had grown to $115 million."
> (Pages 340 -341)

The sum of $115 million in 1968 dollars would be the equivalent of at least one and a half billion dollars in 2006.

Where did Johnson spend this kind of money and what did he get in return?

We will show where that kind of money was going shortly, but first, we want to use Johnson's own words to demonstrate again a very important consideration that all readers must keep in mind when studying the history of those times…and probably continuing today. That consideration is this: *one just cannot completely trust even the most respected media sources on any matter, but one must rigorously hold all evidence suspect until other evidence has been gathered and taken into careful consideration.*

For example, as we can see in Johnson's own words, when he entered office population control expenditures and hence population control activities were negligible. Despite Johnson's claim, Arthur M. Schlesinger, Jr. has this to say on page 604 of his account of Mr. Kennedy's administration, *A Thousand Days*:

> "The Kennedy years thus further strengthened the American attack on world poverty by preparing the means to keep population growth from nullifying the development effort."

In evaluating this statement, one needs to know two things; first, Schlesinger was a wartime member of the CIA-antecedent spy agency, the OSS. Second, many of Mr. Kennedy's most intimate administration members were drawn from the very establishment with which Mr. Kennedy found himself 'battling'. Schlesinger's mis-representation of history is subtle and insidious. Note that he attributes the movement towards population control to the Kennedy 'years', rather than to John F. Kennedy, the 'man'. However, Schlesinger was a clever wordsmith and he knew how the average reader would read the statement as 'Kennedy supported population control'. A lie!

This subtle and insidious deception was picked up by author Donald Gibson:

> "The actual development of population control policy indicates that Schlesinger (Page 604) *was really stretching things* when he claimed that it was President Kennedy who laid the groundwork for population control efforts. President Kennedy's views were essentially at odds with this movement, and his concessions to it were tiny when compared to the aggressive commitment of Johnson." (Page 100, Battling Wall Street)

Gibson's astute awareness of Schlesinger's *dishonesty* (we won't use nice linguistic shadings and refer to it as 'stretching things') demonstrates other considerations which must be kept in mind. One of these is that even Schlesinger, who publicly professed (like Robert McNamara) to be a loyal supporter and friend of John F. Kennedy, was playing a role evidently at odds with his genuine, deeply-held convictions. To demonstrate this we refer not only to the above misrepresentation of the facts, but turning back a few pages in his book, *A Thousand Days*, we note the following:

> "This *problem** (population growth rate—Ed) had nagged the consciousness of foreign aid people for some time. In the very long run, industrialization and affluence might bring down the birth rate (though even this was not certain; the United States, after a period of decline in the thirties, now had as high a rate of population growth as India); but in the short run the situation seemed to require a more specific and purposeful *attack**. In 1959 one of the recurrent blue - ribbon* reviews of aid policy, this one chaired by General William H. Draper, *courageously** recommended that the United States assist birth control programs in developing countries."(*Emphasis added—Ed)

This paragraph (and others that space does not allow us to quote) expresses sympathetically, a position totally alien to the philosophy of John F. Kennedy, the person that Schlesinger was purporting to reveal to the world. Note Schlesinger's rhetorical devices: population growth is a 'problem', not a subject of study; 'attack' suggests the need for a war; 'blue-ribbon' (like the Warren Commission) suggests superior and moral minds; while 'courageously' means that the population control advocates (like the Rockefellers) are heroes and, by inference, non-advocates are cowards. Subtle and insidious…like Anthony's speech to the people of Rome the non-advocates are all honorable men!

Finally, before leaving this consideration of Schlesinger's 'love' of Kennedy, we need to point out that when an important and early book, which questioned the findings of the *Warren Report*, was published in Britain, Allen Dulles contacted Arthur Schlesinger and asked him, sight unseen, to write a critical review and disparage the book as unworthy of consideration. Schlesinger, as a former member of the CIA-antecedent OSS, obliged. Once a spook, always a spook.

An Interlude of Martin Luther King and Robert Francis Kennedy

Martin Luther King

Space does not permit us to develop the evidence that our research has accumulated about the murder of the Rev. Martin Luther King, Jr. Here, we can only summarize the main points of that research to establish its links to the deep politics of America.

First, Rev. King was assassinated because he had begun a program against the Vietnam War. Since a very significant percentage of the fighting men in Vietnam were made up of Black military personnel, no such effort could be tolerated by the Chiefs of Staff, the industrial/oil complex and the other components of the deep politics of America.

Second, there is sufficient evidence to demonstrate the fact that the power of the deep politicians of America extended into Canada, and Europe, where James Earle Ray first sought refuge. The aliases and documents provided to Ray could only have been acquired with the help of Canadian allies, possibly within the Royal Canadian Mounted Police or the Ontario Provincial Police.

Third, under attorney-general Ramsay Clark, Ray was essentially blackmailed by the threat of the death sentence, to go along with the story that he was King's murderer. This shows the profound depth of influence that the establishment could bring to bear through the official agencies of government when required.

Robert Francis Kennedy

The murder of Robert Francis Kennedy followed immediately upon his winning of the 1968 Democratic Primary (as well as other less critical state primaries the same night). The winning of the California Primary virtually assured that Robert Kennedy would be the Democratic candidate for President in November of 1968, and would also virtually ensure that he would win that election.

If he had not won the California primary, our evidence (which includes Sirhan Sirhan's pre-assassination diary) suggests that he would not have been assassinated. The evidence (which we present in much more detail in the book version of this study) shows that Sirhan Sirhan had been carefully prepared to kill Mr. Kennedy if the latter won the primary. The preparations included significant deep hypnosis wherein Sirhan was programmed to act when he received some sort of triggering signal on the evening of the primary.

Our further evidence makes it clear that Sirhan, in front of Mr. Kennedy when shots were fired, did not fire the fatal bullet. That was fired by a part time security guard who shot Mr. Kennedy from behind at very close range when everyone's attention was directed to Sirhan.

Sirhan has never been pardoned because it is absolutely vital that the deep politicians of the U.S. keep him clearly out of the reach of psychological experts who might be able to de-program him.

Regardless of these tragic details, the fact remains that the murder of Mr. Kennedy meant that the Vietnam War would be continued after the 1968 elections.

End of an interlude

PART FOUR

THE DEPLOYMENT

Chapter Thirteen

1966: WHO IS WORKING ON SMALLPOX?

Trade Your Old Diseases for New

In May 1966, the World Health Organization (WHO), nominally an agency of the United Nations, but realistically a Rockefeller fiefdom, was authorized to begin a worldwide effort to eradicate smallpox by vaccination. WHO had let on as far back as 1959 that such an eradication program was being undertaken, but their early efforts were sporadic and more limited in target countries selected for attention. So, the 1959 WHO sponsored smallpox eradication program faded from view.

Then, seven years later, the smallpox vaccination program was re-newed with unusual vigor. WHO contacted Dr. Donald A. Henderson, then at the Centers for Disease Control in Atlanta, and asked him to take charge of the new and better effort. At first, Henderson demurred, but his boss, the surgeon general of the U.S. Public Health Services told him that he had to take the job. The United States had decided at some level in the shadows to make worldwide smallpox eradication their top health priority. Period. The CDC was to put together about seventeen teams of doctors, technicians, support personnel and equipment and get over to Africa and selected other countries as quickly as possible. In these countries they were to encourage, bribe and coerce as many people as they could get their vaccine needles into, and under Henderson and with a certain amount of other nations helping, they worked for approximately ten years.

But, tragically, although the smallpox eradication program worked and on April 17, 1978 Ali Maow Maalin, a hospital cook in Somali was identified as the last person in the world to become naturally infected with smallpox, a funny thing happened on the road to world health: an even worse epidemic broke out. At first it was a sporadically appearing mix of opportunistic illnesses, many not previously thought to be particularly harmful to humans. Then the numbers began to swell. And strangely enough, they began to swell most noticeably in Third World countries that had just recently been the recipients of WHO vaccine largesse. Just what was going on?

Before we answer this question, we must say a word or two about Dr. Henderson, and that mirror image of AIDS that was suddenly to pop onto the scene in 1981, chronic fatigue syndrome.

In 1956 Henderson was the chief of the Epidemic Intelligence Service at the Communicable Disease Center of the U.S. Public Health Service. In this role, Henderson undertook to investigate a mysterious epidemic in Punta Gorda, Florida. In this small town one morning in early 1956, the citizens started out on their usual round of activities - going to school, teaching school, doing laundry and hanging it out in the backyard. Some were walking to work in stores and others were planting gardens. But, most noticed something very unusual: there were millions and millions of mosquitoes!

Now, it was one thing for Punta Gorda to have mosquitoes, but on this spring morning it was ridiculous. Everyone doing anything outside was being bitten by mosquitoes. One local resident even phoned the U.S. meteorological office and reported the infestation. The person answering the call seemed ready with an answer! The mosquitoes, it seems, had fled from a fire in the Everglades some thirty miles away, and had sought shelter in Punta Gorda! Now, according to entomologists, mosquitoes are so insensitive to their environs that they wouldn't flee if they were on one side of a barn and the other side was burning. But, the Punta Gorda mosquitoes evidently knew that there was a fire somewhere nearby and they headed over to the latter city…strangely enough, by-passing other small villages along the way.

Then another unusual thing happened: about a week later the first few cases of chronic fatigue syndrome ever seen in Punta Gorda, struck some of the residents. Before the year was out over 150 persons reported the symptoms of the disease, and this brought Donald Henderson to town.

But, there was something else doing with mosquitoes at the time. Up in Canada, at the Dominion Parasite Laboratory in Belleville,

Ontario, the Federal Government was busy breeding one hundred million mosquitoes a month. These mosquitoes were then being transferred to one of Canada's prestigious old universities, where, in the biology department, a Dr. Guilford B. Reed was contaminating them with experimental pathogens provided to him by the Canadian and American Militaries. When the mosquitoes were suitably disease-laden, Dr. Reed transferred them to the Canadian Military to share with their American counterparts. Then, in selected towns in Canada and the U.S., the military took on the job of turning them loose in the middle of the night by a variety of means. Then, a week or two later people from the Army and from the newly Nelson Rockefeller organized Public Health Services would turn up to see how the folks were making out.

Was this why Dr. Henderson went to a great deal of trouble to evaluate the effects of CFS on Punta Gorda citizens? We don't know, but we do know this: our studies indicate that if some agency is conducting tests in an area, the person(s) that they send to 'investigate' already know what is going on. It would be terribly risky to send in a naive outsider.

However that may be, we know that Dr. MacArthur of the Pentagon was able to report to Congress on June 9, 1969, that one of the Pentagon's new pathogenic disabling agents could be transmitted by primary aerosol and by a mosquito vector! Now how did he know that for sure unless it had been tested somewhere on someone.

Another thing to note: by 1956 the Huebner mycoplasma research was well under way and it also had to be tested on someone, somewhere.

So, this is the Dr. Henderson who is tagged by WHO, through the CDC, to get over to Africa and vaccinate millions of Blacks. Then, sad to relate, some five plus years after getting the smallpox vaccine, millions and millions of Blacks began to present with HIV/AIDS.

Summary

What was going on? Here is our summary timetable of events:
  1942 to 1950: Huebner identifies immune suppressing PPLO later recognized as a species of mycoplasma

1946: George Merck of Biowar research reports to Secretary of Defense that his researchers have isolated the 'disease active principle' from bacteria in crystalline form

1946-1947: the immune compromising mycoplasma tested on school children in Iceland under the well-trained Rockefeller researcher, Bjorn Sigurdsson

1947-1959: Bjorn Sigurdsson turns major research efforts to the retrovirus that presents as Visna/Maedi in sheep

1950-1960: (especially 1959) a variety of tests on human guinea pigs, including children accessed through the Henle's, prisoners in various jails and prisons, nurses and hospital staff who were subject to directed vaccine programs from time-to-time, and even whole communities, exposed to the disabling mycoplasma-based co-factor, by insect vector and vaccines. Koprowski moved from Lederle to Wistar, and co-operates with the Belgian and Portuguese militaries and medical administrators to conduct vaccine tests in selected areas of Africa, wherein the immune suppressing co-factor of the mycoplasma is united with the retrovirus of sheep in various vaccines…including in a major way, oral polio vaccines. Sporadic deaths reported in Africa, Manchester, and other places of African women vaccinated earlier by Koprowski; of David Carr, vaccinated in the Royal Navy as a 'pretreatment' for something; and, others.

1960-1963: a hiatus in many activities following the election of John F. Kennedy who opposed all talk of eugenics and population control.

1963: Mr. Kennedy assassinated; succeeded by liar and eugenics-minded President Lyndon B. Johnson. LBJ appoints John D. Rockefeller lll as co-chair of a government population control committee and boasts that expenditure for population control programs grew from $6 million annually to $115 million under his administration. The secret CIA MK-SVLP moved into official government activity category as Special Virus Leukemia/Lymphoma Program

1964: A trial run of mycoplasma/visna pathogenic co-factors is undertaken in certain African countries under aegis of US International Development Agency with LBJ approval. President Johnson makes 'mysterious' statement to the staff and students at Ann Arbor, Michigan: "Within your lifetime powerful forces, already loosed, will take us toward a way of life beyond the realm of our experience, almost beyond the bounds of our imagination." (Gibson; 1994 Page 99) Was he talking about 'a crime beyond belief'?

1966: All systems are 'Go' for worldwide population growth-rate control action.

1966: Henderson placed in charge of vaccinating millions of Blacks against smallpox.

1969: Richard Nixon elected President. As a result of a pre-election political deal with Nelson Rockefeller, Nixon appoints Henry Kissinger, arch-criminal, as his National Security Advisor. SVLP turned into SVCP…and millions of dollars made available for Nixon's 'war on cancer'.

1969, on June 9, Dr. Donald MacArthur tells Congress that by 1980 the Pentagon will have two new biowar agents in place: AIDS to kill and CFS to disable.

1981: MacArthur's promises come true: AIDS and CFS spring into being; but, not because they were developed according to Dr. MacArthur's promised timetable, but because the seeds had already been planted in the early 1950s and then planted with an all-out campaign following Dr. Henderson's appointment in 1966.

Chapter Fourteen

VO to SVLP to SVCP to VCP to HTLV

*From Cancer to Lymphadenopathy and back to Cancer
Now that we've beaten Polio, let's tackle Cancer*

The Special Virus Cancer Program

We noted earlier, in our discussion of Johnson's immediate changes to Mr. Kennedy's unsigned National Security Action Memorandum #273, that Johnson already had his own agenda for rapid departure from the Kennedy agenda, and he began to put these into effect on November 23, 1963.

As with NSAM #273, Johnson was ready to continue with MKULTRA, and MKDELTA, but with the latter officially being terminated by order of the Inspector-General, the activities had to be carried on, hidden in plain sight, as a 'Viral Oncogenic' (VO) Program and some parts hidden in a 'Special Virus Leukemia/Lymphoma Program' (SVLP). We here begin our commentary of this program with a careful look at key parts.

For emphasis we re-state: the research into the Huebner PPLO or mycoplasma, with the latter pathogen's capability of reducing the human immune system, which was begun as covert Nelson Rockefeller/Allen Dulles projects, (MKULTRA, MKNAOMI, and MKDELTA) were brought out into the government mainstream under the guise of being an effort to discover a viral cause of cancer.

A certain level of confusion enters into the study of this (or these) program(s) because apparently much documentation was ordered shredded by CIA Director, Richard Helms, following the Watergate scandal.

At any rate, the first surviving 'Progress Report' in the undertaking is numbered "Eight" and is dated "July, 1971" Thus, if the eighth annual report is dated 1971, the first must have been 1964. So, despite any planned confusion, we can say that after a brief interruption introduced by the unexpected election and administration of John F. Kennedy, things are back on track with LBJ as of 12:31, November 22, 1963.

History demonstrates that the truth of current *events* is often not known to history until many years after the event when it becomes evident that the events as depicted at the time were falsely reported to the world.

Larry Speakes, a press secretary for Richard Nixon has been quoted as saying that, "History is history, whether fact or fiction." Such a flexible view may serve for the likes of Mr. Speakes and his boss for whom telling lies was very easy.

The definition, however, will not do for all those for whom history is the honest record of what has happened in the past…to the conspiracy buffs, that is. If it is not true, it is not history. What is presented as facts at one point in time can often be seen at a later point in time, to be lies. So it is with Lyndon B. Johnson. From his autobiographical account of his presidential years (*The Vantage Point*: see Bibliography) the reader gets one version of his activities related to population control measures. Some of his account is honest, but a great element of dishonestly is present, but that was not discernible at the time nor for many years that followed.

To get to the truth of Johnson's role in the development of AIDS one must start by turning to page four of a document dated August, 1973, and titled '*the virus-cancer program*'. The publisher is listed as the "Division of Cancer Cause and Prevention; National Cancer Institute". The NCI, in turn operates within the *U.S. Department of Health, Education, and Welfare*, [HEW] (emphasis added—authors) Public Health Service; National Institutes for Health. (Just in passing, note that Nelson Rockefeller spent 18 months in 1953-54 as Undersecretary of HEW.)

When one turns to page four of this document, one is beginning one's fall into the rabbit hole and is about to begin an Alice-like exploration of a medical wonderland. Or, as Hillary Johnson calls it, a 'labyrinth'.

The critical part on page four is titled "FUNDING HISTORY - SVCP CONTRACTS."

Right off the bat there is a problem...like the edge of a wedge to begin with...What is described as the 'Virus Cancer Program' on the title page is suddenly and without explanation presented on the next page as the *Special Virus Cancer Program*. Alright, that's not a big deal, just one more word...possibly just an editorial oversight. But, it turns out to be a hint of the insidious way with words so characteristic of the whole 'war on cancer' enterprise. We'll demonstrate what we mean as we follow the trail.

In the table below the above heading are six columns in ten rows, dated from Fiscal Year (19)64 to (19)73. Thus, the Table professes that the SVCP had, by 1973, been running for ten years from 1964 up to and including 1973. But wait a minute...the SVCP is President Richard Nixon's much touted War of Cancer, which didn't begin until 1971 when Nixon announced that the U.S. was going to beat swords into ploughshares and that he was going to convert the bioweapons base at Fort Detrick into a cancer research facility. How does one explain how a program announced in 1971 had actually begun in 1964?

Again, there is a possible explanation to be seen in the 'Funding History Table' under discussion. It shows that the War on Cancer which was announced in 1971 actually had been funded since 1968 (as we had deduced earlier) when Nixon came to office. However, as we have already seen, the funding table dates from 1964!

How is that explained? Simple. As we have already reported, the program supposedly started in 1964, but under the name of 'Viral Oncology' (VO), then, in 1965 it was augmented with a department titled 'Special Virus Leukemia/Lymphoma Program' (SVLP). Then, in 1968, when Nixon took over, it switched from being a 'leukemia' program to being a 'cancer' program and was titled the *Special Virus Cancer Program* (SVCP), which it still was in 1971 when Nixon declared his war on cancer, and was in 1973 when *Progress Report Number 10* was issued and when, in 1978, the whole shambles was closed down. Mission accomplished: AIDS and CFS were well on their way and the presence of both would be clearly seen in 1981, after being planted in millions of Africans and the poor of other Third World countries and in thousands of homosexual men in New York, San Francisco and Los Angeles. The pathogenic mycoplasma was, as we shall develop from incontrovertible evidence, seeded in the smallpox vaccine in the Third World, and in a hepatitis vaccine in three American cities.

Now, we can return for a further look at the 'Table of Funding History - SVCP Contracts.'

As noted, the Table states that funding began in 1964. (We will develop an anomaly in this date further on.) It is important to note that it was in 1964 that Lyndon Johnson began his first full term as President in his own right. It is also important to recall that Johnson had told the world that when he had come to office, the U.S. was spending $6 million on population control, but that when he left office they were spending $115 million. (*The Vantage Point,* Page 340)

Johnson's figures in *The Vantage Point,* correspond within logical limits for rounding to the figures revealed in 1973 in the Virus-Cancer program; *Progress Report Number 10.*

1964   *The Vantage Point:*$6 million   —   SVCP:$4.9 million
1967   *The Vantage Point:*$115 million—   SVCP:$166 million

What these sources and these figures reasonably and clearly demonstrate is that, after John F. Kennedy's murder, Lyndon B. Johnson wittingly brought the MKULTRA, MKDELTA, and MKNAOMI CIA projects out of the realm of covert criminality, where their financing was covert and he made them a part of the United States official population control activities, with the financing under the budget of the Department of Health, Education and Welfare.

Furthermore, Johnson knew that pilot programs of pathogen-laced vaccines were already being tested by the program planners in certain countries under the aegis of the USAID.

How do we know this? It is obvious from a study of the peripheral details in other sources.

This effort was apparently advanced by Johnson in Nigeria under the aegis of the U.S. Program known as the Agency for International Development (AID). On page 340 of his book he tells how he had advanced a program already in existence by altering the rule that governed AID. Here, he was probably referring to earlier tests begun in 1959.

The allusion we refer to was in his May, 1964 speech at Ann Arbor. In that speech, and not a part of any obvious context, Johnson had suddenly said: "Within your lifetime powerful forces *already loosed*, will take us toward a way of life beyond the realm of our experience…"

What was he talking about? What were the powerful forces? When and where had they been 'loosed'?

We suggest that under the guise of vaccinating certain Nigerian peoples for rubella and smallpox in 1959, there had been a test run of the biological products of MKULTRA and MKDELTA. That test run was probably what Donald Henderson was referring to in the December, 1978 issue of *National Geographic* when he wrote:

> "In 1959 an initial attempt by WHO to eradicate smallpox was begun, but the effort failed. Most countries had too few resources, and WHO could offer little help."   (Page 798)

Of Donald Henderson and smallpox vaccination programs, more later.

A few paragraphs above, we referred to an anomaly in the date of **1964** as the date that funding for SVLP had begun. Here is that anomaly: on pages 249 and 250 of The Virus Cancer Program, Progress Report Number 15, there is a report upon a contract given to Litton Bionetics, Inc. (Contract #NO1 - CP - 6 - 1006). The title of the contract is: Operation of a facility to Provide and Maintain Subhuman Primates for Cancer Research. At the end of the two-page report is this notice: "Date Contract Initiated: February 12, **1962**."

Thus, a program purportedly funded from 1964, was issuing contracts as early as 1962!

Again we feel that it is necessary to remind our readers that the confusion engendered when one attempts to find one's way through the AIDS/CFS labyrinth is not a result of our confusion, but is a natural consequence of the secrecy and obfuscation intentionally employed by those who were working in the shadows, and, in the case of Lyndon B. Johnson, when he was bringing such covertly-funded programs into the mainstream government funding.

We didn't plant the heavy cedar hedges of this labyrinth. Someone else planted the cedars and tended their growth; we are just trying to lead you through it.

Gajdusek and Gallo... and Litton Industries

The above mention of Litton Bionetics makes it appropriate at this point to say some more about Litton, and about Gajdusek whom we introduced in Chapter One. At that point, we had noted that Carleton Gajdusek had turned up in New Guinea in 1957 to study the Fore native tribe which was being decimated by a strange disease that they called 'Kuru'.

Well, Gajdusek turns up again in 1966 working for Gallo and Litton Bionetics. On page 286 of the *Special Virus Cancer Program, Progress Report #8*, it is cryptically reported that:

7. Gajdusek - Gibbs, 4/66 - 5/66   H: Kuru   4   8   4

Just what does this mean?

The seven (7) numbers one of 49 studies that had been completed by the time of the Report. The studies in question involved the inoculation of various primate species with a wide range of inocula including bovine leukemia, lymphoma, influenza, kuru, and a mycoplasma species. These potentially pathogenic agents were derived from a number of sources, including birds, cattle, cats, and humans.

Next to the #7 are the names of Carleton Gajdusek and his longtime working partner, C. Joseph Gibbs. The dates indicate that this particular study began in April, 1966 and was completed in May of the same year.

The 'H' means that the inoculum came from a 'human' and consisted of the pathogenic agent involved in the disease which had been decimating the Fore tribe of New Guinea: Kuru. The source of the pathogen was from a 'tissue mince' and eight (8) primates (probably chimpanzees) were inoculated, of which four died or were transferred.

Simply put: Carleton Gajdusek was working with Litton Bionetics and Robert Gallo in 1966, two years after Lyndon Johnson had launched his 'leukemia/lymphoma' Program. Part of Gajdusek's activities included the mashing of brain tissue from Kuru victims in New Guinea and injecting this mash into primates. At this point one should recall the activities of Gen. Ishii Shiro and Einosuke Hirano in 1942 in New Guinea. (See: Yuki Tanaka: *Hidden Horrors*)

Another point reported by Gallo in the *SVCP, Progress Report #8*, is the list of people who were working with him at the time. Referring again to pages 273 to 289 here are just five of the people referred to who, as early as 1962, were busy inoculating primates with various unusual or even exotic inocula with a brief comment by us to help place them in perspective.

On page 284 Gallo reports:

1. Ablashi, 10/70   S; H. saimiri   1   22   9

This item means that in October 1970, Veterinarian Dharam Ablashi inoculated twenty- two primates with a tissue-culture simian-derived herpes virus saimiri. This work by Ablashi fits chronologically with research reported by Robert E. Lee (See Bibliography). However, the important points about this reference include: (1) Dharam Ablashi was working with Robert Gallo in 1970; (2) Ablashi later turns up in Johnson's book, *Osler's Web*, where he is cited nine time and where his role is as Johnson suggests 'mystifying'; (3) Ablashi later went on to become a key figure in the story about chronic fatigue syndrome and the devious role of the Public Health Agencies; (4) finally, Ablashi was antagonistic to Dr. Elaine DeFreitas upon whom we report later.

Also on page 284, Gallo reports:

3. Levine, 6/69   H; BL   1   38   8

Paul Levine, like Dharam Ablashi, is cited in Johnson's *Osler's Web*, (in his case, it was 22 times) and like Ablashi, he seemed intent on making the life of Dr. Elaine DeFreitas difficult. Also, like Ablashi, it turns out from the above citation that he, too, was working with Robert Gallo, studying how certain primates reacted to certain unusual pathogenic agents. However, in his case he was testing the effects of 'BL' or 'Burkitt's lymphoma.' derived from 'H' - humans!

Burkitt's lymphoma is itself, a very intriguing disease agent because when it was first recognized as a pathogenic agent, it was being seen in children in Central Africa. A question that comes immediately to mind is: how did it get from Africa to America? In 1992, in an intriguing, but very difficult to read study by Dr. Eva Lee Snead titled, *Some call it "AIDS" – I call it murder!* The author suggests with convincing evidence, which it was brought by American researchers.

Another unusual question about Burkitt's lymphoma arose in San Francisco in 1982…Just one year after both AIDS and CFS arrived officially on the world's medical map. At that time nine gay men in San Francisco were diagnosed with BL, and, according to Hillary Johnson:

> "...a disease so rare that statisticians for the California Tumor Registry expect to find only two or three cases of the disease in the entire state every two years. The surge among gay men in San Francisco so impressed that city's infectious disease specialist, Selma Dritz, that she instructed the Centers for Disease Control to assume in the future that 'Burkitt's lymphoma is a form of AIDS.'" (Johnson; Page 92)

On page 317 of the SVCP there is another link between Ablashi and Levine. Besides the fact just noted, that both were working with Gallo and Litton Bionetics, we see that Levine had co-operated with Ablashi and others to write a paper published in the journal *Cancer* in 1971 titled "Elevated antibody titers (sic) to Epstein-Barr virus in Hodgkin's disease" (See Bibliography: Levine, P.H., *et al.*)

Page 287 brings us back to none other than Dr. Robert Huebner, who, as we have already seen, got the whole thing started back in the late 1940's when he noted that a PPLO caused the spontaneous degeneration of lymphoid tissues! It is reported by Gallo as follows:

13. Huebner - Coates, 8/64 - 3/68	H. Ad7	1	3	3
	H. Ad 12	1	6	4
	A; S	1	3	2
	M; S	1	4	3
	S & H; A12S40	1	4	3

We have been unable to trace Huebner's co-researcher (Coates), but it is significant to note that Huebner worked with Gallo from August 1964 to March 1968. It is also worth noting that the Huebner - Coates team drew tissue cultures of their pathogenic agents from human, avian, murine (rats and mice), and simian species. From these sources, they drew adenovirus species number seven and twelve, (Ad 7 and Ad 12); plus sarcoma and an unusual combination of simian and human adenovirus 12 and simian virus 40!

From their work, Huebner and Coates, working for Gallo and Litton Bionetics, produced a prodigious number of scientific papers, Huebner alone being listed with sixty-two in *SVCP, Progress Report #8.*

And what is the critical factor in these? Just this: Huebner, who started out in the 1940's with his serendipitous discovery that cells could be caused to degenerate when infected with a mycoplasmal species, had, by 1968, parlayed this into something very significant, if one is to judge by the amount of work that he did with Robert Gallo.

And not only was he working in the same 'inoculation program' with Gallo (the world 'expert' on AIDS) he was also working with Dharam Ablashi and Paul Levine…later to be heralded as 'experts' in CFS.

Further down page 287, we encounter another familiar name:

16. Koprowski - Jensen   4/66 - 6 - 66H; Ad 7   1   2   2

Hilary Koprowski is just cited once by Robert Gallo! Yet, in Hooper's *The River* (a history of AIDS) he is cited enough times to take up a full page-length column of the index, and in Johnson's *Osler's Web* (a history of CFS) he is cited 30 times. But, right in the middle of his work with ties to both AIDS and CFS, he co-operates in just one project with HIV 'discoverer' Robert Gallo? He and Jensen for just three months in 1966 take a sample of Adenovirus 7 and inoculate two primates with it.

There are two points that need to be made about this citation. First, although there is just one reference to Koprowski in Gallo's report, Gallo and Koprowski had worked together for years but very little of what they were doing ever became public. In his fanciful account about his 'discovery' of the AIDS virus (HIV) Gallo writes:

> "…[Salk] was to be of help to me in other kinds of advice - as Hilary Koprowski has been for many years."
>
> (Gallo, 1991 Page 316)

Second, it is to be noted that Koprowski was inoculating the primates with 'adenovirus 7' and that the adenovirus was originally identified in human adenoid tissue by none other than Robert Huebner (see above). Furthermore, the adenovirus links two important diseases as an etiological agent: respiratory diseases such as catarrh, influenza and 'respiratory distress syndrome' and malignant tumors! Thus, although one reference to Koprowski seems relatively insignificant, it is important because it ties Koprowski to Gallo and to Robert Huebner, as well as to respiratory diseases and cancer and, to Litton Bionetics. It is a keystone in the edifice of AIDS.

We will return to Litton Bionetics shortly, but before we do we must refer to the following paragraph from page 289 of the *SVCP—Progress Report #8*:

> "In 1965, twelve rhesus monkeys were transferred from Brooks Air Force Base to Bionetics for continued maintenance and observation. These animals had undergone irradiation treatments from 1957 to 1960. In 1966, one animal developed sarcoma of the femur, basal cell carcinoma of the skin, and two kidney tumors. In another member of this group, a seminoma of one testicle, a meningioma, and a kidney tumor were found."

This paragraph is significant because it, too, serves to establish links in the medical, political, military labyrinth that we are exploring.

Brooks Air Force Base was the military station to which Dr. Jose Rivera had been assigned during the period 1 April 1954 to 30 September 1957. Rivera, in turn, had mysterious links to Lee Harvey Oswald in early 1963 and he had later links with the Centers for Disease Control/Dr. Brian Mahy and Dr. Elaine DeFreitas in the latter's study of retroviral fragments in the blood of CFS victims. These strange linkages extend those already cited above in Chapter 11.

The paragraph has an added significance in the fact that it links Brooks Air Force Base to Bionetics and hence to Litton Industries who are working with Robert Gallo. Again, this is a complicated series of links, but all must be cited since each played a part in both the development of the AIDS co-factors and in the murder of President John F. Kennedy.

However, at this point we will give further attention to just who and what Litton Bionetics was and who its principal figures were and how they are tied to the Rockefeller apparat for what reason. To answer these who, what, how, and why questions in the most succinct manner we will quote Dr. Leonard Horowitz:

> "At the time Ebola first broke, the president of Bionetics - a medical subsidiary of the mega-military weapons contractor Litton Industries - was Roy Ash. Mr. Ash became director of American industry by appointment of his personal friend, Richard Nixon, beginning in 1969. That year, Nelson Rockefeller's protégé, Dr. Henry Kissinger, received the

> position Nixon also considered for Mr. Ash - National Security Advisor overseeing CIA, FBI, and foreign policy."
>
> "Foreshadowing the Rockefeller family's involvement in global genocide that is evidenced in the pages ahead, author G. Edward Griffin, in *World Without Cancer*, cited Litton's strong direction from Rockefeller's 'pyramid of power'. A spider' web of connections best describes the suspicious outbreaks of AIDS in New York and Ebola in Uganda, the alleged (West Nile Virus) WNV outbreak in New York, Rockefeller links to the cancer industry directed from New York, and Rockefeller ties to the manufacture of carcinogens, particularly Malathion by American Cyanamid, and Anvil, Malathion's replacement, by Rockefeller's own Chevron Corporation, as well as owner of Lederle Labs. Dr. James B. Fisk, director of American Cyanamid, Dow Corning, and Rockefellers Chase Manhattan Bank, was also, during the last half of the twentieth century, on the Board of Overseers of the Sloan-Kettering Memorial Cancer Center (SKMCC) in New York City." (Horowitz, 2001 Pp. 4-5)

Sorting through this confusing cluster of people and institutions is difficult, but needs to be done if one is to get the picture of strange fellowships linked in a cabal to create the AIDS pandemic. To start this sorting let's restate them in a linear format, then we'll comment upon each of them to demonstrate their relationships: Bionetics; Litton; Roy Ash; Nixon; Rockefeller; Kissinger; American Cyanamid; Lederle; Chase Manhattan Bank; and Sloan-Kettering.

We have already noted that Bionetics Research Laboratories, Inc., a Division of Litton Industries, contributed 16 pages to the *Special Virus Cancer Program, Progress Report Number Eight*. It turns out that Robert Gallo, who was working with both the National Cancer Institute (NCI) and Bionetics was serving to create a very important partnership between the U.S. Government and private industry. How is it that the two got linked in the first place?

The answer to that question starts with a quotation from Gallo's book *Virus Hunting*:

> "It was largely because of my friendship with **Bob Ting**, then a well-established NCI investigator, that I first began

even to think about viruses. He and I had known each other socially before becoming colleagues. We had met in 1966; shortly after I arrived at NIH…He introduced me to **(Robert) Huebner**, both the man and his ideas."(Gallo, 1991 Pp. 64-66)

Here, then, we see a link between **Robert Gallo and Robert Ting…as well as Robert Huebner.** Now let's look at a quotation from Horowitz' *Emerging Viruses*:

"A Bionetics contract summary disclosed that Dr. John Landon served as the director of Litton Bionetics along with David Valerio and Robert Ting. Ting had co-authored numerous Gallo research publications." (Horowitz, Page 420)

There is another important linkage mentioned in the Gallo quote (above): "He introduced me to Huebner!"

We're back to where we started with Robert Huebner who had discovered that the PPLO or mycoplasma could cause the spontaneous degeneration of human cells? Now, he's working with Robert Gallo of the National Institutes of Health and with Litton Industries…a leading war weapons contractor.

From VO to SVLP to SVCP to VCP by way of HTLV
From Cancer to Leukemia/Lymphadenopathy and back to Cancer

If the above string of V's and L's and C's and P's and that lone T confuse you, it was probably meant to by the National Institutes of Health. All the V's deal essentially with the same thing…viruses… and all the C's and L's deal with same disease…cancer…(The L is for leukemia which is a cancer of the blood) and all the P's are really one: a Program.

But, as the late great Serge Lang (we've referred to him before) stated in his book *Challenges*, (Page 392) the first technique of obfuscation is to describe the same thing with multiple names…or in this case with multiple initializations.

Those who coined these initials were all working on one thing that they wanted to be able to talk about without giving away what that thing was: a pathogen to kill (or disable) 'enemies'. But the best way to work on something that is going to kill people is to call it something that is going to help those people. If you don't obscure it this way, then someone will try to stop you. So, to look for a virus that will kill on demand, tell the world that you are looking for a virus that causes cancer, and, with that virus identified, you will be able to control it. To the public's great advantage. Or so you say. If you have the support of a pliant media (see Part Six), you can get away with it...for a while at least.

An example of such Orwellian Newspeak is seen in the fact that Dr. Donald MacArthur who was the Deputy Director (Research and Development) for the Department of Defense in charge of programs developing biological weapons (see Ch. 15) to 'kill' and to 'disable' was introduced to certain Congressmen as the person in charge of 'applied research' in the *life* sciences! Further, his earlier weapons research work at Westinghouse had him listed as manager of the '*Life* Sciences Research Center.' Newspeak!

With our confusing string of initials for a single program spread over a period of years (the first few of which were in top secret CIA-sponsored research) we have a group of the same scientists searching for a virus that will cause cancers...including cancer of the blood, leukemia... And, to help that or those virus(es) along in the body of their victim, we will want to suppress the victim's immune system. A good way to do that is to introduce a sterol dependent mycoplasma that will take up *cholesterol* from target cells and kill those cells which are the key mediators of cellular immunity. (See Ch. 23: **1971; Rottem, *et al.***)

The latter would result in an acquired immune deficiency.

The biological reality of such a destruction of cellular immunity is a very complicated sequence of events within the victim and the best we can do for our readers is to summarize a few key points from pages seventy-nine and eighty of Dr. Steven A. Rosenberg's book: *The Transformed Cell*.

In passing we must point out that in his book Dr. Rosenberg gives a very interesting and important account about his research into cancer, however, we are somewhat concerned with the fact that he is listed in the *Special Virus Cancer Program, Progress Report #8*, (Page 299) with two of the articles that he co-authored cited. As we have already acknowledged, a 'cover' story has to be genuine if it is to be a good or believable cover and, if the SVCP is, as we believe, a 'cancer' cover for the development of the AIDS co-factors, the cited cancer researchers must be genuine. However, as we have also pointed out, MKNAOMI is one of the subprojects under MKULTRA, the DOD/CIA covert program for the development of AIDS. Here is our question: did Dr. Rosenberg know that he was a part of the MKULTRA/MKNAOMI/MKDELTA covert programs, or was he one of the many legitimate cancer scientists employed as cover? We are suspicious because Rosenberg says of his year with the SVCP "In many ways, this experience at NIH was the best time of my life" and he named his youngest daughter 'Naomi'. (Rosenberg, 1992 Page 83) We are inclined to give him the benefit of the doubt, but we must put our concern on the record.

In *The Transformed Cell*, Rosenberg says this of Gallo and two of Gallo's co-workers:

> "Their interest was *leukemia - cancer* of blood cells - and they had been trying to grow long-term cultures of human leukemia cells for use in future experiments. But to their dismay, they found that instead they were growing healthy human T *lymphocytes*. They explored this phenomenon enough to identify a protein that they believed caused the growth and called it 'T Cell Growth Factor,' which later became known as Interleukin - 2 or IL-2 ...T lymphocytes are the more common of the two chief kinds of lymphocytes, beginning development in the bone marrow before maturing in the *thymus* and accounting for approximately 70 percent of all lymphocytes. B lymphocytes, which begin development in the bone marrow and mature there, account for about 25 percent of all lymphocytes; when stimulated they transform themselves into antibody-producing factories...T cells divide into two major sub-types: killer cells and helper cells. Helper cells regulate activity in *cellular immunity*, which primarily involves T cells, and control the ability of B cells to make antibodies. (The *AIDS virus destroys helper T cells, preventing the body from defending itself against infections*.) Killer T cells of course kill, and they do so by binding highly specific receptors on their surface to antigens...T cells emerge from the thymus fully

mature, fully differentiated, themselves an end product..."
(Pp. 79-80)

We quote Rosenberg because his passage unites so many of the factors that are emerging in our study: leukemia; cancer; lymphocytes; thymus; cellular immunity, and ties in with the work of Huebner, but nowhere does Rosenberg mention the **mycoplasma** with which it all got started! And the article therefore links the VO to the SVLP to the SVCP of the NIH.

MKULTRA and its many subprograms, including MKNAOMI and MKDELTA were hastily terminated at the end of 1963...just weeks after the murder of President Kennedy. There were persistent rumors that MKULTRA had an "executive action-type assassinations" component. (Richelson; 2001 P. 45) Interestingly enough parts of the program were taken over by a "Dr. Stephen Aldrich, a graduate of Amherst and Northwestern Medical School who had served in the agency's Office of Medical Services and O.S.I.'s Life Sciences Division..." Note two things here: the use of the euphemistic 'Life Sciences' to identify activities associated more with death than with life. Also, note the doctor's name: 'Aldrich.' We have been unable to determine whether he was a member of the Aldrich side of the Rockefeller extended family.

Of more importance to this study is the fact that the secret, very expensive, CIA MKULTRA project ended in fiscal year 1964 and in the next year, under Lyndon Johnson, there suddenly sprang in to being the Special Virus Leukemia/Lymphoma Program -SVLP! Not only did SVLP spring into being, but $8.7 million in contracts were awarded in that year.

A question that must be asked is how could over eight million dollars worth of contracts be issued in the very first year? One answer, and the one most logical is that work which was previously being done (up to 1964) under the CIA covert programs MKULTRA, MKNAOMI and MKDELTA, was simply switched to the National Cancer Institute (in 1965) to continue the work.

Chapter Fifteen

NOVEMBER 1968:
ENTER NIXON AND AGNEW…STAGE RIGHT

"Nixon: '…but the basic thing is the establishment. The establishment is dying, and so they've got to show that the…despite the successes we have had in foreign policy and in the election…they've got to show that it is…just wrong just because of this.'"

On page 83 of *The New York Times* edition of The White House Transcripts the following conversation between President Richard Nixon and White House Legal Counsel, John Dean is reported:

"**Dean**: On the '68 thing…he said that Hoover had told Patrick Coyne…Coyne had told Rockefeller…Rockefeller told Kissinger…
"**President**: Hoover to Coyne to Nelson Rockefeller to Kissinger. Right?
"**Dean**: That's right.
"**President**: Why did Coyne tell it to Nelson Rockefeller?"

Here one has the very image of democracy in America.

Dean and the president have been trying to track down the route by which conversations exchanged in the confidence of the Oval Office have become known to persons who were not present at the time they were made. They return to the 1968 election campaign to see if that will provide any hints for their present problem…understanding and limiting the damage from the Watergate break-in and the problem of leaks from the Oval Office to the media.

The presence of Hoover, the Director of the Federal Bureau of Investigation in 'the loop' is no surprise to Nixon. After all, this corrupt and evil guardian of the law in the United States at the time was known to have spies and sources everywhere so that he could maintain his blackmail files and keep his great Washington power. And 'Coyne', probably Ed Coyne of the *Wall Street Journal*, was no great surprise…he was known to have back channels to many Washington insiders, but, the fact that Coyne brought Nelson Rockefeller in to the loop seems to catch Nixon by surprise: "Why did Coyne tell it to Nelson Rockefeller?"

The exchange between Dean and the president is significantly informative on a number of fronts. First of all, the fact that not only had Hoover learned of the matter under review, he had shared it with a member of the media. Then, not only did the media member have the information as background for any stories that he might see fit to use, he had also passed the information to none other than Nelson Rockefeller!

In other words, the information had been passed up the ladder to a key member of the Rockefeller power center, demonstrating just who it was in the democracy of the United States that was at the center of the shadow government, which was really running things. Even Nixon didn't know…but he had some inkling.

Then, it is important to note where the information went when Rockefeller had it: Henry Kissinger. Up to the top, Nelson Rockefeller, then out to the Rockefellers' man: Henry Kissinger.

We introduce this chapter with this snippet from history to demonstrate where the real power lies in American politics: the money interests who have corrupted senior administration officials (Hoover); who have representatives of the fabled 'free press' as intelligence gatherers(Ed Coyne); and who control the president's senior executor in all matters dealing with National Security (Henry Kissinger).

The power core of the United States is built upon wealth, which controls the media, the medical establishment, the pharmaceutical industry, the military industrial complex, the 'public' politicians, American foreign policy (including that instrument of foreign policy…the making of war).

And the core of the wealthy establishment is the Rockefeller network.

In the same conversation Dean alludes to an FBI operative named Mark Felt:

> "**Dean**: …The other person who knows and is aware of it is Mark Felt, and we have talked about Mark Felt before…"

Little did Dean know at the time that Mark Felt was "Deep Throat", the source of Watergate leaks to Woodward and Bernstein which they in turn were publishing in the *Washington Post*. Nixon was being sabotaged every step of the way...and he had no real idea who was pulling the strings...except that it was in the 'Eastern Establishment' who, he knew, were the core of the CIA.

A few days earlier he had speculated to Dean:

> "**President**: ...the basic thing is the establishment. The establishment is dying and so they've got to show that despite the successes we have had in foreign policy and in the election, they've got to show that it is, just wrong just because of this. They are trying to use this as the whole thing." (*Ibid*, Page 120)

And they succeeded! Because of the Watergate Nixon was out and suddenly the 'establishment' (especially as represented by Nelson Rockefeller) were in.

Henry Kissinger

Although this chapter focuses upon President Richard Nixon and his Vice- President Spiro Agnew, we begin it with a brief summary of Nixon's National Security Advisor, Henry Kissinger. We do so because although Nixon has the title of President and although he thinks that he is in charge, actually there is that Establishment that we introduced in chapters one and nine. The 'shadow government' in the Oil > Wealth > Rockefellers > Establishment > Media > Political Power > CIA > Hidden Wars sequence. In a sense, Kissinger was the Trojan horse within whose belly the Rockefeller apparat is carried into the White House.

In Kissinger, the Rockefeller rubber of eugenics theory meets the road of political population control. Or one might say, the rubber of evil finally meets the pavement of power. The insidious presence of the Rockefellers is translated into the realpolitik of the Nixon administration and a number of threads of science and power lay the ground for the advent thirteen years away when in 1981 a disabling pathogen and a lethal pathogen are officially in the human family and the rate of world population growth begins to slow.

Although President Nixon is the passenger in the limousine and thinks that he is giving the orders, and Kissinger is the chauffeur at the wheel, the route has been set by Nelson Rockefeller and his family, through his friends in high places.

President: "Hoover to Coyne to Nelson Rockefeller to Kissinger. Right?"

Henry Alfred Kissinger was born on May 29, 1923, in Germany. In 1938 his family fled Germany for Britain and shortly after immigrated to the United States. In 1943 he was drafted into the U.S. Army and was sent to Germany where he played an unusually successful role as a district administrator in the occupation of his birth state. His major move towards a significant role in world affairs came in 1956 when Nelson Rockefeller appointed him a director of a Rockefeller Brothers Fund special project to study the major domestic and foreign problems of the United States. Essentially, he was to develop political positions for Nelson Rockefeller's bid to become president of the U.S.

However, all of Rockefeller's money and duplicity together with Kissinger's insidious skills in manipulating those whom he targeted, were not enough to defeat Richard Nixon in the latter's bid for the job. Early in 1968 it had become evident that Nixon was going to be the Republican Party's choice as their candidate, and Rockefeller met with Nixon to strike a deal. Essentially the deal was this: Rockefeller would withdraw from the race and devote his money and media strength to the election of Nixon, if, in turn, Nixon would appoint Kissinger as his head of the National Security Council [NSC] when he had won the election. Nixon agreed, mainly to get Rockefeller into his tent during the campaign.

Thus it was that Kissinger became the Rockefeller's man in the White House. Nelson Rockefeller had added the key stud to his stable of talent. As head of the NSC, Kissinger essentially controlled the Pentagon and the CIA and the great eugenics plan of the Rockefeller family became official (although publicly unstated) United States policy. The MK-SVLP sub-program of MKULTRA had become The Special Virus Leukemia/Lymphoma Program [SVLP] under Johnson when he appointed John David Rockefeller lll co-chair of his Population Control Committee, ending the Kennedy era opposition to the concept. Johnson had moved population control from the basement to the back kitchen. With Nixon's designation of Kissinger as head of the NSC and as the president's special assistant for security affairs, population control moved from the back kitchen to the living room. Under the guise of a great war against cancer, the Rockefeller man in the White House, Henry Kissinger, launched an all out attack upon the Third World's people.

As we have seen, the WHO smallpox vaccination campaign, initiated on a trial basis in the mid-1950's, and revived and extended by the Johnson administration with its John D. Rockefeller lll and Wilbur Cohen Population Control Committee in 1966 went all out in late 1968 when Henry Kissinger came to dominate United States foreign policies on behalf of his Rockefeller patrons. Thus it was that on **June 9, 1969**, Dr. Donald MacArthur of the Pentagon was free to share in secret Hearings with several Congressmen the fact that 'eminent scientists' were ready to launch a double-barreled assault on the world's population growth rate. One barrel would fire a disabling pathogen at the White population of America [CFS/ME] and the other barrel would fire a lethal pathogen at the Black population of Africa. [AIDS]

An Interlude For Justice

At this point, we want to make sure that all of the people involved in this greatest crime in history, the death and disablement of millions of people from AIDS and CFS/ME, is not laid completely at the door of Henry Kissinger. Kissinger was and is part of the executive branch of the eugenics war against humanity in general. He is not alone. In the core are the Rockefeller dominated industrialists, militarists, and media moguls. Around that core are the descending orders of support for the evil policies now at work. And, finally, there are the people of the United States who by a mix of mental lethargy, disinterest, misinformation, disinformation, 'kick-butt' mentality and self-centeredness have allowed themselves to become mankinds' greatest enemy rather than mankinds' best friend.

As part of this total plan are people such as Christopher Hitchens who, while appearing to condemn the evil, singles out Kissinger as the criminal for punishment. Hitchens, in his book, *The Trial of Henry Kissinger* alludes to Nelson Rockefeller only three times en passant and David Rockefeller only twice. If one were to judge by Hitchens' disinformation, Kissinger is the heart of darkness, was literally working alone, and he alone should be put on trial.

Don't buy that! As we demonstrate in the next section of this chapter Kissinger was and is just one stud in the Rockefeller stable. The stable owners (the Rockefellers and their cohorts); the pliant media assets (including *The New York Times, Time, Readers Digest,* and *Science*) which misinform and disinform; the bought politicians; and the public at large are all to varying degrees, complicit in making the United States of America the real 'evil empire'. In other words blame the deep politics of the United States.

End of an Interlude

We have presented the evidence that a deep-rooted and well-hidden part of the Central Intelligence Agency is the administrative agency where *the evil conceived by those who are part of the 'deep politics of America* (certain members of the Rockefeller apparat together with the dynastic Morgans, Whitneys, etc. who are colloquially, variously and collectively labeled 'the Establishment', the 'Secret Government', the 'Deep Politics' of America, etc.) and individuals such as the late John J. McCloy—one of the seven "august" gentlemen on the Warren Commission—and the late Leon Jaworski of Watergate Special Prosecutor fame—*are translated from concepts to actual evil deeds carried out in the real world among human victims.*

As an example of such links between those in the deep recesses of American politics where the overthrow of President Mossadegh was plotted and the Shaw restored to the throne of Iran are people such as Kermit Roosevelt, who with CIA money, translated the plot into covert, illegal, terrorist crimes.

A more significant example of the *link* between the deep politicians of America who plotted the invasion of Vietnam or the murder of a president or the overthrow of a foreign government and the administrative machinery necessary to carry out the plotted crimes is to be seen in the career of Henry Kissinger. Kissinger has all the qualities necessary to represent the deepest and darkest of American politics. First off, he is a protégé of the Rockefeller apparat. He is, therefore, well familiar with the Rockefeller apparat's eugenics schemes [the starting point of AIDS]. He is also sufficiently amoral to play (secretly) on two opposing sides at the same time, as in 1968 when he appeared to be supplying counsel to the Humphrey presidential campaign, while actually working for the Nixon campaign. Kissinger was, therefore, ready, willing, and able to serve whichever side turned out to be the winner in any power struggle.

He is also a liar, as is well demonstrated by several researchers. And finally, he is personally evil…capable of ordering the abduction, or murder of perceived opponents such as General Rene Schneider of Chile (while planting a paper trail of denial on the record) or giving the go-ahead (with President Gerald Ford) to President Suharto of Indonesia to invade East Timor and murder hundreds of thousands of East Timorese.

We have depended upon many sources such as *Kissinger*, by Marvin and Bernard Kalb (1974) and Kissinger; *The Uses of Power* by David Landau (1972), but our main source has been *The Trial of Henry Kissinger* by Christopher Hitchens. (Verso, 2001)

The latter book is essentially a brief for the prosecution in a hoped for trial for crimes against humanity, since it focuses upon the many international crimes of Henry Kissinger…and in truth, it is these crimes that have distinguished the Kissinger career. Here is our summary of Hitchens' brief.

In his *Preface*, Hitchens summarizes 'the identifiable crimes that can and should be placed on a proper bill of indictment, whether the actions taken were in line with general "policy" or not.

These include:
   The deliberate mass killings of civilian populations in Indochina.
   Deliberate collusion in mass murder, and later in assassination, in Bangladesh.
   The personal suborning and planning of murder, of a senior constitutional officer in a democratic nation—Chile—with which the United States was not at war.
   Personal involvement in a plan to murder the head of state in the democratic nation of Cyprus.

The incitement and enabling of genocide in East Timor.
Personal involvement in a plan to kidnap and murder a journalist living in Washington, DC.

These six points are an adequate summary of a reasonable case for crimes against humanity such as the recent trial in Chile against that country's former dictator, the late Augusto Pinochet. Unfortunately, that trial came to a halt when Pinochet died in mid-trial at the age of ninety-one.

It is appropriate that at this point we make a major point: *where Chile finally got around to charging, arresting and trying Pinochet in a court of law for his role in the murder of many hundreds of innocent persons, the United States in stark contrast, insists on holding Henry Kissinger up as a great national statesman.* Whenever the occasion requires, the major all-news TV channel of America, CNN, (which touts itself as 'the most trusted source of news in America') will interview 'elder statesman' Henry Kissinger for his analysis of the crisis.

The stark *contrast* between Chile and the United States, demonstrates just how evil the United States is. A public servant in the United States who is involved in great crimes is touted as an 'elder statesman'; where, in a country that still has some degree of moral strength, such criminals are placed on trial for their crimes.

This profound saturation by evil of the body politic of the United States is demonstrated in other ways that we have reported so far in this study. One of which we will allude to briefly, and to which Hitchens also refers briefly. We will start with a quote from the latter:

> "…Nixon and Kissinger decided to aggrandize the notion of 'hot pursuit' across the borders of Laos and Cambodia. Even before the actual territorial invasion of Cambodia, for example, and very soon after the accession of Nixon and Kissinger to power, a program of heavy bombardment of the country was prepared and executed in secret. One might with some revulsion call it a 'menu' of bombardment, since the code names for the raids were 'Breakfast', 'Lunch', 'Dinner' and 'Dessert'. The raids were flown by B-52 bombers which, it is important to note at the outset, fly at an altitude too high to be observed from the ground and carry immense

tonnages of high explosive; they give no warning of approach and are incapable of accuracy or discrimination because of both their altitude and the mass of their shells. Between 18 March 1969 and May 1970, 3,360 such raids were flown across the Cambodian frontier. The bombing campaign began as it was to go on - with full knowledge of its effect on civilians, and with flagrant deceit by Mr. Kissinger in this precise respect."

(Hitchens, 2001 Pages 34-35)

This paragraph provides us with the opportunity to make several points that need to be made. The first point is that Hitchens, like so many other writers, politicians, and historians, tries to dump all of the blame for the evil of these attacks (and many other crimes dealt with in Hitchens' book) on one man: Henry Kissinger.

This is a cop-out! In general terms, the blame rests with the United States and that means with the people of the United States. Of course, there were voters who did not vote for Richard Nixon, but these people, too, must share the blame because they did not take to the streets in protest when the news came out. The blame must also be shared by the media, especially the large networks such as ABC, CBS, NBC and CNN. There is ample evidence that the crimes being committed against the innocent victims in Laos and Cambodia were well known to many reporters and other observers, but this information was not shared with the public of the United States.

You will note that in the final paragraph of the quoted passage, Hitchens mentions Kissinger alone. At least in the first sentence of the quoted paragraph, the author has the decency to mention not just Kissinger, but he also mentions Kissinger's nominal boss: Richard Nixon. In this we see the first hints of the 'flaw' in Hitchens whole work, which we will develop in detail at the conclusion of this chapter.

But, before we do that, some further comments are necessary in order to make our major point: the crimes of the United States devolve upon the people of the United States.

Note the description of the bombing of Laos and Cambodia. Millions of pounds of high explosives being dumped upon the rice paddies and hamlets of marginal agricultural peoples (not to mention the dumping of Agent Orange and cluster bombs.) The planes are so high as to be practically untouchable by any defense from the ground.

However, when one plane, that flown over Vietnam rather than Laos or Cambodia, by the current Senator from Arizona, John McCain, happened to get hit by a high altitude rocket and the pilot taken prisoner, the pilot is hailed as an American 'hero.'

John McCain is nothing like a hero. He is a terrorist who happened to have a high flying plane to deliver his bombs. He didn't have to strap the bombs onto his body and go to his certain death in delivering them. Being shot down was, for McCain, an unforeseen accident.

Then John McCain is confined to a Vietnamese prison camp to which the American media refer as the 'Hanoi Hilton.' It is depicted as a place of torture and of brain washing, and McCain and all his 'hero worshipers' lament the cruel conditions to which the captured American terrorists in high flying planes were subjected. Yet, some years later, McCain supports President George Bush in maintaining a far worse American detention camp at Guantanamo, Cuba.

And the American people go along with this hypocrisy!

Now, we can address the major flaw of Hitchens' case for the prosecution of Henry Kissinger. That flaw is simply this: no single person can be pointed to as the criminal of America in all of the crimes that Hitchens' cites in his book. The crimes are American crimes, and the criminals are those Americans who range all the way from ardent supporters of the evil, to those who merely shrug and accept the official media interpretation of that evil as Orwellian 'good'.

In other words, Hitchens and his book are examples of a subtle media shift of blame from the people of America who are always talking about 'kicking butt' to one or two specific people. That way, the criminals of America (the people…whether they vote or not) can feel good about themselves while condemning the people who were their servants in the committing of those crimes.

This quality can be seen in the present case of President George W. Bush. Admittedly, his first 'election' was not an electoral victory, it was stolen from Vice-President Al Gore by the likes of Chief Justice Rehnquist and retired justice Sandra Day O'Conner, but this crime against democracy was ratified by the American people in 2004 when they re-elected George W. Bush.

Henry Kissinger is just one of the people in the shadows who appear to be serving the elected representatives of the people of the

United States, but who are in reality, serving the deep politicians of America. Kissinger is one of the people who translate the deep evil spawned by illicit wealth into covert crimes that advance the wealthy few at the expense of humanity. He is one of those whose actions are the rubber of evil that meets the pavement of 'realpolitics.'

The effect of such duplicity by Hitchens is to make Kissinger out to be a lone 'crook'...aided and abetted at times by Richard Nixon. The evil of the United States thus becomes (according to Hitchens) just one loose cannon (Henry Kissinger) rolling around unhindered on the deck of the ship of state. Nonsense!

Hitchens is working to hide the truth, while pretending, as the one-time *Harper's Magazine* token 'socialist' writer; now, a contributing editor of Vanity Fair, to expose it. Just as Vice-President Nelson Rockefeller pretended to 'expose' crimes of the CIA after he and Gerald Ford had been jockeyed into office to replace Nixon and Agnew.

Now, what does this have to do with AIDS and that great crime against humanity?

Just this: AIDS is the product of United States criminality (with lower level allies in Canada, Great Britain, Australia and Israel) and that criminality is a consequence of the self-deception most Americans labour under. Only when the people of America (and to a very great degree the equally self-deceived other citizens of the world) open their eyes and face the reality of their representatives' actions, will the truth be made known, and humanity can get on with the task of being human.

By citing several specific examples of crimes against humanity, and by attributing these to one man (Henry Kissinger), Hitchens hides the real criminals (the deep politicians of the United States, including his patron Nelson Rockefeller) by failing to acknowledge their presence, and he hides the crime beyond belief (the development and deployment of the co-factors involved in AIDS and the Rockefeller eugenics mission.) Hitchens refers only once to 'biological weapons' and that *ironic* reference appears on page 138 of his book when he *quotes* none other than his subject in a letter Kissinger wrote to *The New York Times* on November 5, 2000.

In that letter, Kissinger touts some of the 'good' things Nixon did as President. We quote:

> "4. The Nixon administration concluded the first strategic arms control agreement and the first agreement banning biological weapons; opened relations with China…" etc.

Wherein lies the 'irony' that we have noted?

It is ironic that Kissinger touts 'the first agreement banning biological weapons' when he knows full well that the first official U.S. Government allusion to the most hideous biological weapon devised to date had occurred on June 9, 1969 (Section 2 below) when Dr. Donald MacArthur had promised the Black Budget Committee of the House of Representatives a new microorganism, one which did not naturally exist, and one which promised to be 'refractory' to the human immune system…**AIDS!**

And, Kissinger knows full well that he, as Nixon's National Security Advisor, was in charge of the research into biological weapons being done at that time by MacArthur's researchers.

Does Hitchens not know this? If he doesn't, then shame on him. If he does know it, then why does he not include this crime in his indictment?

Hitchens does not include the development and deployment of biological weapons, including the co-factors of AIDS, under Nixon, Kissinger and the rest, because by focusing upon the crimes known to the world, he helps to hide the crime of genocide.

Hitchens is a 'media asset' of the CIA. His call for a trial of Henry Kissinger simply detracts attention from the real criminals…those deep politicians in the shadows who, through a well-hidden faction of the CIA, run the nominal democratic government of the United States.

AIDS: And the Deep Politics of the United States of America

We acknowledge that the above title derives from the work of Dr. Peter Dale Scott whose careful, even-handed study of the murder of President John F. Kennedy opened up a vast new area of study. We have been greatly influenced by Dr. Scott's work, and that influence has grown much greater as we have proceeded with this evolving work. Our research has finally brought us to the point where the "deep politics of the United States" must be treated as the critical center of any historical/political/medical study of the United States from 1952 to the present, including as we have demonstrated in Chapter Ten, the assassination of John F. Kennedy. As we said in Chapter Eleven, 'it is all of a piece.'

The study of AIDS discovery/development and deployment was to continue during the administration of Richard Nixon, but it was on a new track. The pathogenic co-factors of the immune suppressing mycoplasma and the visna retrovirus had already been seeded during the administration of Lyndon Johnson, and the program had moved into high gear with the assignment of Dr. Henderson in 1968 to head the WHO smallpox vaccination program. Beginning about 1968 the task for the U.S. researchers was to research and understand how the co-factors worked. In other words, the powers of deep politics had turned the epidemic loose even before they knew how it did its damage, and now they needed to learn its secrets…if they could.

So, while Robert Gallo and Robert Ting *et al.* were engaged in that task, Richard Nixon assumed the presidency, with Henry Kissinger as his National Security Advisor. The AIDS epidemic was on its way, and the CFS/ME epidemic was following close behind and Kissinger was preparing for the twin horrors of a lethal biological weapon and a disabling biological weapon by having Dr. Donald MacArthur of the Pentagon bring Congress on board in secret Hearings on June 9, 1969, and by writing a National Security Study Memorandum #200 (NSSM #200) warning of the dangers of the looming world population growth problem. Kissinger was bringing Congress into the loop so that when the epidemics hit, Congress would be muted under the mistaken belief that they shared culpability.

Because of the June 9, 1969 Hearings and the NSSM #200, Nixon has received undue blame for the AIDS epidemic, but he had been in the Eisenhower administration when the CIA got the whole thing started and his friend Roy Ash had founded the Litton Bionetics and other culpable agencies so we wont waste any time trying to exonerate him.

Rather, we will examine Nixon's entanglement with the deep politics of America and how and why these forces brought about his resignation.

The Nixon Presidency

Richard Nixon was elected President of the United States in November 1968 and was sworn into office on January 20, 1969.

As President, Nixon did not begin his term with a clean slate, either personally or in terms of the government operations, which he had been elected to direct, administer and control.

As we have noted, he had been a Congressman, with a number of 'shady' friends, and then a Senator and finally Vice-President during the administration of Dwight D. Eisenhower where he held important control over defense contracts. During this early period of his career he had established tenuous links with key figures in the Federal Bureau of Investigation, especially its Director, J. Edgar Hoover (who provided Nixon with back channel intelligence and gossip on 'communists and Negro agitators') and a variety of somewhat shadowy operators in the world of finance such as Roy Ash of Hughes Aircraft (which he later left to found Litton Industries…the industrial arm of the AIDS development enterprise), and John Mitchell of the law firm Caldwell, Trimble and Mitchell (where Mitchell had helped Governor Nelson Rockefeller skirt the law in New York State finance). Along with these two (Ash and Mitchell) who made it into Nixon's first Cabinet, were other equally shifty characters such as Robert Abplanalp (who financed Nixon's San Clemente, CA, home) and Charles (Bebe) Rebozo (who helped arrange a Howard Hughes 'loan' to Nixon's brother, Donald) who never made it into Cabinet. This was some of Nixon's personal baggage.

In terms of inherited government operations, Nixon undoubtedly had some knowledge of the earlier CIA plot to set up John F. Kennedy so that the latter would have to use American military force to rescue the Bay of Pigs invaders. Just how much Nixon knew about this scheme is hard to determine, but he seems to have had more than an inkling of what was going on. In addition, Nixon seems to have had some knowledge of the CIA's role in the murder of Mr. Kennedy. Again, how much he knew cannot be determined, but his later determination to down grade the CIA suggests that he possibly knew that the CIA was involved. Finally, Nixon knew some details about the plans to develop biological weapons, especially the two-pronged effort to develop the immune-compromising 'mycoplasma' of Robert

Huebner and the retroviral visna 'scrapie' of Bjorn Sigurdsson, which were essential components of the AIDS co-factors. This linkage can be safely assumed from the close links between Nixon and Roy Ash, one of the founders of Litton Industries, which as we have noted, acted as the industrial arm of the AIDS program conglomerate. It was Robert Ting of Litton who worked hand in glove with Robert Gallo of the National Cancer Institute in the scientific work that had to be done to achieve an understanding of the new microorganism which would be refractory to the human immune system, which Dr. MacArthur said was possible, all the time knowing that it had already been deployed.

This is a sketch of the mix of personal and public baggage that Nixon carried when he assumed office in January 1969. What was *added* to the 1968 existing 'mix' of the Rockefeller/CIA/Lyndon Johnson 'eugenics' programs, and industrial 'contract' corruption that had grown out of the early discovery of Dr. Robert Huebner that an unusual microorganism called the 'mycoplasma' could cause the spontaneous degeneration of certain living tissues (such as the adenoids) by the election of Nixon *was the fact that Henry Kissinger was named to the critical post of National Security Advisor to the President.*

This appointment of a Rockefeller apparat protégé meant that the whole enterprise of research into the potential use of the mycoplasma as a biological weapon was moved one step further from the covert CIA/Military/Rockefeller-establishment activities to the highest levels of the United States Government Administration bureaucracy, with Kissinger managing the whole enterprise on behalf of his masters, the Rockefeller apparat.

In the meantime, Kurt Vonnegut's public 'farting and tap dancing' of politics as usual went on in the United States while the on-going drive of the serious business to develop and deploy AIDS to the world had now become a main stream, although still covert, American enterprise. To keep that enterprise on track meant that the real powers behind the scenes had to keep the Central Intelligence Agency strong. Such a CIA role was, as we shall point out seriously threatened as Mr. Nixon began to find his feet and attempted to become his own man and not just a pawn of the power people. Protecting the CIA required the deposition of President Richard Nixon, just as it had required the murder of Mr. Kennedy. Hence: Watergate!

Here we present an alternative view of Watergate to weigh against the folk-myth of Carl Bernstein and Bob Woodward in their book: *All the President's Men*. As far as we can determine, no previous historical research analyst has identified the real reason behind Watergate. Yet, that reason is present for all to see if only they would look.

Aye! There's the rub isn't it? The truth is sitting there waiting for thinking people to recognize it, and that's the tough part, for who wants to think when we can read *All the President's Men* and view the movie over and over again on late night TV?

Add to such flashy disinformation the gobble-de-gook of the mainstream media and you get the world we are living in!

The Election of 1968 — Richard Nixon and AIDS

Shortly after Richard Nixon was sworn in as President, in January 1969, there was a secret meeting held in a room in the Congressional Buildings of Washington. The date was June 9, 1969. That date may well be seen as the most critical date in the history of AIDS or even as the most critical date in the history of humankind on earth for it was on this date that after all of the secret, publicly unwritten efforts of the Rockefeller apparat in particular and the eugenics crowd in general, to convert the scientific knowledge developed over the past four decades by Oswald Avery, the Henle's, Hilary Koprowski, Reinhardt Dietrich, Thomas Merigan, Robert Huebner, Robert Channock, and others that we have encountered thus far in our study into a workable biological weapon which would limit the rate of world population growth (especially in the vast, illiterate masses of Africa) and to make this cult doctrine of mass murder a critical part of United States deep political policy without the people of the United States knowing it, was finally and definitively placed on the written records of Congress.

June 9, 1969

Stop all the bullshit and all the ballyhoo. Turn to page 129 of the Minutes of that Meeting on June 9, 1969 and face up to the truth: AIDS was made in American laboratories! The crime beyond belief.

May the crime beyond belief someday finally be faced up to by humanity as the solid, incontrovertible evidence justifies and may *The New York Times* and the *Washington Post*, and *Time* magazine, and the Toronto *Globe and Mail* and International AIDS Conferences stop their Kurt Vonnegut 'farting and tap dancing' with silly stories about a green monkey biting a black woman who later had sex with a white airline steward who then 'gave it to the whole frontier', and may they say for all to hear: "Acquired Immune Deficiency Syndrome was conceived and carried through to deployment in the laboratories of the United States, and financed by the United States Government and by private interests who were part of the deep politics of America."

Let us now begin a careful analysis of this infamous page 129 from the U.S. Congressional Record. Start six lines down from the top of page 129:

> "…eminent biologists believe that within a period of 5 to 10 years it would be possible to produce a synthetic biological agent, an agent that does not naturally exist and for which no natural immunity could have been acquired."

There you have the first official description of the biological co-factors, which now present as a disease syndrome called AIDS. These co-factors, according to MacArthur, have not yet (*i.e.* in June of 1969) been 'synthetically' united as a new 'biological agent' but can be within 5 to 10 years.

We shall see that in this time frame of '5 to 10 years', MacArthur is lying, but first let's note what he has said, and then we'll get back to his lie. First, he refers to 'eminent biologists.'

Who are the eminent biologists to whom he refers? We suggest that this question can be answered with assurance by looking at the scientific, largely peer-reviewed literature and U.S. Government Documents which were published and by looking at just which scientific researchers and institutions were financed by U.S. Government agencies…including the Pentagon. When one searches such sources it becomes clear that the people we have listed in paragraph one of this section were the 'eminent biologists' who were being consulted and financed by the U.S. Government.

However, we do not have to speculate about this important point! The answer will be found in the records of the Pentagon.

In other words, if the Members of the House of Representatives (current or those to be elected at any point in the future, including November, 2008) want to know from their own written records and from the written records of the Department of Defense over which they constitutionally have control, just who it was that MacArthur depended upon for guidance in developing the tragic biological weapon known as AIDS, all they have to do is screw their courage to the sticking place and go after the answer. All the Congressmen have to do is to establish an "AIDS Committee" with the sweeping power of the people behind them, and go after the Truth!

But, back to this later. Let's continue our look at what MacArthur told the dozen Congressmen who were on the secret budget committee, which financed biological weapons research, on that critical day in June 1969.

Note that MacArthur refers to a 'synthetic' biological agent. That means it would have to be made in a laboratory and by being passaged in the bodies of research animals. (Actually it was already made and had long since been tested at places such as Huntsville Penitentiary in Texas, by Drs. Channock and Couch but MacArthur had his reasons for not telling the Congressmen.)

This is where the co-factors of the visna retrovirus of sheep and the mycoplasma immune system suppressant were united. The critical statement in MacArthur's presentation is this:

> "No natural immunity could have been acquired."

There it is: AIDS—Made in America to kill millions of people worldwide!

However, there appears to be some problem with the projected dates which MacArthur gives the Congressmen. Note, in the middle of the page, the following:

> "2. Within the next 5 to 10 years, it would probably be possible to make a new infective microorganism which could differ in certain important aspects from any known disease-causing organisms. Most important of these is that it might be refractory to the immunological and therapeutic processes upon which we depend to maintain our relative freedom from infectious disease."

Now, MacArthur is speaking on June 9, 1969. He is asking for a budget allowance to become payable in the fiscal year 1970. If the maximum projected period required for the development of this new microorganism is ten years, then it will not be until 1980 that the biological weapon described will be available.

Yet, we know from other sources, that the first official recognition of AIDS came in 1981 (along with the mirror-image disease, epidemic chronic fatigue syndrome). In the case of AIDS, with its visna virus (lentivirus, or retrovirus) component developed by Dr. Bjorn Sigurdsson for the Rockefeller apparat, an infection would not show on average for at least five years. That means it would have to have been deployed by a vaccine in at least 1975. The figures wouldn't fit.

How does one account for this anomaly?

Plain and simply, MacArthur was lying to the Congressmen.

The new microorganism had already been developed under Lyndon Johnson's administration and had been deployed first in Nigeria and later in other African nations receiving aid from the Agency for International Development. (Remember Johnson's boast that he had raised the money spent upon 'population control' from five million to $300 million during the period 1964 to 1968?) Johnson had test run the AIDS genocide, and then, with the help of Belgium and Portugal, and the World Health Organization, and under the direction of Johns-Hopkins School of Medicine Dr. Donald Henderson, and the Atlanta-based Centers for Disease Control had begun a world wide vaccination program against smallpox. But, the smallpox vaccine was laced with the new microorganism MacArthur described, and million of Black citizens of Africa were infected with the AIDS co-factors.

Why would MacArthur lie?

MacArthur had to lie because the program had gone ahead without even the black budget committee of the Congress knowing of it. Now that the Rockefeller apparat was firmly in power, with Henry Kissinger effectively in charge of the Military and the CIA. No need to make any great effort to obscure the reality...so MacArthur brings the concept into the official realm of Congressional oversight.

What does he achieve by this move at this time? Essentially, he helps create in the minds of the members of the Committee the impression when the epidemic hits that *they were guilty of the great crime against humanity*.

Finally, note the first two and a half lines of paragraph three of section four:

> "It is a highly controversial issue, and there are many who believe such research should not be undertaken lest it lead to yet another method of massive killing of large populations."

The Committee approved the requested budget of ten million dollars and AIDS was officially on the way, although it had actually been a part of the deep politics of United States biological weapons development since the administration of Dwight D. Eisenhower.

And the beauty of it for MacArthur and the DoD was that the Congressmen thought that they were the initiators…all the more reason to go along with massive cover-ups and mis-information in the years ahead.

A footnote to demonstrate that AIDS was already well under way can be seen in the fact we have already noted that Dr. Robert Merigan (and colleagues) of Stanford University, one of the institutions and one of the people involved in the whole process, wrote an article in 1971…Just one year after the budget request of MacArthur went into effect, titled: *Viral Diseases of Man and Acquired Immunological Deficiency States (AIDS)*!

Merigan later helped in the early cover-up of chronic fatigue syndrome. For a fuller account of this sister tragedy, see Hillary Johnson: *Osler's Web*.

At this point we must take a further look at Dr. MacArthur's phrase: 'no natural immunity could have been acquired.'

If one has no money, one has a deficiency of money. If one has no immunity to certain diseases, one has a deficiency of immunity; or, put another way: one has an 'immune deficiency'. Furthermore, note that MacArthur is speaking about a deficiency of an **acquired** immunity which according to Elgert (1996) is the immunity which… "develops during the host's lifetime and is based partly on the host's experience." (Page 7) That is, a human being starts off with a level of immunity against certain diseases but at some point there develops a deficiency of such a defence and that deficiency is something foist upon him. Thus, he is more readily disabled or killed.

If MacArthur's eminent biologists have told him that within '5 to 10' years they could have an agent that does not naturally exist, it would, of course, be one which they would have to engineer in their laboratories. And, it would be available between 1975 and 1980.

When was AIDS initially diagnosed in the United States?

And is it an agent for which no natural immunity could have been acquired?

Of course it was and is!

But, MacArthur has some other details for the peoples' representatives in Congress. He tells them that this new agent… "might be refractory to the immunological and therapeutic processes upon which we depend to maintain our relative freedom from infectious disease."

What infectious diseases might he be talking about?

Well, he could be referring to something like Kaposi's sarcoma, a disease affecting the skin and mucous membranes and was formerly limited to elderly men, especially in certain North African countries.

Or, he might be talking about *Pneumocystis carinii* pneumonia, which shows up in infected lung tissue as cysts, containing six or eight oval bodies, and that attacks especially the interstitium of the lungs with marked thickening of the alveolar septa and of the alveoli.

And, of course, he could be talking about *lymphadenopathy*, which was what Luc Montagnier found in the blood of an early AIDS victim. When Luc was studying his samples of blood from the AIDS victim, the virus-like particles that he spotted were like those that he in his experience as a leading microbiological researcher associated with lymphadenopathy. The latter is a disease characterized by the abnormal enlargement of the lymph nodes so Luc named his discovered particles "*Lymphadenopathy Associated Virus*" or "**LAV**." Thus the first acronym to be used to label what is now labeled as AIDS was LAV.

At this point, Luc Montagnier made a mistake. He sent a summary of what he had discovered to the American researcher, Robert Gallo. Gallo promptly used Montagnier's work to re-produce the LAV particle in his own lab and he re-named it HTLV-111, or Human T-Cell Leukemia Virus, third species.

If you haven't followed the above paragraph, here is what it means: Gallo had stolen Montagnier's intellectual property. Period.

Montagnier sued for damages.

Thanks to pressure from President Ronald Reagan, Gallo and Montagnier got together in a secret session wherein they agreed that *both* had discovered the disease agent which caused illness by lowering the victim's immune system. Furthermore, they would share in any profits to be made from this dramatic discovery, and Luc would drop his legal suit against Gallo. Later they agreed that the newly discovered organism should be called a Human Immunodeficiency Virus [HIV] and the LAV and HTLV-111 labels should be dropped.

To summarize to this point: In **1969** Dr. MacArthur of the U.S. Military biowar research folks, told some devious Congressmen that eminent biologists were almost ready with a new infectious organism which would be refractory to the human immune system. This new organism would make humans infected with it subject to diseases that they otherwise would have been able to fight off as part of their natural immune defence system. Diseases such as Kaposi's sarcoma; *Pneumoniae carinii pneumonia*; lymphadenopathy; and others.

Such a masterpiece of biological engineering could be ready between 1975 and 1980, if Congress approved. Well, Congress did approve and work by MacArthur's 'eminent biologists' continued with re-newed vigor. However, as you will have learned from the evidence that we have already presented, *MacArthur already had the new microorganism and it had already been used to infect thousands of people in Africa! MacArthur was just getting the Congressmen on side, and in the process, getting a boost in his budget.*

Then, in 1981 there appeared a new disease organism which Luc Montagnier of France called a Lymphadenopathy Associated Virus (LAV) and which when stolen from Montagnier by Robert Gallo, had been re-named a Human T-cell Leukemia Virus (HTLV-111) but which by agreement between Montagnier and Gallo became known as Human Immunodeficiency Virus (HIV) and which, it is now claimed, is the cause of AIDS.

We have already noted that AIDS, whether caused by LAV or HTLV-111 or HIV, and which presents as various opportunistic diseases such as described in chapter one, had turned up in the scientific literature ten years before it had been 'officially' announced in the article by Thomas Merigan and David Stevens already discussed.

Critical dates to remember:
>   1969: the Pentagon promises AIDS
>   1971: Merigan and Stevens write about AIDS
>   1981: AIDS announced to the world!

Take a moment to study this chronology:
1. The promise of AIDS (1969)
2. A reference to an AIDS-like condition in the medical literature (1971)
3. An article about signs and symptoms now common as AIDS indicators (1981).

Then ask yourself these questions: Is the AIDS that MacArthur promised Congress the same AIDS that by 2007 has already killed millions and is going to kill millions more? If it is, then ask: Were Merigan and Stevens's part of the group of 'eminent biologists' to whom MacArthur had referred? *In other words, were they and others already involved in the creation of the most deadly weapon of war ever devised by man? A crime beyond belief?*

We will take a closer look at Merigan and Stevens and the tantalizing article they wrote in 1971 in Chapter 23: The Scientific Paper Trail to AIDS.

In Chapter Two, discussing William Blum's important book, *Rogue State*, we promised to reveal what Mr. Blum had to say about AIDS. Here it is in *full* from page 156:

"A final thought…What if?"

On June 9, 1969, Dr. Donald M. MacArthur, Deputy Director, Research and Engineering, DoD, testified before Congress.

> "Within the next 5 to 10 years, it would probably be possible to make a new infective microorganism which could differ in certain important aspects from any known disease-causing organisms. Most important of these is that it might be refractory [resistant] to the immunological and therapeutic processes upon which we depend to maintain our relative freedom from infectious disease."

Well, we have an answer for Mr. Blum's question: '**What if?**'
The Answer: Acquired Immunodeficiency Syndrome — AIDS.

On 'June 9, 1969', almost exactly five months after Richard M. Nixon took office as the President of the United States, an important official in the Department of Defense is telling twelve key Congressmen that a microorganism that does not naturally exist, can be created in a laboratory and that this new pathogenic organism can by-pass the human defense system. AIDS!

Keep in mind that these Hearings are taking place in 1969, hence, any money voted by Congress will be spent in 1970 and then results will be reported (in secret or otherwise) in 1971. This chronology is important as will become evident shortly.

The two pages presented above, rank among the most important printed pages from all those pages that have, over time, recorded aspects of humanity's history on this earth, for the page numbered '129' puts into words the essence of the co-factors which between them present in human victims as 'acquired immunodeficiency syndrome', and the title page clearly establishes the role of the United States Government in launching the AIDS epidemic.

MacArthur is telling the Congressmen that a new organism, which can induce a deficiency of acquired immunity because it will be refractory to the immunological and therapeutic processes upon which humans depend to maintain a relative freedom from infectious diseases, and can thus allow any of many illnesses which ordinarily cannot have their way in a human body, to assault that body, can be manufactured in laboratories operated or controlled by the Department of Defense, and be available as a weapon of war.

A population control fanatic's dream pathogen. And here was the top man in the Pentagon bioweapons development hierarchy telling twelve elected members of the United States House of Representatives that they could have such a pathogen in 5 to 10 years if they would vote the necessary $10,000,000.

We now know from Dr. Leonard Horowitz's detective work, that the money was voted to Dr. MacArthur, and that the program got under way.

Or was it already well under way?

It is necessary to study page 129 carefully to answer that and certain other questions. By going back over the records that are available to us, many of which we have already presented...records that are cloaked in the mantle of 'scientific' or 'medical' research into deadly diseases such as pneumonia, cancer, leukemia, polio, and hepatitis, authorized and paid for by the Department of Defense and the American Public Health Agencies, the National Cancer Institute and the Centers for Disease Control, we will establish that the AIDS epidemic had its genesis in the minds of wealthy Americans who seized covert control of the U.S. Government during the Eisenhower Administration, then, following the assassination of John F. Kennedy, with the records hidden in plain sight, where no one would think of looking, advanced the research to deployment. First, let's ask some questions about page 129.

Line six of that page refers to 'eminent biologists.' As we have asked already, who were the eminent biologists who believed that the new 'synthetic biological agent' could be created?

Could one of them have been Dr. Robert Huebner who, some thirty years earlier had discovered that a microorganism called a mycoplasma could reduce the human immune system's functioning by causing the 'spontaneous degeneration' of lymphatic tissues?

The answer is 'Yes.' Dr. Robert Huebner was undoubtedly one of the eminent biologists whose counsel Dr. MacArthur had sought. After all, Huebner had started his move into the study of the mycoplasma (he called it a PPLO) while working with the United States Navy in the late 1940's. Furthermore, by 1969 he was well established at the Infectious Disease Institute. Then, a few months after MacArthur had received his $10 million from Congress, and Nixon had declared his 'great war on cancer', Huebner moved from the Infectious Disease Institute to the National Cancer Institute, where he was to work with Robert Gallo.

Now, if MacArthur has been in discussions with certain 'eminent biologists' about the laboratory creation of a new microorganism which would be refractory to the human immune system, and he is reporting on these discussions on June 9, 1969, *and* if (as they did) Congress secretly approves the expenditure of the $10 million to start in 1970, *the earliest report on progress would be in 1971.* That's the year that Nixon took the advice of Henry Kissinger and 'declared a great war on cancer'!

Furthermore, it seems self-evident that with the program approved and the money voted, MacArthur would get started in 1970 with the help of the people that he had been consulting. And that is just what he did. And the results of that 1970 work would be reported the *next year*, in 1971 that is. And again, that is just what happened: a Progress Report was issued in May, 1971, then up-dated a bit in July, then presented to the 'Annual Joint Working Conference, SVCP' at the Hershey Medical Center, on October 24 - 27, 1971.

An Interlude on the mechanics of AIDS and the research of: Rottem, Pfendt and Hayflick

An article in 1971 by Drs. Rottem, Pfendt and Hayflick requires special mention at this point since it demonstrates the mechanics of how one of the AIDS co-factors, a species of Mycoplasma works.

The authors are S. Rottem, E. A. Pfendt, and L. Hayflick. (It is important to know that as far back as 1962, Hayflick had been contracted by the NIH to establish a national Mycoplasma Laboratory. The significance of this will become apparent as our study develops).

> "T-strain mycoplasmas are very sensitive to digitonin, amphotericin B, and progesterone. This sensitivity and the relatively high content of cholesterol found in the cells indicated a possible requirement of T-strain mycoplasmas for sterols. This suspected requirement was demonstrated directly in a lipid-poor medium and *can be met by cholesterol.* [Emphasis added...authors]...Because of their sterol requirement and their unique requirement for urea, T-strain mycoplasmas might be classified as the third genus of the order *Mycoplasmatales.*"

Now, we know that this scientific data will not mean much to most of our readers, however, we feel that it is important to share the scientific underpinning of just how various mycoplasma species play a critical role in the activity of the mycoplasma as a co-factor in AIDS, and as the critical factor in chronic fatigue syndrome, fibromyalgia, rheumatoid arthritis, Parkinson's Disease, multiple sclerosis, diabetes type one and many other diseases.

What the article says (in plain street language) is this: The mycoplasma, patented by the U.S. Government, uptakes pre-formed sterols (including cholesterol!) from cells which it invades, and causes the cell membrane, made up of 25 percent cholesterol, to disintegrate. Thus, the infected cells cease to produce the enzymes they normally produce or otherwise cease to function as a healthy cell should. If the cells so destroyed, such as the beta cells in the pancreas or the substantia nigra cells in the brain stem, insulin or dopamine production is reduced or lost altogether and the diseases diabetes or Parkinson's will present. Not only that, but cholesterol supplies in the body will be reduced and the hormones which are manufactured by certain secretory glands, will be reduced, causing sexual impulse loss, or various body functions to be interrupted. Since the lymphoid tissues are particularly affected by this mycoplasmal effect upon cells, the immune system will be greatly reduced.

It is this loss of immune protection, which allows the visna retrovirus of sheep to enter the human body and as a co-factor with the mycoplasma, present as AIDS.

We cite Rottem, *et al.* only to demonstrate that there is a solid scientific basis for our conclusion that Pentagon-directed scientists created or engineered the new microorganism that Dr. MacArthur referred to on June 9, 1969. We cite many more critical scientific, peer-reviewed articles in Chapter 23: The Scientific Paper Trail to AIDS.

Evidence...stick to the evidence, which can be verified, not to Internet babbling.

End of an Interlude

North Atlantic Treaty Organization (NATO)— The CIA's Overseas Arm

At this point in our study we must draw attention to the North Atlantic Treaty Organization (NATO).

The North Atlantic Treaty Organization between the United States, Great Britain, Canada, the Netherlands, France and other neighbouring states was created in 1949 as what was promoted as a defensive alliance against the perceived aggressive intentions of the Soviet Union. France withdrew from the military side of the alliance in 1966.

With the collapse of the Soviet Union and the Warsaw Pact in the 1980s, the raison d'etre for NATO ceased to exist, but, instead of being dismembered in a move towards a less confrontational world order, the United States took the opportunity to convert NATO into an armed branch of the CIA, and the latter's hidden wars...now more and more blatant wars.

There had long been subtle links between the CIA- and the covert powers in the shadows of the United States—the Establishment—but after September 11, 2001, the subtlety gave way to direct action when the United States called upon NATO members to help it 'resist' terrorist aggression, and join in the invasion of Afghanistan.

Most NATO allies have responded to this totally spurious and criminal appeal, and under the guise of 'protecting' their ally (three hundred million population, armed-to-the-teeth Americans) from sixteen million Afghans who lack an Air Force, a Navy, and are very poorly armed, have joined in the attack. The criminality of the CIA has gone world-wide.

In respect to the 'subtle links' between NATO and the U.S. Establishment mentioned two paragraphs above, we draw attention to the fact that in 1970 Robert Gallo of the NCI reported to NATO on scientific work linked to the development of AIDS-like viruses:

> "Here was documented evidence that senior investigator Robert Gallo presented the methods and materials used to produce AIDS-like viruses before NATO military scientists at 'the NATO International Symposium on Uptake of Informative Molecules by Living Cells" in Mol, Belgium, in 1970."   (Horowitz; 1996, Page 72)

As we have said before, the criminality is of a piece. As we fit together the many and varied pieces of this study, it is more and more evident that Jackie Horowitz' intuitive speculation about a link between the murder of President John F. Kennedy and ..."the orders to develop AIDS-like viruses" is accurate.

National Security Study Memorandum - 200 (NSSM-200)

On December 10, 1974, Henry Kissinger submitted a commissioned study to President Richard Nixon of the effects of an increased growth rate of the world's population upon the economy and security of the United States, which he titled National Security Study Memorandum 200. (NSSM 200)

To quote from Horowitz' account of the Memorandum, Kissinger wrote:

> "…there is a major risk of severe damage to world economic, political, and ecological systems and, as these systems begin to fail…urban slum dwellers may serve as a volatile, violent force which threatens political stability."

He thus recommended these and other people in lesser developed nations be culled through a variety of methods involving the United States Agency for International Aid (USAID), the World bank, and other organizations serving to protect "our humanitarian values."

In other words: do something about the increasing rate of world population growth.

Now, if 'doing something' had actually already begun in 1952 when as we have seen, Eisenhower was elected President, and Nelson Rockefeller got his chance to apply the Rockefeller apparat's eugenics philosophy, why would Kissinger, a Rockefeller protégé, feel obliged to issue NSSM 200 in 1974?

The answer is logical: although the Establishment got things under way with MKULTRA, MKDELTA and MKNAOMI in 1953 and 1954, it had taken the intervening two decades to get AIDS fully developed and deployed. In fact, as we have shown in chapter thirteen it was 1966 before trials in countries being 'helped' had established their efficacy that the World Health Organization was brought fully into the operation and 1968 before Dr. Donald Henderson was placed in charge of the smallpox eradication (with AIDS co-factors included) program.

Kissinger knew that about 1975 to 1979 would see the first breaking of the AIDS epidemic worldwide, and by suggesting in 1974 that the U.S. should 'think about' what it should or could do, he was closing the door to the possibility of anticipated rumours that the epidemic had been engineered by the U.S.

"Look", he is saying, "in 1980 when AIDS hits, as we know it will after all of those millions of vaccinations, and if there is any suspicion or inadvertent hint that the disease is man-made, we can always point to NSSM-200 and say 'we had just got around to talking about the problem of over-population in 1974!'"

An Interlude on Crimes and Criminals

In Section One, Chapter One of this study, we parsed our title (*AIDS: The Crime Beyond Belief*) and there we defined a 'crime' as a purposeful act or failure to act in such a way as to deprive another person of generally accepted inherent rights.

We then undertook to establish that the intentional laboratory development, testing and deployment of a human immune suppressant pathogen was indeed a crime since it was designed and destined to deprive infected victims of their inherent right to life and health.

Over the fourteen chapters of this study to this point we have presented evidence to establish the fact that this crime had indeed been committed. We have presented medical, scientific, and political evidence to support our thesis. In this interlude we want to move specifically from the crime to those who have committed this 'crime beyond belief': the criminals.

In general terms we have already cited what we have variously referred to as the 'establishment' or the 'secret government' or the 'shadow government' or the 'Rockefeller apparat' as the principal criminal coterie that gave rise to, and continues to covertly promote, the crimes under review. Members of this coterie include Allen Dulles, John J. McCloy, William Casey, Richard Cheney and certain members of families such as the Rockefeller family and the Bush family.

In more specific terms there are those who act or have acted as the executive arm of the prime movers. These include people that we have already specifically looked at such as David Ferrie in chapter eleven.

In this Interlude we will develop in more detail two further criminal 'go-fors' upon whom the powers behind the crimes have depended to get the actual deeds done. The two are E. (Everett) Howard Hunt and Alexander M. (Meigs) Haig. After establishing their credentials for being identified as go-fors for the prime criminals we shall identify their sponsors specifically.

E. Howard Hunt: Foot Soldier in the Hidden War

A researcher into the role of E. Howard Hunt first encounters him in Korea in 1955. There he is a member of the North Asia Command of the Central Intelligence Agency. The CIA in turn, was involved in the covert use of biological weapons against the Chinese and the North Koreans.

The evidence available today is very convincing that, even though the use of such weapons was vigorously denied by the U.S. government and its media assets such as *The New York Times*, they were indeed being used, and E. Howard Hunt and his employer, the CIA, were part of the crime. And, although much is now known about these criminal actions, there are hints that there are even more crimes deeply hidden which have not yet come to light. We get a hint of them, however, when we read the White House Transcripts of the tapes Nixon had secretly recorded. On page 190 of the N.Y. Times edition of these tapes we read:

> **Dean**: 'Hunt has now sent a blackmail request directly to the White House.'
>
> **Ehrlichman**: 'That he would hurt the Eastern Asian Defence. Right there. That is blackmail.'
>
> **Haldeman**: 'For example, where does that take you? That takes you to your support, the other people who are not fully aware of the DC (probably 'District of Columbia') end of it. But then, we didn't know about it either.'"
> (Conversation between Nixon, Dean, Haldeman and Ehrlichman on March 21, 1973)

So what is the 'it' which would somehow compromise the U.S. and about which Hunt knows and will reveal to the world if he is not paid the one million dollars hush money he has demanded? Was it the use of some more dangerous and evil biological weapons in 'Eastern Asia' (*i.e.* Vietnam) that even the 'DC' component of government didn't know about? The conversation is enlightening, since Hunt's presence in Korea in 1955 was due to his role in the CIA's use of biological weapons. An inference that what he might tell the world had to do with biological weapons use in Vietnam is reasonable. And how about Haldeman's suggestion that the release of whatever secrets it is that Hunt is using would affect Nixon supporters who don't know whatever 'it' was? The inference is that Nixon would lose such support.

It is important to realize that at some level of power, the United States was engaged in covert and obviously immoral activities that were not known to the legal government, but were known to a person such as E. Howard Hunt! Who were those powers? Obviously they included Hunt's former employer, the CIA. And who was giving the CIA their marching orders? Orders which involved the Eastern Asian Defence? The source of marching orders has to be the 'establishment', or the 'secret government' by whatever name one wished to identify them.

But the most important implication in this conversation is that E. Howard Hunt in 1973 is still privy to top-secret information from the 'Eastern Asian Defence.' That is, he still has channels to the top of the CIA. And, although superficially working for the Richard Nixon White House, he is working at a deeper level for someone else! Who is signing his paychecks?

And here we must state our conclusion clearly: E. Howard Hunt is a foot-soldier in a hidden war. A war with many battles fought covertly from Korea to Guatemala, to Cuba, to Dealey Plaza to the 'Eastern Asian Defence' (Vietnam?) to the Watergate break-in. On the one side in this hidden war were and still are all those nations which stand in the way of the other side's imperialist ambitions to control the basis of modern wealth: oil and other raw resources. E. Howard Hunt had bosses in all of these undertakings and those bosses were the same whether in the Bay of Pigs or the Watergate break-in.

It is also critical to our present study to emphasize that Hunt's activities in Korea involved biological weapons, and that means that biological weapons had already been developed to the point where they were capable of deployment and were indeed being deployed despite all denials to the contrary.

The next time that E. Howard Hunt is noted in the pages of history is in the Spring of 1954 when the CIA is engaged in a 'major covert-action operation designed to remove the leftist president of Guatemala from power...' (Richelson; 2001, Page 31) Hunt is assigned a major role in this action which is clearly a crime under international law. This is, in other words, a hidden war which the establishment of the U.S. is waging through the agency of the CIA.

The success of the Guatemala operation won the admiration of Eisenhower, and encouraged the CIA to undertake an illegal invasion of Cuba. Always, however, without the overt hand of the U.S. being shown. Eisenhower had made it clear that he did not object to such criminal activities as long as the guilt could not be fixed upon the guilty.

That worked fine until Eisenhower himself was duped into the Cuban invasion. In 1959 he was encouraged to sign an authorization to land a group of armed Cuban ex-patriots in Cuba to foment a rebellion against Fidel Castro. Then, Eisenhower, ill and tired and at the end of his term as President, essentially phased himself out of the action, and Allen Dulles placed E. Howard Hunt in charge of a greatly enhanced Cuban invasion program. In place of the Eisenhower authorized 50 or 60 invaders, the CIA secretly recruited, trained and armed a Brigade of dis-placed Cubans. Nixon, who was running to succeed Eisenhower as President, knew what was going on, but his opponent, John F. Kennedy, did not.

After winning the election, Kennedy was assured that Eisenhower had authorized the invasion, and he reasoned that if a great war general such as Eisenhower thought the move was proper and that it would likely succeed, then he had to reluctantly agree.

Kennedy did not know that the plan as sold to Eisenhower required only 50 to 60 men. He also did not know that once the landing had begun, the CIA planners and their Establishment sponsors were confidant that U.S. forces (Marine, Army, Navy, and Air Force) would be landed in support of the Brigade. This scenario evidently had the agreement of Vice-President Nixon, but Kennedy had made it clear that he would not allow U.S. military involvement when he gave the go-ahead.

Kennedy had also been assured by the so-called 'intelligence gatherers' in the CIA that the people of Cuba would rise up in support of the U.S.-backed Brigade.

When the invasion at the Bay of Pigs failed miserably and thousands of pro-Castro supporters flocked to the beaches to repel the invaders, and Kennedy refused to be blackmailed or embarrassed into sending in the U.S. military, the essential insidiousness and stupidity of the CIA was revealed, Kennedy vowed to break the Agency into a 'thousand pieces and throw them to the wind.'

If the president broke up the CIA, the establishment would lose its secret army and would be unable to wage its secret wars against countries and ideologies that it wanted destroyed.

Allen Dulles and Richard Bissell were fired, but E. Howard Hunt managed to hide himself within the shelter of the CIA bureaucracy until November 22, 1963, when he turned up dressed as a tramp riding on a freight train leaving from behind Dealey Plaza in Dallas after Mr. Kennedy had been killed.

It is obvious that Hunt was involved in the assassination of President John F. Kennedy, but he was never charged with involvement because those who control the mechanics of Government in the United States take their directions from the powers in the shadows.

During the night of June 16, 1972 five men were arrested by Washington, D.C. police for illegal break and enter at the Watergate complex offices of the Democratic Party. The word 'Watergate' was now on the pages of U.S. political history. Address books were found on two of the burglars, and each book contained the name Howard E. Hunt, with notations of 'W. House' and 'W. H.'

A reporter for the *Washington Post*, Robert (Bob) Woodward tracked the name Howard Hunt to the White House, and then to a Washington public relations firm, Robert R. Mullen and Company. As Woodward and his partner, Carl Bernstein, later tell the story in their book, *All the President's Men*:

> "Woodward called the Mullen public-relations firm and asked for Howard Hunt.
>
> 'Howard Hunt here,' the voice said.
>
> Woodward identified himself.
>
> 'Yes? What is it?' Hunt sounded impatient.
>
> Woodward asked Hunt why his name and phone number were in the address books of two men arrested at the Watergate.
>
> 'Good God!' Howard Hunt said. Then he quickly added, 'In view that the matter is under adjudication, I have no comment,' and slammed down the phone."   (Page 24)

That, at any rate, is the way the call went according to the Watergate mythology, but there was a lot more to it than that. According to the mythology, Bernstein and Woodward were two diligent, determined investigative reporters just doing a superb job. Our research reveals that actually, Woodward was a plant at the *Washington Post* designed to remove Richard M. Nixon from the Presidency.

It had all started in 1969! Just months after Nixon had taken office as President. As told by Kathleen Woodward, Robert's first wife:

> "...Bob announced quite suddenly that he was taking a 'good assignment [that] involved this work at the White House.'...After Bob left, Kathleen remembers, 'I tried to visualize what he was doing in the basement of the White House.'" (Colodny and Gettlin; 1991, Page 80)

So, E. Howard Hunt was not alone in working in the basement of the White House! And both Woodward and Hunt knew another White House basement 'go-for' named Alexander Haig!

Just what was going on?

Clearly this: with Woodward's assignment to the office of Admiral Moorer with a job which involved frequent visits to the White House to deliver vital, courier only deliveries and occasionally to brief certain White House personnel on matters of extreme sensitivity, the Joint Chiefs of Staff had 'eyes' and 'ears' in the heart of the Nixon Administration. Nothing official, but an effective link to others who worked there.

As Fletcher Prouty described the kind of job Woodward had:

> "'...one of the most interesting and effective roles is that played by the behind-the-scenes, faceless, ubiquitous briefing officer who sees the important people 'almost daily'. Moreover, the briefer 'comes away day after day knowing more and more about the man he has been briefing and about what it is that the truly influential pressure groups at the center of authority are trying to tell these key decision makers.'" (*Ibid*, Page 83)

So, Robert Woodward in June 1972 is not a fresh-faced deep-digging investigative reporter for the *Washington Post* who just happened to become involved in the removal of Nixon from the

Presidency. But more of this later. In the meantime, how about the other person we spoke of above: Alexander M. Haig?

There's another story of double-cross and deceit in high places: Alexander M. Haig.

Haig got his start up the ladder of power when, as a mediocre graduate of West Point, he was sent to Tokyo as a first lieutenant at the end of 1948. There he did what many junior officers wished they could do: Haig married General Alonzo Fox' daughter Patricia.

General Fox, in turn, was deputy chief of staff to the supreme commander, Allied powers (SCAP), Douglas MacArthur. Soon Haig's new father-in-law managed to get Lt. Haig assigned to MacArthur's headquarters, where he had his first taste of the intrigue, plotting, scheming and other elements of the MacArthur command. As Roger Morris describes it:

> "Much of the seething in that 'vortex,' Haig neglected to recall, was the jealous, ceaseless jockeying and maneuvering of high-level aides around MacArthur, staff politics of the sort described in William Manchester's MacArthur biography American Caesar as 'more appropriate in Medicean Florence.' Ever competing in flattery as well as suspicion of SCAP's enemies in Washington and elsewhere, MacArthur's twin insatiable appetites, they poured it on,' said one eyewitness, 'and the general ate it up.' They were an uncommon group, these headquarters courtiers for and around whom the young Haig worked. Of those closest to MacArthur, one openly extolled military dictatorship, another lionized Franco and his Spanish dictatorship, while a third spied on his fellow staff officers." (Morris; 1982, Pp. 22-3)

In this cesspool of high command, as we noted earlier, many things were going on. MacArthur had double-crossed the Allied prisoners of war who had been used as biological weapons test subjects by Japanese Dr.-General, Ishii Shiro, and who had on his staff Major General Charles Willoughby who was later to figure in the assassination of President John F. Kennedy. (For more details on the role of Willoughby in the assassination see Dick Russell's The Man Who Knew too Much and Peter Dale Scott's Deep Politics and the Death of JFK.)

A series of adventures followed, but the point and time where we will now focus is February, 1962, when as a newly anointed Lt. Col. he was (in Morris' words) 'assigned…to a staff job in the murky reaches of the Pentagon.' (Page 58) It is important to note that Haig entered the Pentagon as a Lt. Col. whose job evolved in to being that of a 'courier' along the lines of the 'briefer' role of Bob Woodward a few years later, leading up to Watergate. That is, Haig took oral messages from one of the Chiefs of Staff to others in comparable roles and carried their response back to their source. Nothing was put on paper and only one man…Haig…officially knew what was being hatched. Haig probably shared his covert knowledge with his father-in-law, Alonzo Fox, who probably shared it with his fellow general, Charles Willoughby, who we have reason to believe shared it with General Douglas MacArthur (retired) and a small circle of other top military brass. And just what secret messages flowed among the joint chiefs and a few inner sanctum former Tokyo alumni? It is our opinion that Haig was the channel of communication in the Pentagon for those who were involved to various degrees with the CIA planning to assassinate President John F. Kennedy.

And what was to be Haig's reward for this insidious but crucial role? Knowledge. Haig knew of enough incriminating crimes in high places (including the staging of a *coup d'etat* on November 22, 1963) to ensure that he would rise through the ranks from message-carrying Lt. Col. to four star general in a dramatically short period of time. But, before this rapid rise had been achieved, it helped him in December 1968, when the newly-elected President, Richard Nixon, introduced his new national security adviser, Henry Kissinger. It helped because Kissinger would shortly phone Alexander Haig and 'magically' summon him to the inner sanctum of the White House.

How would Kissinger know of the obscure colonel?

Kissinger was a part of the Nelson Rockefeller 'loop', cited above. From the Watergate tapes: Nixon asks Dean: "From Hoover to Coyne to Rockefeller to Kissinger. Right?" (*White House Transcripts - N.Y. Times Edition*, Page 83)

Thus, shortly after Richard Nixon took office, the U.S. military had Bob Woodward in the White House basement; the Rockefeller apparat had Kissinger and Alexander Haig there as well; and, the CIA had E. Howard Hunt there on the White House payroll.

When it became evident to the establishment that Nixon had to go…he had let down the Seven Sister's oil coalition as represented by John J. McCloy (who you will recall, served to frame Lee Harvey Oswald) by reducing their depletion allowance; he was taking steps to pare down the CIA; he was largely ignoring the Joint Chiefs of Staff; and he was investigating the role of drug smuggling by the CIA…everything was in place to burglar the Watergate office of the Democratic Party, sabotage that effort, and hang E. Howard Hunt out to dry.

Then the *Washington Post*, which had by now hired Robert Woodward as a 'reporter', was able to assign the latter to the Watergate break-in story. Woodward, in turn, had a secret source he would only identify as 'Deep Throat' who was in a position to provide information from inside the White House. It turned out that Deep Throat was actually FBI Assistant Director, Mark Felt. And, as Nixon's presidency was essentially destroyed, Alexander Haig was in place to keep the office functioning.

Before too long, Nixon was retired in California (interestingly enough for an unindicted co-conspirator, on a United States Government pension recommended to Congress by Ford, while the other conspirators sat in jail); Gerald Ford…a CIA 'go-for'…was President; Nelson Rockefeller was Vice-President; Woodward was a 'famous' reporter; and Haig became the Supreme commander on the North American Treaty Organization, and E. Howard Hunt was also in jail.

So, who was in charge of all of this? Certainly not Nixon who had no idea what was happening to his administration. Certainly not E. Howard Hunt who had dutifully recruited some Bay of Pigs survivors to break into the Watergate. The obvious powers in the shadows, including Nelson Rockefeller and John J. McCloy and others of the establishment, were in charge and the foot soldiers, such as E. Howard Hunt, Alexander Haig and Robert Woodward, carried out their orders.

And it was the establishment powers in the shadows that had sponsored the Bay of Pigs and had murdered John F. Kennedy and had developed, tested and deployed the pathogenic co-factors that present as AIDS and kills 8,000 people a day. And although the results of the Establishment planning are to be seen in all manner of evil acts, it takes people like E. Howard Hunt, Tracy Barnes and Alexander Haig to get the jobs done.

End of an Interlude

The Election of 1972 — Watergate

> "The analogy of Watergate is helpful here: the Erwin Committee, *though it never fully established the reasons for the original Watergate break-in*, was able from documentary evidence to expose many of the principals in the ensuing conspiracy to cover up. By focusing on some initially technical details, we can pick up a trail that leads to the conspiratorial involvement of army intelligence, not just in the cover-up, but in the circumstances surrounding the assassination itself."
> Peter Dale Scott: *Deep Politics and the Death of JFK*, Page 267

> "There is a principle, which is proof against all argument, and which cannot fail to keep a man in everlasting ignorance. That principle is: 'Condemnation before Investigation.'"
> H. Spencer

Peter Dale Scott's masterful study of the assassination of President John F. Kennedy, *Deep Politics and the Death of JFK*, does something most such studies fail to do, it draws attention to the wealth of evidence which exists that demonstrates that the narcotics trade in the United States was not in the 1960s (and, as we shall establish, continues to this day) just an activity of Mafia-linked criminals, but that it is an essential part of the functioning of the Central Intelligence Agency, other American intelligence agencies, and the U.S. Defense Establishment, as well as the functioning of organized crime. Dr. Scott devotes parts of four chapters of his book to this aspect of the President's assassination and cover-up. (i.e.: chapter 8: 'Ruby and Narcotics: the Heart of What Was Suppressed') He also shows how the Justice Department of the United States participated in that cover-up, even when such cover-up allowed the murderers of Mr. Kennedy to go unpunished.

In addition to the important theme of mob/CIA/Justice Department/military/establishment collusion in the all-pervasive U.S. drug trade, Scott also presents evidence that many of the people, who were involved in the murder of President Kennedy, were also involved later in the Watergate break-in and the removal of Richard Nixon from the office of President. Chief among these people was E. Howard Hunt, who as we have seen, was arrested, but never charged, booked or finger-printed, in Dealey Plaza, Dallas, minutes after the murder of the president. The late John Kenneth Galbraith has suggested that Hunt and his ilk were 'luminously insane'. If not insane, Hunt was at the least a bungler and this is seen in the fact that not only was he arrested in Dallas, but he was also one of the chief 'planners of the Bay of Pigs' fiasco, and later, while casing the Watergate prior to the botched break-in, he managed at one point, to get himself locked in one of the Watergate banquet halls overnight. He had to remain locked therein until morning when someone opened the place up and he was able to sheepishly exit. (Bruce Oudes: *Richard Nixon's Secret Files,* Page xi)

Bernstein and Woodward's imaginative tale of Watergate, *All the President's Men,* is to the historic break-in of the Democratic Party's National Committee Headquarters in Washington, D.C., what the *Warren Commission Report* is to the assassination of President John F. Kennedy: it is the official myth about a historic event which *appears* to answer questions.

But the fact is that both the *Warren Report* and *All the President's Men* are still just myths: fanciful tales where certain facts are strung together to the exclusion of other critical facts to create an easily told fiction that hides the truth.

Fortunately, The *Warren Report* myth was significantly corrected by Oliver Stone's movie, JFK. Unfortunately, *All the President's Men,* was itself presented as a movie with attractive actors playing the parts of intrepid reporters searching for the truth. Both the book and the movie were received with popular and critical acclaim, thus the myth was converted to folklore and Richard Nixon emerges as 'tricky Dicky' who planned a cheap burglary and got caught.

End of story.

Or is it?

It is not. Let's set the record straight.

In chapter one of *All the President's Men*, Bernstein and Woodward tell a truth and then that truth is dropped from sight, never to be referred to again by mythmakers Bernstein and Woodward. What is that 'truth' and why would it be dropped down the Orwellian memory-hole?

The **truth** to which we refer occurs at the top of page 25 of the 1974 hard cover edition of *All the President's Men* written by Carl Bernstein and Bob Woodward and published by Simon and Schuster, New York. Here is the paragraph with the critical words in italics:

> "An hour later, Clawson called back to say that Hunt had worked as a White House consultant on declassification of the Pentagon Papers and, more recently, on a *narcotics intelligence project*. Hunt had last been paid as a consultant on March 29 (1972- Ed.) he said, and had not done any work for the White House since."

There it is: 'a *narcotics* intelligence project'. Mentioned...then dropped from their book by Bernstein and Woodward for good.

There isn't even a reference to this 'project' in the Index of their book. Nor is there any reference to heroin or cocaine or the Drug Enforcement Agency. Nothing more about narcotics! The whole book focuses upon the break-in of the Democratic National Committee's offices in the Watergate complex in Washington, D.C. on the evening of June 16, 1972, and Nixon's heavy-handed, bungling efforts to cover-up the relatively innocuous crime.

Should there have been some reference to just what 'a narcotics intelligence project' consisted of and why E. Howard Hunt had been hired to participate in that project?

It is the view of the authors that this narcotics intelligence project was the crux of not only the break-in of the Watergate but of the deposition of Richard M. Nixon as President of the United States, just as the narcotics trade, as Prof. Scott has shown, was a critical factor in the cover-up following the murder of Mr. Kennedy.

Furthermore, it is our belief, supported by the research that we have done into the whole affair, which Bernstein and Woodward intentionally left out any further references to the matter in the next 300 pages of their book. It is a further example of the critical significance of what Peter Dale Scott has referred to as a 'negative template.' That is: pay more attention to the things that are hidden from view or are not reported than to the things that are shown if you want to find the truth. Especially the truth about the discovery, development, and deployment of the co-factors that present as AIDS and the truth about why this great crime was a factor in the murder of one president and the deposition of another.

Bernstein and Woodward are 'media assets' who tell you what the powers in the shadows want you to believe and they don't report what you need to know if you are to learn the truth about the murder of one president and the deposition of another. Let's look at what they have left out of their critically acclaimed book and movie.

We'll start with a Memo written by H.R. Haldeman on behalf of President Nixon on September 22, 1969:

September 22, 1969

TO: Mr. Ehrlichman
Attorney General Mitchell
Dr. Kissinger
Secretary Richardson (in Rogers' absence)

FROM: The President

I feel very strongly that we have to tackle the heroin problem regardless of the foreign policy consequences. I understand the major problem is with Turkey, and to a lesser extent with France and with Italy.
In any event, I want the group included in this memorandum to give me a recommendation as to what we can do.

HRH 228
(Oudes: *Richard Nixon's Secret Files*, Page 51)

This is a very critical *Memo* for many reasons, some of which are: (1) it was written in 1969, just eight months after Nixon was sworn into office; (2) it is a working *Memo*, not a statement designed for public consumption; (3) it reflects a tremendous Nixon naivete about the role of narcotics in the deep politics of America, especially the role of the CIA as later revealed by Peter Dale Scott. (Admittedly, it is a *naiveté* that would have been shared by practically all Americans of the day, but one would assume that the man who had been Vice-President for eight years, and who had worked, at least peripherally, with the CIA planners of the Bay of Pigs would know about. The fact that he apparently did not know suggests just how far 'out of the loop' he functioned in respect to the real power-people of the United States.)

Nixon was a loner.

Nixon, in the earliest days of his administration, wanted to do something about the drug problem in America, especially the growing problem in the U.S. Military. Stephen Ambrose, in his biography of the President, notes on page 371 of Volume Two that some 40,000 U.S. soldiers out of 400,000 in Vietnam, were heroin addicts!

In the above Memo that we are considering, Nixon specifies, 'heroin' from Turkey, France and Italy. He apparently isn't aware of the heroin from Afghanistan and Vietnam, nor the cocaine from Colombia. In other words, his sources, whatever they were, had given him only the shallowest of briefings. But, by wanting to do something about even this limited part of the 'drug problem', Nixon *was unwittingly wanting to do something about cutting off the life-blood of the CIA* (If we accept Professor Peter Dale Scott's careful, well-documented evidence that the narcotics trade not only kept the mob going, but it was an essential part of the financial under-pinning of the CIA. Another essential part of such intelligence financing includes large-scale fraud such as the Savings and Loan scandal and the Bre-X scandal, which we will examine.)

A Brief Interlude on Central Intelligence Agency Finance

At this point we must pause to clarify the role of the CIA in drug running, the savings and loan industry scandal (in the mid 1980s), the collapse of Bre-X (in the late 1970s) as well as other huge financial fraud cases where vast sums disappear yet no one seems to know to whom they have gone.

Briefly we advance the following theory based upon our research.

Initially, when the CIA was signed into law by President Truman, he apparently believed what he had been told about the rational for such as agency: it would draw together foreign intelligence from the numerous intelligence agencies operated by the Navy, the Army, the Air Force, the State Department, and others. Then, the collected and rationalized intelligence would be used by the President to reach decisions on foreign policy questions. There was to be **NO** domestic involvement of the new Agency. Its modest budget was to be fractioned off that of the Department of Defense.

That, at any rate, was what Truman appears to have been told by advocates such as John J. McCloy, William Donovan, Nelson Rockefeller, Allan Dulles and others.

The truth is now evident. Actually, the CIA was to be the secret military arm of what Eisenhower came to label (albeit with the help of his speech writers) the 'military-industrial complex', or what Nixon called 'the secret government', or what others prefer to call 'the Establishment', and which we have now come to identify as 'the deep politics of America.'

In or out of office, this shadowy power structure had foreign policy and financial goals which were its own and which it wanted to advance by all possible means. Sometimes, those means corresponded with official, U.S. Government policy. At other times the latter had one set of announced goals, while the power behind the scenes (by whatever label you wish to identify it) had other goals. Thus, it was necessary that the secret arm have sources of finance beyond the whims of an elected body which was subject to change. Thus, it was necessary that the money officially voted to the Agency by Congress (See above: **June 9, 1969**) through the 'Black Budget' committee be complemented by the freest of free enterprise activities, including drug running, bank looting, industrial fraud, etc.

This whole enterprise seems to have got under way in late 1945 when Allan Dulles (then of the OSS) together with the help of the United States Navy and the Treasury Department found and surreptitiously incorporated Nazi 'Gehlen' gold into their own resources. Part of the spoils were divided with the founding state of Israel to permit its purchase of modern arms. The other part was used to influence politics in Italy and to finance a secret war on communists.

Allies in the Mafia, some recently deported to Sicily, were used to help move into the drug trade.

Then, as the secret government decided to replace the flagging powers of France in Vietnam, the CIA began drug trading in a major way.

However, even the Black Budget money from Congress and the drug money from East Asia would prove too little for the growing ambitions of the CIA and it was necessary to co-operate with the New York financial barons in huge fraudulent ventures such as the looting of the Savings and Loans industry and the Bre-X scandal to find ways to supplement their budget.

More of this, when we consider the terms of Ronald Reagan and George Herbert Walker Bush as Presidents.

End of an Interlude on CIA Financing/Drug Running

In addition to the Memo cited above about Nixon's desire to do something about the drug trafficking, which was an important illicit source of CIA finance, there are even more dramatic Memos in the Nixon library, some of which are presented by Bruce Oudes (cited above). One of the most critical of these is dated May 18, 1972, and was sent from Nixon to Bob Haldeman(Pages 448-9 of Oudes). The Memo includes the following, "I want a study made immediately as to how many people in CIA could be removed by Presidential action…I want action begun immediately…for a reduction in force of all positions in the CIA of 50 percent…"

That Memo and subsequent Memos and actions sealed Nixon's fate and started his removal from office. He was on the same track that Mr. John F. Kennedy had been on when the latter vowed to break up the CIA into a thousand pieces and throw those pieces to the wind.

Nixon was going to reduce the CIA and he was going to purge it of existing Ivy-league aristocrats. Unfortunately, Nixon shared his intentions with Henry Kissinger, and hence with the deep politicians and thus began Nixon's rush to the door!

There was another reason that Nixon was marked for removal from office and that reason can be summarized in one word: oil.

During his first term in office, Nixon had grown increasingly independent of what Anthony Sampson called, *The Seven Sisters*, the great oil companies and the world they shaped. In his book, Sampson writes:

> "…The oil companies, while trying hard to change U.S. foreign policy, were faced with a heavy disappointment: most of all after the inauguration of President Nixon in 1969."

> "Nixon had always been regarded as a likely friend of the oil companies…But soon after his election, Nixon agreed to the reduction of the depletion allowance from 27.5 to 22 percent." (Sampson, 1975 Page 245)

The seven sisters were represented by John J. McCloy, himself described by Sampson as '…part of that discreet *"supragovernment"* which remains while Presidents come and go.' (*Ibid*, Page 1980)

The 'supragovernment' that Sampson speaks about is the 'shadow government' that we noted in Chapter Nine of this study, and is another name for the 'establishment' that Nixon identifies as the force that was trying to destroy his presidency in his March 13, 1973 conversation with John Dean. (*White House Transcripts*, Page 120) Nixon probably had no idea just how right he was and just how powerful that 'establishment' was.

Thus, Nixon's early struggle with the oil interests followed by his plans to reduce the CIA substantially sealed his fate. He had to go.

Cut off CIA illicit drug financing and purge the Ivy-leaguers! Not if they struck first and they did. First of all, though, they had to get rid of Spiro Agnew who would succeed Nixon if the latter were turfed. They needed a Gerald Ford in the line of succession…so a number of people were put to work to protect the CIA. Frame Spiro Agnew and get him to resign, then stage the Watergate break-in and replace Nixon with someone more pliant.

1975: Exit Agnew and Nixon…Stage Right

We do not have the space to detail Spiro Agnew's departure from the vice-presidency, nor are those details relevant to our major thesis. Enough it is to say that powers in the shadows framed him and using Alexander Haig as the hatchet man, gave him no choice but to leave.

Agnew himself expressed it this way:

> "It is possible that I lost not only the vice-presidency, but the presidency. For if I had carried on my battle for vindication through the impeachment process and the courts, I would still have been Vice-President at the time Nixon resigned. If he had resigned, I would have become President. This was the one event, as I have stressed, which Richardson was determined to prevent no matter what happened."

> "[Nixon's] enemies had to get rid of me first, then move a malleable man into the vice-presidency (Gerald Ford admirably filled the bill), then shove Nixon out and Ford in." (Agnew, 1980 Pp. 202-3)

As important as the fact that Gerald Ford (who, like McCloy, had been a Warren Commissioner) was the fact that the new Vice-President of the United States was Nelson Rockefeller! (See Ch. 16)

Chapter Sixteen

GERALD FORD

Pardon?

Gerald Ford's main *raison d'etre* in history was to act as a safe way for the deep political powers of the United States to get rid of Richard Nixon, who, as we have seen, was threatening the overt political arm of the deep politics, the Central Intelligence Agency. The threat was two-fold: first, Nixon, as we have seen, naively wanted to act against the drug trade in the United States, little realizing that the drug trade was one source of the life blood of the Agency; and, second, Nixon was moving to cut the CIA in half, and any replacements for those deposed, would be from outside the 'Eastern Ivy League School Establishment.' Nixon seemed to understand intuitively, that this clique was the source of much of his trouble.

When it became obvious that Spiro Agnew was on his way out, and that his replacement would soon be President of the U.S., a very safe Vice-President had to be found. One who was to be counted on by the Establishment, and at the same time, someone who Nixon could manipulate to save himself.

The ideal person for the job was Gerald Ford. Bland, apparently clean, devious, an early ally of Nixon, and, perhaps the most important feature of the man was the fact that he was completely trusted by the power people. An early list of Congressmen that the CIA wanted to have re-elected in an early campaign was none other than Gerald Ford. The choice of Ford as the front runner for this honor reflects how loyal he was behind the scenes to the FBI (he had acted as J. Edgar Hoover's conduit to the Warren Commission) and had always supported the Rockefeller apparat's CIA initiatives.

Ford had been elected to Congress with Nixon, and had soon tied himself closely to Nixon's entourage of unprincipled neophyte

Congressmen who were in search of a leader to give their group some cohesion. Nixon rose to the occasion and obviously earned Ford's loyalty.

Thus, with Agnew gone and a successor needed who met the dual qualities noted above, Nixon settled on Ford. Later, as impeachment loomed, Nixon extracted a promise from Ford that the latter would pardon the former in return for Nixon's early resignation without a constitutional crisis.

There were other considerations, such as Presidential pension rights, but these were secondary. The main factor was Ford would pardon Nixon for all crimes and misdemeanors known and still to be discovered.

Ford did the job, and so sacrificed the good will his initial appointment had generated.

NELSON ROCKEFELLER

From the CIA basement to the Oval Office by Proxy
Revealing CIA Mis-deeds

With Vice-President Ford established as President of the United States, it was time to select a 'safe' vice-president. Who better for the job that Nelson Rockefeller, former Assistant Secretary of HEW and later special consultant on CIA activities under President Eisenhower?

Rockefeller wanted the job for several reasons. First, he apparently felt that since Ford had said that he would not run for President when his appointed time was up, the way was open for a Rockefeller run for the White House. Of course, Ford, as insidious as ever, changed his mind about running, but that it not of concern here.

Another reason Rockefeller sought the job (needed it in fact!) was that following Watergate there was a great clamor in Washington for everybody to investigate everything…including the CIA. Since Rockefeller had been the initiator of so much of the evil whose odors seeped through the Halls of Congress and around the world, someone very, very dependable, discreet and knowing had to do the job. Rockefeller would investigate the CIA 'excesses'. To do the job, Rockefeller persuaded Ford to appoint several other insidious gangsters such as Gen. Lyman Lemnitzer to the Commission. He rounded the group off with right wing ideologues such as Ronald Reagan.

When Ford was asked why his 'Rockefeller' Commission had so many right wing, shadowy military/intelligence members on it, he replied in a private off-the-cuff answer that it was to make sure no embarrassing questions were asked. When asked what subjects he meant by 'embarrassing subjects', he replied 'Assassinations for example.'

Rockefeller did the job, and by hanging out some totally unexpected dirty laundry he caught his critics off guard with the 'Rockefeller Report on CIA Excesses' and so took the edge off demands for an even more rigorous investigation of CIA mis-deeds.

As with the Warren Commission, appoint the main gangsters to investigate a crime if you want to cover it up!

By the time the next election rolled around in 1976, Rockefeller had shot his bolt; Ford had decided to run, but the odor of the Presidential pardon reeked through the land. The electorate in disgust turned to an earnest, highly moral, fresh-faced, smiling candidate from Georgia, and Jimmy Carter was elected President. But he committed a grievous error right at the outset and was soon removed from the scene by the power people.

JIMMY CARTER

Jimmy Carter managed to defeat Gerald Ford because the latter had pardoned Richard Nixon for all crimes, presently known, and any which might subsequently come to light, following the Watergate break-in. Although Ford had been greeted by the public for the apparently refreshing move away from 'the old style of politics' only a few months before, the pardon took much of the luster from his candidacy.

In the first months of his administration, Carter won approval for his down to earth approach, returning for example to the Franklin Roosevelt style 'Fireside Chats' wearing a sweater instead of a business suit and tie.

In terms of real life politics, however, he early on sealed his fate when he charged his newly appointed Director of the CIA, Admiral

Stansfield Turner, with the task of investigating programs engaged in by the CIA between 12 and 25 years earlier. (These time frame limits were specified by Senator Daniel Inouye when he called the first meeting of a joint Hearing by the Senate Select Committees on Intelligence and Human Resources to order on August 3, 1977.) That is, programs dating from 1952 (the year that Eisenhower began his presidency) to 1965 (the year that the Special Virus Leukemia/Lymphoma program was launched under Lyndon Johnson.)

The main interest of the joint committees was the institution and activities of three particular CIA programs that we have already noted at several points in this study. The programs were code named MKULTRA, MKNAOMI and MKDELTA. Interest in these programs had been heightened by the fact that the CIA records had been shredded and burned by Dr. Sidney Gottlieb on orders of CIA Director, Richard Helms. After his appointment as CIA Director, Admiral Turner had ordered that all CIA files were to be reviewed to determine whether any records had been missed by Dr. Gottlieb in the latter's efforts to conceal what had gone on from 1952 to 1965.

The search turned up 64 pages of what had been thousands of pages of information about what the MK programs were all about. The 64 pages were published in August 1977 as pages 103 to 167 of a 171-page report of the above referenced Senate Hearing. We will look more closely at those salvaged pages later. In the meantime we will summarize President Carter's four years in office. Those four years can be boiled down to this: fifty-two American employees in the Embassy at Tehran held hostage from early November, 1979 until half an hour after Carter's successor, Ronald Reagan was sworn in as President. As Bob Woodward has expressed it: the hostages "in Tehran had sunk Jimmy Carter's presidency." (Woodward, 1987 Page 23)

The seizure of the hostages had seemed to catch Mr. Carter totally off guard. He had been given little or no indication from the CIA that such an eventuality was about to come to pass as he went about his job as president, spiced up by headlines about the misdeeds of the CIA 12 to 25 years before. At the same time, Admiral Turner was busy paring down the CIA, reducing its strength significantly. At last, the goals of both John F. Kennedy and Richard Nixon to see the CIA drastically reduced were coming to pass.

And then it hit. Student-led activists attacked the U.S. Embassy in Tehran and the hostages were seized. Carter was immobilized and the investigations into the CIA faded from view. A terribly planned attempt at rescue was a total failure, resulting in the deaths of several American special operations personnel and further emphasizing Mr. Carter's impotence.

Woodward, cited above, asks:

> "Could American intelligence have failed as badly as DIA chief Tighe said? (Tighe had said that Iran was 'a ghastly intelligence failure') (Woodward, 1987 P. 101) How had the CIA missed the precariousness of the shah's position, his physical condition, his utter weakness?"
>
> (Woodward, 1987 Page 108)

Our research over the past twelve years now leads us to the conclusion that the CIA had not missed any of this. As with intelligence from Vietnam to President Kennedy, so intelligence from Iran to President Carter was purposefully corrupted. The CIA had taken a lead role in the murder of Mr. Kennedy, and they took a lead role in the Watergate break-in and the sabotage of that break-in and subsequent removal of Mr. Nixon from office and they flanked Mr. Carter's attempts to curtail their activities by letting the Iranian threat come to pass.

Mr. Carter, like John F. Kennedy and Richard Nixon, had been out to clip the wings of the CIA and the CIA had murdered Mr. Kennedy, deposed Richard Nixon and toppled Jimmy Carter from office. The secret army of the establishment was not to be tampered with.

BACK TO MKULTRA

In chapter two we looked at some of the details of MKULTRA, MKNAOMI, and MKDELTA as revealed by Stansfield Turner in 1978. Here we will cite a few further details that support our hypothesis that these three programs were all principally designed to develop, test, and deploy to the extent possible, biological agents. Of course, we suggest that the best evidence of these evil plans lies in the fact that Richard Helms ordered all records destroyed by Dr. Sidney Gottlieb before they could be examined by Congressional or other investigators.

There are those who say that because the records are destroyed, we have no right to accuse the CIA of such a crime beyond belief. We have already acknowledged our high regard for the English common law tradition that a person is innocent of a crime until he is proven guilty. But here we draw the line. The CIA destroyed the evidence and we are therefore entitled to assume that they did so because the evidence would have proven their guilt in a program to murder millions of people with biologically engineered pathogens, based upon the mycoplasmal co-factor and the sheep retrovirus, visna.

Now we will present and comment briefly upon a series of quotations from the MKULTRA report of August 3, 1977. In presenting these we want to alert you to the likelihood that even though the information is more up front than many documents, it is still subtly misinformative. We have already mentioned this earlier (Ch. 1) but must repeat the warning. For example, the report's title is "Project MKULTRA - The CIA's Program of Research in *Behavioral Modification*."

Note the reference to 'behavioral modification'. It is pure red herring. There is little evidence, as we develop below, that behavioral modification had anything worth mentioning to do with what actually went on. The actual goal was to follow up on the promise of biological weapons presented by the mycoplasma of Dr. Huebner and the retrovirus of Dr. Bjorn Sigurdsson. For convenience, we number the quotations, followed by the page number from the Report, then present the quote followed by our comment.

1. Page 5: "...there are 149 MKULTRA subprojects" To give the reader some idea of the scope of CIA activities…149 subprojects allows plenty of room for the wide range of research conducted during the 1952 to 1964 time frame.
2. 6. "Under CIA's Project MKNAOMI the Army assisted CIA in developing, testing, and maintaining biological agents and delivery systems for use against humans as well as against animals and crops." This quote clearly establishes the Army/CIA linkage and must be kept in mind when one reviews the scientific paper trail to AIDS in Chapter 23 below. It must also be kept in mind when one recalls Cuban complaints of that time period when over- flights of Cuba by unidentified aircraft were followed by outbreaks of animal diseases such as African swine fever.

3. 6."...researchers and institutions associated either on a witting or unwitting basis with MKULTRA activities." Note the fact that a number of research projects were conducted without the researchers realizing that their particular assignment fitted in to other witting research. The work was highly compartmentalized so that the ultimate product of such work (i.e. disease co-factors presenting as AIDS) was known to only a small number of people such as Richard Helms and Sidney Gottlieb.
4. 7."The institutions include 44 colleges and universities, 15 research foundations...12 hospitals...and 3 penal institutions."This quote emphasizes the scope of the work required to develop, test and deploy biological weapons.
5. 8."MKULTRA, a project which took place from 1953 to 1964" Note that the work began on Eisenhower's watch and continued on Lyndon Johnson's watch.
6. 11."...there are three subprojects on activities whose nature simply cannot be determined." Consider how sensitive such projects were! They were secret subprojects within a secret project within a secret intelligence agency! Just what evil was so great that it had to be hidden to this extent?
7. 14."To my knowledge, there was no Presidential knowledge of this project at the time." This means that from 1953 to 1964 there was no Presidential knowledge, meaning that Eisenhower and Kennedy at least did not know what the army and CIA were up to. However, after the MK projects were terminated in 1964, there suddenly sprang into being in 1965 the SVLP under Lyndon Johnson. In other words, Johnson was a witting participant behind the back of President Kennedy.
8. 16."...there are perhaps any numbers of Americans who are walking around today...with all kinds of physical and psychological damage....it is significant and severe indeed." The unwitting subjects of tests conducted upon American citizens by their own Central Intelligence Agency! (See Chapter Eight above)
9. 43."...we had two CIA prisoners in China..." This would be a reference to Agents Downey and Fecteau who had been dropping biological agents on China during the Korean War. Their planes had been shot down and the Chinese government said that they could be repatriated if the American government acknowledged

what they had been doing. Rather than admit the truth the U.S. Government let them sit in a Chinese prison for over twenty years!

10. 71. "A special procedure designated MKDELTA was established to govern the use of MKULTRA materials abroad. Such materials were used on a number of occasions. Because MKULTRA records were destroyed, it is impossible to reconstruct the operational use of MKULTRA materials by the CIA overseas; it has been determined that the use of these materials abroad began in 1953 and possibly as early as 1950." The 1953 date fits with the January 1952 approach to Hilary Koprowski by Joseph Smadel of the U.S. Army about doing polio vaccine testing which led to the former's work in the Belgian Congo.

Space does not permit a more exhaustive review of the 171 pages which are all that remain of the huge number of CIA files dealing with the monkey kidney (MK) projects, but even this short look shows that it all fits with our major hypothesis that the AIDS co-factors were developed, tested and then deployed by the CIA. No wonder that CIA Director Helms ordered Dr. Gottlieb to shred and burn all the records! The crime beyond belief!

Of the thousands of pages of documents that were evidently generated over the life of MKULTRA from 1953 to 1964, only a slim booklet of 171 pages is available to historians and researchers. These pages are all that are left of the full records because, after the Watergate scandal hit Washington, all manner of legislators who believed that they had something to gain politically and the relatively few who were genuinely concerned with the rot at the U.S. Government's core, joined forces to begin a study of just what had gone on. In the face of such candor, CIA Director Richard Helms ordered Sidney Gottlieb to gather up all records of MKULTRA and to shred and burn them. Gottlieb did his best and he and Helms believed that MKULTRA was now down the Orwellian memory hole.

However, when Jimmy Carter was elected to succeed the insidious Gerald Ford, Nixon's hand-picked successor, he appointed Admiral Stansfield Turner as his Director of the CIA and challenged the latter to come up with any documentation of MKULTRA that could still be found. Hence we have the 171-page booklet. The full document is available from us (see the note at the end of the Bibliography).

Even the title page of this slim source is dishonest. The dishonesty begins in the first, ten-word, title: "Project MKULTRA, the CIA's Program of Research in Behavioral Modification."

The Project was as Admiral Turner states in his testimony on pages eight to eleven:

> "MKULTRA, a project which took place from 1953 to 1964… was an umbrella project under which there were numerous subprojects for research, *among other things*, on drugs and behavioral modification…" [Note the reference to 'among other things'- authors] there are 33 additional subprojects concerning certain intelligence activities previously funded under MKULTRA but *which have nothing to do with behavioral modifications*, drugs and toxins, or any closely related matter…there are three subprojects on activities *whose nature simply cannot be determined*…there are subprojects involving funding support for unspecified activities *conducted with the Army Special Operations Division at Fort Detrick, Md."*

Thus, to start off with a title that specifies 'behavioral modification' by itself is a lie.

In other words, this 171-page booklet, although it contains a few valuable details, is essentially an example of what is known as 'limited hangout'. Under this technique, a certain amount of new and often startling information, is revealed which draws attention from the fact that there is much more detail not being revealed.

Among the details that are worthy of note are the following:

> "**Mr. Brody**: To my knowledge, there was no Presidential knowledge of this project at the time…there are perhaps any number of Americans who are walking around today on the east coast and west coast who were given drugs, with all the kinds of physical and psychological damage that can be caused. We have gone over that in very careful detail, and it is significant and severe indeed…"

Also worthy of note is the following statement:

> "The institutions (funded by MKULTRA - authors) include 44 colleges or institutions, 15 research foundations…12 hospitals or clinics…3 penal institutions."

It is important to keep these numbers in mind as we proceed with our study.

Finally, we draw attention to the following paragraph of the document on page 71. It is from page 391 of an earlier document and reads:

> "A special procedure, designated MKDELTA, was established to govern the use of MKULTRA materials abroad; such materials were used on a number of occasions. Because MKULTRA records were destroyed,, it is impossible to reconstruct the operational use of MKULTRA materials by the CIA overseas; it has been determined that the use of these materials abroad began in 1953, and possibly as early as 1950."

This is the one and only reference to MKDELTA in the whole 171-page booklet of salvaged records! And that reference is misinformative.

Ronald Reagan in the White House; William Casey in the CIA
AIDS: *Officially on the Record*

The most significant date within the Reagan Years (1981 to 1988) was December 10. On that date *The New England Journal of Medicine* published an article titled *"Pneumocystis carinii* Pneumonia and Mucosal Candidiasis in Previously Healthy Homosexual Men."

This article actually dealt with an acquired immunodeficiency and some of the opportunistic diseases that co-presented with that deficiency.

Thus, acquired immunodeficiency syndrome [AIDS] was officially on the medical map.

Assassination Attempt

On March 30, 1981, just two months and ten days into his Presidency, Ronald Reagan was shot. His purported would-be assassin was John W. Hinckley, Jr., who it later turned out, was an acquaintance of the family of Vice-President, George H. W. Bush! Had the attempt succeeded, the latter would have advanced to the Presidency, just as Lyndon Johnson had succeeded John F. Kennedy.

It is not part of our perceived objective to speculate upon just where and when Hinckley began his planning, and whether there was any Bush family involvement in his selection as a 'controlled' executor of plans developed by the powers in the darkness. However, it must be kept in mind that Reagan was not a first choice of the American deep political faction, and that George H. W. Bush was a former Director of the CIA.

Whether or not the attempted assassination had its roots in plans to unite the overt and the covert bodies of the American political reality by having ex-CIA Director Bush assume the office of President requires other researchers. Our goal is to simply sketch the political background to what was going on in the realm of AIDS/CFS research, and the U.S. government's response to that developing crisis.

However, we must note that the bullet wounds probably triggered the early onset of Alzheimer's disease in President Reagan, and reduced his effectiveness as the Chief Executive, leaving a vacuum for other power people to fill.

It is also important to note that soon after Mr. Reagan was shot, Alexander Haig, Secretary of State, who had quarter-backed the railroading of Nixon out of the White House, had turned up on TV to announce "As of now, I am in control here, in the White House."

As with the Kennedy assassination, when an army communications spokesperson announced, (then backed away from) a claim that "Robert McNamara and the Joint Chiefs are President now", it could well be that the plans to assassinate Reagan were actually envisioned by the planners as only the first step towards a more extreme seizure of power.

GEORGE H. W. BUSH AND THE FIRST GULF WAR

OIL> WEALTH > ROCKEFELLERS > ESTABLISHMENT > MEDIA CONTROL>POLITICAL POWER > CIA > AIDS

"You are a force for moderation in the region, and the United States wishes to broaden her relations with Iraq."

Message delivered to President Saddam Hussein from President George Bush, on February 12, 1990

It began with oil and it moved to control wealth, media and politics and it is still oil which motivates American foreign and military policy.

There are side-shows aplenty: North Vietnamese naval units attack American naval units sailing peacefully in the Gulf of Tonkin. There's no choice but an all out American retaliatory attack on North Vietnam. Dastardly Iraqi soldiers pull premature Kuwaiti babies from hospital incubators and throw them to the floor…then send the incubators to Baghdad. There's no choice but to rally to the defense of Kuwait and those poor kids and on the night of January 17, 1991, send waves of American stealth bombers to shock and awe the people of Iraq. On September 11, 2001 nineteen young Arab men in the United States legally from American allies Saudi Arabia, (17) Lebanon (1) and Egypt (1) do all kinds of aerial acrobatics and blow down the World Trade Center in New York, and blow a hole in the Pentagon in Washington, and at 10:10 am send United Flight 93 into a field near Shanksville, PA. while President George Bush reads a story of a goat to schoolchildren…(He didn't want to agitate the kids by leaving early!) There's really no choice but for the North Atlantic Treaty Organization to attack Afghanistan, and later for the United States to re-invade Iraq with a 'coalition of the willing'.

What a sorry, cruel, tragic, evil mess following upon the murder of President John F. Kennedy at 12:30 pm on November 22, 1963 in Dallas, Texas.

We write this summary with a note of sad and bitter irony because from the Gulf of Tonkin, through the Gulf Wars to the collapse of the Twin Towers and the subsequent deaths of thousands of Vietnam and Iraqi and Afghan civilians and military, not to mention soldiers from the United States, Great Britain, Canada, Australia and other nations, all are based upon a tissue of lies. Lies conjured up in high places and pushed by media assets controlled by those who would dominate the world.

Let's start with the First Gulf War

Saddam Gets Suckered In

The Middle East today is the geographic region of the world where the greed and bullying of a powerful faction within the United States is made most manifest. From 1964, following the Gulf of Tonkin encounter staged by the U.S. as a reason to send the military into Vietnam in great force, until 1975 when the American Embassy in Saigon was over-run by victorious North Vietnamese forces, those qualities of American greed and bullying had been most apparent in Vietnam. As in the latter war, American Middle East aggression had been initiated as a hidden war by covert forces of the CIA in 1953 when the Iranian populist government of President Mohammad Mossadegh was over-thrown.

Quoting Peter Scowen from Barrie Zwicker's book Towers of Deception:

> "Clearly, Iran's political life from 1953 on was a creation of the American government, not the Iranian people. Iranians were manipulated into thinking that their country was in the midst of a homespun political revolution, when in fact it was in the grips of determined CIA agents equipped with a million dollars, a few Photostat machines, and a conscience that allowed them to terrorize people and bomb their homes and make it look like someone else had done it."
> (Zwicker; 2006 Page 263)

Or, as Wesley Wark suggests in his July 21, 2007 *Globe and Mail* review of Tim Weiner's *Legacy of Ashes*:

> "The U.S. intervention in Iran in 1953 continues to reverberate in that country and throughout the Middle East."

From 1953 to the present much of the madness of the Middle East is attributable to the United States within our frequently referred to profit paradigm of OIL > WEALTH > ROCKEFELLERS > ESTABLISHMENT > MEDIA CONTROL > POLITICAL POWER > CIA > RESOURCE CONTROL (including the place where we came in with this study: control of African resources by way of the US /AIDS genocide) > HIDDEN WARS > HOT WAR.

In the case of the Middle East today, we enter with the CIA and Iran in the 1953 hidden war that deposed Mossadegh and brought the Shah back to the Throne.

The 'HOT WAR' between Iraq and Iran which followed was first fought for the US by proxy when in 1980 Iraq was encouraged by the US to invade Iran while the latter country was in the throes of a civil war to depose the America-installed Shah, and turn the government over to the Ayatollah Khomeini. Although there was a terrible mix of religious fundamentalism, tribal loyalties and nationalist populism on display, underneath all of the chaos was the first element of our paradigm: OIL. And, geographically in the midst of it all was the State of Israel…armed to the teeth by the United States, including nuclear weapons developed by Israel in defiance of President Kennedy's opposition, while Iraq was armed with chemical and biological weapons by the United States. (An attempt had been made by France to assist Iraq in becoming a nuclear power, but the Israeli Air Force destroyed that weapons option for the time being.)

At the end of the 'Iraq- Iran' American proxy war (a variant hidden war of the CIA) on August 8, 1988, Iraq was in terrible shape. So was Iran, but unlike the revolutionary government of Ayatollah Khomeini which saw the U.S. as the 'Great Satan', and any debt owed by Iran to the U.S. as a tabula rasa, the Iraqi government, and principally President Saddam Hussein, saw the debts as current obligations which had to be met if Iraq was to survive on continuing U.S. credit and more than that, was to take its place as the leader of the Arab world.

> "At the beginning of the war Iraq had held reserves of $30 billion. Eight years later it was in debt to the tune of nearly $100 billion."   Salinger and Laurent (1991) Page 1

And now the squeeze was on!

> "On August 9, 1988, just one day after Iran accepted the cease-fire, Kuwait took the decision to increase its OIL

> production, in violation of the agreements signed within the Organization of Petroleum Exporting Countries (OPEC). In particular, it intended to extract more from the wells at Ramailah, which is situated in a border region long claimed by Iraq and the subject of bitter diplomatic debate.
>
> "For Saddam Hussein the Kuwaiti move was an act of betrayal and provocation. It would make the present situation of overproduction and falling prices even worse. Iraq's revenues, which were 90 percent dependent on OIL, would fall to $7 billion a year, while the cost of servicing the country's debt would rise to $7 billion. Iraq would be slowly strangled."   *Ibid*, Page 2

Saddam was being suckered in. On the one hand he was being portrayed in the U.S. by Congress and the media, as a violent, cruel, bully…which he was. But on the other hand he was being courted by President George Bush as 'a force for moderation in the region.' (*Ibid*, Page 4)

> "(T)he Foreign Affairs Committee of the House of Representatives proposed the adoption of a resolution condemning Iraq for its 'gross violations of human rights.' The Bush administration protested vigorously against the move and blocked its adoption."   *Ibid*, Page 5

What, in effect do we have here? We have a schizophrenic U.S. Government bargaining with the psychotic Iraqi madman, Saddam Hussein. (Mad psychologically as well as figuratively…at one meeting with his military general officers, Saddam Hussein listened while one audacious general spent several minutes criticizing Saddam's policies. When the audacious general had finished, Saddam drew a revolver and shot him dead.) And the madman, Saddam, forced to choose which of the two U.S. personalities he should respond to, chose the George W. Bush personality and received a delegation sent to him by Bush:

> "On April 12, just ten days after the Iraqi President's violent diatribe, a group of five American senators arrived in Baghdad on an official visit. The delegation was led by a

> senator from Kansas, Robert Dole…Saddam Hussein was thus to address a man whom he considered important and influential and, more significantly, whose views were shared by President Bush." *Ibid*, Page 23

And:

> "On April 25, as an indication of this new-found peace of mind, George Bush sent a message of friendship to Saddam Hussein…" *Ibid*, Pp. 25-6

Isn't it nice to have friends in high places?

Emboldened by such a positive response to his saber rattling, Hussein mobilized the Iraqi army on the Kuwaiti border. Then, just to make sure that he had been hearing George Bush correctly, on July 25, Saddam summoned the American Ambassador, April Glaspie, to a meeting, where he delivered to her a long, coherent and rational summary of the affairs in the Middle East.

Ambassador Glaspie responded positively, and then she added:

> "But we have no opinion on Arab-Arab conflicts, like your border disagreements with Kuwait" *Ibid*, Page 58

In other words the message from the U.S. was: 'go ahead and invade Kuwait if you have to.'

As for Kuwait, the Kuwaiti Foreign Minister, Sheikh Sabbah said:

> "If Saddam comes across the border, let him come. The Americans will get him out." *Ibid*, Page 67

Which would you believe: the American Ambassador or the Kuwaiti Foreign Minister? Saddam chose to believe the American Ambassador:

> "In Kuwait City Crown Prince Saad was awoken at 1:30 a.m. by an anguished call from the Defense Minister, speaking from army headquarters. The Minister informed him that Iraqi forces had crossed the border." *Ibid*, Pp. 81-2

Saddam Hussein had taken the bait in a trap laid by the United States of America. He had been suckered in.

The First Gulf War

Following upon Iraq's invasion of Kuwait, there was a desperate frenzy of diplomatic activity from August 1990 until January 16, 1991 when, at 11:30 p.m. London time, allied bombs began to fall on Baghdad, and Iraqi military installations. The bombing campaign was augmented by a ground war on February 24, 1991 and essentially in four days 'the military capability of Iraq had been crushed,' *Ibid*, Page 219

A summary of the diplomatic activity is beyond the scope of this study, and the reader is directed to the aforementioned Salinger - Laurent book, Secret Dossier for a fuller account. For our purposes it is enough to cite two passages from that source.

The first deals with the United Nations' support for an American-led coalition to use force to expel Iraqi forces from Kuwait:

> "When UN Resolution 678 was adopted on November 29, 1990, it became clear that war had become a serious option in the Gulf crisis. If the United States and other coalition powers had felt a negotiated solution was possible - some experts believed that they did not want a negotiated solution - this resolution would not have been adopted."
>
> *Ibid*, Page 200

Note the interjection in italics: "...some experts believed that they did not want a negotiated solution."

The other passage is a statement by King Fahd of Saudi Arabia:

> "I trust George Bush. I've known him for years, since the time when I was Interior Minister and he was Director of the CIA."

The latter passage explains the former passage for it demonstrates what we have learned over our twelve years of study and have been reporting over the previous pages in our study of AIDS: there is a government of record in the United States, and there is the hidden government of the Establishment with its foreign policy arm...the Central Intelligence Agency.

It is obvious from a careful reading of the activities of August 1990 to February 1991, that the hidden government of the United States did not want a negotiated Middle East solution. It wanted full and unfettered control of Middle East OIL.

But there was one unexpected hitch to this anticipated outcome: biological weapons. What really happened when Iraq seemed to have collapsed?

On February 28, 1991, President George Bush announced to a surprised world that the Coalition Forces had reached a provisional agreement for a cease fire. Air attacks had been stopped and the land forces would cease their attack in Iraq at midnight Washington time.

Within weeks all Coalition forces were on their way home after an apparent decisive victory. The war was over…or so it appeared, but, for some unknown reason Saddam Hussein was still in power in Iraq! For some reason the 'victorious' Coalition Forces were heading for ships and aircraft out of 'defeated' Iraq.

There was something President George Bush had not revealed to the world. He had failed to reveal that the Coalition forces had been defeated, and that full and unfettered control of Middle Eastern oil would have to be put on hold for a while.

Yes, you have read that right: In the first Gulf War the Coalition Forces had been defeated! They didn't recognize it, and the world didn't know it…but George Bush and the biological weapons experts in the CIA knew it! Allow us to explain.

Gulf War Illnesses and the Riegle Report

> "Florence Nightingale, near death at the age of 90, lay upon her bed. Her nurse whispered to her 'Are you alright?' And Florence Nightingale answered 'I am watching at the altar of murdered men and I shall be fighting their cause.'"
> Quoted from a conversation with Karen Seay of Hamilton recorded in Steve's *Dreamcatcher* (1999 Page 8)

Murdered men. To which group we now add: murdered 'women and children.'

Captain Louise Richard

Captain Louise Richard, R.N., of the Royal Canadian Navy, volunteered to serve as a nurse in Canada's military contingent sent to Saudi Arabia in the fall of 1990, initially as a part of Operation Desert Shield and subsequently as a part of Desert Storm. With the launching of the ground war in February her forward Field Hospital came under attack from an Iraqi Scud missile.

We take up the story with the following excerpt from Steve's Dreamcatcher (Scott, D.W. 1999).

> "No damage appeared to have been done and (Capt. Richard) and her fellow medical personnel went on with their work. It was not many hours later that she began to experience nausea, fatigue, headaches, and muscle pain… and soon after her hair began to fall out by the handful.
>
> "Louise Richard was one of the first victims of Hussein's biological weapons attack on Desert Storm Forces."
>
> (Page 81)

What had happened? How had defeat of the U.S. - led Coalition been snatched from the jaws of victory? The answer was as simple as it was when expressed by Shakespeare in Hamlet nearly four hundred years before: the United States and its tragically deceived Coalition had been 'hoist on its own petard.'

Defeat of the U.S.-led Coalition in the First Gulf War

To explain this defeat and to further explain why this is probably the first time that most readers have seen the outcome of the first Gulf War described as a defeat, we will quote five further paragraphs from Steve's Dreamcatcher:

> "The facts are simple: there is a fine young lady named Louise Richard who came under SCUD attack in the Gulf War. Following that attack she became sick and all of her hair fell out."
>
> "The Pentagon had been developing biological weapons since at least 1942 (and probably longer than that) using mycoplasmas and brucellosis in their research. They had sold some of the weapons components to Iraq from 1985

> to 1989. (During the administrations of Ronald Reagan and George Bush!)"
>
> "Iraq had and used skyburst SCUD missiles over Desert Storm forces. No cascade of shrapnel followed the skyburst…does that mean that Iraq fired empty SCUDs or were they armed with biological agents capable of covering a 500 square kilometer area?"
>
> "The only logical answer is the latter."
>
> "In sum: Allied personnel were subjected to biological weapons attack. But because of the culpability of the Pentagon in creating the potential for this attack, a vast conspiracy of silence and disinformation had to be undertaken…"
> (Page 103)

When the SCUD skyburst missiles began to explode overhead, biological weapons detectors were activated over many miles of the front lines, yet biological weapons intelligence officers sent the word to Coalition Forces in the area. "The alarms are simply malfunctioning. There is no cause for worry."

Officers such as Louise Richard believed them, but within hours the first signs of illness began to show as we have described above in the case of Captain Richard. However, there were some who knew the truth: President George Bush and certain of his Command officers and biological research officers…including medical personnel, knew that disabling biological weapons were being used against them.

Furthermore, President Bush and his select insiders knew that if Saddam Hussein could deliver disabling biological agents by SCUD attack, he could just as readily deliver other more deadly agents such as anthrax the same way. And, where the disabling agents could present with the disabling signs and symptoms already beginning to show in Captain Richard and her affected colleagues, anthrax would produce fatalities at a rate as high as ten percent of the Coalition ground forces…There would be up to 50,000 dead allied troops on the desert of Iraq and Saudi Arabia!

There was no choice for George Bush: the attack must stop; the Coalition forces must be withdrawn; Saddam Hussein must be left in power…and the truth about Gulf War Illnesses must be kept hidden from victims and the public alike.

And how do we know much of this? We know it from a Report titled "United States Dual-Use Exports to Iraq and their Impact on the Health of Persian Gulf War Veterans." for sale by the U.S. Government Printing Office, Washington, D.C.

The Report was written following Hearings held under Chairman Donald W. Riegle, Senator from Michigan. It is 551 pages long and demonstrates the dishonesty, duplicity and shallow concern for the welfare of Coalition Forces, as well as a breach of all international standards of war conduct.

We cannot summarize the 551 pages of testimony and evidence presented by the Riegle Report but we can give a couple of examples. In respect to the chemical/biological weapons detectors that were sounding all up and down the front following the SCUD attacks such as that experienced by Captain Louise Richard, and which were being described as simply 'malfunctioning' by biological intelligence officers, Chairman Riegle has this to say:

> "These alarms went off for a reason, and I think it's clear, in my mind because the things they were designed to detect came into that zone and set them off. I mean, they didn't go off ahead of time, they didn't go off afterward; they went off during the time that things were going on in the war zone [i.e. SCUD attacks - Ed] that they were designed to detect."
>
> Page 55

And what were the detectors designed to detect? They were designed to detect all manner of chemical and biological agents that the United States Defense Department had reason to believe they might face.

As for what the Department of Defense had reason to believe Iraq possessed that could be used against the invading Coalition Forces, we turn to page 265 of the Riegle Report:

> "According to the Department of Defense's own Report to Congress on the conduct of the Persian Gulf War, released in April, 1992; 'By the time of the invasion of Kuwait, Iraq had developed biological weapons. It's (sic) advanced and aggressive biological warfare program was the most advanced in the Arab world…The program probably began

late in the 1970's and concentrated on the development of two agents, botulinum toxin and anthrax bacteria…Delivery means for biological agents ranged from simple aerial bombs and artillery rockets to surface-to-surface missiles [i.e. SCUD missiles-Ed]"

The Riegle Report also tells us where Iraq was able to purchase botulinum and anthrax: they purchased these and other deadly and disabling disease agents from the United States of America between 1986 and 1989…almost right up until the outbreak of war during the Presidency of George H. W. Bush! On pages 267 to 275 there are listed a vast range of such deadly and disabling agents, including brucella bacteria. And, on page 266 the Report tells us that *Brucella Melitensis* "…can cause chronic fatigue, loss of appetite, profuse sweating when at rest, pain in joints and muscles, insomnia, nausea and damage to major organs." The symptoms presented by Captain Louise Richard after she came under attack by surface-to-surface missiles.

There is no doubt in the mind of any thinking and honest researcher who studies the Riegle Report and evaluates that Report against the biological weapons' research as we have presented it in this study that President Saddam Hussein had been armed with deadly and disabling biological weapons during the administration of President George H. W. Bush . And there is no doubt that several Coalition units came under missile attack and that many of those so exposed developed all or most of the disabling symptoms seen in Captain Richard after such an attack.

There can also be no doubt that in addition to such disabling disease agents, Hussein had also been supplied with deadly disease agents such as anthrax.

If Hussein could disable Coalition Forces, as he was doing…he could also kill them…and George H. W. Bush knew that. He had no alternative but to stop the attack; withdraw all troops; leave Hussein in power; and betray the veterans of the First Gulf War by denying that they were ill. All of which he did.

The effort to gain total U.S. control of Iraqi OIL would have to wait a few more years, until the eleventh of September, 2001, when George Bush Jr., would try again.

(See Section 10, below: 'G.W. Bush Jr. and the World Trade Center')

Major Timothy Cook

When Captain Louise Richard returned from the First Gulf War she was a tragically disabled veteran. By fortuitous good fortune the present authors of this study met Captain Richard and learned from her the tragic story that we have summarized above. We say 'good fortune' because it has been an honour and a privilege to come to know her. She was ready to serve Canada when given the opportunity to do so. And her service in a forward field hospital tending to the needs of wounded allies and Iraqis alike was the same type of service given by Florence Nightingale to British veterans of the Crimea some 150 years before.

But, where Florence Nightingale was to be honoured by her nation for the rest of her life and where she was able to use that adulation to advance the cause of her fellow veterans, Captain Richard was essentially bullied and left to carry her heavy burden of illness with little help from her fellow Canadians. And that is where the fate of Captain Louise Richard enters this study of American biowar research and the criminal use of science to kill and disable humans rather than to advance the lives of all.

It happened this way.

Captain Richard had turned to the Commanding Officer of Canada's Armed Services, General Baril (now retired). She shared with General Baril the results of research that she had done into Gulf War Illnesses, and the role of various mycoplasmal species in those illnesses. General Baril followed up on her presentation by asking Major Timothy Cook, M.D. FRCPC, Head Medical Services, if indeed the mycoplasma might be a key factor in Gulf War Illnesses. Major Cook replied with a superficial and misleading Memo wherein he pooh-poohed any idea that the mycoplasma was a possibility.

A copy of this Memo came to us and we noted that in addition to sending his reply to General Baril, Major Cook had 'cc'd a copy to a 'Craig Hyams.' We recognized the surname 'Hyams', since a Kenneth C. Hyams of the United States Naval Research Branch had written a number of contrived articles putting down the idea that there was such an illness as Gulf War Illnesses. We say 'contrived' because Kenneth C. Hyams' articles were full of the mocking clichés which characterized articles by other deniers of Gulf War Illnesses and remarkably also denied the reality of chronic fatigue syndrome and fibromyalgia as done by Edward Shorter and Elaine Showalter.

We decided to see if there was a link between the 'Kenneth C. Hyams' of the U.S. Naval Service and the 'Craig Hyams' on Major Cook's Memo to General Baril. We phoned the Naval Research offices in Bethesda, Maryland and asked if there was a Kenneth C. Hyams on staff. The operator immediately said, "Yes, I'll put you through."

"Captain Hyams here," someone said after the first ring.

"Captain Hyams, this is Donald Scott calling. Do you know a 'Craig Hyams'?"

"That's me. My full name if Kenneth Craig Hyams and my friends call me Craig. Why?"

"I just needed to know if 'Kenneth C.' and 'Craig' were related. Thank you."

So, Major Cook of the Canadian Military felt some need to send a copy of a Memo to his Commanding Officer to a Captain in the U.S. Naval Research Branch! A Memo which put down Gulf War Illnesses in line with the United States need to also put down such illnesses!

We immediately wrote the following letter to General Baril.

February 28, 1999
General J. M. G. Baril,
Chief of the Defence Staff
National Defence Headquarters
North Tower, 13th Floor,
101 Colonel By Drive,
Ottawa, Ontario, CANADA
K1A 0K2

Dear General Baril,

I am in receipt of a copy of your letter of October 8, 1998, to Ms. Louise Richard, RN (Lieutenant, RCN. Ret'd) and the Memorandum from Major T. Cook, Head Medical Services. I will limit my comments to the latter Memorandum.

The Memorandum is Titled GULF WAR ILLNESSES & MYCOPLASMA - BRIEF TO CDS, and is dated August 1998, and is intended to be "…a summary overview of data related to Gulf War Illnesses and any causative role Mycoplasma infections may have in them." Some of my concerns are simply details, but I feel that I should refer to them in the interests of complete accuracy. However, the other concerns are substantive because they deal with important questions of our Canadian Veteran's health, and the nature and quality of the response afforded to these questions by the Department of National Defence, by Health Canada and by the Department of Veterans Affairs.

I shall quote excerpts from Major Cook's Memorandum directly and comment upon each particular.

"Mycoplasmas…were first identified and classified in the 1960's."

I would suggest, in the interests of accuracy that this statement is in error. Because the mycoplasma has no cell walls and hence can adapt itself to its environment, it is extremely hard to locate. This has led to its being largely overlooked or even unknown to the average medical professional. However, it has been known for many years to military research facilities which could afford the time and money necessary to understand its pathogenic qualities. Rather than the "1960's", mycoplasmas were first identified and named by B. Frank in 1889. (Frank, B. Int. Journal Syst. Bacteriol. 23, 62 (1973))

"…common pathogens of the upper and lower respiratory tract and urinary tract."

I suggest that this summary fails to do full justice to the pathogenic range of the mycoplasma, of which there are approximately 69 recognized species. (Brock and Madigan, Biology of Microorganisms 1991, Page 780) Major Cook's brief allusion to a couple of species of mycoplasma tends to contribute to the view that the pathogen is insignificant. Actually, there is an extensive range of infections associated with *M. fermentans incognitus* including, but not limited to, "…AIDS or ARC, chronic fatigue syndrome, Wegener's disease, Sarcoidosis, respiratory distress syndrome, Kibuchi's (Kikuchi's) disease, autoimmune diseases such as Collagen Vascular Disease and Lupus and chronic debilitating diseases such as Alzheimer's disease." (Lo, Pathogenic Mycoplasma, United States Patent #5,242,820; September 9, 1993 Page 20)

I have added the emphasis to "chronic fatigue syndrome" for reasons I shall develop later in this review.

"There has been considerable controversy regarding the pathogenicity of other strains of Mycoplasma including *M. fermentans*."

I am not familiar with any serious challenge to the 'pathogenicity' of certain strains of mycoplasma. Certainly, some strains are more virulent than others, but I don't think it is advisable to include *M. fermentans incognitus* in this group. Two points should be made: (a) "When silver leaf monkeys are inoculated with *M. fermentans incognitus*, the monkeys show wasting syndromes and die within seven to nine months after inoculation. At necropsy, the monkeys do not show evidence of opportunistic infections, acute inflammatory lesions or malignancy." (Lo, *op cit*, Page 20) (b) Dr. Lo also approximated Koch's postulates when he took mycoplasma from AIDS patient's tissues and injected them into animals. [It is necessary to stress that it was the mycoplasma transfer that seemed to meet Koch's postulates, not the AIDS retroviruses. Lo makes this point on page 3 of his Patent, citing the work of Carleton Gajdusek.] The animals so injected became ill and died of a wasting illness (Ostrom, America's Biggest Cover-up; 1993 Page 17) (very closely resembling the consequence of the Visna virus in sheep; 'visna' is the Icelandic word for 'wasting'.) (Dignum, S., The Shepherd, August 1991 Pp. 18-20)

It is also important to stress that the AIDS virus and the Maedi/Visna (OPP) virus are closely related, and sheep are a much more likely source of the AIDS virus than are any simian species.

I would suggest that the prudent position to take is that mycoplasmas are very pathogenic and hence it is appropriate to respond to those who test positive with great care. The test results should not be dismissed out-of-hand, as in the case of Lt. Louise Richard.

"…this organism has been proposed as the causative agent of Chronic Fatigue Syndrome, Fibromyalgia and Illnesses in Gulf War Veterans."

In point '2' above, I quoted Dr. Shyh Ching Lo to the effect that *M. fermentans* has been isolated from chronic fatigue syndrome patients.

Although this does not establish that the mycoplasma caused the CFS, it does require that we take the linkage very seriously.

It is also important to note that Major General Ronald Blanck of the Walter Reed Army Medical Center is on the record to the effect that the symptomology of Gulf War Illnesses is analogous to chronic fatigue immune dysfunction syndrome. (Blanck, R. M. & Schmidt, P. Gulf War Syndrome and CFS, CFIDS Chronicle, Vol. 8; 1995 Pp. 25-27) If, as Dr. Lo has established, the *M. fermentans* is clearly linked with CFS and as Brig.-General Blanck has suggested, the symptoms of CFS and GWI are 'analogous' then it is reasonable to assume a possible mycoplasmal factor in Gulf War Illnesses.

There are now several other peer-reviewed articles in various journals which support this thesis.

"The principal proponents of this latter theory are the husband and wife team of Garth and Nancy Nicolson…"

In the light of the professional status of Brig.-General Blanck, Dr. Lo and others, I would like to suggest that Major Cook's reference to Drs. Garth and Nancy Nicolson as the 'principal proponents of this latter theory' is inappropriate. This reference is dismissive and suggests that these well-qualified researchers lack the agreement of professional colleagues. This tone is evident throughout Major Cook's paragraphs 3 and 4 where Major Cook places certain terms in quotation marks ("patients", "cured", etc.) with an apparent intent to suggest an ironic use of the term.

"…take moderate exercise and have a sauna once or twice per day! (See ref. 3)"

Since I do not have 'ref. 3' I cannot assess Major Cook's accuracy in attributing the suggestion '…a sauna once or twice per day!' to the Nicolson's. However, I do have a two-page document by Dr. Nicolson titled, Additional Considerations when undergoing Treatment for Gulf War Illness/CFIDS/FM" as released by The Institute for Molecular Medicine, March 15, 1997. In the latter document Dr. Nicolson states: "Dry saunas help rid the system of contaminating chemicals, and saunas should be taken at least 3 - 5x per week. Moderate exercise, followed by 15-20 minutes of dry sauna and tepid shower. The sauna can be repeated, but not more than two per day."

We have on file a variety of ameliorative protocols which suggest that many Gulf War veterans have experienced noticeable relief from pain from dry saunas. I had always taken Dr. Nicolson's comment above as a warning not to overdo the sauna experience, rather than a suggestion to have such 'twice a day!' as Major Cook's source appears to suggest. There is a big difference between recommending a sauna twice a day and a warning against such. Perhaps Major Cook would provide us with the relevant 'ref. 3'?

Although the above are of varying significance, Major Cook's fifth section with its sub-sections a. to g. merits very careful consideration. I will have to quote substantial portions of these sub-sections in order to comment in a meaningful way.

"a. *M. fermentans* would be an unlikely candidate for a biological weapon as it causes, at most, a chronic illness arising late after exposure rather than an acute, disabling or fatal one desirable of a weapon."

Apparently Major Cook is not familiar with significant aspects of biological warfare. I will cite some of these for the record:

Dr. Donald MacArthur, Deputy Director (Research and Technology), Defence Research and Engineering in the office of the United States Secretary of Defence, who was responsible for the development and testing of biological weapons for the Pentagon, had this conversation on June 9, 1969 with Congressman Daniel J. Flood of Pennsylvania:

Flood: Why do you emphasize and lay so much stress on the stockpile and speak so highly of the killer rather than the disabling agent...

MacArthur: Incapacitating agents are a more recent development and are largely in the R. & D. phase. In fact, the prime emphasis in agent R. & D. is on developing better incapacitating agents...We are synthesizing new compounds and testing them in animals. [Probably at the Plum Island Laboratories to be mentioned below] I should mention that there is a rule of thumb we use. Before an agent can be classified as incapacitants we feel that the mortality must be very low. Therefore, the ratio of the lethal dose to the incapacitating dose has to be very high. Now this is a very technical job. We have had some of the top scientists in the country working for years on how to get more effective incapacitating agents. It is not easy."
        (Hearings before a Subcommittee on Appropriations,
                                 June 9, 1969 Pp. 116-7)

Dr. MacArthur later makes the point that such 'incapacitating' agents (Not Lethal) are 'strategic rather than tactical'. (*Ibid*, Page 121) He also makes the critical point that a disabling agent "… imposes a greater logistic burden on the enemy when he has to look after the disabled people." (*Ibid*, Page 114)

It is well known from the Riegle Report (Senate Hearings of May 25, 1994 Pp. 103-900) that the United States had supplied Iraq with both disabling and lethal weapon components between 1985 and 1989 (including Anthrax), their Chiefs of Staff could well surmise that if the disabling pathogens were ignored and the attack maintained, the next Scuds could be armed with lethal weapons.

Additional weight can be given such a hypothesis when one considers the fact that the 'Mycoplasma Research Project' at the University of Baghdad was under the direction of Dr. Jawad Al-Aubaidi. Dr. Al-Aubaidi had taken his graduate research training in the United States at Cornell University and at Plum Island.

Cornell University is on the record as having received biological warfare contracts from the Pentagon. (Hearings before the Subcommittee on Health and Scientific Research of the Committee on Human Resources, March 8 and May 23, 1977 Page 84) However, of even greater significance was Dr. Al-Aubaidi's acceptance at the top-secret Plum Island Research Station. It is now common knowledge that this Plum Island facility was devoted to research into biological warfare with emphasis upon mutating certain animal pathogens so as to be more infective and contagious and to jump species to humans.

There is compelling evidence that one of the research projects involved the attempt to infect ticks with a pathogen developed from the active agent of brucella toxin to present in humans as Lyme disease. It is undoubtedly not a coincidence that the first known case of Lyme disease was diagnosed in 1975 in a youth in Old Lyme, Connecticut which is just about 12 miles across Long Island Sound from Plum Island.

The most important point about Plum Island, however, is that under American law at the time, mycoplasmas could not be experimented with on mainland United States. Plum Island was the designated research station for this pathogen, and Dr. Al-Aubaidi was doing research there.

It should be noted that Dr. Al-Aubaidi's University of Baghdad requested and was shipped a supply of Candida species yeast cultures on June 25, 1985. Candida has been implicated in several Gulf War veterans' symptoms.

Dr. MacArthur reported during the June 9, 1969 Hearings that the 'incapacitating' pathogens could be delivered by aerosol diffusion carried to the enemy by aircraft or missiles [i.e. Scuds] and would be 'effective over relatively large areas (greater than 500 square kilometers…)'

Finally, in addition to several primary state symptoms, mycoplasma can present with learning disability, cognitive disorder, memory loss, fatigue, myoclonus, abdominal pain, painful granulomas under armpits, headaches, nose-bleeds and hair loss.

Lt. Richard experiences practically all of these symptoms… including hair loss. When this is considered together with the fact that a skyburst Scud missile exploded within sight of Lt. Richard during the Gulf War [putting her well within the 500 square km. area] the most logical conclusion is that the missile was armed with a biological 'cocktail' which included the *Mycoplasma fermentans* incognitus, brucella and Candida with a trace of mustard gas.

"b. Dr. Nicolson has not published any of his diagnostic or therapeutic studies in peer-reviewed journals…"

I have Dr. Garth Nicolson's 32-page curriculum vitae. It lists several hundred articles, most of which were published in peer-reviewed journals. Among the peer-reviewed articles are:

Mycoplasmal infections and Chronic Fatigue Illness (Gulf War Illness) associated with deployment of Operation Desert Storm (with M. Nasralla), Intern. J. Med. 1998 1 Pp. 80-92

Diagnosis and Treatment of chronic mycoplasmal infections in Fibromyalgia Syndrome and Chronic Fatigue Syndrome: Relationship to Gulf War Illness (with M. Nasralla and M. Hier), Biomed. Therapy 1998 16 Pp. 266-271

I suggest that Major Cook's emphasis should be upon the science involved and not upon attempts to misrepresent the work of Drs. Garth and Nancy Nicolson.

I also think it is appropriate to ask whether Major Cook has read these articles and is so, was he moved to write to the editors of the respective journals to take exception with any of the Nicolson's, *et al.* findings?

"c. ...The Presidential Advisory Committee made an independent inquiry into Garth Nicolson's research and deemed it not credible."

We have had occasion to study the summary findings of the Presidential Advisory Committee on Gulf War Illness and we find it to be superficial in the extreme. In this conclusion we are not alone. The General Accounting Office of the United States studied the Report and were critical of the Committee for "...virtually discounting any link between biological agents and troop complaints."

"d. ...a second lab in California is using his technique and finding the same results - it is a laboratory started by him."

Dr. Nicolson comments as follows: "The statement that we started this laboratory is a complete lie…"

I think it is incumbent upon Major Cook to identify the source of this claim. But more to the point, I would suggest that since the gene tracking technique was published in the peer-reviewed journal, International Journal of Occupational Medicine, Immunology and Toxicology, Volume 5, Number 1 (1996) Major Cook should read and critique the technique for himself.

Again I must suggest that it is not professional to focus upon imagined inadequacies by personal innuendo rather than focusing upon the science involved.

"e. …the evidence for chronic mycoplasma infection in GWV, Chronic Fatigue Syndrome, Fibromyalgia, etc. is weak…There are significant risks associated with antibiotic regiments such as those described by the Nicolson's. These include side-effects to the patient & production of drug resistance organisms not to mention the cost. (Emphasis added)

I suggest that the evidence for mycoplasma infection is not weak. What is weak has been the response of the parties responsible for responding to the tragic illness of many veterans. For example, when I interviewed Lt. Col. Ken Scott in Ottawa on April 23, 1997, he advised me that even though he was (and may still be) Head-Gulf War Clinic and a Member Canadian Gulf War Illness Advisory Committee, he was not familiar with the work of Dr. Garth Nicolson. This was a stunning admission, given the fact that Dr. Nicolson had already published one of the few scholarly articles on the subject up to that time.

Furthermore, Dr. Scott advised that he had not and did not intend to order any MRI's of Gulf War veterans. Since there is compelling evidence to suggest that GWVets may well present with the punctate lesions characteristic of 80 percent of CFS patients tested, such a diagnostic tool should be utilized. The fact that this is not the case reflects upon the weak approach of the Medical Services and not the weakness of the case for mycoplasmal involvement.

In passing, I must observe that when the health and lives of Canadian veterans are at stake, it is improper for Major Cook to suggest that the cost of an intensive diagnostic approach should be a consideration.

As to the risks involved in the Nicolson protocol: which is better - to leave the sick veterans untreated and sick or to offer them a chance to at least test a proposal by a well-qualified scientist?

"f. …No double-blind placebo-controlled, randomized controlled trial of antibiotic therapy in these individuals has been completed …" and "funds and research resources have been allocated by the American government for this purpose."

To the first part of the above: I suggest that as Head Medical Services, it is Major Cook's responsibility to institute such a study. Just what level of effort should the Head Medical Services expend in trying to cure sick Canadian veterans?

However, it is appropriate to report at this point that in the United States the "VA Cooperative Clinical Study #475" at 18 VA Medical Centers is being developed using the Nicolson protocol.

To the second part of the above: Perhaps Major Cook had not learned by the time he had completed his Memorandum that on August 13, 1998, Dr. William Reeves of the National Institutes of Health confessed under the protection of the "Whistle Blowers Act" that the majority of funds voted by Congress for research in Chronic Fatigue Syndrome had been misappropriated and that no significant research had been done.

Again I must make the point that Major Cook has spoken to the issue of resources allocated by the American government. Since this is Canada, I suggest that it is inappropriate to allude to what is happening in the United States. Tell us what Canada is doing!

"g. Both the CDC & Canada's LCDC have allowed veterans to donate blood on the strength of numerous studies confirming that they do not carry infectious disease (ref. 4)."

Again I am handicapped by not having Major Cook's references. However, I must state unequivocally that allowing persons with CFS, FM or GWI to donate blood is reckless in the extreme. Not only has it been established that persons with these diseases have a reduced blood volume level to begin with, but practically all of the persons with one of these diseases tested by Dr. Les Simpson of the Department of General Practice, Otago Medical School, Dunedin, New Zealand and whose reports I have seen, present with a grossly exaggerated number of hardened and distended red blood cells. This latter condition causes reduced blood circulation through the capillaries to the brain and all major organs as well as the extremities, and could well present as a variety of illnesses including Raynaud's phenomenon and mytral valve prolapse.

In the case of Lt. Richard it is pertinent to know that she has 71.0 % flattened discoid cells. This is in contrast to healthy female controls who have on average, 43.5 %.

Our current research suggests that allowing CFS, FM and GWI victims to donate blood is equivalent to allowing someone with sickle cell anemia to do so.

Major Cook's final paragraph is a very poor commentary upon those responsible for our Gulf War veteran's health. He suggests that we should wait "…until reproducible, rigorous, controlled studies provide evidence…we should consider Dr. Nicolson's theories highly suspect." Is Major Cook reflecting the will of the people and Government of Canada that until someone else tries to cure our sick veterans that we should sit around on our hands and do nothing? Surely we can do better than that if we are concerned about the lives and health of young men and women who served Canada in the Gulf War.

I am copying this letter to several persons who have a need to know what is happening to our Canadian veterans. In particular, I copy this to the Hon. Fred Mifflin who said in a speech in Halifax on August 17, 1998 that Gulf War veterans will receive "…the benefit of the doubt" in applications for "benefits that are their due." (Fred J. Mifflin, Minister of Veterans Affairs speaking to the Army, Navy & Air Force Veterans of Canada Annual Convention, [August 17, 1998] Page 3)

Given the facts that:

The United States devoted great effort to develop disabling biological weapons;

The United States provided huge quantities of biological warfare weapon components to Iraq between 1985 and 1989;

The Republic of Iraq had and used Scud skyburst missiles over Desert Storm Forces;

The Director of Mycoplasma studies in Iraq, Dr. Al-Aubaidi at the University of Baghdad had studied in the United States at the Plum Island Research Laboratory where mycoplasma applications for biological warfare were being developed;

Lt. Louise Richard was within the target area of such a skyburst Scud explosion and she has tested positive for *M. fermentans incognitus* strain;

Lt. Richard presents with all the major symptoms attributable to mycoplasma infection, including loss of hair;

In a letter dated 05 October 1998 from the Veterans Affairs Canada, Pension Services, Lt. Richard was denied the benefit of the doubt. Her pension application was denied and she was told that "Mycoplasma: Not pensionable under Section 21 (1) of the Pension Act, Special Duty Area (Persian Gulf) service."

I had the privilege to join the Royal Canadian Navy at the age of 17 and to serve for seven years and nine months. Since my termination of service I have never had occasion to require any health service extended by the Department of Veterans Affairs. However, should that day ever arrive I hope that I will be treated with dignity and respect, something that has been lacking in the treatment of Canada's Gulf War veterans…

Finally, I am very concerned to note that the Head Medical Services in the Canadian Armed Forces, Major T. Cook, in his Memorandum to the Canadian Chief of the Defence Staff, copies his reply to (among others): 'Capt. Craig Hyams' and 'Dr. Fran Murphy'. Unless there is a remarkable coincidence in names here, both of these people are American government employees!

I have reason to believe that the 'Capt. Craig Hyams' is actually Captain Kenneth Craig Hyams of the United States navy. I also have reason to believe that this is the same Kenneth C. Hyams who serves in the U. S. Naval Research Institute, 12300 Washington Avenue, Rockville, MD, and is the principal author of the article titled, War Syndromes and Their Evaluation: From the U. S. Civil War to the Persian Gulf War published in the Annals of Internal Medicine, Volume 125; No. 5 in September 1996.

Given the fact that the U. S. Naval Research Institute has been heavily involved in biological warfare research, it would be to the advantage of the Naval Medical Research Institute to obfuscate the truth about Gulf War Illnesses. Therefore any communication from this Institute is suspect.

Even if this were not so, and I have confidence in our evidence, I think that it is highly inappropriate for the Head Medical Services of the Canadian Armed Forces to copy a Memo to the CDS to the United States Military.

I also have reason to believe that the 'Dr. Fran Murphy' named on Major Cook's Memo is Dr. Frances Murphy of the United States Department of Veterans Affairs. Just what reason could possibly exist for involving such an American functionary in Canadian military communications?

A likely scenario is as follows:

In response to your request, General Baril, for information on the 'Gulf War illnesses and any causative role mycoplasma infections may have in 'them', Major Cook turned to Dr. Frances Murphy and Captain 'Craig' Hyams for his information. Major Cook did this because of the almost complete lack of independent, comprehensive Canadian Military response to Gulf War Illnesses.

Dr. Murphy and Captain Hyams responded with the personal innuendo about Drs. Garth and Nancy Nicolson, and the superficial and frequently erroneous information about the *M. fermentans incognitus*.

On the basis of Major Cook's Memorandum you wrote to Lt. Richard on October 8, 1998 and told her: "…I cannot authorize testing or administration of antibiotic therapy as described by Dr. Nicolson."

So we the citizens of Canada, continue to deny the sick veterans a full, proper, honest and scientific response through our Government and our government agencies largely on the basis of insidiously dishonest United States military input.

If we are truly concerned with the health of our tragically ill veterans then we should provide as follows:

Every sick Gulf war veteran and affected members of his/her family who agree should be diagnosed using the following techniques:

A blood test for flattened red blood cells by Dr. Les Simpson

A blood test for *Mycoplasma fermentans incognitus* by Dr. Garth Nicolson.

A blood test (concurrent with #2) to determine whether there is evidence of brucella nucleic particles by Dr. Garth Nicolson.

An MRI to determine whether the punctate lesions characteristic of 80 % of chronic fatigue syndrome patients tested are present in Gulf War veterans.

In respect to #3 above, it should be stated that the ancient disease known as 'brucellosis' which has largely disappeared in North America because of the near total milk pasteurization, presented with damage to the brain (neurobrucellosis), the heart, the lungs, the digestive system, the genito-urinary system and the bone/muscle system.

There is compelling evidence (and some of it from Capt. Hyams Naval research Institute) that brucellosis was involved in extensive biological warfare weapons development.

It must also be emphasized that *Brucella melitensis* and *Brucella abortus* were among the biological warfare components sold to Iraq between 1985 and 1989. For example, in the Riegle Report the following shipments to Iraq are listed on page 41:

"21. *Brucella melitensis* Biotype 1 (ATCC 23456)
Batch #02-08-78 (2 each)
Class 111 pathogen
"22. *Brucella melitensis* Biotype 3 (ATCC 23458)
Batch #01-29-68 (2 each)
Class 111 pathogen (*Just two out of over 100 shipments)

And, the Riegle Report also makes the following point:

"*Brucella melitensis*: a bacteria which can cause chronic fatigue, loss of appetite, profuse sweating when at rest, pain in joints and muscles, insomnia, nausea and damage to major organs." Combine this with the *Mycoplasma fermentans incognitus* and you have Gulf War Illnesses.

Captain Kenneth Hyams might be a source of further information on this aspect of biological warfare research since some of his Naval Service antecedent personnel (including Lt. C. Howe, USNR and Lt. Emily Kelly, USNR) participated in a study of laboratory researchers who became ill from brucellosis while trying to create a weapons grade pathogen. Reported in *The New England Journal of Medicine*, May 15, 1947

In conclusion, Lt. Louise Richard who courageously volunteered when Canada asked, came under Scud fire while in the Gulf. She became desperately ill with all the symptoms of the mycoplasma and the brucella pathogens. However, she came home to neglect and very superficial treatment from the Department of Defence and the Department of Veterans Affairs.

Our veteran's deserve much better treatment than the superficial insidiously dishonest response afforded them thus far.

Yours sincerely,
Donald W. Scott, M.A., M. Sc.,

President, The Common Cause Medical Research Foundation
Adjunct Professor - Medical History, The Institute for
Molecular Medicine
Life member, OSSTF

Military Decorations: 1939-45 Star; North Atlantic Star; Burma
Star with Clasp; Canadian Volunteer Service Medal; Victory
Medal
Co-author (with William L. C. Scott), *The Extremely
Unfortunate Skull Valley Incident* CFS, AIDS and GWI
Co-author (with William L. C. Scott), *The Brucellosis Triangle*

cc: Lt. Louise Richard, RN (RCN Ret'd)
Dr. Garth Nicolson
Dr. Donald Philbin
The Right Honourable Jean Chrétien, MP, Prime Minister
The Honourable Arthur C. Eggleton, MP
The Honourable Allan Rock, MP
The Honourable Fred Mifflin, MP
The Honourable Preston Manning, MP Leader of the
Opposition
The Honourable Diane Marleau, MP Sudbury riding
The Right Honourable Joe Clark, Esq. Leader - Progressive
ConservativeParty of Canada
Ms. Judy Wasylycia-Leis, MP - Health Critic, NDP Caucus
Ms. Pauline Dicard, MP - Health Critic, BQ Caucus
Mr. Greg Thompson, MP - Health Critic, PC Caucus
All Executive Members: The Common Cause Foundation
The Editor: The Toronto Star
The Editor: The Montreal Gazette
The Editor: The Ottawa Citizen
The Editor: The Globe and Mail
The Editor: The National Post
The Editor: The Sudbury Star

General Baril declined to answer our letter, but he had another
General Officer in the Canadian Military answer for him, stating that

General Baril had no objection to having Memos to him being sent to officers in a foreign service!

This exchange confirmed for us the fact that there was a deep-set and covert level of co-operation between certain branches of the Canadian military with their opposite numbers in the U.S. in matters dealing with biological weapons development, deployment and denial such as we had seen when Canada undertook to contaminate mosquitoes at Queen's University, in response to an American request! It was the kind of co-operation we had seen when Pershing Gervais of New Orleans was given covert sanctuary in Canada as we have already described.

In other words…there is a Canadian arm of the American shadow government at the military, national police, deep political and intelligence levels that betrays Canadian standards of human rights and acceptable international activities. A betrayal seen in the cases of Maher Arar and Omar Khadr, two young Canadian citizens who have been badly betrayed by the RCMP and the Canadian Security and Intelligence Service (CSIS) and also seen in the development of immoral biological weapons.

To develop the case of Omar Khadr as an illustration of the fundamental evil of the shadow government of the United States and hence make clearer the reality that this government in the shadows is evil enough to develop and deploy biological agents (including the co-factors involved with AIDS) as weapons of war we will summarize Mr. Khadr's situation briefly.

Omar Khadr was raised in the home of an ardent Arab nationalist father who was a strong supporter of al-Qaeda chief Osama bin Laden. Children do not pick either their homes or the politics of their parents, but they are certainly inclined to be influenced by both. At the age of fourteen, Omar left Canada and traveled to Afghanistan to attend an Arab private school to study religion and language. While there Afghanistan came under attack by the United States and its NATO allies for obviously trumped up charges of terrorism stemming from the activities of September 11, 2001. Objective study of the latter charges demonstrates that the terrorists in the case were the United States operating under the influence of the OIL > WEALTH paradigm.

The claim was made by the U.S. that the attacks of September 11, 2001 were planned and promoted by Osama bin Laden who was living in Afghanistan. The Taliban government of that nation offered to arrest bin Laden and send him to an Islamic nation for trial under Islamic law if the U.S. would supply their evidence that bin Laden was involved in the attacks. The United States refused this offer; probably because, as the evidence now shows, [and will be developed later in this study] the attacks were planned and carried out by elements within the United States itself. The American-led Forces invaded Afghanistan and many Afghani citizens and soldiers fought back, including students from the school attended by Omar Khadr. In the fighting, Omar Khadr is alleged to have killed an American soldier and was captured. At the age of 15 he was sent to the Nazi-style American concentration camp in Guantanamo Bay, Cuba where for six years he has been held and tortured by the Americans.

The whole action by the Americans reeks of evil cruelty and ranks with the worst of Hitler's Germany or of Stalin's Stalag prisons. Only a Republican Party administration, run by mentalities and philosophies the equivalent to Eisenhower's administration which got the whole Middle East agony under way (see above…Wesley Wark) could tolerate such a situation, with, unfortunately, little opposition from the Democrats. The *Globe and Mail* published an editorial on June 5, 2007, wherein they made some of these points, adding that 15 year olds in "Rwanda, Sierra Leone or in the former Yugoslavia" had not been treated in such an evil manner.

In response an American reader of the 'kick butt' school with little or no effort to evaluate the evil of the American actions or for the rights of Omar Khadr to defend his host country against foreign attackers, wrote a letter to the editor as follows:

> "Love your idea, folks. As a periodic visitor from the United States, I read your paper on occasion. I agree entirely with your editorial 'Give Omar Khadr A Ticket to Canada' (June 5). If your lobbying efforts bear fruit, you could invite him into your homes for a celebratory lunch. Anything that would take his attention away from killing U.S. military personnel would be good news as far as your neighbours go.
>
> 'Keep up the good (chortle) work.' Greg Inman, Golden, CO"

Typical.

President William (Bill) Clinton

Bill Clinton defeated George Herbert Walker Bush in November 1991, and served as President of the U.S. from 1992 to 2000. He won the election despite the efforts of *The New York Times* to discredit him because he had participated in a failed land development plan called the Whitewater Development.

As President he supplied a welcome relief from the idiocies of the Reagan/Bush years, and established an excellent record, except in the area of health where his cabinet secretary, Donna Shalala, managed to down play the effects of chronic fatigue syndrome and Gulf War Illnesses. Unfortunately, President Clinton was stuck with his chosen Attorney-General, Janet Reno, who was in turn cowed by the Republican Congress and allowed the appointment of Ken Starr as a special prosecutor to investigate the Whitewater affair. Ms. Reno was also pressured into adding Mr. Clinton's silly sexual peccadillo with a Ms. Monica Lewinski to Mr. Starr's inquisition.

In articles to impeach Mr. Clinton in a charade that held the United States up to the ridicule of the world, Mr. Clinton was able to withstand the republican's efforts to remove him from office.

Despite the latter nonsense, Mr. Clinton's administration was far more sound and beneficial than most administrations since John F. Kennedy.

When one considers that the Republicans would try to impeach a President on such trumped up evidence, and would defend his successor George W. Bush who is arguably the most disastrous President in the history of the Union, one gets some idea as to the extent to which evil in the government of the United States is institutionalized. And such institutionalization is seen in the cruel fact that George W. Bush was elected for a second term in 2004, thus the American people validated the evil and inhumanity of the administration.

The Ken Starr/Linda Tripp/Monica Lewinsky Diversionary Tango would not have reached such absurd heights of public interest were it not for the American media. Madeleine Albright in her important biography, *Madam Secretary*, recounts an anecdote which illustrates the media role. Ms. Albright recounts an incident where, after meeting with Palestinian leader Yasser Arafat, President Clinton opened the meeting to questions from the press. All hell broke loose as reporters from all major media began shouting questions about Monica Lewinsky while Chairman Arafat sat ignored:

> "The eyes of the world were on Washington, but they weren't seeing a debate on the great issues of war and peace. Instead they were witnessing the creation of a new era - entitled "All Monica, All the Time." (Albright; 2003 Page 300)

On a similar note, Ted Koppel on *Nightline* would be almost beside himself with vicarious excitement when he had some Starr/Tripp gossip to report.

This pattern of media nonsense reflects our paradigm of OIL > WEALTH > ROCKEFELLERS > ESTABLISHMENT > MEDIA > POLITICAL POWER…

Back to the Paradigm: Get Control of the Gulf OIL

President George H. W. Bush's first Gulf War gambit had failed miserably when Saddam Hussein fired the biologically-armed SCUDS across his bow. But, Hussein had been chastened by the overwhelming defeat of his Republican Guard and by the brutal bombing of Iraq. This led the latter to reluctant and at times defiant co-operation with the United Nations' biological and chemical disarmament team, but the latter were able by the end of President Clinton's administration to report that Iraq had little or nothing, with an emphasis on the likelihood of the latter, in weapons of mass destruction.

The latter assurances were not enough to deter Mr. Clinton's successor, George W. Bush, Jr. from looking for an opportunity to re-new his father's failed campaign to gain complete control of Iraqi OIL. The opportunity was presented when on September 11, 2001; several attacks were mounted against mainland United States. The latter quickly blamed Osama bin Laden, and al Qaeda, and focused their media assets' propaganda attention on the country that had provided him with a refuge when he fled from his native Saudi Arabia…Afghanistan and its religious fundamentalist government of the Taliban.

From then on to the present, the whole effort has been a classic study in an OIL driven scenario cleverly disguised as a 'crusade' against nations which shelter 'terrorists' and stone adulterous women.

The public of the United States has been led by the nose with the co-operation of the pliant media into an era of evil that rivals the evil periods in Nazi Germany and Stalinist USSR.

The rest of the world was initially not far behind, but as the lies, dissembling, and brutality of the whole effort have become known, slowly the United States has become isolated along the path as a lunatic, criminal state. The 'war on terror' all emerges as one colossal lie, beginning with the attacks of September 11 themselves!

Gulf War Mark Two

As Linda Tripp milked Monica Lewinski for all the salacious details about the latter's sexual peccadillos with U.S. President Bill Clinton, and while the Republican Congress bullied the well-meaning but inept Janet Reno into extending the nonsensical mandate of Special Prosecutor Ken Starr's "endless investigation into Whitewater related (and unrelated) matters" [as Madeleine Albright puts it - Albright, 2003 Page 300], the United Nations slowly, effectively and finally oversaw the removal of biological and chemical weapons from Iraq, most of which had been supplied by the United States.

Saddam Hussein tried to limit his compliance, "but the combination of sanctions, inspections, military pressure, and possible air strikes had placed him in a box." (Albright, *Ibid*, Page 276) By 1990 (the beginning of G. W. Bush's first administration) it is reasonable to state that Iraq no longer posed a serious threat to its neighbors in the Middle East. Neither did Afghanistan on the opposite side of their mutual neighbor, Iran.

Therefore, if the shadow government's hopes to dominate Iraqi, Kuwaiti, Saudi Arabian and United Arab Emirates oil were to be realized and if the oil of the Caspian basin was to be diverted geographically from the pipeline flow west to the Mediterranean and (hence) the European economic zone, and politically from Russian control, the need existed for a reason to invade Afghanistan and Iraq.

That reason emerged on September 9, 2001 when certain vital commercial/military/political/symbolic sites within the United States were attacked. The Twin Towers of the World Trade Center in New York City—the pride and joy of Nelson Rockefeller's younger brother David—and the Pentagon in Washington, D.C. (A third attack appeared to have been planned against an unknown target - probably the White House - but was prevented by the crash (?) of United Airlines Flight 93 into a field near Shanksville, Pennsylvania.)

The best evidence in all three instances points to just one logical conclusion: the attacks on the United States of 9/11 2001, were planned and executed by powers within the shadow government with some level of fore-knowledge and co-operation from within the official government itself. The latter cabal almost certainly contains Vice-President Richard Cheney and quite likely extends to President George W. Bush.

In our research into the source of the AIDS/CFS/ME epidemics we have amassed many volumes of scientific, historic and political evidence that establishes that many of the great tragedies of the past six decades have not been isolated acts of lone lunatics. They have been the deliberate albeit covert politically motivated acts of a unified and powerful force outside of the apparent and overt government of the United States. The same force that executed one President, deposed another together with his Vice-President, almost succeeded in assassinating a third and attempted to impeach a fourth, overthrew the populist President of Iran, plotted the invasion of Vietnam, attacked Panama and put together the development of biological factors presenting as AIDS/CFS and ME under the cover of developing a polio vaccine and of discovering a viral cause and a cure for cancers, found it necessary to plot a "terrorist attack" on innocent American citizens. All because the terrorists "hated our democratic institutions."

For millions of people world-wide, the cover story for 9/11 worked. However, almost immediately the cover story began to unravel. Had it not been for a pliant media the cover for the 9/11 events would have totally collapsed within two months. Instead the cover has largely stood for six years, and has seen hundred's of thousands of Iraqi and Afghani citizens killed or crippled; over four thousand soldiers of the "Coalition of the Willing" in Iraq and of NATO in Afghanistan killed and thousands wounded; a moronic President elected to a second term in the U. S.; all while the world environment faces unprecedented challenge; and billions of dollars worth of non-renewable world resources are consumed forever in the process. And it all started as another element in our OIL > WEALTH > ROCKEFELLER > ESTABLISHMENT > MEDIA > POLITICAL POWER > CIA > HIDDEN WAR > HOT WAR paradigm.

It is not within our self-imposed mandate of tracing the discovery, development and deployment of the AIDS co-factors to establish the validity of the assertion that the shadow government of the United States covertly mounted the 9/11 attacks upon its own citizens and assets. However, as with the murder of John F. Kennedy, and the other tragic horrors that we have adduced in support of our thesis that these horrors are not random acts of lone criminals, but are part of the paradigm of the times, we will cite just three obvious pieces of evidence that the popular media have not cited or examined rigorously and suggest where support for our allegations can be found.

	Took Off	Crashed	Hit
American Airlines Flight 11, Boston	0759	0846	North Tower WTC
United Airlines Flight 175, Boston	0814	0903	South Tower WTC
American Airlines Flight 77, Washington	0820	0937	Pentagon
United Airlines Flight 93, Newark	0842	1006	Shanksville, PA

According to available evidence, United Airlines Flight 175 hit the South Tower of the World Trade Center at 0903; nearly fifteen minutes after American Airlines Flight 11 hit the North Tower. There were several broadcasts of a large plane arcing to its left and flying approximately into the south buildings ninetieth floor where it exploded into a huge ball of flames.

This dramatic and tragic impact was seen that day by millions of TV viewers and has been seen by millions more since. However, the authors of this study were able to view a stop-action frame-by-frame DVD of the event in August 2004, at the Annual conference of the Common Cause Medical Research Foundation in Sudbury, Canada. The DVD, "*In Plane Site*" had been edited by broadcaster Dave vonKleist and was shown by his co-host, Joyce Riley of the radio show: The Power Hour. A subsequent DVD by Dave vonKleist, titled *The Ripple Effect*, elaborates on the evidence further.

The stop-frame photography of *In Plane Site* reveals a large grey-looking plane with no passenger windows along its fuselage and it has a large pod slung beneath it. In the fraction of a second before the nose of the plane hits the wall of the Tower, there is a distinct flash, then the great explosion. As we and the other Conference attendees watched in horror and surprise (we had never heard so much as a whisper that there was any plane other than high-jacked passenger planes involved), CCMRF-member Richard Loyer who had flown commercial passenger flights as a pilot for Air Canada for over twenty years spoke out in shock: "That's not a passenger plane!"

Every thinking citizen of the world—let alone of the U.S.—should view this startling DVD and/or its sequel. (They may be readily purchased through Executive Services Limited, Box 133, Station 'B', Sudbury, Ontario Canada P3E 4N5 for $20.00 each.)

Special Flights to Saudi Arabia

The next question all concerned citizens must ask is: "Why did the U.S. Government organize 'a special flight out of the same airport' [Boston, Ed] and "whisked 11 members of Osama Bin (sic) Laden's family [among several others—Ed] off to Saudi Arabia?" (Ahmed, 2002 Page 184)

The reader should consider carefully the fact that the "attack" on September 9 was supposed to have been planned and financed by family member Osama bin Laden! Even if other family members were not involved in the attack, that does not mean that they would not have had critical information which might come to light if they were carefully interrogated. Furthermore, one should note carefully the alliance of the bin Laden family, the Bush family and former Defense Secretary Frank Carlucci in the Carlyle group.

Here, again, we have the "same old gang" turning up in tragic and criminal events. Consider the following paragraph quoted in *The War on Freedom*:

> "[D]ocuments recently uncovered through Judicial Watch's FOIA to the Department of Defense shows that the Carlyle Group has high-level access to the U.S. Government. The documents include a February 15, 2001 letter on the Carlyle Group letterhead to Defense Secretary Donald Rumsfeld from former Defense Secretaries Frank Carlucci and William Perry, both now with Carlyle Group. The documents also include Secretary Rumsfeld's April 3 response to Messrs: Carlucci and Perry. The letters seemingly discuss the restructuring of the Defense Department. The Carlyle Group is listed as Defense Department contractor."
>
> (Ahmed, *Ibid*, Pp. 182-3)

Now, go back to Leonard Horowitz' critical book: *Emerging Viruses*:

> "A key player in administering CIA operations in Sub-Saharan Africa was Frank C. Carlucci, III. Carlucci, while advancing through the ranks of military intelligence, became the point man for CIA-infested 'healthcare' programs in various parts of Africa." (Horowitz, 1996 Page 353)

Frank Carlucci was not just a member of the Bush family/bin Laden family/September 9, 2001 activities. He had earlier in his career been a key player in the "Establishment" plan to conquer the resources of Africa by killing off that continent's people with AIDS:

> "According to the Church Commission hearings, *Henry Kissinger*, and by association Elmo Zumwalt or Melvin Laird, and *Sidney Gottleib* ordered or administered the development and/or stockpiles of biological weapons, including immune-system-destroying viruses functionally identical to HIV, and the deployment of systems necessary to administer these viruses to large populations. *Frank Carlucci*, Joseph Califano, and *Alexander Haig* may also have been involved." (Horowitz, *Ibid*, Page 494)

Note especially the role of the people whose names appear in italics!

So now, (September 9, 2001) Frank Carlucci is a part of the Carlyle Group which is looking for an excuse to re-new the Gulf War for the control of the Middle East oil. That excuse was provided by the "attacks" on the Twin Towers and the Pentagon!

The Krever Commission

The Whole Truth — Up to a Point

On October 4, 1993, the Privy Council of Canada received the approval of the Governor General to appoint the Honourable Horace Krever, a Judge of the Ontario Court of Appeal, as a Commissioner to

> "review and report on…all activities of the blood system in Canada, including the events surrounding the contamination of the blood system in Canada…"

This Royal Commission was a consequence of the tragic fact that several hundred people in Canada had 'in the early 1980s' received blood transfusions which were contaminated with 'HIV' and hepatitis 'C', and had gone on to sicken and die from these diseases.

Horace Krever turned out to be a very thorough and committed Commissioner and he began a careful and thoughtful study of every aspect of the system of blood retrieval and storage and transfusion.

In the meanwhile, two years before they were to begin their study of chronic fatigue syndrome, the present authors noted the Commission appointment and the occasional news story about its work, but had no other concern about it…until 1996 that is.

By the latter year we had slowly come to the conclusion over a seventeen-month period of study that not only were AIDS and hepatitis transmitted by blood, but also there was sufficient evidence to support the claim that many other diseases were also likely to be transmitted. Thus it was that we decided to communicate our findings to Commissioner Krever with the following letter:

November 25, 1996

Dear Justice Krever,

Re: Blood tainted with CFS, FM, and ME

We, the undersigned, have recently completed a seventeen-month study into the nature and origin of chronic fatigue syndrome. We feel that it is important to summarize some of our research findings for your Commission. Although we are aware of the fact that your specific mandate is to focus upon HIV and hepatitis B contamination of Canada's blood supply, we also believe there is an implicit duty for your Commission to alert the public and its governmental, health, and other agencies to the general risk to human health posed by an unsafe blood supply from any source.

Our research has led us to the conviction that there is a very significant threat to the health of any person who requires a blood transfusion. This is not only the threat posed by blood contaminated by HIV and hepatitis B, which your Commission is currently addressing. We refer to the more subtle threat posed by blood provided to any transfusion service by persons carrying the agents which sooner or later manifest their presence in the form of chronic fatigue syndrome (CFS); fibromyalgia (FM); and, myalgic encephalomyelitis (ME). There is some evidence that this same pathogenic agent can cause other degenerative brain diseases such as Parkinson's disease and Alzheimer's disease.

Let us assure you at the outset that we are not medical doctors. We began our research from a social, not a medical, basis. We were concerned by the fact that victims of CFS, FM, and ME were: (a) far more numerous, (b) much more disabled than generally recognized and were also: (c) bullied by bureaucratic agencies (d) superficially responded to by a large part of the medical profession (e) often mistreated and misunderstood by employers, unions, family members and society at large.

In the course of our research we interviewed in person or by phone such authorities as Dr. D. Carleton Gajdusek (Nobel Laureate); Dr. Garth Nicolson (formerly) of the University of Texas Medical School and the M.D. Anderson Cancer Research Center; and others at the Aaron Diamond AIDS Research Center, the Dana-Farber Cancer Research Institute of Harvard Medical School, etc.

The gist of our findings *apropos* your Commission mandate is:

- CFS, FM, ME and other degenerative brain diseases are "mirror images of AIDS"
- Although transmission originates primarily by the inciting pathogen being transported by air, the evidence is very compelling that the pathogen is also carried by blood transfusion or other blood mingling
- The pathogen is not capable of being detected by ordinary blood and tissue assay and is in the form of a mycoplasma that possesses the HIV-env. gene
- Although transmitted by blood, the pathogen works by affecting the shape of the red blood cells so that circulation through the capillaries to the limbic system of the brain is severely compromised, causing a shortage of oxygen and nutrients to the affected parts of the brain
- The affected parts of the brain develop lesions, ranging from punctate to larger size and similar to those found in the brain of victims of multiple sclerosis, AIDS victims, Parkinson's disease and Alzheimer's disease
- Ancillary effects cause a reduced blood supply to other body parts producing symptoms of chronic pain, non-restorative sleep, etc.

These blood-related diseases are, we strongly believe, directly linked to AIDS in that all the diseases are aspects of immune system dysfunction. Our research drew heavily upon the secret testimony of Dr. Donald MacArthur of the U.S. Department of Defense Biological Research Branch to a group of United States Congressmen on June 9, 1969. During that testimony, which was only released under Freedom of Information order, Dr. MacArthur revealed that new synthetic viruses could be created which would be "refractory to the immunological and therapeutic processes" of the human body. He also revealed that there would be a "new infective microorganism which differ in certain important aspects *from any known disease-causing organisms.*" These are direct quotes from HIS testimony and the microorganisms which he alludes to strongly suggest the mycoplasma discovered in the blood of many victims by Drs. Garth and Nancy Nicolson.

Dr. MacArthur's testimony also alluded to two types of pathogen: one which would be fatal (AIDS?) and one which would be disabling (CFS?).

There is more that we could share with you in your Commission's study, such as the very suggestive role of Dr. Gajdusek in the research into AIDS and hemorrhagic fevers and the role of blood as the conveyor of the inciting pathogen. However, this letter is not meant to summarize our research, but to share with you the fact that although AIDS is the center piece of concern, the disabling diseases of CFS, FM, and ME are communicated in blood transfused to patients.

There are at least five million victims of CFS in the United States and Canada and there are indications that it could be spreading exponentially. We can either ignore what is happening or take steps to avert a disaster.

We cannot anticipate the conclusions which you will publish in your Report, but we imagine there will be enough responsibility to share among several people who played a role in the past tragedy.

What we wish to emphasize is that by taking steps now to investigate the nature and origin of the degenerative brain diseases such as CFS, FM, and ME and the role of the blood in their transmission, we may preclude the necessity of a further Royal Commission in ten years time being set up to examine the tragedy of these diseases.

For your information, the title of our book is, *The Extremely Unfortunate Skull Valley Incident*.

Thanking you for the great efforts that you are making on behalf of the Canadian people, and looking forward to your Report, we are yours sincerely,

Donald W. Scott and William L.C. Scott

We sent our letter by hard copy in the mail and by fax on November 25, 1996. We thought that we might hear from Judge Krever or his staff sometime in the next few weeks. We were, therefore, somewhat taken aback to receive a phone call from his Executive Co-ordinator, Penny Chan, Ph.D., and MHSc. the next morning! Dr. Chan said that she had shown our letter to Judge Krever and that he wanted to include it as part of the record of the Commission that would be available to the public if we would agree. We said that we would be happy to see our research on the public record. Dr. Chan said that she would send written confirmation to us that same day.

At the time, although we were well aware of the fact that we were dealing with something important to human health, we had no idea of what we would come to realize over the next few years. Fine! Our information, flawed as it was we now recognize, would be placed before people caring enough to read such things as a Report of a Royal Commission on the safety of the blood supply. And they would learn (probably for the first time) that there was such a dangerous pathogen as the mycoplasma. But, we were to learn something else very soon.

In the meantime, within two days we received Dr. Chan's letter. It read:

November 26, 1996

Dear Messrs. Scott:

Justice Krever has asked me to respond to your letter dated November 25, 1996.
Thank you for taking the time to communicate with us.

The terms of the inquiry are to review and report on the mandate, organization, management, operations, financing and regulation of all activities of the blood system in Canada, including the events surrounding the contamination of the blood system in Canada in the early 1980s. I have attached a copy for your information. Certainly the greatest concern in the early 1980s was the contamination by HIV and hepatitis C virus. From the review of the current blood system that was the subject of Justice Krever's Interim Report, however, it is clear that there are other risks to the blood supply. Justice Krever's final report is to contain recommendations on an efficient and effective blood system in Canada for the future. A major aspect of any system involved with health care is the ability to identify, assess and either avoid or control risks. Effective systems integrate scientific, medical and research to ensure that there is a rapid response to new, emerging or existing threats to safety.

Justice Krever has requested that your letter be treated as a public submission and form part of the record of the Commission that will be available to the public. Please let me know if you wish your correspondence with us to be kept confidential.

Thank you for your interest in Justice Krever's work.

Yours very truly,
Penny Chan, Ph.D., MHSc.

We replied:

December 5, 1996

Dear Dr. Chan:

Reference your letter of November 25, 1996

Thank you for your letter and Justice Krever's request that our earlier letter of November 25, 1996 be treated as a public submission.
We are pleased to agree to Justice Krever's request, and we are willing to co-operate in any way that you may feel would be helpful.

Yours very truly,
Donald W. Scott

That was the last we ever heard from them…Justice Krever, Dr. Chan, you name it…no further word.

In the meantime, we sent copies of our correspondence to Sudbury's Canadian Broadcasting Corporation's News Department.

No word from them, either.

After a couple of weeks we phoned the CBC and asked about our correspondence and Justice Krever's interest in it and the News Director said something to the effect of: "Mr. Scott, I've been broadcasting the news for 'X' years (he gave a figure, but we forget it) and I know my Northern Ontario audience and they're not interested in the safety of the blood supply."

From then on we have referred to the CBC as the 'Make Believe News Department.'

Then something else happened. Out of the blue, without apparently talking it over with Justice Krever, the Government of Canada shut down the Royal Commission on the Safety of the Blood System in Canada. Justice Krever issued his final report…but he didn't send us a copy. And we learn from the internet that in some sort of index it is noted that Donald W. Scott and William L.C. Scott had made a submission. Period.

So much for our research and findings about the mycoplasma being made available to the public. The government and the media were informing the Canadian public about serious health issues.

Then we learned that something else that was very funny had taken place. The government announced that it was presenting new legislation to protect the blood supply without waiting for Justice Krever's Report.

Financing the CIA: Bre-X

In his important book, *Deep Politics and the Death of JFK*, Professor Peter Dale Scott makes one of several very important observations: it takes money to be a crook. Here is one relevant quotation:

> "The fact remains that Rothman did avoid imprisonment, along with his fellow defendants Sam Mannarino of Pittsburgh and Giuseppe Cotroni of Montreal, despite their having been caught red-handed for illegally pledging *$8.5 million worth of securities stolen from a Canadian bank, in what the FBI then called 'the biggest burglary in the world.'"* (Page 200)

As we gathered data and evaluated the evidence presented in this book about the scientific, medical and other research that was needed to produce AIDS, one of the factors that we tried to track was the cost of doing what was being done and where the money was coming from. We realized that there was the private money put up by families such as the Rockefellers and the Morgans, and there were the vast sums put up by the various Foundations such as the Ford Foundation and the Rockefeller Foundation. Then there was the public money that went into research initially put up illicitly by the CIA and other intelligence organizations under programs such as MKULTRA and MKDELTA, which continued even after Lyndon Johnson brought the research out of the covert shadows under the guise of it being a special leukemia/lymphoma viral study (SVLP) and Richard Nixon made it even more open by calling it a great war on cancer (SVCP). And even with all of this money, we detected an apparent shortfall that had to be made up from somewhere, just as Rothman and Cotroni had found it necessary to rob a Canadian bank to finance their life of crime. And that was the answer. Did the CIA need more money? Steal it.

There was ample evidence of precedents. For example, following WW ll millions of dollars were stolen from the Allies by the U.S. when under Allen Dulles and Secretary of the Navy, James Forrestal, captured Nazi gold was shipped from France to the U.S. and turned over to the U.S. Treasury to finance covert operations. There is much public chatter about 'where did the Nazi gold go at war's end?' But it is spelled out in 'in plain sight' as it were by Hoopes and Brinkley in their biography of Forrestal, *Driven Patriot*.

Then there was the already cited precedent of Rothman and Cotroni, and as we continued looking it became evident that the family of George H. W. Bush and someone still unknown had profited to an extraordinary extent from the Savings and Loan scandals of the 1980s. But such fraud as that involved with Silverado in no way accounted for the billions of dollars that were siphoned from that industry when Reagan loosened the regulatory bonds that had previously protected the investors. It was at this point that we determined to look more deeply into one of the greatest fraud cases of recent years: the Bre-X scandal. We asked who were the principals? Who had made the most money from the fleecing of thousands of investors? Who had made that fleecing possible?

We learned of the deep involvement of people such as Henry Kissinger, and of the intelligence operatives of Australia, and the role of J.P. Morgan, and (again) of George H. W. Bush…former Director of the CIA and latterly President of the United States, as well as that of Brian Mulroney, former Prime Minister of Canada. To quote Douglas Goold and Andrew Willis about the latter:

> "Newspaper accounts of the bid mentioned that former Prime Minister Brian Mulroney, a Barrick director, was part of the lobbying effort. Former U.S. president George Bush was in there, pushing Barrick as well. Charlie Harper said Mulroney's presence made everyone nervous, including their broker at Richardson Greenshields, The game was changing in Indonesia and they didn't know the rules. When Cropper told his clients it was time to sell, he had no trouble convincing the GM workers. "When Brian Mulroney and those big boys appeared on the scene," said Charlie Harper, "I knew it was time for a little guy like me to head out."
>
> (Goold and Willis, 1997 Page 238)

However, our concern was not with Brian Mulroney…it was with the confluence of George Bush (whose family and others unknown had profited so greatly from the fleecing of the Savings and Loan investors) and Henry Kissinger and the firm of J. P. Morgan. With heavy hitters such as these who had ties going a long way back in the affairs of the CIA (George H. W. Bush had once been the Director of that agency) and their links to Australian intelligence apparat colleagues, the idea that '…a bright young Filipino geologist named Michael de Guzman' could hype a $5 million scam into a $3.5 billion promotion was just not credible.

As one experienced executive was to put it:

> "However, the magnitude of tampering with core samples that we believe has occurred and the resulting falsification of ore values at Busang, is of a scale and over a period of time and with a precision that to our knowledge, is without precedent in the history of mining anywhere in the world."
> (Goold and Willis, 1997 Page 218)

Who would have the understanding, the operatives, and the financial clout necessary to strip at least $3.5 billion from investors? Given the principals involved as noted above, we suggest that the CIA was the likely beneficiary of the fraud. We summarized the story earlier and published it in *able* magazine and reproduce it here.

Question: What do you have when you put the now-deposed President Suharto of Indonesia; Henry Kissinger, former U.S. Secretary of State (under President Gerald Ford); former CIA Director and later President George H. W. Bush; Freeport McMoRan Copper & Gold President, Jim Bob Moffett; former Prime Minister of Canada, Brian Mulroney; Peter Munk of Barrick Gold Corp.; David Neuhaus of J.P. Morgan; and Tim Scott, former Australian secret service officer and later Peter Munk/Barrick Gold's commercial manager in Indonesia into the same room?

Answer: A Meeting of the Board of Directors of the Bre-X Fleecing Society.

Bre-X: Do you wonder where the money went?
The CIA Tries Free Enterprise, and Finds that it Works!

If one believes Douglas Goold and Andrew Willis, among the principal writers for the *Globe and Mail* in covering the rise and fall of Bre-X, then there is little room for doubt that Michael de Guzman, a Filipino geologist, devised and carried out the plan that fleeced free-world investors of some eight billion dollars.

In their self-serving book, *The Bre-X Fraud*, which ends with a pithy two-word summary: 'Fantasyland indeed', Goold and Willis are at their *Globe and Mail* best in drifting from objective data into subjective fantasy. Their chapter seventeen starts briskly with most of the newsman's five W's: who, what, where, when and why:

> "His name is Salin. He's thirty-five years old, a member of the Dayak tribe, and a familiar face to anyone who pans gold from the rivers near Busang. Salin buys gold grains from the locals, many of whom are also Dayak. He buys them behind the counter in the store he runs in the village of Mekar Baru…" [Pages 251-252]

From there it is all downhill as far as objectivity is concerned. Without troubling us with the details, nor with their sources, Goold and Willis suddenly reveal that for three years Michael de Guzman 'was a regular customer of Salin's', and that he had been buying the river gold to salt the Bre-X drill core samples that were on their way to assay labs for testing. These seasoned *Globe and Mail* writers then move rapidly to the point where on page 258 they ask rhetorically '*Why did de Guzman do it?*' Not '*Did de Guzman do it?*'

The answer to this critical question is immediately forthcoming as Goold and Willis tell us:

> "It seems likely that he was driven by a compulsion to gain acceptance for his theories and by greed. For a while, he was successful in finally winning the approval he craved. And before his death he cashed in $4 million worth of Bre-X options."

Thank you, Doug and Andy, for this incisive observation. But tell me, if as you suggest, greed was one of his two major motives for the fleecing of all those free-enterprisers, why did de Guzman only cash four million dollars worth of his nine million dollar stake? After all, his boss, John Federhof had cashed forty-two million, four hundred thousand dollars worth in just 1996 alone! And David and Jeannette Walsh, titular leaders of the Bre-X 'team', had cashed thirty-four million, nine hundred thousand dollars worth of paper.

In all, eight billion dollars disappeared down the great sinkhole in Suharto land, but de Guzman's take was only 0.0005% of that! Who got the other 99.9995% or $7.996 billion?

This rather naive question is based upon the hypothesis that for every dollar lost by someone in a transaction, there is a dollar found by someone else.

This is just one of several problems that crop up when one examines the *Globe and Mail* 'de Guzman' theory of Bre-X fraud.

Kissinger the Venal

Anyone who encounters a story of a crime with the dimensions of the Bre-X swindle, and who then discovers that the name of Henry Kissinger figures in that story, should immediately re-consider any thoughts about that crime being the creation of Michael de Guzman.

When there is a lion in the cage and a kitten in the cage and one or the other has killed and eaten the family pet terrier, start any investigation with the lion.

Always, down the line, there may be a role for the Filipino geologist that requires review, but before one gets to consider that possibility, one must remember what an insidiously evil creature Henry Kissinger is, and then one must take a second look at all the players in the Bre-X scam with which Kissinger had ties. There may be answers to be found in this approach that wont be found by a *Globe and Mail* investigative team who had themselves, just months before, been touting Bre-X as a good investment opportunity.

In fact, Douglas Goold had once sat on critical negative evidence about Bre-X for over a month before attempting to verify his data. We'll talk about this and 'propaganda assets' later.

How does Kissinger's name come up in the story? Plain and simply, Henry Kissinger was a director of Freeport McMoRan Copper and Gold.

And why should that exercise any student of crime? Because Freeport McMoRan is an evil empire of money grubbers under the direction of Jim Bob Moffett whose links to shady international rip-offs date back to the 1960's. Furthermore, Jim Bob had long been a partner of President Suharto.

First to the Freeport Story

Freeport Sulphur was born in Texas in 1912. The Company had a rather devious history which encompassed more than simply mining sulphur, but we'll skip over that to consider Moa Bay Mining Company, Freeport's Cuban nickel mining subsidiary.

In 1957 Moa Bay won significant tax concessions from Cuban President Batista, and at the same time won a U.S. Government contract to buy up to $248,000,000 worth of nickel for stock-piling. Things were coasting along swimmingly until two setbacks occurred: Fidel Castro overthrew Baptista in 1959 and John F. Kennedy was elected U.S. President in 1960.

Cuba tried to pressure Freeport-Moa Bay into re-negotiating the Baptista tax concessions, but Freeport would have none of it and began planning to assassinate Castro. The company was aided in their efforts by virtue of the fact that high-ranking CIA operative, David Attlee Phillips, was fronting as the Freeport-Moa Bay President. [*Probe*, V.3, #3, Page 20]

Then Freeport came under attack from the United States Senate which had begun a review of the stock-piling policies at the request of President Kennedy who felt that the drain of government money was simply a prop for the wealthy mine owners.

Meanwhile, against this public background of trouble, Freeport was engaged less publicly in two shady ventures. In North America the company, through Charles A. Wight, President of Freeport Sulphur, was engaged in a covert effort to have a front company in Canada buy the Cuban nickel and then trans-ship it back to Freeport's New Orleans smelter for processing, thus circumventing the U.S. trade embargo.

On another front, in August 1959, Freeport Director and top engineer Forbes Wilson met with Jan van Gruisen of the East Borneo [*i.e.* Indonesian—Ed] Company who told him of the rumored mineral wealth in West Iran, formerly Dutch New Guinea. A joint venture was signed February 1, 1960 and Freeport was in business in Indonesia.

Indonesia was at that point in time a nation of 13,677 islands and islets and over one hundred million citizens spanning five time zones. One significant island (Timor) was divided between Indonesia and Portugal. Another European presence was the Dutch who were determined to retain their hold on West New Guinea. In addition to these challenges, there was the challenge of many indigenous peoples who did not consider themselves a part of any central Indonesian administration.

Into this confusing mélange moved the CIA, dominated by the Rockefellers who were intent on protecting their Standard Oil and Socony Mobil interests in Indonesia, at the same time expanding their holdings in other interests, including mining.

The founding President of Indonesia, Sukarno, was just as determined not to exchange one form of colonialism for another, and in 1958 was able to marshal enough forces loyal to him to crush a CIA fomented rebellion.

On January 20, 1961, when John F. Kennedy took the oath of office as President of the United States, he thus had Freeport Sulphur on two flanks: in Cuba where the company was willing to co-operate with the CIA in an effort to assassinate Fidel Castro and in Indonesia where the same CIA had already attempted to assassinate Sukarno. All of which led Kennedy to observe:

> "No wonder Sukarno doesn't like us very much. He has to sit down with people who tried to overthrow him."
>
> [*Probe*, V.3 #4 Page 21]

The world knows about the Bay of Pigs fiasco, and we won't cover it here. However, to put Freeport into perspective in the Bre-X scam, we must précis the less well-known saga of Sukarno, Kennedy, West Iran, Suharto, Kissinger, Gerald Ford, George Bush Sr., East Timor and then McMoRan. With this saga well and truly set down, the full irony of Goold and Willis' comment below will be evident:

> "Of the players, Jim Bob Moffett's Freeport-McMoRan was the most successful at keeping its reputation in Indonesia intact."

To paraphrase Winston Churchill: "Some success…Some reputation."

The Précis

When Kennedy became President in 1961, he was determined to dis-entangle the United States from foreign struggles of emerging nations. He also sought to encourage other imperialist nations to shed their control over territories acquired during the European period of colonial expansion in the 12th to 19th centuries.

This led him into reasonably friendly discussions with Indonesia's founding President Achmed Sukarno, and into stressful relations with certain foreign factions such as the members of the French Military who were determined to retain their hold on Algeria.

In Indonesia, the first major challenge for Kennedy was to settle the dispute between Indonesia and the Netherlands over the status of Western New Guinea or as it is now known, Irian Jaya. With the considerable help of Robert Kennedy and Ellsworth Bunker, a peaceful accord was achieved, and a Dutch Vietnam was avoided.

When Sukarno had achieved his goal of uniting Western New Guinea to his new nation, he turned his attention to the Dutch approved Freeport agreements. His intention was to exercise a stronger role in the development of national resources. In this objective he stood to profit from an $11 million aid package approved by Kennedy on November 19, 1963. [*Probe*, V.3 #4, Page 22]

Three days later that all changed when President Kennedy was assassinated in Dallas.

Under the insidious and, indeed, traitorous Lyndon Baines Johnson, the CIA was again free to operate its own Rockefeller-biased policies in Indonesia, which included plans to depose Sukarno.

Days of Living Dangerously

On October 1, 1965, a group of young military leaders in Indonesia killed a bunch of older, centrist leaders who, they claimed, were going to—with the help of the CIA—stage a coup against Sukarno. [*Probe* V.3 #4 Page 24] Under this banner, General Suharto joined with

General Abdul Haris Nasutin to 'protect' Sukarno by isolating him in a suburban palace, and essentially stripping him of his power.

Then, while Sukarno remained as titular President until 1967, Suharto and the CIA conducted a massive murder campaign against 'communists', 'agitators', and 'leftists' throughout Indonesia. For Freeport Sulphur, the climate had changed dramatically in their favour.

The change showed when under a new Foreign Investment Law which extended more generous benefits to the new imperialists, Freeport's contract was the first signed. The agreement was a joint venture between Freeport and the Suharto military government.

Fast Forward to 1975

On December 7, 1975, there were four men in high offices in the United States and Indonesia. Three of these would later figure in the Bre-X scam.

First, there was Gerald Ford, Richard Nixon's hand-picked successor as President of the United States. Next, there was President Suharto of Indonesia who owed his high office to the CIA. Next, there was Henry Kissinger who by 1975 had emerged as Gerald Ford's Secretary of State. Finally, there was George Herbert Walker Bush, who had just been nominated by Gerald Ford as the Director of the CIA.

On December 7, 1975, President Ford and his Secretary of State, Henry Kissinger, left Indonesia for Hawaii after a day and a half visit with President Suharto and the latter's Military Chiefs.

While Air Force One was winging its way serenely towards the east, Suharto's armed forces began crossing from West Timor into the Portuguese colonial remnant of East Timor.

The timing was obviously more than coincidental. Before leaving for Hawaii, Gerald Ford and Henry Kissinger had given Suharto the green light to invade its neighbour. With this tacit approval would go the co-operation of the still sizeable CIA presence in Indonesia? George Bush's CIA, with the considerable support of the Australian Secret Service would be monitoring it all.

Following the occupation of East Timor, over 200,000 Timorese were slaughtered with Suharto's express consent. And the United States said nothing and did nothing.

Obviously, Kissinger and Bush would have some chips to pick up from Suharto at some later date.

When Shall We Three Meet Again?

Suharto, Kissinger and Bush were to meet again during the balmy days of Bre-X exploration, development and collapse. A collapse that left hundreds of investors fleeced and a hidden few very, very rich.

1988

In early 1988 a Calgary hustler, entrepreneur, stock dealer, or whatever title fits best, David Walsh of Calgary and his wife Jeanette founded Bre-X Minerals Ltd. He was Chairman, Chief Executive Officer and President. Jeanette was the corporate secretary. The Company did not take off, but it did limp along with Walsh dabbling in all manner of speculative ventures.

The following year (1989) Freeport McMoRan, with its links to Suharto still firmly in place, found it necessary or at any rate useful, to invite another Suharto ally, Henry Kissinger, to become a Freeport Company 'advisor' for a total of $800,000 plus 2% on earnings, and a Freeport Company Director.

To seal their new 'business' relationship, Kissinger and Jim Bob Moffett of Freeport McMoRan made a 1991 trip to Indonesia, where they toured some possible mine sites, but where they mainly met with their mutual friend, President Suharto.

In the meantime, by a rather circuitous route, David Walsh of Calgary brought his mining expertise to Indonesia and by May of 1993 had bought an option on a property on Indonesian Borneo near a village named Busang. The area had been drilled for mineral deposits some seven years before by an Australian team which, although finding some traces of gold, abandoned the property as being of insufficient promise. It is important to emphasize that the initial exploration of the site had been done by an Australian team, whose activities would be very well known to the Australian Secret Service, who were CIA allies in Indonesia skullduggery.

Unthinkable Thoughts

In the same year American Barrick Resources- renamed Barrick Gold Corp. in 1994- took an interest in David Walsh's Busang property and Barrick's head of exploration, Paul Kavanaugh, arranged for a tour of the site. He was, or at any rate let on that he was, impressed with the potential of Bre-X's Busang.

Then, a little square dance took place. Kavanaugh recommended that Barrick take a position in Bre-X. He pressed this recommendation upon his successor, who agreed to take it seriously. Then Kavanaugh retired from Barrick and accepted a job as an 'outside director' with no pay from Bre-X. He was to work 'behind the scenes' to find funding for Bre-X and was to be rewarded with Bre-X options.

One might well entertain the thought that this whole square dance had been carefully choreographed in order to put a Barrick operative on the Bre-X 'team'. But, more of that later.

Another 1994 Item

In November of that year a powerful newsletter writer, Michael Schaefer of the *Global Gold Stock Report* wrote that David Walsh of Bre-X was "one of the sharpest executive officers that we have ever encountered in this business. He is also one of the most honest and dependable."

The major problem with this glowing assessment was that Schaefer had never met Walsh, and a couple of years later he could not remember what had inspired him to write it!

Besides his Bre-X puffery, Schaefer took a chunk of the offering in the Company at $1.20 a share and held it until it reached $250.00 before cashing in…before the fraud was exposed.

One might well entertain another thought to go with the Kavanaugh square dance: Michael Schaefer was either a 'propaganda asset' or a shill working to pump up the Bre-X share values on behalf of clients whose names he could not recall just two years later.

Enter an Australian Spook

Tim Scott had been in Indonesia for over thirty years. He had been assigned to that country from his native Australia by the Australian counterpart to the CIA. Australia had entered into an agreement with the United States to share intelligence and to co-operate in areas of mutual interest. This agreement was based upon the model signed between Britain and the U.S. in 1947.

Over and above the intelligence sharing agreement between the CIA and the Australian Secret Service for which Tim Scott had worked, there was a large element of U.S./Australian mutual concern about communist incursions into the whole Far East area. Australia had co-operated fully with Britain in putting down the communist led post-war revolution in Malaysia, and was one of the only Commonwealth countries to support the lunatic U.S. efforts in Vietnam.

Tim Scott had been in Indonesia in 1965 when Sukarno was effectively isolated in a Jakarta palace, and when the CIA -with the most probable support of the Australian Secret Service- had overseen the massacre of hundreds of thousands on Indonesians. Tim was also there when the George Bush CIA of 1975 had followed (or quite likely led) Suharto's forces into East Timor with the further blood bath that saw 200,000 Timorese slaughtered.

Well, as luck would have it, by 1995 Tim Scott had 'retired' from the Australian Secret Service (keep in mind the spook adage: ('once a spook, always a spook') and was looking for consulting work in the realm of mining. What a stroke of good fortune for Peter Munk and Barrick Gold, for in 1995 they were looking for someone to run an office that they were about to open in Jakarta.

No reports exist as to how Peter Munk whose Barrick Gold Corp. featured former CIA Director George Bush and former Canadian Prime Minister Brian Mulroney on its Board of Directors came to meet Tim Scott, late of the Australian Secret Service, but somehow Barrick and Scott united forces when Scott was hired to run the new Barrick operations.

One might well entertain the thought that Tim Scott with his CIA ties to all the murders of the past thirty years was the necessary link between the CIA and Suharto and Barrick Gold as they all participated with George Bush and Brian Mulroney in the fleecing of America.

Tim wasted no time in getting to work for Barrick. Shortly after coming on board the Barrick band wagon, he met with two lawyers sent to Jakarta by Peter Munk to prepare an offer to Haji Syakerami to buy the latter's interest in the Bre-X Busang property.

The three men - two shysters and an ex-spook - labored all day drafting an offer to Syakerami. Finally, their proposal was finished and was already for delivery to their targeted customer. Delighted with their long day's work, the shysters and the spook left for the local bar to celebrate their craftsmanship. But silly, silly fellows…they forgot their hard work and left it sitting on the desk in open and unsecured view.

Again, as luck would have it, an unsavory Indonesian geologist on the Barrick pay-roll happened by, saw the hard-worked agreement proposal, pocketed it, and carried it post-haste to Minorca Resources Inc. another Canadian company [Note: there is a very sound reason why it went to another 'Canadian' company, but we'll get to that in our summary—Ed]

Minorca couldn't believe their good fortune and, with the proposed agreement hot in hand, they rushed off to Haji Syakerami and signed him up. Thus, Minorca had a Munk style hold on a Bre-X partner.

Despite their king-sized boo-boo, the shysters and the spook stayed on the Barrick Gold Corp. payroll!

One might well entertain the thought that the over-looked agreement was not accidentally left in full view and that the unsavory Indonesian geologist was not acting upon an impulse when he pocketed it. Further, one might entertain the thought that the a-fore-mentioned unsavory geologist didn't just find Minorca Resource's address in the phone book. It is much more likely that the 'stolen' draft contract had been delivered to Minorca as part of a well-planned enterprise.

Well, enough with thoughts that one might entertain which never seem to occur to *Globe and Mail* or *New York Times* experts. Sufficient to note that by the end of 1995 there were real, although carefully hidden links between corrupt President Suharto, former CIA Director George Bush [once a spook always a spook], Australian Secret Service retiree Tim Scott, and Peter Munk of Barrick Gold Corp. with his Canadian Director Brian Mulroney. All that is missing from the mix at this point is Jim Bob Moffett of Freeport McMoRan and his star 'consultant' Henry Kissinger.

Good Corporate Citizenship

We should note in passing that concurrent with the gathering of the Bre-X major players as noted above, Henry Kissinger's employer, Freeport McMoRan was having a simply awful time in Irian Jaya (formerly West Irian). Their huge insurance policy with the Overseas Private Investment Corporation (OPIC), 'a Federal body that exists to help US companies overseas', cancelled Freeport McMoRan's investment insurance and it took the help of Henry Kissinger to clear up that problem.

Then, in 1996, large scale rioting broke out around the McMoRan cash cow mine in Irian Jaya. Despite the fact that in 1995 alone Jim Bob Moffett had paid himself $47 million in cash and stock options, his Company was determined to wreak havoc on the environment and to brutalize the original residents of the area.

A thoroughly rotten company that only a Suharto/Kissinger/and Bush team could love. But then, these people have a different standard of human values than most others do.

Back to Bre-X Basics

While the above coincidences were falling into place, Bre-X was basking in the glory of glowing assay results...and was selling holdings to a variety of enthusiastic buyers.

All of this activity was, if you can believe the *Globe and Mail*, built upon salted core samples which were up-graded in gold content by Michael de Guzman who was busy buying river gold from a Dayak tribesman named Salin and then sifting it into the sample bags on their way to the assay laboratories. Just who managed the store for Michael when he was away making speeches or accepting awards, no one has yet said. Is it possible that the Bre-X scam wasn't a one-man job after all?

Let's continue to review all the critical evidence.

Enter J. P. Morgan

In September 1996, Bre-X got another big boost...this time from J.P. Morgan & Co. Inc. of New York, who agreed to act as Bre-X financial and strategic advisers. This gave Bre-X a boost in two ways.

First, it opened the door to some of J. P. Morgan's network of big American stock underwriters who could buy into the young company's shares and options and then hold until a moment came when it was wise to sell out their interests.

Second, it could add credibility to a very junior Canadian company, which, except for its rather tenuous hold on the Indonesian Busang property, had neither a pot nor a window worth speaking about.

And J. P. Morgan rose to the occasion admirably. One of their chief analysts, David Neuhaus, had made a trip to Busang and came away bubbling with excitement, announcing that "150 -million ounces is a conservative guess as to what Bre-X will ultimately come up with."

Nor was the J. P. Morgan love affair an over-nighter. In 1997, when Bre-X was beginning to show the first signs of faltering, Leslie Morrison of the Wall Street giant weighed in with some very misleading data. As Goold and Willis were to put it:

> "The powerful Wall Street bank was doing a stellar job of putting the faltering Bre-X story in its best light."

Just enough time was bought to allow those of J. P. Morgan's early insiders who had not already moved on, to cash in their low cost investment and take their share of the huge, eight billion dollar scam.

And who might such insiders be? We won't anticipate too much at this point, but keep in mind the fact that the CIA was chafing under new Clinton-imposed budget constraints and would welcome some money through the back door.

When the Kids Can't Get along, Dad Has to Settle the Quarrel!

When Bre-X first found itself holding what it thought was a ninety percent share of a mining property in Busang, the local folks who knew the score suggested that they had better get a member of President Suharto's criminal family onto their team.

Bre-X brass responded to the advice by hiring none other than Mr. Sigit Harjojudanto who turned out to be President Suharto's eldest son. They made their announcement on October 28, 1996.

Not to be outdone in their 'struggle' to gain control of Bre-X, Peter Munk and his ex-spook adviser (but terribly inefficient as a file clerk) Tim Scott, had put Suharto's daughter, Tutut, on their team as an 'adviser'. Obviously, when push came to shove, Dad would have to settle any disagreement…which wasn't long in coming.

Bre-X, with Sigit in tow, and Barrick, with Tutut in tow, began a long struggle to arrange for full legal control of the Busang site.

Finally, President Suharto himself had to enter the fray, and to everyone's great surprise, he opted to call in the expertise of his buddy, Jim Bob Moffett of Freeport McMoRan to get the mine into production.

Jim Bob, presenting a *noblesse oblige* front, reluctantly agreed to provide the necessary production heft. Now things were ready to start bringing all of that gold out of them thar hills.

McMoRan sent in its drill teams to begin their operations planning, and Michael de Guzman flew to Toronto to be honoured by all of his investor fans who held interests in Bre-X.

Sorting Out Who's On First

When two teams are playing any game, it is necessary to determine not just who's on first, but who indeed is actually playing.

One team we are relatively sure of. It was Bre-X with David and Jeanette Walsh and their geologists, John Felderhof and Michael de Guzman. Tied to these relative babes in the woods were all manner of hangers-on…but the team that mattered are the ones just named.

Who was the other team that wound up with Jim Bob Moffett of Freeport McMoRan named by Suharto as the starting pitcher? As Goold and Willis of the *Globe and Mail* say, in one of their few statements that suggest they suspected that there was another team: "The old Indonesian hands couldn't figure out who the brains was (sic) behind Busang."

The Phone Call

In late August 1996, Douglas Goold of the *Globe and Mail* received a mysterious phone call:

> "Bre-X now has a market capitalization of more than $5 billion and is up for the renewal of its exploration permit," the caller whispered. "The company already knows it hasn't got the permit, because it was cancelled by the corrupt Indonesian government." The caller then offered the phone

number of one of the most prominent members of Canada's business community, who had agreed to provide details first thing Monday.

Shades of Watergate and Deep Throat!

Sure enough, on Monday this unidentified 'prominent' member of the business community shared much of the Bre-X challenge with Goold...who then sat on the information until October 4 when the *Globe and Mail* reported Bre-X's SIPP cancellation.

This stunning revelation had some shake-out effects on Bre-X shares, but David Walsh and his 'team' were largely successful in patching up the damage.

They were still in their 'holding' mode when (1) Suharto appointed Jim Bob Moffett to take over the property and (2) when Michael de Guzman attended at the Royal York for the accolades being heaped upon him and (3) when Freeport McMoRan geologists phoned de Guzman and (4) when de Guzman headed back to Busang to show the McMoRan folks where they were going wrong in their drilling on the property.

However, after Michael de Guzman boarded a chartered helicopter (being flown by an off-duty Indonesian military pilot) for the flight from Samarinda to their Busang site, the Filipino geologist suddenly [choose one of the following]:

❏ Fell out of the helicopter
❏ Jumped out of the helicopter
❏ Was thrown out of the helicopter
❏ None of the above

By whichever way, he left the flight, we will never really know. (He may, indeed, have disembarked from a landed helicopter, with the rotting de-composed body found some days later in the wet, hot, steamy jungle being that of some one else...well, if one is going to entertain possibilities why not consider all that are available?)

But we do know that thousands of Bre-X innocents who had taken money from socks and from under mattresses and out of pension funds, suddenly found themselves fleeced and holding worthless paper, and the 'investigative media' had a fall guy for it.

And Michael de Guzman was to blame, said Goold and Willis of the *Globe and Mail* after a brief trial they had conducted in their book on the subject.

Hypothesis

We are now prepared to state the following as its hypothesis based upon much more evidence than has ever crossed the desks of media analysts and J.P. Morgan experts (or, at any rate, been acknowledged by them):

The Bre-X scandal was a carefully crafted plan developed by certain powers in the shadows which include the top level operatives of the CIA, wherein a Canadian corporate non-entity would be set up to find a promising gold property in Indonesia.

The 'finders' of this property of great promise would be Canadians to put them outside of the reach of any subsequent U.S. Senate or Congressional enquiry.

The Canadians, with the help of a Filipino geologist, would ipso facto, stumble upon a 'promising' gold property and would scrape together enough money to start extracting drill core samples to be sent several miles under very loose security to an assay lab.

The assay reports would be very heartening, and various propaganda assets would promote the company and its management. Some would even buy in themselves for (say) $1.20/share and sell for $250/share 'before the de Guzman/Bre-X fall.'

As part of the plan, a mock struggle would ensue between Bre-x and Barrick Gold (who, we remind you, had a former Australian spook on staff who would accidentally leave behind a 'plan' to buy into the property). Another Canadian company (Minorca Resources who would also be beyond U.S. Congressional reach) would get a chance to 'see' the Barrick Gold proposal and would take that proposal over lock, stock and barrel.

Meanwhile, the prestigious Wall Street firm of J.P.Morgan would be completely fooled by Michael de Guzman's assay results, and they would rush in to help Bre-X reach the masses…through intermediaries who would also buy in for about $1.20 and sell before the crash.

In all of this it seems apparent to able that Bre-X was a genuine patsy, and Minorca a likely patsy.

When Bre-X and Minorca and Barrick 'clashed' over who would do what to whom in relation to the gold find, President Suharto, friend and cohort of Henry Kissinger, would step in to settle the squabble: Jim Bob Moffett, taking time off from his Irian Jaya environmental degradation and his rioting local neighbours, would ride into the arena to restore order and credibility. As Goold and Willis and their employer the *Globe and Mail* were to observe, only Jim Bob and McMoRan would succeed in emerging from this unsightly scam with their reputations intact.

McMoRan would then discover that their drill samples were no way as good as those found by Michael de Guzman, so the latter would be invited to return from Toronto where the brains of the mining community were hailing him as a hero.

Guzman started his flight back, pausing to buy a new suit of clothes and then catching a helicopter ride with the peace of mind that comes in the Borneo jungle when one knows that one's pilot is an off-duty Suharto Airforce officer. To listen to music while flying, he plugged in the jack, and then suddenly he left the helicopter. (See possible choices above.)

Bre-X would collapse. Thousands would lose billions…which someone else would, again ipso facto, have found. And the finders would be: President Suharto, Henry Kissinger and the American CIA, David Neuhaus of J. P. Morgan, Jim Bob Moffett of McMoRan, and Peter Munk of Barrick Gold Corp. with his star employee Tim Scott and his Directors, George Bush and Brian Mulroney.

All of these parties would not be equally complicit, with the latter two perhaps unwittingly along for the ride and their Barrick director's fees. However, the readers of able now have a choice between the *Globe and Mail* culprit, Michael de Guzman, and the clutch of sturdy rogues and able-bodied beggars that our research has found clustered together in J. P. Morgan's Board Room, toasting their mutual but absentee friend, President Suharto without whose help none of this would have been possible.

Bre-X: A Postscript

In setting out to write this study of *AIDS: A Crime Beyond Belief*, we, in a sense, stepped on to a treadmill. In this undertaking there is no set, static point where, finally, we can rest; step off the moving belt of events and, pointing to some fixed point as a 'milestone of history', leave off our labors.

This analogy applies to all aspects of our study from the historical - the assassination of John F. Kennedy where we had to include a brief postscript reference (see Ch. 10) to Vincent Bugliosi's new book Reclaiming History through to the requirement that we include a summary and comment upon the events of September 11, 2001 et sequent to the scientific where we included letters to *Harper's Magazine* (May 2006) in response to Celia Farber's article of March 2006, and all aspects in between.

Our treadmill is the treadmill of history - and history didn't start in 1952 as we have started this study, and it won't end when we deliver this work-in-progress to our publisher.

Thus it is that we here must add this postscript about the fate of John Felderhof, of Bre-X Minerals Ltd.

We begin with a story from The *Globe and Mail*, titled 'The end of the trail', and dated August 1, 2007, by Paul Walde and Janet McFarland. The teaser reads:

> "Ten years ago, $6.1 billion vanished when tests found next to no gold in an Indonesian mine. Now, the only man to stand trial has been cleared of $84- million in insider-trading charges. Civil suits are pending, but for many investors, yesterday's ruling means just one thing: 'The end of the trail.'"

The ruling was made by Mr. Justice Peter Hyrn of the Ontario Court of Justice and it is fully reasonable and right. The allegations of wrong doing had been taken to court by the Ontario Securities Commission and the main reason for charging Mr. Felderhof would appear to be like the reason Sir Edmund Hillary gave for scaling Mt. Everest: "Because it was there." Felderhof was there, while David Walsh, a former colleague was dead of a brain aneurysm since June, 1998, and Felderhof's chief geologist, Michael de Guzman was dead of a sudden fall from a helicopter in Indonesia in March, 1997.

And, the Ontario Securities Commission, together with the major media have given no indication that they even know that, while OSC barks up a tree at a bedraggled cat, there are (or have been) people in the background prowling like jungle tigers such as Henry Kissinger,

J.P. Morgan Ltd., Jim Bob Moffett, George Bush Sr., Godfrey Rockefeller, Brian Mulroney, and Robert Lovett and many of the principals cited in this study. And, where Felderhof sold some $42 million of Bre-X shares, some of which he re-invested in Bre-X, the cats in the background sold some six billion dollars worth of shares.

PART FIVE

WORLD HEALTH

Chapter Seventeen

AIDS, CFS, AND COLLATERAL DAMAGE: THE COMMON CAUSE

HIV belongs to the family of retroviruses. By a remarkable stroke of timing, they were discovered in 1970 and first cultured in laboratories in 1978, just as the AIDS pandemic was starting."

(Arno Karlen: *Man and Microbes* (1995) Page 187)

And if you believe that, we have an ocean front lot in Arizona…

Part One: AIDS and CFS

A reprise of some of the people and some of the key elements in AIDS (Robert Gallo) and CFS/ME (Brian Mahy)

Robert Gallo and AIDS

Robert Gallo's attempt to claim Luc Montagnier's LAV as his own discovery under the name HTLV-lll is well-known. His experiments upon children aged as young as two years [and to whom he referred as 'informed volunteers'] are on the record. In our chapter on Hilary Koprowski, we have already noted Gallo's 'father/son' relationship with Koprowski. Less well-known, is Gallo's 'friendship' with Dr. Carleton Gajdusek.

When Gajdusek was arrested for sexually molesting one of his adopted 'sons', it was Gallo who put up the bail money. We reviewed Gajdusek's role in AIDS in chapter one, Section 9 but at this point we want to make it clear that Gallo has critical links with all the main players in the tragic story of AIDS.

When the eugenics evil came to dominate the minds and social goals of the Rockefellers and they in turn used their inherited wealth [much of it criminally acquired by the family patriarch John D. Rockefeller, Sr.] to buy the media and the politicians, they needed someone in science, who had one foot in the public sector camp of government health agencies, and another foot in the camp of the private capital pharmaceutical industry who would convert the science of Koprowski and his colleagues into the vaccines of the WHO smallpox campaign.

Developing and deploying such vaccines was well under way by the time Gallo joined the NIH in 1965, but to refine scientific understanding of the pathogens that were being set loose among the human family required the recruitment of many promising scientists by the powers that be. Such recruits had to be not only very intelligent, but they had to manifest qualities of character such as arrogance and a desire to exercise power and probably acquire wealth and powerful friends. Such possible recruits would be identified through agency contacts in colleges and universities and as an added inducement the potential recruit would be allowed an exemption from or preferential treatment in the military services that carried with it no risk of being shipped to Vietnam.

An example of just such a recruit was Philip Agee who was recruited into the CIA. Alternate plum postings to military tasks were to include Charles Radford's posting to the Joint Chiefs of Staff as one of Admiral Wegener's staff, and the 1969 posting of Bob Woodward (later to be one of the *Washington Post*'s Watergate investigative reporters) to the Pentagon.

The NIH and CDC offered similar favored treatment to their recruits.

In Robert Gallo the NIH had their man to continue their biological research into the AIDS co-factors and to advance the lunacy of eugenics into the crime beyond belief. AIDS and its mirror image…CFS/ME. And, in the process, do the collateral damage described in Part Two of this chapter.

In Gallo's self-serving account of his career, *Virus Hunting*, some of what he writes is apparently true. Let's start with one of those truths quoted from page 20:

> "In Providence College I majored in biology, helped in a research project on **cholesterol** biosynthesis…and became interested in the **thymus gland**…As a strange coincidence,

the focus of my research team twenty years later would be on the thymus-derived T-cells."

A strange coincidence, indeed.

To the average reader, this quote of 42 words appears to be making note of one or two simple facts of Gallo's career. However, when one has spent the last twelve years as we have trying to plumb the murky depths of AIDS and CFS/ME the words 'cholesterol' and 'thymus' are very suggestive.

When Robert Huebner found the mycoplasma in the spontaneously degenerating adenoids of some Naval recruits, [Ch. 3] he realized that the mycoplasma was apparently capable of doing great damage to living tissue. But he didn't know how it all worked.

The science of how certain species of mycoplasma acted was explored by other scientists, and in the work of three of the latter, we find our first intriguing detail linking AIDS to Robert Gallo in Providence College. The three scientists, S. Rottem, E. A. Pfendt, and L. Hayflick, released the results of their research in 1970 in an article titled "Sterol Requirements of T-Strain Mycoplasmas". [Ch. 22] The researchers demonstrated that the T-strain mycoplasmas had an absolute growth requirement for the up-take of pre-formed sterols from host cells. Such sterols included **cholesterol**.

Cholesterol! Take another look at what Gallo was doing when he was a student at Providence College: "...a research project on the biosynthesis of **cholesterol**." He was off to an early start. The question is: was it just a co-incidence (as he labels it) that one of the critical factors in mycoplasmal-instigated diseases happened to be the subject of early Gallo study? Or, was Gallo being prepared very early on to work in a field that required knowledge of cholesterol biosynthesis?

Your guess is as good as ours, but we believe that there is a very strong possibility that Gallo had been identified early on for work in the 'relevance of this field of [molecular biology] to biological warfare' as Dr. MacArthur was later to suggest to the Congressmen (June 9, 1969) and that in 'the mid-1950s' Gallo was being prepared while still a college student for a future role in that warfare. We do not have the space to develop this theme here, but we refer the reader to the recruitment of college students for service in certain government agencies in lieu of being drafted for military service. The story of people like Philip Agee is an example. [See Agee, 1975]

Gallo himself acknowledges the appeal of becoming a clinical or research associate since the 'war in Vietnam made an appointment even more desirable…as service in [NIH] was accepted in lieu of a military obligation.'

Not only had Gallo been given an early start on the role of cholesterol in the degenerative diseases, but he also had the good fortune to develop an early interest in the thymus gland. The latter glandular structure of largely lymphoid tissue with its critical role in the maintenance of the immune system was the key to a growing understanding of how that immune system could be compromised and so opens the victim up to assault by opportunistic and normally innocuous diseases. It was to become a part of the *Special Virus Leukemia/Lymphoma Program* [SVLP] which finally emerged as SVCP. (Ch. 13). A co-incidence? Most unlikely.

Following Providence College, in 1965 Robert Gallo joined the National Institutes of Health. Things were beginning to boom at NIH. The effects of the Lyndon Johnson drive towards population control, with his appointment of John David Rockefeller lll as a co-chair of a special committee was accompanied by dramatic increases in funding for activity in that field. It was in 1965 that the SVLP got its official funding with $8.7 million and this shot up to $13.5 million by the next year. Something dramatic was going on and in *Virus Hunting* Gallo does his best to obfuscate just what that something was! In fact, trying to follow the action as Gallo recounts it is something like trying to track footprints through a bog.

An Interlude

In 1964 NIH launched what they officially called a 'Viral Oncology Program' [VCO] but NIH labeled it simply 'VO' in their public references and funded it with $4.9 million. This program was apparently initiated so that there was an executive agency which would lay the foundation for bringing all the pieces of the Gajdusek, Koprowski, Huebner, Deinhardt, Sigurdsson, Henles' research together and translate them into a program to produce a vaccine as a carrier for Huebner's mycoplasma and Sigurdsson's visna virus. The visna having been passaged through cows to emerge as bovine leukemia virus. [BLV]

As already noted, the VOP lasted for four years, but in its second year an off-shoot called The *Special Virus Leukemia/Lymphoma Program* [SVLP] (note BLV above) was created with the noted budget of $8.7 million. The 'leukemia/lymphoma' emphasis of course, ties together much of what the listed researchers were 'publicly' working on. SVLP lasted for three years, but in 1968 was converted to the *Special Virus Cancer Program* [SVCP]. At this point we can repeat a quotation from Lyndon Johnson:

> "When I entered office we were investing $6 million annually for population control. During my last year in the White House (1968) that investment had grown to $115 million."

In that last year that Johnson refers to, the official spending on the Special Virus Programs totaled $18.7 million. Where did the other $100 million (approximately) go? In response to this question, one needs to read further in Johnson's autobiography. In the same chapter [15] he tells how he was able to funnel funds through the Agency for International Development [AID] which had been working with the CDC on African 'health' projects. Here it must be noted that Bill Foege of the AID-CDC African health projects, became a key administrator when Donald Henderson launched the revived 1966 WHO program to eradicate smallpox from the world.

Convoluted? Yes, indeed, but one doesn't set out to kill off 8,000 people a day in broad daylight (as is happening today) without doing everything possible to cover one's tracks.. So, bear with the VOP to VO to SVLP to VCP to SVCP labyrinth. It was meant to confuse you, but don't let it! Follow the money.

End of an Interlude

Now, back to Gallo.

In 1965 when Gallo joined the NIH, Robert Huebner who had got a lot of the action under way in the late 1940s when he tied the degeneration of adenoids to the mycoplasma, was already a member. Later, Huebner transferred to Gallo's National Cancer Institute (NCI) in 1971.

Not only was the NCI of the NIH growing in terms of personnel, but there was a physical plant growth as well which coincided with Gallo's arrival. It was decided in 1964 to build another office/laboratory complex to be called 'Building 41' (all NIH buildings were numbered for their place in the sequence of additions to the campus). Here again, there is a small detail to be noted: corresponding as it does with the launch of the SVLP, it is significant that Building 41 was referred to by NIH staffers as **"The Germ Warfare Facility".** (Weinberg, 1996 Page 80)

Despite the fact that Bldg. 41 was commonly referred to as the 'germ warfare facility' and is even referred to that way in Robert A. Weinberg's book *Racing to the Beginning of the Road*. There is no hint in *Virus Hunting* that Gallo had any clue that the building was even there nor had he any clue as to what was going on inside.

The NCI/NIH interest in Huebner's mycoplasma is also evident in the outside research that they financed. For example, in 1965 the NIH awarded a contract to Michael Gabridge and William Murphy of the University of Michigan [Contract SVLP: PH43-65-639]. The subject of the Gabridge/Murphy research was "Toxic Membrane Fractions from *Mycoplasma fermentans*"! For more detail on why this research is critical to any study of AIDS, see chapter one, Section 4: 'Shyh-Ching Lo'. In a Patent that Lo filed for the U.S. Government this **mycoplasma** is postulated as a co-factor in AIDS.

Also relevant was the fact that at this same time Dr. Leonard Hayflick, over at the Wistar Institute produced a study called "The Mycoplasma and Human Leukemia".

Another important personnel addition to the NCI/NIH research group was Sol Spiegelman who joined in 1969. We cannot go into detail about Spiegelman's work, but to give you an idea we refer to the SVCP Progress Report #8, page 324. Here it is noted that Spiegelman co-authored a research report titled: "DNA polymerase activities in virions of **VISNA VIRUS**". We noted in Chapter Four the work of Bjorn Sigurdsson on the visna/maedi/rida virus of sheep. However, the literature prior to 1981 has no record that we can find of this disease of sheep jumping species to human kind. Why is Spiegelman studying the visna virus?

Another Gallo-Spiegelman link that is significant to our study is a biologist named Arsene Burny. Gallo introduces Burny as a 'member' of the Spiegelman 'group'. For our purposes we need to note that Burny had first worked in Belgium [Ch. 7] His special field was bovine leukemia virus [BLV], which is what Gallo was working with, but which he disingenuously named HTLV-1. Furthermore, Burny was a co-author with Spiegelman on the visna article noted above.

We could add more examples about the Gallo years at NIH, but we've made our point: when one looks behind Gallo's obfuscating and selective details, one finds solid links to the *mycoplasma and the visna virus* that we started with, and the scientific trail to AIDS. [Ch.25]

'Negative template' could be Robert Gallo's middle name.

In 1970 Gallo co-authored an article with Stringner S. Yang and Robert C. Ting. The title of the article is *"RNA Dependent DNA Polymerase of Human Acute Leukaemic Cells"*. Gallo, in his *Virus Hunting* alludes to Ting, but makes no mention of Yang. No apparent problem there.

However, there is a problem in the fact that both Yang and Ting worked for **Bionetics Research Laboratories** and at the time Bionetics was a biological weapons contractor to the United States Government. Nowhere in the *index* of Gallo's misinformative book does Bionetics or its principal, Litton Industries, appear. Again, Gallo deals with suggestive material simply by leaving out all possibly compromising references to such.

The fact is this: all the evidence that we have been able to seek out makes it clear that Robert Gallo was the man with one foot in the government camp (NCI) and one foot in the industrial camp (Bionetics Research) where he was charged with the responsibility for monitoring the effects of the smallpox vaccine program for WHO, and determining the scientific mechanics of the AIDS co-factors whose damage would soon be apparent to the world. He was charged with the task of making all the research sound something like a great war on cancer, while he was actually carrying out a secret Rockefeller/Kissinger eugenics war on humanity.

But, when, in 1983 Dr. Luc Montagnier of the Pasteur Institute in Paris identified a particle in the blood of AIDS victims which he believed was related to the disease agent which causes lymphadenopathy in humans and which he linked to a retrovirus, he called it Lymphadenopathy Associated Virus [LAV] and so pushed Gallo to claim that he had already isolated the disease agent. Typical.

But, our focus is upon the negative templates that Professor Peter Dale Scott suggests we look for, and in Gallo's career one can hardly see the forest for the templates!

Brian Mahy and CFS/ME and Collateral Damage

Money Goes Missing, but Brian Stays Put

First, as we embark upon this study of Dr. Brian Mahy formerly the Director of the Centers for Disease Control in Atlanta, Georgia, we want to pose a 'Hypothetical Situation'.

> "An eighteen year old boy in the mail room of a large office is also in charge of collecting money from all staff members for the coffee fund. He collects the money once a week and on Saturday morning he goes to the mall and buys coffee, filters, cream, sugar and diet sweetener which he takes back to the office lounge and stores appropriately, to be available for Monday morning.
>
> One Monday morning he tells certain members of the staff that he had not bought any decaffeinated coffee on Saturday because he did not have enough money. The office manager calls him aside and learns that on Friday the boy had collected $90 from staff members. He also learns that on Saturday he had bought and paid for $40 worth of supplies, and has receipts for these. He also has receipts showing that he had paid for a movie ticket, a bag of popcorn and a large soft drink. Total: $10. The boy is short $40 of what he had collected for the coffee fund, and he can not account for the shortage.
>
> So there is a hypothetical situation, now we want you to suggest what should be done about the $40 shortfall, and what should happen to the mail room coffee break eighteen year old boy."

Once you have carefully thought it over, **forget about it** for the time being, as having been just an idle diversion from this study of AIDS and CFS.

Dr. Brian Mahy, the Director of the viral diseases division of the Centers for Disease Control, had been given, during his tenure, somewhere around $24 million by vote of Congress to investigate chronic fatigue syndrome. Many members of Congress may personally have been inclined to dismiss the disease because they had read such trivial junk as Dr. Edward Shorter's *From Paralysis to Fatigue*, but they also held elected office and the growing numbers of CFS/ME victims made it prudent to go along with the appropriation of research money.

Thus, into the hands of Director Mahy there was delivered $24 million of U.S. taxpayers' money. And Brian made a big thing about how the money was being spent to make great progress in the search for CFS/ME disease answers. However, like Kurt Vonnegut's spacemen in *Breakfast of Champions* who communicated by farting and tap dancing, Mahy never managed to give a clear picture of how his expensive research was progressing.

Then one day Dr. William Reeves, who was also a researcher at CDC and whose department was supposed to be getting some of that $24 million, called a press conference under the protection of the *Whistle Blowers' Act*. At the press conference Dr. Reeves alleged that his boss, Dr. Mahy was misspending the money voted by Congress.

Congress had no choice but to act. They temporarily relieved Mahy of his title, but kept him on payroll. Then, they asked for an audit of where the $24 million had gone.

The auditor's report was damning. It seems that Mahy had spent about $12 million on what might be termed CFS/ME research if, that is, one were to interpret 'CFS research' in the most liberal way. Then, said the auditor, Mahy had clearly misspent $8 million on things that in no way could be called CFS research. Finally came the 'coffee fund' clinker (see 'Hypothetical Situation' above). The auditor reported that, try as hard as he could; *Dr. Brian Mahy was not able to remember where the remaining $4 million had gone.*

This, of course, was very serious stuff and Congress took appropriate action. First, they appointed a new Director. Then, to punish Mahy for the loss of $4 million, they moved him to a smaller office down the hall from his previous large director's office. There, to our current knowledge, he still sits. Doing what, we are not sure. We tried to phone him to ask, but the telephone receptionist at CDC to whom we spoke told us that we would have to speak to CDC's public relations people. Dr. Mahy, she told us, was not being forwarded any phone calls.

After we had posed our 'Hypothetical Situation' above and had asked what you would do about the boy and the forty missing dollars, we said 'forget it'. We take that back. What would you do? Chances are that a number of you would say "Fire the coffee boy".

Now to the crux of this whole affair: **Why was Mahy not fired or even criminally charged for the loss of $4 million?**

Answer: *Dr. Brian Mahy knew too much about the development of the AIDS/CFS disease pathogens to be fired. Furthermore, Congress has been given their marching orders by those who give such orders from the shadows: "Do not press the Mahy loss of $4 million. Period."*

And that is where it sits.

Before we leave this aspect of the Brian Mahy story, we must make one passing reference to the media assets who cover up the truth about AIDS and CFS/ME.

When Mahy was revealed to have lost $4 million, *Science* magazine suggested two possible explanations. First, they suggested, Mahy is a scientist and not an accountant. Maybe he had just got mixed up when he did his bookkeeping. Or, said Science perhaps Mahy, being a scientist, knew better where to spend the money from Congress than did the Congressmen who had voted it to him.

Science is, by and large, a magazine devoted to reporting news about science. However, at some high level of its administration there is a knowledge and acceptance of certain subjects that must be kept from their readers. Such subjects include, and indeed especially include, any reference to the truth about AIDS and CFS/ME.

What Does Mahy Know, and When Did He Know It?

There are different places in the human body where organs or other sites function as defenders of that body. As we have noted in our chapter on Huebner (Ch.3) one of the first sites of defence are the adenoids and the tonsils. These clusters of lymphoid tissue sample air heading for the lungs and food heading for the stomach. If the adenoids pick up air-borne mycoplasmas they can react by degenerating spontaneously.

But, there is another important line of defence, and that is to be found in each individual cell of the body: that is *cell-mediated immunity*. This line of defence in the human immune system looms awfully large when one reads certain literature such as the Progress Reports of the *Special Virus [Leukemia/Lymphoma] [Cancer] Programs*. For example, in *Progress Report #9*, on page 39, the researchers report that they had been busy studying 'host immunocompetence', and how that competence might be compromised. When the cell loses its ability to intercept pathogens, a major part of the defence system is lost. If this happens, then retroviruses, which normally cannot access a cell, are able to do so and once inside they are able to do their damage.

So, one must first destroy the cell's defence if one is to get a retrovirus such as that of sheep visna, into the targeted-cell where the latter's own DNA is taken over by the RNA of the invader. One must access the reticuloendothelial system comprising all the phagocytic cells and put them out of action. Phagocytic cells in turn are those cells that sweep through the body consuming foreign and hence potentially hurtful invaders. If these cells are compromised, the cell's defence is compromised.

Enter Brian Mahy a way back in the early 1960's where he is found to be studying an unusual virus called 'lactic dehydrogenase elevating virus' [LDEV] and its association with leukemia. Keep in mind that the whole focus at the start was the 'leukemia/lymphoma' consequences of immune system compromise, as triggered by the mycoplasma. In 1954 D. G. Edward had built upon the work of Huebner with a study titled "The pleuro-pneumonia group of organisms: a review together with new observations." The PPLO is the mycoplasma, and Mahy was attempting to understand the process by which cellular defence is destroyed by LDEV effects upon the reticuloendothelial system.

Taken in isolation, such research could appear innocent enough. However, fitting in as it does with the related research going on at the time under the SVLP and with the related scientists such as Guy de The [Ultrastructure of the lactic dehydrogenase virus and cell-virus relationships] and J. B. Moloney [The rodent Leukemias: Virus-induced murine Leukemias] and considering the fact that Mahy was recruited into the CDC and rose to be a major officer therein, all hints of innocence evaporate. (Moloney, by the way, was a friend of Robert Gallo.) Of their relationship Gallo has this to say:

> "Although my lab was then part of the Cancer Treatment Division of the National Cancer Institute, John Moloney, who was then running the Virus Cancer Program in the Division of Cancer Cause and Prevention, passed funds from his program to our laboratory, hoping our work might help his."

In other words, Moloney and Gallo were conspiring to have money voted to one area, actually go to another area. This is called 'conversion', in the legal sense of unauthorized use of property belonging to another. It was only one part of the financial sleight on hand that was designed to make it difficult if not impossible to trace what was going on.

Another important part of this financial trickery lay in the fact that President Nixon was to be the sole approving signatory for money handed out under SVCP, and it was to Nixon alone that Moloney was responsible.

The adage 'follow the money' was, therefore, very difficult to do in practice and it showed in the way Mahy handled the money entrusted to him.

Why would Mahy not use the money voted by Congress for the purpose of researching CFS for that purpose? The answer is clear: as a part of the vast conspiracy that brought the SVLP/SVCP program into being with its twin pathogens as the product of millions of dollars expended, *Mahy already knew what caused CFS and by extension, he knew full well where and how AIDS came to invade the human family.*

There was a great danger for Mahy if he actually paid out this money to genuine and moral researchers. They might well, indeed probably would, discover and report the truth: AIDS and CFS/ME had been developed in United States Government and Government-controlled private laboratories and for the former (AIDS) were deployed by the Centers for Disease Control overseas as a smallpox vaccine, and at home as a Hepatitis vaccine, while at home and in certain co-operating countries such as Canada, Britain and Australia /New Zealand the CFS/ME pathogen was deployed by insect vector (Punta Gorda and the St. Lawrence River Valley); by aerosol (Tahoe-Truckee High School) and in the food chain (Lyndonville, New York) among other sites.

And that is why Mahy still works for the CDC. He knows too much to be fired.

We are greatly indebted to author/researcher, Robert E. Lee for the information on Brian Mahy's early work.

Collateral Damage

An overview of the pathogenic effects of the mycoplasma as a factor or co-factor in various diseases; the potential for damage to the human body by certain species of mycoplasma: a summary review.

The most important thing to keep in mind about the role of certain species of the mycoplasma and the human body is this: certain species of mycoplasma have an absolute growth requirement for pre-formed cholesterol.

An important source of cholesterol drawn upon by the mycoplasma is found in the membrane of cells. Approximately twenty percent of the membrane of the roughly 50 trillion cells in the average human body is made up of cholesterol while the other eighty percent is made up of phospholipids. Two layers of phospholipids packed with cholesterol between them to give the membrane fluidity, face in two directions in each cell…one layer faces out from the cell and the other layer faces in and together they create the barrier which at one and the same time keep foreign elements out of the cell and keeps the cellular contents within.

If a sufficient quantity of mycoplasma pulls a sufficient amount of cholesterol out of the protective membrane, the cellular integrity is destroyed and the contents are spilled into the surrounding milieu, and the cell is killed. As Huebner discovered with his coughing recruits, mycoplasma-infected cells may 'spontaneously degenerate'. So there is one level of potential damage.

Among the cells which may thus be destroyed are the essential lymph cells which act as an essential part of the immune system. Existing lymph cells are overloaded with foreign elements, are not replaced by new lymph cells, and swelling and lymph cell death can result…presenting as lymphadenopathy. The compromised immune system is rendered less effective than is normally required and previously innocuous disease agents can opportunistically take advantage of the weakened defence. Normally inconvenient distress is converted to life threatening damage.

The next level of damage occurs when the contents of the damaged cell are spilled. Among those contents is a quantity of glutamate, which in the right place at the right time and in the right amount, is essential for the functioning of the cell. It is a neurotransmitter which passes messages from one cell to another cell. Because it is so active the body has a defence system to rein it in. A free molecule of glutamate is neutralized by the uptake of an ammonia ion and is thereby converted to the more passive glutamine. The free glutamine can be carried safely around the body until its glutamate is required for some metabolic activity, at which point it sheds its ammonium ion and reverts to its original, dynamic self.

The loss of certain cells can cause the loss of neurotransmitters or enzymes that are largely produced by those cells, with a consequent deleterious effect upon the infected patient. See Parkinson's disease and Diabetes Type One below.

But in the body defence system lays a great danger. In the process of up taking ammonia, the glutamate can derive that ion from a molecule of urea, and this in turn, liberates an ion of cyanide. And therein lies the next level of damage initiated by the mycoplasma. The liberated cyanide, which in the normal case would be rendered harmless by the red blood cells which are sometimes called 'cyanide sponges' by researchers, is too much to be handled and does serious damage to the cell it happens to be in. It finds its way to a mitochondrium of the cell, and at the fourth complex of the cell's Krebs cycle, uptakes the energy being produced. Extreme fatigue, unrelieved by rest, is a consequence.

There is another level of damage done by the mycoplasma. Since cholesterol is up-stream of many of the secretory glands which take it in as cholesterol, then modify it to become a particular messenger, a shortage of cholesterol causes a reduction of essential hormones, hence messages from one part of the body to another part are not delivered, and many essential functions of life are not performed.

The same principle is at work with cholesterol and vitamin D. A supply of cholesterol near the surface of the skin is modified by ultra violet energy from the sun and becomes vitamin D. Then, a portion of that vitamin D is transported to bone marrow where it forms one of the essential ingredients of new blood. If the vitamin D is in short supply, there is a consequent reduction in the supply of new blood. Like the assembly line of an automobile factory, if one of the essentials of a car or of a red blood cell is missing, the production line stops.

Not only is the supply of new blood curtailed by mycoplasmal infection, but the existing red blood cells, in some instances, are directly destroyed. We quote Krause and Taylor-Robinson:

> "*M. pneumoniae* is capable of catabolizing glucose or mannose but will not hydrolyze arginine as a carbon and energy source. Tetrazolium reduction occurs anaerobically or aerobically, and hydrogen peroxide and the superoxide anion are by-products of glucose catabolism, *resulting in complete hydrolysis of erythrocytes* when overlaid in agarose on mycoplasma colonies."   (Maniloff, 1992 Page 420)

We have referred earlier to the fact that mycoplasma are living microorganisms at the very balance point between the living and the non-living world. At one point the mycoplasma in solution can function as a participant in the dynamics of life. However, given certain changes in concentration, temperature, pressure, and pH, the mycoplasma can revert to a crystalline form. This quality can be the source of many disease symptoms.

All of these qualities of the mycoplasma can under certain conditions of lowered immunity and genetic inheritance present as lethal or disabling disease in the infected individual. No wonder that Dr. Shyh-Ching Lo and Carleton Gajdusek and other skilled researchers have at one time or another, listed many diseases with the mycoplasma as the critical factor or perhaps as a co-factor. The signs and symptoms (and hence the damage) may differ, but we suggest that the cause is common to all: the mycoplasma.

Related to the latter suggestion, we feel that Gajdusek's interpretation needs to be noted:

> "In some of these diseases the host genetic composition is crucial to the type of pathogenesis that occurs, as is the age of the host at the time of infection, and the immune system may be involved in different ways…"
>
>   (Nobel Lecture, Pp. 174-5)

The Common Cause Hypothesis

This possible factor could explain the illnesses of say a husband and wife. He has Parkinson's disease and she has Alzheimer's disease. We suggest that they are both ill with a mycoplasmal infection, but that the genetic vulnerability of each was genetically determined. In our files are hundreds of letters such as the following:

> April 16/02
>
> Dear Mr. Scott,
>
> This is my letter to let you know about the illness I have, to see if we can make sense of this nonsense.
>
> I was in Kingston in 1970 till 1978. My husband went to Queen's University before that doing his MBA and his MD. We met in 1971. We both lived near the university and spent a lot of time camping around Belleville and Picton. He was diagnosed in the late 80s with ALS and died in 1992. In 1994 I was diagnosed with MS. It started with optic neuritis where my eyes were blurry and I thought I hadn't eaten enough glucose..."
>
> Name withheld at authors' discretion.

Please see below, the sketches on ALS and MS, also, note Chapter 19 and the 'mystery disease' of the Kingston to St. Lawrence Valley.

At this point we summarize the nature of the damage done in many well-known diseases. We will begin with a re-statement of a quotation from Dr. Shyh-Ching Lo's Patent of the Pathogenic Mycoplasma to which we alluded in Chapter One, Section Four.

> "Some of these patients who are infected with *M. (ycoplasma) fermentans incognitus* will be patients who have been diagnosed as having AIDS or ARC, Cchronic (sic) Fatigue Syndrome, Wegener's Disease, Sarcoidosis,

respiratory distress syndrome, Kibuchi's (Kikuchi's) disease, autoimmune diseases such as Collagen Vascular Disease and Lupus and chronic debilitating diseases such as Alzheimer's disease." (U. S. Patent #5,242,820 Page 20; lines 47 to 54)

Please note that although these lines were written by the leading medical doctors in the U.S. Government Medical hierarchy, the average medical doctors seeing, diagnosing and treating thousands of patients daily have no idea that such a claim has ever been made, and if they are asked 'Where does Alzheimer's come from?' (or lupus or sarcoidosis or other of the above) they likely will reply: "I'm sorry. No one knows where these come from." Or "There's no known cause." Yet, Dr. Shyh-Ching Lo and his associates who researched and patented the pathogenic mycoplasma state quite openly that the latter infection is likely to be present in all of the patients diagnosed as above. We place three asterisks after each of these in our summary below. We have also added other diseases which our research strongly suggests are linked to a mycoplasmal infection. All of these are collateral damage to humanity resulting from the work done to isolate the mycoplasma and to enhance its ability to infect humans. The immunity developed over thousands of years of human evolution has been suddenly and seriously reduced by the biological warfare weapons researchers working under the direction of the United States Government. (See Chapter Fifteen, Section Two above: June 9, 1969)

1. **Adenoids:** We encountered adenoids in chapter three when we looked at the work of Dr. Robert Huebner and the 'coughing recruits' of the U.S. Navy. The pleuro-pneumonia-like organism (PPLO) which he found, turned out to be a species of mycoplasma and its damage, seen as spontaneous degeneration of the adenoidal lymph tissues gave rise to much biowar weapon research, ultimately, with its great damage to the human immune system, led on to AIDS and CFS.

2. **Air Rage:** If a certain level of concentration of mycoplasma in the blood is achieved, or there is a drop in pressure or pH or temperature then there is no logical reason why the mycoplasma would not act like any other crystal undergoing such alteration in its environment…it will lose its fluidity and present as crystals. Such crystals will be infinitely small, but they are crystals all the same and thus the passage of blood through the capillaries of the brain will be seriously impaired. The loss of

full blood flow and the consequent reduction of oxygen in the brain can produce aberrant and uncharacteristic behavior, which is reversed when the environmental factors return to normal, and the crystals return to a fluid state.

3 **Alzheimer's Disease:** ** When certain mycoplasmal species are carried by air into the nasal chamber, and hence past the adenoids to the lungs, a trace of that air will be picked up by the olfactory nodes just in front of the adenoids and transported via the olfactory passage to be identified as particular odors and in the process, depositing their burden of mycoplasma in the brain. Over many years and under particular circumstances and also dependent upon pre-disposing genetic factors (some familial) the deposited mycoplasma burden, usually triggered by a trauma such as a fall, will convert from a semi-fluid to a crystalline form, causing a loss of cognitive skills.

4 **Amyotrophic Lateral Sclerosis:** Messages from the cortex of the brain are required to travel along neuronal axons to synaptic gaps before activating muscle responses. At the synapse, neurotransmitters such as glutamate bridge the space to the muscle receptor. However, with time and/or often toxic influences and usually triggered as a consequence of a trauma, the synapses fail and the messages are not delivered as they would normally be. The synapses in turn, are maintained and renewed by cholesterol generated by astrocytic cells. When the latter are damaged by a mycoplasmal infection, insufficient cholesterol is produced to maintain the synapses and progressive paralysis results.

5 **NvBrucellosis:** ** A disease caused by a bacterium of the genus *Brucella*, characterized initially by undulant fever, extreme weakness, and chronic fatigue and often followed by focal point infections of any of the main organs. Evidence now suggests that the bacterial toxin is a crystalline form which presents as the ancient disease, but with none of the traditional bacteria evident. In effect, it is a bacterium-less bacterial disease presenting as Chronic Fatigue Syndrome/Myalgic Encephalitis (CFS/ME)/Fibromyalgia.

6 **Collagen Vascular Diseases:** ** Collagen, which comprises about one-forth of the body's total protein, is essential in the

building and the maintaining of the body's structure. All tissues and muscles, as well as the matrix of collagen forming the bones, provide the framework within which the heart pumps, the blood circulates, and the brain receives and transmits energy… in other words the structure within which life is expressed. The fact that Dr. Lo includes 'collagen vascular disease' in his list of *M. fermentans* diseases often diagnosed as one of the CVD variants warrants our careful consideration, for included in these diseases are rheumatoid arthritis, systemic lupus erythematosus, polyarthritis nodosa, scleroderma and dermatomyositis.

It must also be noted that like most of the other diseases specified, it is said of all of the CVD's that "…the etiology is unknown."

7   **Crohn's Disease:** Ileitis that typically involves the distal portion of the ileum, and capable of spreading throughout the digestive track. Our research has led us to the conclusion that a mycoplasmal infection is sited initially in the lymphoid tissue cells of the intestines known as the Peyer's patch, similar to the siting of the mycoplasma in the adenoids. The infectious mycoplasma is normally pacific until triggered by a trauma at which point it begins to uptake cholesterol from the intestinal membrane, leading to the degeneration of the latter. Hence, a trauma is usually involved in the onset of Alzheimer's, CFS/ME, Fibromyalgia, Crohn's and other mycoplasmal-related diseases.

8   **Creutzfeldt-Jakob (CJD):** This is the disease that was discovered among the Fore peoples of Papua-New Guinea in the early 1950s and called by them 'Kuru' which was subsequently investigated by Dr. Carleton Gajdusek of the U.S. Army and the NIH. Dr. Gajdusek links CJD or Kuru to familial Alzheimer's disease in humans and to 'Scrapie' or Visna Virus in sheep and goats. (See Gajdusek's Nobel Lecture, Page 167).Our research has established the strong likelihood that during the 1942 Japanese occupation of the Fore territory, a number of the people were inoculated with a sheep-derived pathogen to establish the latter's effectiveness as a biological agent. However, before the Japanese could learn anything about

it, they were driven from the area by the Australian defenders. Dr./General Ishii Shiro revealed what his unit was doing in the area in return for war crimes amnesty from General Douglas MacArthur. The Americans have never released what they learned, but in the early 1950s Gajdusek arrived to investigate the disease. (Ch. 1, Section 9)

9 **Diabetes Type One:** (aka Diabetes Mellitus) This disease results when the Beta cells in the pancreas fail to produce enough of the hormone insulin to regulate the body's use of GLUCAGON. The essential question seldom addressed is what causes the failure of the beta cells in the first place? There is a strong familial factor, but given that predisposition, there has to be an operative disabling agent. It is our view that a likely disabling agent is a species of mycoplasma which uptakes the preformed cholesterol from the beta cell membrane, killing the cell. In this respect it resembles the damage to the cells in the substantia nigra by a mycoplasmal species and the reduction of dopamine production. The loss of dopamine results in Parkinson's disease. We have noted that many families where the male has Parkinson's, the female will have Diabetes Type One. A reasonable therapeutic response might address the possible mycoplasmal damage, with stem cell treatment to replace the lost beta cells.

10 **Kibuchi's (Kikuchi's) disease:** ** Kikuchi's disease is also called histiocytic necrotizing lymphadenitis or Kikuchi-Fujimoto disease. It is an uncommon, idiopathic, generally self-limited cause of lymphadenitis. Kikuchi first described the disease in 1972 in Japan. Kikuchi disease (KD) most frequently manifests as a relatively acute onset of cervical adenopathy associated with fever and flu-like symptoms. Other symptoms include headache, nausea, vomiting, fatigue, weight loss, night sweats, rash and thoracic/abdominal pain. The most common clinical manifestation is cervical lymphadenopathy, with or without systemic signs and symptoms. Studies report that women are affected more often than men by a ratio of approximately 3:1. It typically affects young people.

11 **Lupus:** ** Lupus is a disease in which the body's own defenses

are turned against themselves. It affects the joints, muscles and other parts of the body such as the heart, kidneys and brain. Complications from Lupus can be life-threatening. Symptoms such as extreme sensitivity to light, sunburn after short exposures, skin ulcers on the tongue or inside of the mouth or nose, joint pain, stiffness and swelling are common. Women are nine times more likely than men to develop Lupus. In addition, African-American women are three to four times more likely to develop Lupus than Caucasian women. Lupus is not curable but it can be managed with drugs. Because Lupus is a systemic problem, patients can at best manage the disease by generally taking better care of themselves. Lupus victims have to improve the function of their immune system by getting proper rest, exercising lightly and regularly, refrain from smoking, limit their alcohol use and by reducing stress.

12 **Sarcoidosis:** ** Sarcoidosis involves inflammation that produces tiny lumps of cells in various organs in the body. These lumps can grow and even clump together thus affecting how that organ functions. It usually begins in the lungs or the lymph nodes (especially in the lymph nodes in the chest cavity.) Sarcoidosis almost always occurs in more than one organ at a time. The course of Sarcoidosis varies dramatically among people and even within the victim themselves. In many people, Sarcoidosis is slow and mild. However, in some victims it slowly gets worse over the years causing permanent organ damage resulting in death. According to the official literature there is no known way to prevent Sarcoidosis. It affects people of all ages and races worldwide. Sarcoidosis may also cause more general symptoms, including an overall feeling of ill health, severe fatigue, loss of appetite, fever, weight loss, night sweats and sleep problems. Currently, the main treatment for Sarcoidosis is Prednisone, an anti-inflammatory drug.

13 **SARS:** ** (We strongly believe that 'Severe Acute Respiratory Syndrome is the same infection Dr. Lo calls 'respiratory distress syndrome'.)

14 **Wegener's Disease:** ** Wegener's granulomatosis is an uncommon disease that can affect persons of any age and presents with an inflamed mass in the mucous linings of the

nose, throat and lungs. It affects twice as many men as it does women. The disease may present suddenly and severely or it may take years to develop. Wegener's can begin with flu-like symptoms or a general feeling of not being well. Early indications of infection include fever, joint pain, loss of appetite and congestion of the nose and sinuses. This leads many physicians to mistake Wegener's symptoms for chronic sinusitis. Other symptoms may also appear such as rough, bumpy skin rashes, eye problems including redness and eyestrain. It is not known what causes Wegener's granulomatosis. While it appears similar to an infection, no bacteria or virus has been identified as a cause. We suggest that there is a role in the onset of this disease in the mycoplasma. Eventually the disease spreads to the blood vessels and causes serious complications such as fluid leaking into the lungs and especially inflammation of the tiny capillaries of the kidneys. Some long-term patients with Wegener's granulomatosis will develop bladder cancer.

** Listed in Shyh Ching Lo's Patent

An Interlude on the Amyloid, the Prion and the Mycoplasma with a Comment on Cyanide

In Section Nine of Chapter One of this study we referred to the package of literature sent to us by Dr. Carleton Gajdusek. In one piece we encountered a puzzling statement that we have come to believe re-enforces our hypothesis that at some level of the scientific hierarchy there are persons who intentionally foster false scientific dicta to obscure certain realities that are deemed to be best kept from general knowledge.

The puzzling statement is in Gajdusek's "Infectious Amyloids: Subacute Spongiform Encephalopathies as Transmissible Cerebral Amyloidosis". The article was published as Chapter 91 in *Field's Virology*, 1996; Pages 2851 to 2900, and the statement which puzzles us is the following from pages 2861-2:

> "Since the unconventional and atypical viruses of SSVE [Subacute spongiform viral encephalopathies - Ed] (kuru - CJD - GSS - scrapie - BSE) have been identified as infectious

amyloid molecules, our laboratory has slowly switched to designating them as infectious amyloids instead of unconventional viruses. Others have accepted the term *prions* for these agents."

Why should such a statement puzzle us?

It should puzzle us because we have been searching for the disease agent or agents which cause the brain diseases Gajdusek has listed (kuru, CJD, GSS, scrapie, BSE) and to which we have added Alzheimer's, Parkinson's, Huntington's, and AIDS dementia complex, and the evidence as we have presented in this study strongly suggests that a species of mycoplasma is that agent or, more likely, a co-agent in that disease process.

Does Gajdusek's statement suggest that we are wrong? That the unconventional virus known as an infectious amyloid molecule, rather than the mycoplasma, is really the cause?

Then, to compound the puzzle, Gajdusek introduces the startling possibility that the unconventional virus, later called the amyloid, is really the protein particle called the prion?

First, to deal with the so-called prion this has been thrown into the mix. The prion was supposedly 'discovered' by Stanley Prusiner who received a Nobel Prize for his work. We say 'supposedly' discovered because in our twelve years of research we have been unable to locate any definitive evidence that it exists.

The Webster's *New Explorer Medical Dictionary* defines it as:

> "prion \ n: a protein particle that lacks nucleic acid and is sometimes held to be the cause of various infectious diseases of the nervous system (as scrapie and Creutzfeldt-Jakob disease) Page 557

This is a very tenuous and imprecise definition of an agent that is supposed to be involved with such critical animal and human disease conditions. The human body is full of protein particles, especially in the lymph system and subsequently in the blood and urine and how such protein particles can, as Prusiner hypothesizes, misfold to create "severe neurological disease called scrapie in sheep and kuru in humans" (Gallo, 1991 Page 54) is a mystery that no one has been able to clear. And yet, Dr. Prusiner received the Nobel Prize for his "discovery." This fact has led us to further question the possible political considerations which may motivate the Swedish learned societies in their selection of the person or persons whose work in physics, chemistry, physiology or medicine is deemed most significant in their field.

Fritz Haber (1868 - 1934)

The prime example of this possibility is to be seen in the award of the Nobel Prize in chemistry to Fritz Haber for his work in the development of mustard gas in 1918. This horrible chemical weapon of war was used by Germany against allied armies in Europe in World War I and the award set an unfortunate precedent for later work in biological weapons research by Frank Brunet and Carleton Gajdusek. (The same political consideration may extend to the selection of the Nobel Prize for Peace by the Norwegian Parliament with laureates such as Henry Kissinger and Menachem Begin, but our focus is on the listed sciences.)

In the sciences listed laureates include Carleton Gajdusek and Frank Brunet, both of whom figure prominently in any study of biological weapons research. When Prusiner is added to the Nobel laureate triumvirate of Kissinger, Gajdusek and Brunet, one may reasonably speculate about the possible political aspects of certain Nobel awards.

Did the Nobel selection committee choose Prusiner simply to validate the very questionable theory of the prion; and hence lead enquiry away from the mycoplasma? Consider the following:

> "As early as 1911, it was discovered that the Rous sarcoma virus causes tumors in birds, but decades of searching for microbes in human cancers ended in failure."
>
> (Karlen, 1995 Page 201)

Now consider the following:

> "Rous never named his RNA chicken sarcoma virus 'a virus' but rather 'a filterable transmissible agent.'"
>
> (Cantwell, 2005 Page 69)

And also consider:

> "In 1966 Jackson [Eleanor Alexander -] demonstrated in Growth that the Rous virus was actually a filterable virus-sized form of the cancer microbe ('*Mycoplasma* [PPLO]

isolated from Rous sarcoma virus'). In 1970 another of her papers was published in the Annals of the New York Academy of Sciences that demonstrated (by use of spectograms obtained with the ultraviolet spectogramic microscope) that the RNA Rous sarcoma agent contained traces of DNA - thus indicating the Rous 'virus' was essentially related to bacteria that Eleanor [Jackson] had consistently isolated from cancer." (Cantwell, 2005 Page 70)

How does this all add up? We believe the following summarizes the situation.

Gajdusek's 'amyloid' is not the cause of degenerative diseases such as kuru (CLD) and scrapie; it is a product of the actual cause, which is the microorganism we have described in this study as a species of mycoplasma.

This interpretation would fit with Gajdusek's definition of **Infectious Amyloidosis** on page 2,853 of his article:

> "Amyloids are insoluble deposits of polymerized fibrils of crossed-beta-pleated sheet configuration of host-precursor proteins…"

This also fits with the fact that certain species of mycoplasma have an absolute growth requirement for pre-formed sterols including cholesterol. The latter cholesterol is up-taken from its host cell, leading to cellular degeneration while creating the polymerized fibrils that Gajdusek has observed. The degenerated cells present as the subject diseases, which vary in observed effect as the loss of cell function resulting in deficits such as reduced dopamine when cells of the substantia nigra are lost.

The mycoplasma is the cause; the amyloid is a product; a disease is the subsequent loss of function.

Where does that leave Dr. Stanley Prusiner and the prion? Our initial hypothesis expressed above, that the Nobel Prize to Dr. Prusiner is simply an attempt to validate an unlikely theory to lead enquiry away from the mycoplasma.

It should be noted before leaving this Interlude that among the other papers sent to us by Dr. Gajdusek was a re-print of an article titled simply, "Kuru" co-authored by Dr. V. Zigas. The article had been published in the March 1959 issue of the American Journal of

Medicine. On page 464 of the Journal the authors write the following very important paragraph:

> "In sheep exposed to a phalaris - dominant pasture a staggers syndrome called 'phalaris staggers' is produced and this neuro-muscular disorder involving hyper excitability, tremors, ataxia and in-coordination, loss of ability to rise and progressing usually to death is in its clinical picture akin to Kuru [which is known as Creutzfeldt - Jacob disease - Ed] It has been found that frequent oral administration of soluble cobalt salts to sheep will completely protect [but note: not cured - Ed] the animals against phalaris staggers …"

There is much of critical importance in this paragraph. Note that it is "sheep" that the authors refer to (although there are similar diseases in other animals). Also note that sheep had been used for "experimental" purposes at Japanese biological weapons test sites (see Chap. 1, Sec. 8 of this study). The symptoms of the ill sheep apply almost exactly to cattle with what is now known as "mad cow" disease.

Note further that the cobalt salts have a strong chemical relationship to nickel and copper (it is usually obtained as a by-product of nickel and copper mining). In this respect it also has links to gold and iron mining. All the minerals cited (cobalt, copper, nickel, iron, silver and gold) have important medicinal uses. To quote Dr. Andre Voisin:

> "The mineral elements of the soil are in fact transformed by the plant into organic compounds which have a dietetic value very different from the same element under its mineral form."   (Voisin, 1959 Page 101)

The question arises: Why does cobalt (and according to Voisin, copper) protect sheep from phalaris staggers?

In the twelve years of our research into the origin of AIDS and collateral damage diseases such as cancer, Parkinson's disease, Alzheimer's, and others we have formulated the theory that the actual doer of damage is cyanide and that damage is either prevented or reduced as the presence of the cyanide is reduced.

In the Sudbury area of Ontario where we are pleased to reside, we see the fundamental reality of cyanide reaction with minerals applied all the time in the mining operations upon which the City of Sudbury is based. Mineral- containing ore is crushed to a powder and is then mixed with cyanide. The gold and the cyanide have a strong chemical affinity for each other and when so mixed quickly bind. The bonded mineral and cyanide can then be readily drawn off and then separated.

Here we see one of the fundamental truths of cyanide and minerals at work. We see the same reality in the case cited by Dr. Gajdusek and Zigas. The cobalt added to the pasture neutralizes the cyanide and hence prevents phalaris staggers.

In the Canadian Medical Association Home Medical Encyclopedia there appears the following:

> "Antirhueumatic drugs, such as gold or penicillanine, may be used to arrest or slow the progression of the disease [rheumatoid arthritis—Ed] (Morgan, 1992 Page 874)

How does this chemical reality relate to the degenerative diseases is the focus of this study?

There are several ways, but we will cite one as an example of the many.

The mycoplasma infects the body and sequesters in certain cells.

A trauma of some kind activates the mycoplasma into action which begins to up-take the pre-formed cholesterol of its host cellwall.

The cell is ultimately killed and the glutamate in its nucleus is spilled into the blood and lymph fluid.

The glutamate with its high affinity for ammonia combines with the latter taken from urea to form the less dangerous glutamine. However, the latter action liberates cyanide from the urea molecule.

Normally, the cyanide is up-taken and neutralized by the red blood cells; however, when the quantity of cyanide is excessive due to extreme cell damage the cyanide is free to do its harm.

It is at this point that certain minerals can unite with the free cyanide, neutralizing the latter to be removed as urine.

Hence gold or silver or vitamin B12 (which is manufactured from cobalt by an actinomycete named *Streptomyces grisens*) work against the cyanide and reduce disease.

It is not our purpose in this study to go into specialized technical studies of the biological malfunctioning in plants and animals. After all, we are tracing the many factors which have entered in to the laboratory-engineered disease agents of biological strategic war against population growth. However, we present such interludes as this to demonstrate the scientific basis of the whole effort and to ensure our readers that our major thesis has a fundamental scientific basis.

PART SIX

THE MEDIA

Chapter Eighteen

THE MEDIA: INTRODUCTION

Living creatures including humans, to different degrees varying with species and age, learn from experience. Humans have a particular advantage in the learning process over other living organisms because the human brain is capable, again to various degrees and varying from one individual to another, of learning from another's experience. A sign at the side of a road which has printed upon it the message, 'Caution' will lead some humans to move more carefully along that road than they normally would. They exercise caution because apparently someone else has had an unfortunate experience and has attempted to prevent others from experiencing the same consequence by putting up the sign.

The sign is a medium of communication. If the medium is accurate, one person's bad experience will not be repeated by those who see and understand the message and then act upon it. Unfortunately, there are false media, including human speech, which do not communicate true messages. There is a loud cry in a crowded theatre 'Fire!' and patrons stampede for the exits. Some are trampled by others behind them.

Some false messages are intentional; others are learned on the basis of the authority of the teacher. Both the intentionally false messages and those which are part of religious or political dogma are devices to control the learner.

In 1996 we were just completing our first year of research into CFS/ME, and were puzzling over the many allusions to an apparent relationship between CFS/ME and AIDS as noted by Hillary Johnson in *Osler's Web*. (Chapter Nineteen below) In early July of that year we noted two news items about AIDS. Both stories dealt with a new book titled *Emerging Viruses: AIDS and Ebola*, by Leonard Horowitz. The stories were based upon the opinions of two academics, one at the Dana-Farber Cancer Institute and the other of The Aaron Diamond AIDS Research Centre. Both academics were dismissing the major hypothesis of the Horowitz book (that AIDS may have had its origins in American biowar laboratories) as unfounded.

We tracked down the academics at their respective institutions and spoke to each on the phone. We were concerned by the fact that we had recently learned of the June 9, 1969 Pentagon Hearings (Ch. 15) and of Dr. MacArthur's promise to a Congressional sub-committee that the U.S. military could probably develop within ten years a new microorganism, one which did not naturally exist and which would be refractory to the human immune system. We also shared our concern that Dr. MacArthur at the same Hearings had told the Congressmen that the U.S. was developing two pathogens, one which would kill and one which would disable. We asked if it were simply a coincidence that within ten years of those Hearings, a new lethal disease (AIDS) was beginning to present in epidemic numbers and a new disabling disease (CFS/ME) was also appearing. We also asked what had become of the Pentagon research after Congress voted to go ahead with MacArthur's plans. We asked, as well, how it happened that two strains of HIV appeared at almost the same time.

Both gentlemen asked for more time to consider our concerns and promised to answer them if we would put them in writing. We did so and mailed them off.

After about two weeks, having had no reply to our written questions, we phoned each again to determine whether we could expect an answer. Our contact at Dana-Farber assured us that we would receive his answers soon. The call to The Aaron Diamond AIDS Research Center was more interesting. It went something like this (from memory…no notes were kept at the time):

The Aaron Diamond AIDS Research Center

DWS: Is Dr. Moore available?
Operator: Who shall I say is calling?
DWS: Donald Scott of Sudbury, Canada.
Operator: Oh, Mr. Scott, Dr. Ho would like to speak with you. May I put you through?

Now, I had a vague awareness of who Dr. Ho was…he had been named by Time Magazine as their Man of the Year for his work on

AIDS. *I was surprised that a person of his stature would want to talk to me.*

> **DWS**: Alright
> **Dr. Ho**: Mr. Scott. We've been discussing your letter to Dr. Moore. Do you mind if I enquire why you are interested in the origin of AIDS?
> **DWS**: I'm interested in the origins because I believe that if we know the real source, we'll be closer to finding a cure.
> **Dr. Ho**: Well, the source is pretty well established; it's a zoonotic primate disease that has jumped species.
> **DWS**: That's what I've read…but I'm concerned about other possibilities.
> **Dr. Ho**: Wouldn't your time be better spent looking for a cure?
> **DWS**: Finding the source is part of finding a cure. But I'm concerned whether I'll get a reply to my questions to Dr. Moore.
> **Dr. Ho**: Oh yes. We'll answer those for you.

A few days later we received the following letter. We have numbered and italicized certain quotations to facilitate our comments which follow.

> The Aaron Diamond AIDS Research Center
> Affiliate of the Rockefeller University
>
> July 22, 1969
>
> Dear Mr. Scott,
>
> Thank you for your letter of July 19 and the enclosed documents. Rather than filling in your questionnaire, I will respond in this letter, from which you may freely quote. I do hope that you will use your access to Ontario schoolchildren to give them an accurate perspective on the origin of HIV, and (1) *to dispel the ridiculous notion that this virus arose from biological warfare* programs. I would also like to make the point that it seems to me more constructive to inform

children of the great efforts that medical science is making to conquer HIV, by stopping its spread and by treating those infected with it. This is much more positive, and important, (2) *than speculating on old conspiracy theories that are utterly without foundation.*

HIV is a virus that was transmitted into the human species from animals in a perfectly natural process, examples of which abound in the virology literature. Influenza viruses, for example, transmit between humans, pigs and ducks, and the increased genetic diversity acquired during such passages creates new strains to which mankind has relatively limited immunity - hence the great influenza pandemics that arise infrequently, but with serious consequences. (3) *Laurie Garrett's book: The Coming Plague is very good on these issues.*

In the case of HIV, there is overwhelming evidence that HIV-2 arose in humans from a limited number of transmissions of SIV from African monkeys - the two viruses are virtually identical, and SIV has certainly infected an animal researcher accidentally in a laboratory. Relevant species of monkeys are used for food in rural Africa, and it is easy to imagine blood-borne cross-transmission during the hunting and processing of monkeys. The original animal host of HIV- 1 is more obscure, but HIV-1 strains have been isolated from chimpanzees, so it is at least plausible that the virus crossed into humans from these apes.

To turn to your questions. I am quite satisfied that there is no chance that HIV is a man-made virus, whether from a biological warfare program or otherwise.

(4) *Firstly, there are documented, characterized cases of HIV-1 infection of humans dating back to the 1960's, possibly earlier, well before the time frame you consider in the Congressional documents.*

(5) *Secondly, I am convinced that even today after 13 years of*

HIV-1 research, the technology exists to create such a virus de novo, even if anyone were evil enough to want to do this. It certainly could not have existed in the early 1970's, the period you refer to implicitly.

(6) *Thirdly, I know many of the scientists who work in the military HIV research program.* They are fine individuals, as much dedicated to eradicating HIV as are their civilian counterparts. It is inconceivable to me these people would have been involved in something (7) *as evil as you seem to be suggesting.* They are also no more or no less competent than civilian scientists - as I say, I doubt any human could create HIV from scratch, whether a military person or a civilian.

(8) *Fourthly, supposing your hypothesis were true?* HIV would be an incredibly foolish choice for a biological weapon aimed at wiping out human populations. True, it is a lethal virus for which (9) *cures are only now being considered feasible.* But it is also relatively difficult to transmit, and (10) *it takes a decade to kill most of the people it infects.* If one were evil enough to want to use a biological weapon on mankind, are these desirable properties for such a weapon to have? I am sure many more plausible viral or bacterial candidates for genocide are known to science.

To close, you refer to chronic fatigue syndrome. This is not an area on which I feel professionally qualified to comment. But I am not convinced that this syndrome has any true relationship, reciprocal or otherwise, to AIDS.

Yours sincerely
(signed)
John P. Moore, PhD
Staff Investigator
Aaron Diamond AIDS Research Center

Our Comments:
(1) We had not communicated a 'notion'; we had sent Dr. Moore a photocopy of the report made to select Congressmen by Dr. MacArthur of the Pentagon.
(2) 'old conspiracy theories that are utterly without foundation.' The meeting between Dr. MacArthur and the Congressmen was kept secret until revealed under the Freedom of Information Act and it dealt with a new *lethal* weapon that would be refractory to the human immune system. So, our letter had not suggested a 'theory', it had shared facts. Further, such a meeting would fit the definition of a 'conspiracy.'
(3) We had not read Laurie Garrett's book, but we did follow up on HIV-2 and learned that it had only been found in laboratory monkeys, and had never been found in monkeys in the wild! If it had jumped species it was from humans to monkeys, not the other way around.
(4) It was not until much later that we were able to study the question of when AIDS had appeared among humans and had found that Ed Hooper in *The River* had followed up on these claims very carefully. We came to the conclusion that such cases as had occurred were more likely the consequence of early testing of pathogens developed in the laboratories owned or controlled by the U.S. Government.
(5) Dr. Moore seems to forget that it was Dr. MacArthur's statements to the Congressmen that we were questioning. Is Dr. Moore suggesting that MacArthur was lying or badly informed?
(6) Bringing up military scientists who are now studying AIDS is dragging a red herring across the path. We had been asking about the scientists who had advised Dr. MacArthur that an AIDS- like disease was possible. We were not asking about anyone who took up the study of AIDS after the epidemic began to show. Here, Dr. Moore was using a sophomoric rhetorical device.
(7) We had not been 'suggesting' anyone was 'evil'...although the creation of biological weapons that are refractory to the human immune system is in our view, evil. We were talking about Dr. MacArthur's statements made on the Congressional record.

(8) Again, we were not suggesting a hypothesis to Dr. Moore; we were sharing the historical record with him. The question is, was the CIA- Pentagon researching an AIDS-like biological weapon? **That is what Dr. MacArthur said they were doing!**
(9) Having no known cure for a biological weapon would seem to us to be an advantage for such a weapon.
(10) Taking a decade to kill would also be an advantage for a biological weapon such as AIDS. If people got sick and died the day after receiving a smallpox vaccination that would strongly suggest the fact that the vaccine was deadly. Getting sick five years after a smallpox vaccination and dying ten years after would help cover the crime that had been committed.

All in all, Dr. Moore's answers struck us as superficial, and we were in no further touch with him.

The Dana-Farber Cancer Institute

The following letter containing answers to our questions was received by Fax the day after we received the above reply from Dr. Moore. In reproducing this letter, we will comment in italics upon certain points as we proceed:

> 1. Dr. MacArthur spoke in 1970 *[it was actually 1969]* of an agent that in his estimate, would take 5 to 10 years to create. I have no personal knowledge of such an agent being created. As I'm sure you know the Geneva Accord does not allow its signatories to engage in biological weapons research (or the US to engage in biological weapons research except for defensive purposes.) *[The US was not a signatory to the Geneva Accord until 1970. In the meantime it had been researching and using bacteriological weapons against China as early as 1952!]* Public opinion in this (and other) countries was strongly against this type of research by the military, and such research was halted. *[It was halted in public statements only, not in actual fact.]*
>
> All history aside, there are several practical and medical reasons that it is unlikely that this 'synthetic biological

agent' was not HIV. 1. The technology to create a synthetic retrovirus was beyond our means until recently *[this is a case of setting up a straw man and then knocking it down... Dr. MacArthur had not mentioned a 'retrovirus' anywhere in his report. He spoke of a 'new' microorganism. Such could be an old microorganism from (say) sheep, which had been passaged through a bovine species to make it pathogenic to humans. Hence, it would be 'new' to humans.]* For example the means to grow primary T cells, e.g. IL-2 were not discovered until 1978 (ref. Gillis, *et al.* J. Exp. Med 148-1093) If it would take 5 to 10 years to develop, this would not allow enough time to explain the appearance of many cases of AIDS (which has a median incubation of 8 years) to appear between 1978 and 1981 in young men on both US coasts. *[This is the same conclusion that we had reached after considering Dr. MacArthur's suggestion that within 5 to 10 years his laboratory could produce such a 'new' microorganism. If, as we were coming to believe, he already had the pathogen and that it was first seeded in vaccines over ten years before it would begin to present in epidemic proportions within his 5-10 year time frame (i.e. 1975 to 1980) and that he was just trying to get the Congress involved retroactively. Then, when it did begin to appear, the Congressmen would be restrained from demanding action.]* 2) Phylogenic evidence indicates that HIV-1 is at least 100 years old (reviewed by Krause, Science 257:1073-1077) (current unpublished estimates place it at 200years old), and that HIV-2 is much older. Even within the limits of these estimates of their age, HIV-1 and -2 are too old to be the work of modern technology. *[Here our correspondent seems to have gotten mixed up. We had suggested that if such an immune suppressant were already naturally available, why would MacArthur have to develop such as he promised the Congressmen.]* 3) Finally, the same evidence suggests that HIV-2 and HIV -1 share close evolutionary relationships to viruses in monkeys. HIV-2 is related to SIVmac (simian (or monkey) immunodeficiency virus). While SIVcpz (found in chimps) is related to HIV-1. In other words it is likely that the HIV's evolved over time as opposed to being a 'synthetic biological agent.' 4) Finally common sense- it has taken over 15 years and billions of dollars and some of the brightest minds in medical science to only now just scratch the surface of the AIDS problem, it's unlikely that HIV could have been created, much less designed, 25 years ago with the limited technology we had back then.

This speculation still doesn't explain upon what basis Dr. MacArthur could have made his commitment to the Congressmen.

Finally, we should point out that in contrast to tularemia, Q fever, and some of the other biological warfare agents mentioned by Dr. MacArthur, HIV has two drawbacks from a military perspective:

1. There is no way to prevent its spread to an army's troops as there is no vaccine or prophylaxis. *[Even if this were relevant to our question, how would one know that the military did not have such a vaccine? After all, it is no use coming up with a population growth control disease one day, and then announce a vaccine to stop it the next day]* 2. HIV has a long incubation period before it causes disease – on average 8 years for infection to the onset of AIDS (although this period may be prolonged with the exciting new combination therapies discussed in Vancouver).*[As we noted in our reply to Dr. Moore... such a gap between infection and disability could be seen as an advantage.]*

2. It is unlikely that HIV was what Dr. MacArthur was thinking about for the reasons enumerated above. It is unlikely for those reasons that HIV would have been invented. *[Obviously, Dr. MacArthur was not thinking about a naturally occurring immune deficiency disease. He told the Congressmen that it would be a 'new' microorganism, not an old adapted microorganism.]* The question as to why HIV appeared on the world scene now as opposed to several hundred years ago is much tougher. Some have suggested that it is the

rapidity of global travel combined with the encroachment of large numbers of humans on parts of the world only sparsely inhabited by people that puts us into contact with deadly infectious agents like Ebola, or HIV. If there is a human agency involved in the AIDS epidemic this is likely to be a part of it. *[This thesis was rapidly becoming a modern social myth that really can't stand up to logical analysis. Is it likely that an African native would be in the jungle where he kills an SIV-infected chimpanzee which bites him and infects him with the virus, and then the native boards a jet plane and flies to San Francisco where he has a homosexual relationship with several gay white men? Would that account for the heterosexual epidemic back in Africa?]*

3. As an infectious disease physician and a virologist, I am unaware of a specific known infectious cause for the chronic fatigue syndrome. At this point an infectious cause of CFS would be hypothesis. *[Perhaps...but how else could one account for the epidemics of CFS/ME that had occurred in the 1980s without there being an infectious agent?]* CFS obviously requires further study, and individuals diagnosed with this syndrome should be certain to be evaluated for treatable disorder, such as depression and endocrine abnormalities.

4. Since we don't know of an infectious agent for CFS, it would be premature to attribute an incapacitating synthetic virus to its existence. *[Yes, but should some infectious agent not be looked for? And, since it was Dr. MacArthur who said that the Pentagon was searching for a disabling biological agent, might not CFS have started with his research?]*

As we discussed, I don't wish to be quoted *[We believe that by leaving your name and title off the letter, we are meeting our commitment.]*

This correspondence was our first introduction to many of the theories that we were to encounter over the next eleven years of our research. Although we were not, at the time, sufficiently informed to challenge the writers on some of the technical details, we did reach the conclusion early on that the mainstream medical researchers were not doing much to challenge the early stories about green monkeys or chimps, biting Black people who then gave a simian virus to huge numbers of victims by way of gay white male promiscuity. The answers didn't help us much, but they did alert us to the kind of response many so-called scientists were making to two tragic diseases. The answers didn't seem very scientific to us.

They only stimulated us to do as Dr. Harvey Caldwell of Guelph University had urged us to do in the face of any great human problem: gather more facts. We did that by ordering the book that both the above correspondence had panned as nonsense...we ordered Leonard Horowitz' *Emerging Viruses: AIDS and Ebola*...

Media and Science Magazine

Even in media, which are supposedly objective reporters of established evidence, the effects of the official mythologies can be found. A case in point can be seen in the June 9, 2000 issue of *Science* magazine. Let us explain.

Every day over 8,000 people world-wide are dying of AIDS. And, as we have seen, the evidence that has been secured by courageous researchers such as the late Ted Strecker (he died mysteriously of gun shot wounds a few months after securing the document from the Pentagon) is beyond question: the AIDS pathogen was developed in laboratories across the United States by several of the world's top biological researchers and was deployed by the United States in several of the world's poorest countries under the direction of Henry Kissinger.

Despite the solid, unchallenged government-printed documentary evidence upon which we have based our major theses, as to the true source of AIDS, the establishment powers-that-be continue to promote a weird and fantastic tale of humans infected with a monkey virus. These powers, with their media assets such as *The New York Times*, *The Washington Post*, *Time*, etc. have kept up a steady stream of 'evidence' that they claim proves their story. Almost every six months there will be a new report from some obscure biological institution in Alabama or Mississippi or New Mexico about some research group which has found the AIDS virus in some monkey cadaver.

Well, on June 9, 2000, (a date exactly thirty-one years after Dr. MacArthur's Hearings before the Congressmen) a new piece of evidence was adduced by a group of mathematicians and microbiologists from New Mexico, England, Illinois and (you guessed it) Alabama, that 'proved' statistically that the 'Ancestor of the HIV-1 Pandemic Strains' had leaped from chimpanzees to humans in 1931! Nowhere in the story do they suggest the day, date and specific time… but if you asked for this information, they could probably come up with it. They had used 'parallel supercomputers'. If there is one thing that impresses the unwary (and uninformed) it is to be told that the computers say it is so.

The report of B. Korber, *et al.* was published in *Science*, V. 288, #5472, on pages 1789-1802, and the media grabbed the story and ran with it. Papers across the nation, and probably much of the world, picked it up and trumpeted it to the masses. A member of our Common Cause Medical Research Foundation in Atlanta, GA, sent us a clipping from page A-16 of the *Atlanta Journal-Constitution* and another member from Ingersoll, Ontario, sent us a clipping from *The Toronto Star*. 'Study traces AIDS to 1930's' claimed the heading from Atlanta, while the *Star* informed its readers: 'HIV originated in Africa in 1931: Study.'

When our copy of *Science* arrived in the mail, we turned to page 1789 and read the evidence which so precisely established the year that some darn chimp had bitten some poor African. We first read the introductory abstract and were re-assured to read that the researchers had '…validated our approach by correctly estimating the timing of two historically documented points.' Great! We would be able, finally, to find a point that was documented, and we could then look up those documents and compare them with the government documents that indicated quite clearly that AIDS hadn't come from some monkey bite, but from some NIH laboratory. We were also somewhat concerned when we read that these scientists-mathematicians had employed "…a method that relaxed the assumption of a strict molecular clock…" Relaxing an assumption means that if something in your theory doesn't fit with some previously determined position, and then ignore the latter!

As we struggled through the pages of mathematical jargon, we kept recalling the old computer GIGO dictum: 'Garbage in; garbage out'.

At last, we reached the place in the text where the authors introduced their 'two historically documented points.' We carefully underlined the four sentences which we reproduce in full below: (the numbers in parentheses are endnotes from the original article)

> "AIDS was first identified as a clinical syndrome in 1981 (47). Twelve AIDS cases were retrospectively identified in 1978-79, and by the first quarter of 1983, there were already 1299 cases of clinical AIDS reported in the United States, spread over 35 states (48). In both Haiti and the United States, scattered cases of HIV-1 infection or AIDS were identified in the late 1970's with a handful of possible and probable cases noted in the United States and Haiti between 1972 and 1976 (48,49). Thus, our timing estimates for an ancestral sequence are plausible…"

We didn't feel challenged by the first claim, identified as endnote #47…after all, our *Cambridge Factfinder* says right there on page 161 "1981 First reports of AIDS", so we could chalk that up for Korber, *et al*. We next turned to their next 'historically documented' point, and here we began to run into trouble.

First, we noted their dependence upon 'L. Gazzolo, N. Eng. J. Med. 311, 1252 (1984).' We were rendered a trifle uncomfortable by the fact that Gazzolo is listed in the *"Special Virus Cancer Program" Progress Report #8*, as one of the researchers working at Nixon's War on Cancer back in 1971. Given the strong evidence that the SVCP was a cover for the laboratory development of the AIDS pathogen that had been promised to the US Congress by the Pentagon in 1969, it struck us as a possibility that Gazzolo might well want to promote the idea that their handiwork had actually come into the world in 1931 when a green monkey or a chimpanzee or other simian species bit an African.

However, we managed to suspend our disbelief in Gazzolo long enough to make our way to the Laurentian University Library where we dug out volume 311 of *The New England Journal of Medicine*, and read Gazzolo's 'historically documented' point. We received quite a shock when it turned out to be simply a letter to the editor! No peer review here. Then we received another surprise…one of Gazzolo's fellow signatories to the letter was none other than 'G. de-The'! Why, you may well ask, should we be bothered by this discovery? We were very bothered by the fact that G. de-The is also listed in the SVCP, Progress Report #8, and he has a total of 18 articles cited therein. He was, in other words, a major researcher in the program. Furthermore, on two of those articles, de-The collaborated with L. Gazzolo.

Our greatest shock came when we read this letter which the authors of the Science piece, so broadly reported by media assets throughout Canada and the U.S., had suggested was a historical document that validated their supercomputer-generated date when a chimpanzee bit a human being and gave the latter the world's first case of human AIDS. It is mind-boggling to report that the letter does not deal, as we are led to believe it does, with either Americans or Haitians. It deals, instead, with 211 residents of French Guiana who had immigrated to that country during the previous 10 years from Haiti. Furthermore, their blood had been drawn in 1983 by the Pasteur Institute, and had been tested, not for HIV, but for HTLV antibodies. This was very misleading!

Enter Jean W. Pape, et al.

Perhaps we'll do better when we refer to the next 'historically documented' evidence cited by Korber, *et al.*, we mused, and we took down volume 309 of *The New England Journal of Medicine* and turned to page 945. Here, we had been led to believe, we would find solid evidence that as Korber and his colleagues had assured us, there was a 'handful of possible and probable cases [of HIV-AIDS] noted in the United States and Haiti between 1972 and 1976.'

Pape, *et al.* makes no such a claim, despite their article being cited in *Science* magazine by Korber, *et al.* In fact, on page 949 of their article, Pape and his colleagues state quite unequivocally: "We do not believe that AIDS was present in Haiti before 1978."

Are the authors (skilled mathematicians and microbiologists) of this *Science* piece, who are so capable of relaxing scientific assumptions, and producing a date so specific as to when AIDS infected our human family, literacy-challenged? Or, are they, like Edward Shorter and Elaine Showalter, willing to misrepresent history to help cover the greatest crime ever committed against humanity?

You have to choose between the clear-cut, specific US government document of June 9, 1969 and all of the media ass*et al.*ternative evidence such as the piece under review.

Oh! Did we happen to mention that for the reported research, four of the authors had received funding from the NIH?

The authors wrote to the Editor of *Science* and pointed out the errors in their story, but we still have no reply.

The point again is clear. The mainstream media are willing to distort verifiable evidence in support of official mythology about the origin of AIDS and CFIDS. The latter characteristic also is seen in many of the conferences, symposia etc. presented by the AIDS establishment—the 2006 International AIDS Conference in Toronto, for example. Following are two articles written by one of the authors (DWS) for *The Journal of Degenerative Diseases*.

The Dog and Pony Show

Try as I may, I can't get over an urge to refer to the recent biennial International AIDS Conference held in Toronto as a dog and pony show. Something of a three ring circus with Bill and Melinda Gates tossing in $500,000,000 over and above the billions that they have already contributed and Bill Clinton blasting George Bush for not doing something that Clinton had failed to support when he was himself President (*i.e.*: establish several 'safe sites' in major drug and AIDS-rampant districts where AIDS-infected addicts could get clean needles and hence reduce 'needle-sharing' and consequent disease spread. To his credit, Clinton acknowledged that he failed in this respect) and Stephen Lewis conducting several of his tear-jerking laments about the tragedy of AIDS, while (according to an op-ed article from the Pembroke *Observer*) 3,000 journalists 'from around the world' reported the proceedings to their readers. My goodness… three thousand journalists…what in heaven's name did they write about?

Perhaps my characterization of this huge event is unfair. Perhaps one should be more respectful of a 'conference' that draws between 24,000 and 31,000 attendees (the reports vary with the reporters). Perhaps I would have seen it differently had I been there, but unfortunately, I could not attend because our Common Cause Medical Research Foundation is so short of money that I had to count on the media (3,000 journalists!) to tell me what went on…and according to my reading of *The Sudbury Star* and the Toronto *Globe and Mail*, the whole affair was a dog and pony show.

None of Bill and Melinda Gates billions has trickled down to us. And, unlike Stephen Lewis, I don't get invitations to speak to Teachers' assemblies or Steelworkers' meetings or Nurses conferences. Stephen Lewis is an effective speaker who generally entrances his audiences with tragic anecdotes about the effects of AIDS upon its victims and upon the orphans and grandparents left behind. Expressions such as 'there was not a dry eye in the room' characterize news reports about Mr. Lewis' presentations.

And well his listeners should get misty-eyed, for over eight thousand people a day are dying from this terrible plague and the world should shed tears of sympathy for the physical suffering of the victims and the social tragedy of the orphans left behind. And Mr. Lewis gets his listeners weeping.

But, **tears are not enough**…how about a little bit of truth and honest science? How about facing Mr. Clinton with the reality of United States genocidal policies and his own failure to rise to the occasion when he had the opportunity?

And how about the Gates' billions contributed to research AIDS and other diseases which afflict humanity such as tuberculosis and malaria? The latter two diseases have been with us for the history of mankind, and we will not comment upon them. The first …AIDS… was officially recognized in the medical literature in 1981, and the research into AIDS is largely dishonest and designed to mislead, not to discover truths.

The Gates are to be thanked sincerely for their apparent efforts, but money paid to the likes of Tony Fauci and Robert Gallo is largely wasted. More of that in a minute.

Of Bill Clinton and Stephen Lewis, the Pembroke Observer has this to say:

> "Bill Clinton, who despite his personal issues will some day be regarded as one of the best presidents the United States ever had, has taken a lead role alongside Gates in advocating for a concerted effort to beat HIV/AIDS."

And

> "UN AIDS for Africa envoy Stephen Lewis is also front and centre at the conference, as the world's leading diplomat in the fight against the disease should be. A more eloquent (spokesperson) for the cause could not be found…"

To these passages of praise I respond: **talk is cheap**. Let me explain.

First, to Bill Clinton. There is no doubt that, especially compared to his successor, George W. Bush, Mr. Clinton was an above average president. However, we are talking about AIDS and Clinton's eight years as president during which time he had a chance, through his administration and his Secretary of Health and Human Services, Dr. Dona Shalala, to do a lot of important work. Here, Clinton and Shalala failed miserably.

I had some first hand experience with Shalala and her totally failed term as Secretary. It is only one example of many because it *is* first hand, and because it explains so many other failures to deal with the emerging crisis of AIDS and it need be noted, with other related diseases such as chronic fatigue and fibromyalgia.

At some point in the Clinton years (1992 to 2000), I was contacted by Dr. Hugh Fudenberg who had learned of our work with brucellosis and the mycoplasma. He phoned me several times with questions that his review had raised and on his second to last call he said to me, "I'm on Bill Clinton's Health Council, and I'm going to raise your evidence at our next meeting." That would have been a very important break through and I looked forward to hearing more from him. No further word was forthcoming and it was not until two or more years later that Dr. Fudenberg phoned me on an entirely different matter.

What had happened? Did he raise the whole question of the mycoplasma and of its possible antecedent, the brucella bacteria, at the Health Council, chaired, I am given to understand, by Dr. Shalala? If so, what was the result?

Who knows? But I have my theory. I can imagine Dr. Fudenberg raising the whole matter and being immediately put down and advised not to raise the subject further. Why do I suggest such a scenario? I do so because Dona Shalala before she became Mr. Clinton's Secretary of Health, had been the Chancellor of Wisconsin University. Furthermore, the U. of W. was one of the universities listed by the Department of Defense as co-operators in their biological warfare weapons development research. She would know of the source and purpose of much government money into the University. She would know what questions must not be asked, let alone answered.

I assume that Dr. Fudenberg was told to shut up…and he did.

Furthermore, it was during this time frame that even though all manner of professional microbiologists were down-playing the significance of the mycoplasma, one of Dr. Shalala's underlings, Dr. Shyh Ching Lo, of the American Institute of Pathology, was busy applying for and receiving a patent on none other than a 'Pathogenic Mycoplasma'. In the Patent, on page 22, Dr. Lo states that patients infected with the mycoplasma will include patients diagnosed as having AIDS, or ARC (AIDS-Related Complex) chronic fatigue syndrome and other diseases.

Dr. Shalala would know which lines of enquiry to shut down, and she was appointed to office by Bill Clinton. Why would he appoint her? Because he was told that she would be a 'safe' appointee.

Now that he is out of office, Mr. Clinton can make all of the impassioned speeches he wishes without fear of stumbling upon or exposing the truth.

Talk is cheap.

Now to Stephen Lewis…In words reminiscent of a vaudeville song and dance routine: 'After you my dear William.' 'No, after you my dear Stephen' and to quote from an article by Andre Picard, public health reporter for the *Globe and Mail*, August 16, 2006:

> "Mr. Lewis spoke of the former president and his foundation in glowing terms. He said that most international groups in the field work with 'supernatural acceleration, from inertia to paralysis.' but that Mr. Clinton is a man of passion and action."
>
> "'What has filled my soul with admiration for the Clinton Foundation is their belief that in the battle against the virus every minute lost is a life lost. That quality of urgency is desperately needed' Mr. Lewis said." (What about the eight years of his presidency lost? Ed)
>
> "Mr. Clinton, in turn, lavished praise on the Canadian icon, calling him the conscience of the world on HIV-AIDS."

> "'I thank him for a lifetime of public service,' Mr. Clinton said and then turning to Mr. Lewis, he added: 'The world is in your debt.'"

My oh my, pass the Kleenex. Don't you get warm and fuzzy feelings when you read this drivel? One would think that between these two, great progress was being made in the struggle against acquired immune deficiency syndrome. Nothing could be further from the truth. There are still 8,000 people a day dying from AIDS and that figure gives every indication of going still higher. The Clinton-Lewis song and dance team make some contribution with their high-profile lamentations, and there is some value in Mr. Lewis handing out condoms across Africa while Mr. Clinton's Foundation negotiates lower prices for drugs being shipped to third world countries [*The Sudbury Star*, Jan.12, 2006, Page B5], but add all of these initiatives together and they amount to only a few drops of rain during a severe drought.

Let me elaborate. And here we move from the warm and fuzzy stuff to the cruel, hard reality of AIDS.

Three days after Mr. Picard presented the above report on the Lewis-Clinton mutual admiration society meeting, he was back with another article: "Investment must be made to save lives, Lewis warns." by Andre Picard public health reporter.

In this piece Mr. Picard illustrates what is tragically wrong with the struggle against AIDS, but he also illustrates what is tragically wrong about the reporting of that struggle.

> "Mr. Lewis was equally harsh on developing countries, in particular the government of South Africa, which has been reluctant to accept that HIV causes AIDS, slow to offer drug treatment and whose senior officials tout bizarre treatments such as lemon juice"

> "It is the only country in Africa…whose government is still obtuse, dilatory and negligent about rolling out treatment. It is the only country in Africa whose government continues to propound theories more worthy of a lunatic fringe than of a concerned and compassionate state,' Mr. Lewis said."

Mr. Lewis' statements and Mr. Picard's unqualified reporting of them demonstrate that Mr. Lewis certainly, and Mr. Picard possibly, are either very uninformed on the history of health issues, or are intentionally withholding critical facts. These latter, unstated facts start with simple, school-days history and extend into the vast, unstated reality of AIDS: a tool for global genocide, which, as the United Nations special envoy on HIV-AIDS (Mr. Lewis) and as the public health reporter for the *Globe and Mail* (Mr. Picard) should be, *but isn't*, cognizant of. First, to the school-days facts…simple but absolutely vital.

In the 16th and 17th century England was engaged in a great period of global exploration, conquest, and settlement. However, their sea-going enterprises were severely handicapped by a terrible disease that disabled and killed many sailors, and caused many expeditions to fail. The disease was scurvy, which is characterized by spongy gums, loosening and loss of teeth, and bleeding into the skin and mucous membranes. The mucous membranes, in turn, are vital in the production of immune-advancing protection. Secondary diseases resulted from the initial scurvy, and further, more deadly diseases resulted. The British navy and British privateers suffered greatly from the seemingly incurable scurvy.

Then, in 1795 some obscure person in the hierarchy of the Admiralty, suggested a 'bizarre' response: issue a daily lime to each sailor on every voyage. Limes were plentiful in the British holdings of the Caribbean, and soon huge burlap sacks of fresh limes were delivered to each ship prior to its departure for often long and dangerous voyages. And of even more significance, these ships began returning from such voyages with healthy crews. The 'bizarre' lime juice had done its job and scurvy passed as a threat to sailors' health.

Now, just imagine if you will, what would have happened had that obscure Admiralty employee who first proposed such a bizarre treatment had been compelled to get the permission of Stephen Lewis as First Lord of the Admiralty?

Doesn't Stephen Lewis know the story of limejuice and scurvy, and of equal importance, doesn't the *Globe and Mail* public health reporter know that story? And, if either or both know that such a bizarre treatment worked in 1795, why do they not acknowledge the fact in their public utterances and reportings?

While I leave you to ponder this question let me quote briefly from a 1987 document titled, *"Problems Associated with AIDS",* by Dr. John Seale and published by the British House of Commons.

> "1. In the face of a lethal disease, journalists and media editors have been frightened to contradict the conventional wisdom being put across by the scientists. There has been no serious attempt at investigative journalism into the wealth of scientific scandals surrounding AIDS" (Emphasis added. I thank Ms. Peg Laurian for bringing this valuable document to our attention.)

We will return to Dr. Seale's article later.

An Interlude on Synchronicity or Things Happening at the Right Moment

"There is a destiny shapes our ends, Horatio, rough hew them how we will..." or something like that said Hamlet to his friend.

And in my almost single-minded search for the truth about AIDS, there have been wonderful comings together of events that have made my search easier. Take Andre Picard, for example, he is listed in many of the clippings I have from the *Globe and Mail* as their public health reporter. As such, a reader would assume that he would be reasonably well-informed on questions of health...especially *public* health. He would know, for example, about scurvy, and lime juice. And, when he reports upon Stephen Lewis' diatribe against South Africa and the 'bizarre' treatment of AIDS with lemon juice, one could hope that he would remind readers about the scurvy-lime juice connection. But no, not a peep. He just reports Mr. Lewis' nonsense as if it were indeed, accepted fact.

When I noted Mr. Picard's treatment of Mr. Lewis speech, I wondered if the reporter just didn't know about the scurvy-lime link, or did he know and just didn't want to bother his readers with an important fact? I thought that it would be helpful if I could ask Mr. Picard to justify his shallow response to an important situation involving public health. I paused whimsically to think over, should I phone Mr. Picard and ask him? After all, I am well aware of how warped the media have generally been in their reporting of AIDS and

AIDS issues and how they seem to favor the high price pharmaceutical response far out of reach for the vast majority of AIDS victims.

I decided not to take the time off from my research to do anything about Mr. Picard's superficial contribution.

It was at this precise point in my work that I decided to take a brief break. I picked up the latest issue of *The Sudbury Star*, delivered just moments before, and there was an enclosure reporting upon the year's accomplishments of the Sudbury & District Health Unit for 2005. Included in that report was the news that none other that Andre Picard, public health reporter at the Globe and Mail, would be a guest speaker in Sudbury on September 20 at 7:00 p.m.!

Synchronicity! If I can't go to Toronto in order to question Andre Picard, Andre Picard will be delivered by synchronized forces neither of us are aware of, to Sudbury, where I will be able to hear him.

As I write this Interlude, it is Monday, September 4, 2006. On Wednesday, September 20 I will attend Mr. Picard's presentation. I intend to ask him if he recalls Mr. Lewis' comment that lemon juice as part of a treatment protocol for AIDS is 'bizarre'? I will then ask if he (Mr. Picard) agrees. I will then mention the scurvy-lime linkage.

I will ask him whether he has studied the Congressional Minutes of the June 9, 1969 Meeting between Dr. Donald MacArthur and twelve Congressmen on the 'black ops' budget committee? If he has, does he agree that MacArthur was describing the United States efforts to develop an AIDS pathogen?

I will ask him if he has studied the Patent of the United States Government American Institute of Pathology of the micro-organism called the 'Pathogenic Mycoplasma'? If he has such knowledge, I will ask him whether he has a response to Dr. Shyh-Ching Lo's claim that 'patients infected with the mycoplasma will be patients who have been diagnosed as having AIDS or ARC' (AIDS Related Complex) among a list of other diseases?

I will then ask him if he could accept the view that the 'respiratory distress syndrome' mentioned by Dr. Lo could be the same disease as the 'Severe Acute Respiratory Syndrome' (SARS)? Or, if there is a difference between RDS and SARS, could the same pathogen be behind both diseases? After all, a 'respiratory syndrome' can be 'severe', 'acute', and distressful all at the same time! In other words, Dr. Lo's 'respiratory distress syndrome' can quite possibly be the 'severe acute respiratory syndrome, SARS. I will ask him in public, out loud, and clearly, and I'll wait for an answer.

You see, we believe that the failure of the world to come to scientific grips with AIDS and all the related mycoplasmal diseases cited by Dr. Lo is due to a combination of humanity's deep psychological resistance to face up to the cruel realities about our species' proclivity for evil, and to the conscious decision by a powerful few to take advantage of this human trait and to create and propagate carefully crafted myths which appear to account for cruel reality while cloaking it in the apparently logical inventions.

I also believe that the so-called leading media of our society are essentially fraudulent in their reporting. They ignore clearly enunciated public truths because they don't know how to explain them without coming to grips with the truth about what's been going on. And the controllers of the media are part and parcel of the gangsters that run their own evil world because the average person is just too chicken livered to demand the truth.

So…on to the synchronicity of Mr. Picard coming to Sudbury so I can ask these questions.

End of an Interlude on Synchronicity

A SPECIAL REPORT TO THE JOURNAL OF DEGENERATIVE DISEASES

A brief burst of reality almost spoils 'feel good' parade

At about six o'clock in the evening of Wednesday, September 20, 2006, I dragged myself out of my comfortable, warm condominium, and into my car. I say 'dragged' because, quite frankly at the age of eighty-two and deteriorating somewhat in health, I would have preferred to stay home. However, Andre Picard, whose business card tells the world that he is a 'Public Health Reporter' for the *Globe and Mail*, was going to address the Sudbury public as part of the 50th Anniversary Meeting of the Sudbury and District Public Health Unit and I wanted to be there. Partly, I wanted to hear what he had to say, but mainly, I wanted to ask Andre Picard some questions.

You see, I had read several pieces by Mr. Picard in recent issues of the *Globe and Mail* about the just ended one week International Conference on AIDS (See article above: 'The Dog and Pony Show') Since I was terribly dissatisfied with the superficial stuff that had made its way into print, I decided that I would take advantage of Mr. Picard's visit to move past the dog and pony stuff and get right to some of the harsh, cruel realities of AIDS specifically, and of public health in general.

For moral support I picked up my son, William, President of the Common Cause Medical Research Foundation, and arrived at Bryston's on the Park in Copper Cliff in lots of time to get the seat about two feet to the right of the public microphone. I was going to ask questions.

I had lots of questions because, quite frankly, the major media in North America have mis-reported, under-reported and generally skewed the truth about AIDS, Chronic Fatigue Syndrome, avian flu and other vital health issues. Led by the *New York Times* with their superficial and dishonest health reporter, Gina Kolata, and followed along by smart alecky *Time* magazine (who had coined the name the 'gay plague' for AIDS and the 'yuppie flu' for CFS) and the *Globe and Mail* here in Canada, the public at large has been lied to for years about what is happening to human health.

I listened, somewhat impatiently because of a twenty-five minute delay in the meeting getting started; to various public-health associated people recite the trivia of the past year. Finally, the moment arrived. Everyone on the stage, including Mr. Picard, had had their time at the microphone and 'question time' had arrived.

The Chair of the Meeting, Dr. Penny Sutcliffe, invited questions and before she had finished her invitation, I was standing at the microphone. I thought I detected a hint of consternation in Dr. Sutcliffe's nod to me to ask my question. I responded, delighted to seek answers from a senior health reporter who worked for a national newspaper. I had read so much garbage in the Globe and the *Times* and the *Post* over the years…now Mr. Picard could be asked something significant (by my standards at any rate) in public. I had boiled my many questions down to two. I began:

> "This question is directed solely to Mr. Picard." Mr. Picard nodded his acceptance. "Mr. Picard, are you aware of and do

you factor into your research and your writings, the United States Patent held by the American Institute of Pathology and sponsored by Dr. Shyh-Ching Lo titled *The Pathogenic Mycoplasma?*"

Mr. Picard had a rather strained grin. Did he look a trifle uncomfortable?

The audience, of course, had no idea what I was talking about. I also doubted that Dr. Sutcliffe knew what I was asking. However, there seemed to be a certain tension in the air, suggesting that, although the question was obscure to practically every one of the 150 people in attendance, it had a significance.

Mr. Picard leaned forward to his microphone, still grinning, and answered "No."

The audience laughed a nervous laugh, and Dr. Sutcliffe spoke (was there a hint of nervousness?) into her microphone. "Thank you Mr. Scott, if you would now sit down and let others ask some questions."

"No, Madam Chair", I replied. "There's no one else in the line and besides I haven't finished my question." I directed my attention back to Mr. Picard.

"You answer 'no' to a question about a scientific, United States Patent, Number 5,242,820 and dated September 7, 1993, granted after several years to one of America's top doctors and biological researchers, who says therein…and I'll quote briefly: 'Those patients infected with the *Mycoplasma* fermentans incognitus will be patients who have been diagnosed as having AIDS of AIDS Related Complex, chronic fatigue syndrome…' (and here I elaborated editorially to try to convey to the audience, if not to Mr. Picard, the absolute significance of the mycoplasma and the Patent …That's AIDS and Chronic Fatigue Dr. Lo refers to. The one disease now killing 8,000 people a day, and the other CFS, disabling other thousands, yet about which many doctors say is all in the patient's head. Yet, you do not know of it, and you do not factor it into your research or your writings."

I thought Mr. Picard looked strained, but he still grinned. Dr. Sutcliffe leaned into her microphone. "Will you leave the microphone Mr. Scott and give others a chance to ask their questions?"

"No," I replied. And I turned back to Mr. Picard: "Dr. Lo continues his list of diseases which are somehow linked to the mycoplasma: '… Wegener's Disease, Sarcoidosis, respiratory distress syndrome (again

I editorialized…'That is respiratory syndrome' I said. 'Could Dr. Lo be referring to severe (an adjective) acute (also an adjective), respiratory syndrome?' SARS? I continued reading the list:'…Kibuchi's Disease, autoimmune diseases such as Collagen Vascular Disease and Lupus and chronic debilitating diseases such as Alzheimer's Disease."

Now…get this! Here was I, quoting one of the highest status medical researchers in the United States about a terrible disease organism. And, I was quoting him in the presence of the highest Public Health officials in Ontario, and the top reporter for what purports to be Canada's national newspaper. And lo and behold— none of them seemed to know what I was talking about!

Some health officials!

Some health reporting!

I rained on a feel-good public meeting about nothing of consequence!

I told the truth and surprised them all!

Denis St. Pierre Reports the News

On the facing page we reproduce a story from a recent issue of the *Sudbury Star* by reporter Denis St. Pierre titled "Man claims he cured AIDS". (see Exhibit 5 in Appendices) Let me tell you my side of the story about Mr. St. Pierre's 'report of news' in respect to our forthcoming Conference. It explains a lot about why the public is so badly informed on so much that is of critical importance to them, their families and indeed, their world. It is another example of the failure of the media to do its job of educating humanity.

Some weeks ago, after months of planning and effort, Bill Scott, Conference Co-coordinator, was able to present the first draft of our Program. Then, our hard working Publicity Co-coordinator, Ms. Marlene Johnson, saw to it that the Program was delivered to the major media in Sudbury. Ms. Johnson also graciously arranged to interview me on her radio program out of Laurentian University's CKLU about the Conference.

Aside from the latter interview there wasn't a peep from any other of the media that I know of. Of course, that is to be expected initially, and continued contact with them would, we were sure, bring results.

In the Program we reported that our guest speakers would include the following persons of international stature and expertise.

We reported upon William Blum, a senior *Washington, D.C.*-based reporter and news analyst who is regularly published in the major media of that world capital. Mr. Blum had recently written a best selling book called *Rogue State* which had been reported upon by none other than CNN and had even drawn a favorable comment from Osama Bin Ladin in one of the latter's taped TV interviews!

We reported upon Dr. Garth Nicolson who with Dr. Singer had developed what is known as the Fluid Mosaic Model of Cell Membrane, an absolutely critical article if one is to understand just how the cell membrane can be destroyed. Drs. Singer and Nicolson were published in the journal Science and their article was later named as one of the top ten of the year. It has since been reported in many if not most of the pre-medical textbooks that aspiring medical doctors must study.

Dr. Nicolson went on to a distinguished career with the Salk Institute and later was simultaneously Director of the world-famous M.D. Anderson Cancer Center and was also Professor in three major medical subjects at the University of Texas. He was nominated for the Nobel Prize at one point. Dr. Nicolson had agreed, at great personal sacrifice to himself to participate in our Conference with a report upon his cutting edge research into autism…a subject of increasing tragedy and concern for parents world-wide. Well, the Sudbury parents were being given a chance to hear first hand a world expert on the subject.

The Program also reported that Dr. Nick Begich of Alaska, would be with us to lecture upon his latest findings into the efforts by the United States to modify the natural weather patterns of the world, using such things as the High Altitude Atmospheric Resonance Pulsing (HAARP) facility built in the home state of Dr. Begich, Alaska, and designed to pull the high altitude jet stream several miles further north than normal. Again, cutting edge, first hand reporting by a scientist on a subject many people are beginning to puzzle over.

We listed other lecturers including a lecture by physicist Basil Wainwright. Now, Basil Wainwright has developed a dialysis-related process wherein he draws blood from people ill with mycoplasmal infections, including AIDS, CFS, multiple sclerosis and other,

(See earlier 'The Dog and Pony Show' and 'A Special Report on Degenerative Diseases,' as well as the following 'Two Cancers...')

Now, I was first contacted about four or five years ago by Wainwright, who phoned me from Kenya. He had read the book that my son and I had written titled *Skull Valley*, and he suggested that the mycoplasma deserved far more attention as a factor in AIDS and other blood-borne diseases. He also suggested that a species of mycoplasma was involved in many if not all cancers, and that he had found that if the microorganisms involved were expose to pure oxygen they could be greatly reduced , if not totally destroyed.

(In this, please refer to the Nobel Prize awarded to Dr. Warburg who demonstrated that the greatest enemy of cancer is oxygen.)

I expressed my interest and he said "I'll send you some literature on oxygen therapy and reports upon my work with patients who have AIDS, CFS and other diseases."

About two days later I received from Kenya, a huge parcel of literature by Federal Express. It cost Wainwright somewhere about $250 to ship it to me at his expense. *There was absolutely no hint of a suggestion that I pay anything.*

Space limits our freedom to develop the material here, but in concluding his conversation with me, Wainwright said... "Of course I am very unpopular with mainstream medicine. My treatments (which he later supported by reports from the University of Kenya) cost only pennies and are as effective as, if not more so, than the hundreds of dollars charged by the chemical messes that the pharmaceutical industry pushes on the gullible public. I am harassed wherever I go."

In the package were also five videos, some of which we will be showing at our Conference.

These four scholars, plus others, we reported in our Program.

Well, as I have stated, for weeks, we heard nothing, then I received a phone call from Denis St. Pierre of *The Sudbury Star*. I assume that he was working with the approval of his editor. We re-produce his article in its entirety on the facing page.

Mr. St. Pierre began his 'interview' with something along the line of "Do you check the criminal or police records of your speakers for your Conference?" I knew full well that he was on the Wainwright track and I answered "No."

I tried to tell Mr. St. Pierre that I had heard accusations, innuendo, gossip and other drivel about Wainwright, but that my concern was not with such garbage, as Mr. St. Pierre's apparently was, but with the science of Wainwright's work.

Mr. St. Pierre went into a brief lecture about criminals and juries and so on, and I tried to make the point that when someone challenged the huge money machine of pharmaceutical company medicine which DOMINATES our medicine in North America, one is bound to encounter resistance at the highest levels.

I thought later, but didn't think to raise with Mr. St. Pierre, of Nelson Mandela who was convicted of sedition and sentenced to life at hard labor. I thought of O. J. Simpson who was found to be innocent of murdering his estranged wife and her friend by a jury of his peers. I thought of Galileo who challenged orthodox garbage about the relation of the sun to the earth and was found guilty of heresy. Guilt? Innocence? Who's to say? But when we are talking about science show us the data and the reports and that is what we at the Common Cause Medical Research Foundation ask for and seek to verify.

Not Mr. St. Pierre and *The Sudbury Star*, at least in his latest article. Mind you, the *Sudbury Star* has been very fair to us when they sent careful, thoughtful, analytical reporters to see our data first hand, or when they have published articles such as that by Carole Mulligan on our Chairman Emeritus, Dr. Harold Clark, or pieces I have submitted as op ed articles. But in the article under consideration, the story is warped and misleading.

Now, I ask the questions: If you are the parent of an autistic child would you like to hear a report by a leading medical researcher on the subject? Or, if you wonder why and how Canada has been snookered into Afghanistan at the cost of forty plus young Canadians and numerous Afghan citizens, would you not like to hear the evidence amassed by William Blum of Washington, D.C.?

How about if you or a friend has cancer, would you at least like to hear how oxygen has been utilized in many medical jurisdictions outside of the baleful influence of the American medical establishment. (See: Two Cancers…this issue) Finally, if you have AIDS or CFS or fibromyalgia, would you like to see scientific data from Basil Wainwright and then hear him questioned by a panel of doctors and researchers?

If you would, you can attend the Conference sponsored by the CCMRF on Nov. 17, 18, 19.

But don't count on Mr. St. Pierre to let you know that you have this chance…and right here in Sudbury which has to stop acting like a rube town and get with those who ask for evidence, not rumor, innuendo, gossip, or Internet downloads.

PART SEVEN

THE DAWNING OF AWARENESS

INTRODUCTION

> "The period between the forties and the early sixties was one of Cold War-driven paranoia, when government officials and scientific experts were considered the final arbiters of ethical as well as logistical conundrums. In times such as these, *times of ordinary madness*, it was but a small matter to stage a vaccine trial in a faraway place, without the process having to be approved by any but the colonial government in charge, and without any checks and balances to ensure the safety of the participants." (Hooper 1999, Page 815)

When Ed Hooper quoted from Bukowski's *Tales of Ordinary Madness*, he was apt as far as the sentiments expressed, but short on the time frame. The times of ordinary madness have stretched well beyond the early sixties and well into the present century and they will be with us for many years to come.

It is, of course, all a matter of degree; however, by the early 1990s there were some early stirrings of suspicion that the gilded gods of accepted wisdom (or baffle-gab) such as we had read in the letters from The Aaron Diamond AIDS Research Center and from the Dana-Farber Cancer Center, had feet of clay.

Between 1990 and 1999 there was a *dawning of awareness* in four writer/researchers, three in the United States and one in Great Britain, that the truth about three critical public issues was not being told. The issues whose 'official lines' they questioned were the truth about the murder of President John F. Kennedy; the nature and origin of the Acquired Immune Deficiency Syndrome (AIDS) epidemic; and, the nature and origin of the Chronic Fatigue Syndrome (CFS) epidemic.

The skepticism was not new in the tragedy of Mr. Kennedy's murder. Right from the first reports of the murder some of which stated that the President had been hit in the throat (hence he was shot from the front) and in the upper back (hence he was also shot from the back) at least two shooters were involved with the logical conclusion that there was a conspiracy of two or more people to execute President John F. Kennedy. And right from the first the 'official line' emerged that a lone lunatic nut had killed the President.

There were early critics of the official line, including the 'dean' of researchers, Harold Weisberg; Editor, Penn Jones; and scholar, Peter Dale Scott. Each of these and several others brought important details and insights to the record, demonstrating to the objective reader that the official line was false. However, it remained for Professor Donald Gibson in his book *Battling Wall Street* (**1994**) to place the murder with all of its contradictions, lies, and obvious distortions that the others were clearly establishing, into a historic, philosophical, economic and political framework, which fitted into those times of ordinary madness.

Two years later two more books appeared…one which challenged the 'official line' about AIDS and one which traced a decade of deceit about CFS.

The former was by Leonard G. Horowitz, *Emerging Viruses: AIDS and Ebola* Nature, Accident or Intentional. Horowitz, a dentist by profession had begun his research in response to the case of an AIDS-infected patient and her dentist, David Acer. The more that Dr. Horowitz studied the nature of AIDS, the more he challenged the official line from the evidence available, the theory that AIDS was an ancient zoonotic disease that had jumped species from a primate to a human. Building upon his work investigating Dr. Acer, Horowitz began to track the syndrome from both a scientific and a political perspective. In 1996 he published his findings. The green monkey-bites Black woman-launches worldwide pandemic was gone forever.

In the same year (**1996**) another critical book on the subject of truth in illness was published. Hillary Johnson, herself a victim of CFS, had begun her research into the syndrome when she began to present with the signs and symptoms which in some ways resembled those of chronic brucellosis and those of various 'mystery' illnesses from 1934 that although differing in specifics seemed to have a common thread and was called 'the disease of one thousand names'. (See; Byron Hyde, 1992) Her first reports were published in 1987 *Rolling Stone* magazine which enjoyed the presence of an enlightened and honest publisher and editor (Jann Wenner) and (Bob Wallace)

Then, in **1999**, researcher/writer Ed Hooper published *The River*:

A Journey to the Source of HIV and AIDS. A fitting end to the decade. It is a magnificent book. One which if the truth were to be recognized, should as the late W.D. Hamilton suggests "…merit for Hooper and Pascal jointly a Nobel Prize." But, the world of science and letters and Nobel Prizes being what it is, that will not come to pass. (If a Nobel Prize can be given to a Henry Kissinger or a Sir Frank Burnet or a Menachem Begin, please spare Ed Hooper such an 'honor'.) Even though our research demonstrates that a major premise of his book is flawed, (that AIDS had its source, like the Congo River, in the Heart of Africa) it is essential reading for anyone who would know the 'many details of the early spread of AIDS'. As Bill Hamilton has said, "I have seen the cost the task has had for him manifested in many stages of tiredness, illness, and despair, which however he has always managed to overcome."

In this part of our study we consider each and how what each has to say relates to our major hypothesis that AIDS is a product of the scientific laboratories largely owned or controlled by forces public and private of the United States.

Chapter Nineteen

HILLARY JOHNSON: A PROSE OF REPORTORIAL CALM

Nowhere in Hillary Johnson's magnificent book, *Osler's Web*, does she state a belief that Chronic Fatigue Syndrome; Myalgic Encephalomyelitis (CFS/ME) had its epidemic origins in American Government-owned or -controlled laboratories. However, she suggests very strongly in her 'Acknowledgments' that this possibility is there. For example, she thanks Charles Ortleb and Neenyah Ostrom of the *New York Native* for their 'commitment to investigating the nexus between AIDS and CFS in the face of *antagonism* from many sources...' Later she thanks her mother, Ruth Jones, who 'railed against the villains, took umbrage on behalf of the long-suffering, erupted with unprintable witticisms, yet counseled a prose of reportorial calm.'

Ms. Johnson responded to her mother's wisdom and did, indeed, write with a reportorial calm, but all the way through *Osler's Web*, starting with the title, there is a tension manifested between the victims of this terrible and tragic illness CFS/ME and those people in positions of power who were supposed to be the agents of health protection in the United States, the National Institutes of Health and the Center for Disease Control.

The subtle oxymoron in the title: '*Osler's Web*', with the name of the great and caring Canadian doctor whose message to medical care givers was the open suggestion that 'The edifice of medicine reposes entirely upon facts...truth cannot be elicited but from those which have been well and completely observed', stands in sharp contrast to the '*Web*' which suggests entrapment and dark and shadowy corners and most of all deceit.

And that is what *Osler's Web* is about: the open reality of the disease of victims of CFS and the deceit of the health authorities who were supposedly responding to their plight, and (in passing) about the insidious role of much of the media in reporting that struggle. Media which had its roots deep in the dank soil of American deep politics.

And, since the media are so critical a part of our thesis, that the reality of laboratory-created AIDS and CFS makes them as much a political study as a medical study, we will begin this chapter with an early (1987) report on a CBS program on CFS, just as seven years later (1994) they did a hatchet job on AIDS. (See below: Ch.20)

In *Osler's Web* Johnson reports as follows:

> "On December 10, West 57th tackled the disease about which so much had been written lately in the lay press: the controversial yuppie flu. The segment led the Saturday night show, with reporter Steve Kroft narrating. As he began his report it was evident Kroft had set out to debunk what he perceived to be a bogus disease. Instead of focusing a journalist's healthy skepticism upon an imperious medical establishment, Kroft turned it on the victims of the disease. In a teaser segment before a commercial, Kroft was seen in a story meeting…The journalist tapped his forehead and, winking at his colleagues, said, 'Some doctors think it's all up here.'…Kroft…introduced their medical expert, Richard Jacobs, an associate clinical professor of infectious disease at the University of California in San Francisco. Jacobs began by saying that 'this is a trend. It's a real fad, just as other things have been trend and fad lately…'"
>
> (Johnson 1996, Page 232)

Note that 'Kroft turned it on the victims.' The victim is to blame.

Johnson's book is characterized by the tension of an ever-present dichotomy between patient reality and public health agency myth-making about that reality. She traces a decade of that dichotomy from 1984 to 1994 through what was happening to victims in various epidemic areas of the United States, but we will only focus upon two epidemics: the one in Tahoe-Truckee High School in 1984 and the other in school-children in Lyndonville, New York, in 1985.

In the summer of 1984 a work crew arrived at Tahoe-Truckee High School and ripped out the old air-conditioning system and put in a new system. The new system had a unique feature unlike that of the old system. Air was drawn from individual rooms, carried by individual systems of ducts to be heated or cooled, and then returned to the same individual rooms from whence it had come. When the school re-opened in the fall, eight teachers were assigned to a small secondary workroom to eat their lunches, have their coffee breaks, prepare and mark their tests. The other twenty-five teachers used a larger, fresher staff room. To make matters worse for the teachers in the secondary staff room, they found that the windows of their workspace were shut and nailed to prevent opening. And soon after school opened the eight teachers began to complain about the air quality. It got so bad that one teacher brought a trailer and parked it nearby and whenever he had a break he went there instead of to his small staff room. Over the coming months the teachers began to experience a variety of 'mystery' symptoms. Nausea, dizziness, sleeplessness at night, night sweats…until by the end of the school year, 'only one teacher among the eight emerged unscathed: Eric Jordan, the outdoorsman who had chosen to prepare his lessons and grade papers in the stillness of his camper'. (Johnson, 1996; Page 28)

What was going on?

Biological warfare weapons testing of a disabling air borne pathogen!

Tahoe-Truckee High School

There is no public record that says so, but the history from June 9, 1969 when Dr. MacArthur promised the Congressmen a new *disabling* weapon that could be spread by aerosol or by insect vector says as much. Consider: the research, MacArthur had said, 'was not easy' but he was sure it could be achieved. There was a flurry of mycoplasmal research contracts until Watergate hit the fan, and then everything slowed to a crawl. Under Carter the CIA was damped down until 1980 when the powers in the shadows through their man in the CIA, William Casey, were able to put a disabling, aerosol weapons agent back on track. By 1984 they were ready for the test and so, just a few miles along the highway west from Dugway Testing Grounds in Nevada, at Tahoe-Truckee High School, through a modified air-conditioning system, a 'disabling' biological agent was released into an eight-person staff room, and was passaged through that room hour after hour. As the testers had obviously expected, seven of the eight occupants of that room became ill with chronic fatigue syndrome. Only one escaped…the teacher who had refused to use the room with its re-circulated and contaminated air.

There was a scattering of others in the school, students and teachers, who also became ill. But these were random and few in number. The aerosol test was a success. (For a more detailed study of this test, refer to our earlier book: *The Brucellosis Triangle*.)

Lyndonville, New York

In October 1985, some school children in this small town in western New York State had an early winter-first snowfall toboggan party, followed by copious quantities of hot chocolate made with local unpasteurized goat's milk. Then, as Hillary Johnson writes "In the next several months virtually every child in both families fell ill with an inscrutable disease" (Johnson, 1996 Page 61) which came to be called 'chronic fatigue syndrome.'

In *Osler's Web* Johnson traces the fortunes of the victims and their medical caregivers, but there were certain factors upon which we focused. First, there were the doctors in the Tahoe-Truckee High School and the Lyndonville school children's CFS/ME outbreaks. In the former there were Drs. Daniel Petersen and Paul Cheney. In the latter there was a husband-wife team, Drs. David and Karen Bell.

In both instances we were interested in the fact that careful, caring doctors were readily available in each locale when the epidemic 'mystery' disease had hit the communities. We were interested because we knew from our research that in all cases of the testing of any new pathogen, the testers would ensure that anyone who became ill would be carefully checked and monitored. To achieve this end, doctors with the necessary qualities would have to be on site.

Doctors Daniel Peterson and Paul Cheney

It turned out in the case of both the Tahoe-Truckee and Lyndonville outbreaks, such doctors were there and ready to receive the ill patients. We recognized, of course, that such good fortune for the communities could be the result of happy coincidence, and we were prepared to learn this and to accept it objectively. However, we also knew that the presence of well-qualified and well-equipped medical doctors would be part of the planning for the testing of any new pathogen. After all, there was the precedent of Dr. Bjorn Sigurdsson being supplied with ample money by the Rockefeller Foundation to establish an Institute for Experimental Pathology in Iceland (of all places!) and the coincidence that shortly afterwards there was an outbreak of a 'mystery' disease (much like those in Tahoe-Truckee and Lyndonville) in Akureyri, Iceland. (Ch. 4). Then there was the chance arrival in the wilds of Papua, New Guinea of Dr. Carleton Gajdusek in time to study an outbreak of a 'mystery' disease, related to the sheep visna disease. (Ch. 1; Sect. 9)

We wrote to Drs. Peterson and Cheney. Dr. Cheney never bothered to reply and even declined to accept our phone queries as to whether he had received our letter. Dr. Peterson on the other hand wrote a short but polite reply. Here is the latter correspondence:

August 2, 2000

Dr. Daniel Peterson
Sierra Internal Medicine
By Fax transmission to 775-832-3046

Dear Dr. Peterson:

Thank you for your August 1, 2000, faxed curriculum vitae by way of your assistant, Ms. Michelle van Rijn.

Continuing my current research, I wonder if you could elaborate upon certain of your career details. I would be grateful for any information in respect to the following:

1. According to Hillary Johnson's *Osler's Web* you received 'government sponsorship' for your medical education (page 18). Would you be good enough to advise which agency of government was your sponsor and over what period of time were you obliged to serve to discharge your obligation?

2. Your CV records 'Internship and Residency: 1976-1979' at University of Utah Medical Center and according to Johnson (supra) you worked in Burley and Nampa, Idaho. Would you advise what dates were covered by the latter service?

3. You apparently invited Paul Cheney to join you in Incline Village in 'early 1983' (page 20) after enquiring who were the 'indentured public health and military internists working in the state'. Why did you look for such an obligated individual, and how would service in Incline Village qualify as service which discharged such an individual's government/military sponsorship?

I hope that you will be able to oblige me with answers to these questions as I continue my research.

                                              I am, yours sincerely,
                                                    Donald W. Scott

Dr. Peterson replied with the following:

August 13, 2000

Mr. Donald W. Scott, President
The Common Cause Medical Research Foundation
405-190 Mountain Street
Sudbury, Ontario
CANADA P3B 4G2

Dear Mr. Scott:

Out of the following response to your questions received by recent fax, I was a member of the United States Public Health Service and in exchange for financial support during my years in medical school, I have fulfilled a two-year obligation with the United States Public Health Service in a migrant health center which had multiple sites including Burley and Napa, Idaho. The service occurred in July of 1979 through June of 1981. Dr. Chaney (sic) had completed his service with the Air Force at the time he was recruited to join the practice in Incline Village.

I hope these answers are satisfactory.

Sincerely yours,
Daniel L. Peterson, M.D.

Actually, Dr. Peterson's reply was unsatisfactory since, among other things, he failed to address the question why had he asked for the names of doctors to join his practice who were 'indentured' to the government, and had been given Dr. Cheney's name. If a doctor was still 'indentured', that would mean that he was obliged to attend for a fixed period at a place he was assigned.

However, that did not raise questions as much as the timetable of his reply. It had been dictated on August 13, 2000 and the envelope was post marked 'airmail': September 24, (forty-two days later!) And it was delivered to my address on October 11, 2000. Another seventeen days for a total delivery time of 59 days! And that by 'airmail'!

There were and still are things that are very suggestive about the background and role of Dr. Peterson, For example, besides having been assisted financially by the U.S. Government, he had co-operated with people such as Dharam Ablashi and Paul Levine in writing research articles, and both the latter are listed as participants in the *Special Virus Cancer Program* (ch. 13) Also, we had just published out first book and we received an order from a patient of Dr. Peterson who said that he had recommended it to her? We were puzzled because to our knowledge, Dr. Peterson had never seen our book. Furthermore, at the time of writing The *Extremely Unfortunate Skull Valley Incident*, we had focused upon brucellosis as a likely precedent etiologic factor in chronic fatigue. At that point there was no sign of *B. brucella* in blood tests of CFS/ME victims. It was only later that we learned that the Department of Defence had earlier learned how to remove the toxic agent from *Brucella* in crystalline form and hence spread it by aerosol or insect vector or food chain. In the meantime, directing patients, doctors or researchers to *Brucella* appeared to be pointing them in a false direction.

Doctors David and Karen Bell

Nine years ago we were planning our first conference of the Common Cause Medical Research Foundation, when we received a phone call from Dr. David Bell of Lyndonville. Dr. Bell wanted to know if the Conference was open to anyone who wished to attend, or was attendance limited? We assured him that it was as open as we could make it, and we invited him to attend and to speak about his early experience with CFS/ME in Lyndonville.

Dr. Bell accepted our invitation and attended with several members of his Lyndonville staff and did speak at the appointed time. However, he seemed very remote from any other aspects of the Conference. He did not attend lectures by Dr. Les Simpson of New Zealand, or Dr. Garth Nicolson or Dr. John Martin of California. He declined to attend for the group picture of Conference presenters. He came, he spoke, and he left. The only further word that we had from him was a query about being paid for his expenses. We were late with these, but did get a cheque off to him. That was the last we heard from Dr. David Bell.

The next year our Conference was in Rochester, New York, and Dr. Bell did not turn up. In fact, he didn't reply to our invitation. However, we had invited Dr. Elaine DeFreitas of Miami with whom we had become acquainted by phone a few months before. Dr. DeFreitas replied that she would have liked to attend but that she had received an invitation from Dr. Bell to visit him that same weekend at his home in Lyndonville and she felt obliged to accept that invitation.

Somehow we got the impression that Dr. DeFreitas had been intentionally diverted from our Conference by design of Dr. Bell. Her companion on her Lyndonville visit to Dr. Bell dropped in briefly at our Conference, introduced himself and said that Dr. DeFreitas would have liked to be with us, but could not decline Dr. Bell's invitation.

Something about Dr. Bell's self-promoted image of a friend of the CFS/ME victims did not ring true.

Like Dr. Peterson's patient who had been advised by him to read our book, long before we knew much about Dr. David Bell, he too, had recommended to a patient in Rochester that she read the book! And, like Dr. Peterson, Dr. Bell had never bought our book. He was recommending it sight unseen. We wondered why. Again, was it that our attention to Brucellosis appeared to be a false trail and were readers being directed to it because we were apparently so far off track?

We went back to see what Hillary Johnson had to say about the Lyndonville epidemic, and were surprised to learn that when the disease had struck the children of the area, Dr. Karen Bell had suspected Brucellosis just as we had. Here is how Ms. Johnson describes it:

> "Karen began a mental inventory of milk-borne infections. Brucellosis, or undulant fever, was at the top of her long list; in the absence of antibiotics, the disease can persist for years. Brucellosis tests were uniformly negative, however."
> (Johnson, 1996 Page 62)

A bacterial disease without a bacterium! Of course… The Pentagon researchers had, as we have already noted, reported just such an accomplishment to a Senate enquiry.

Dr. Elaine DeFreitas

Hillary Johnson devotes over five inches of her index to items involving Dr. Elaine DeFreitas of the Wistar Institute! Wistar! With all of its links to Hilary Koprowski and Hayflick and the Henles and monkey viruses!

We were, therefore, reasonably delighted to receive a phone call one day a few months before Dr. David Bell had called from a lady who identified herself as 'Dr. Elaine DeFreitas'. "I want to order your book *Skull Valley*," she said. "How much should I send?"

We replied that in view of her wonderful work as described by Hillary Johnson, especially her struggle to gain acceptance of her discovery that the blood of CFS/ME patients contained evidence of a retrovirus, we would send her a copy at no charge. After a further brief chat, we rang off and sent the book.

A few weeks later the phone rang again. It was Dr. DeFreitas, and quoting strictly from memory we recall the conversation: "My goodness" she said, "I've finished reading your book, and if I'd known that such things as you report were going on in the realm of biological weapons research, I would have acted a lot different that I did."

We asked her to elaborate.

"Well, Brian Mahy," she said. "When I reported my findings of a retrovirus in CFS blood, he called me up and said 'Elaine, you can't be right. There's no way you can find a retrovirus in CFS blood.' I said that my results had been carefully arrived at and that I'd checked them several times. There was a retrovirus there. Mahy then said 'Look, Elaine. If I send you some blood samples of CFS patients we are following, will you test those for the retrovirus?' I said, 'Yes, I'd be happy to'. Then he said, 'Can I send along an observer who will work with you and follow your protocols?' I said, 'Of course.' Well, the blood arrived and the observer arrived and I did the full process…and not one of them produced any hint of a retrovirus. I was shocked, but now after reading your book I doubt that it was even human blood that he had sent me."

We asked, 'Not human blood?'

> "Yes…it was goat's blood or something, but you see, when I did my original work I had used some healthy controls, and even though they were healthy, there was a small number who had traces of the retrovirus. And in the blood Mahy sent me there wasn't even that incidental show."

We were at a loss for words, and then suddenly we were inspired to ask: "Did you ever know a Mahy associate named Jose Rivera?"

Dr. DeFreitas replied immediately, "Of yes, he was the person Mahy sent with the blood. Why do you ask?"

We said, 'We hesitate to tell you this, but Dr. Jose Rivera had some sort of link with Lee Harvey Oswald, the purported assassin of President Kennedy.'

> "Oh my goodness. What is that supposed to mean?"

We explained the strange links between Rivera and Oswald, and soon after rang off. Later we called Dr. DeFreitas to ask if she would attend our Conference in Rochester and she tentatively agreed… declining later only because Dr. David Bell had urged her to visit with him at his home.

We've had no further contact with Dr. DeFreitas.

The Kingston to St. Lawrence Valley 'Mystery Disease' of 1984

In the period from August to November 1984, there was an outbreak of CFS/ME affecting some 500 victims that ranged from Kingston, Ontario down the St. Lawrence River to somewhere near Montreal. As a consequence of the numbers involved and the similarity of symptoms, the federal health department took a special interest in the epidemic and by 1990 issued an alert to doctors about chronic fatigue syndrome.

Hillary Johnson had promised to write her account of the chronic fatigue web with 'reportorial calm.' She has done that, but below the surface there seethes an intrigue we continue to study. The deep politics of the United States.

Chapter Twenty

EDWARD HOOPER: ENTHUSIASM AND GOOD COUNSEL IN EQUAL MEASURE

> "Claudius: He, being remiss
> Most generous, and free from all contriving
> Will not peruse the foils…"   *Hamlet* Act IV; Sc.vii

One cannot call Ed Hooper 'remiss'. He is obviously and demonstrably one of the most (indeed we think that he is the most) conscientious, fair-mined, hardest working researchers into the origin of AIDS that one could hope to meet. He is, however, like Hamlet, generous in nature and free of all contriving. And, as Claudius says in the lines above, the latter quality has kept him from 'perusing' the foil of biological warfare research in the evolution of AIDS.

In his book *The River*, Hooper devotes pages 151 to 169 to the dismissal of theories, which, he suggests, treat 'AIDS as evidence of Man's evil, as the result of manipulations by scientists and generals in their laboratories of biological warfare.'

Included in his list of dismissed theories is the history that we have been researching and writing about for nearly twelve years. Hooper writes:

> "Not all the *conspiracy theories* are quite so pleasingly transparent. The most notorious of them proposed that American scientists (with, it was *inferred*, the involvement of the U.S. Army and perhaps the CIA) had developed HIV at Fort Detrick, Maryland, as a weapon of germ warfare. This theory has received extensive coverage since the mid-eighties and, for this reason, *its convoluted* history deserves some attention.

> "The *story* first appeared in October 1985 in a Soviet literary weekly, and was then picked up by the wire services. Much of the theory appeared to be based on the ideas of *John Seale*, a British venereologist who, for more than a year, had been arguing that AIDS was artificially created, and that it might be *linked to biowarfare programs*."
>
> (Hooper, 1999 Page 153)

Our present study obviously falls within the 'conspiracy theories' that Mr. Hooper is discussing and we will comment upon the italicized parts.

'Conspiracy theories': We have commented upon the denigration of 'conspiracy buffs' and 'conspiracy theories' elsewhere in this study. We readily accept the suggestion that our major thesis is a theory that a group of powerful people are and have been for some time involved in planning to reduce the rate at which the world's population is growing. As we have said before, one can view an unexpected grouping of events as quite fortuitous or one can suggest that perhaps their grouping was not a matter of coincidence, but rather a matter of planning. For example, one can look back at our account in chapter fourteen about the Hearings held on June 9, 1969 between Dr. Donald MacArthur of the Pentagon and several Congressmen who were on a 'black budget' committee which ruled upon illicit proposals.

Dr. MacArthur asked for a $10 million budget to finance research into a 'new microorganism, one which was refractory to the human immune system.' The Committee and hence the Congress voted their approval.

Our Oxford English Reference Dictionary defines a conspiracy as: "1. a secret plan to commit a crime or do harm, often for political ends; a plot." (Page 308)

Why does Hooper label our theory 'notorious'? Again, with reference to our Oxford Dictionary: "notorious - well known, esp. unfavorably"…Is our theory, built as it is upon twelve years of searching through the scientific, medical and political literature, all that well known? And, well known to whom?

'Inferred: 1. deduce or conclude from facts and reasoning…' We have tried and we continue to try not to infer anything…we search for facts and we state them, then we state our reasonable thesis based upon such facts. It is, as far as we can determine, a fact that there was a biological weapons research section within the U.S. Pentagon; there was a meeting on June 9, 1969 wherein money was approved to develop an new infectious agent, one which does not naturally exist. It is a fact that the CIA was involved and that Dr. Gottlieb of the CIA on orders from Director Helms, shredded all the related documents that he could locate. Nothing inferred here…or elsewhere in this book…we state what we have found and we direct the reader to the sources of our evidence, which is made up mainly of U.S. Government Printing Office documents and peer-reviewed articles from the professional journals. This is not 'inferring' anything. This is stating facts.

'Its convoluted history'? We set out in 1995 to study the nature and origins of CFS/ME. We have been led by clear evidence to our present position that AIDS is a mirror-image of CFS/ME. We have a copy of a Patent by Dr. Shyh-Ching Lo which states that 'people with a mycoplasmal infection will be patients who have been diagnosed as having AIDS or ARC, chronic fatigue syndrome…' etc. There is nothing about our history of exploration that is convoluted.

'The story first appeared…' Is this volume of evidence, which we have struggled to place in an order that makes it evident to readers, a 'story'? No, it is not a story, it is a statement of history, and there is a difference. Again with reference to our *Oxford Dictionary*:

> "story: 1 an account of imaginary or past events; a narrative, tale or anecdote."

A history, on the other hand, is defined in the same source as:

> "history 1. a continuous, usu. chronological record of important public events. 2. a the study of past events, esp. human affairs, etc."

Ours is a history, not a story. Ed Hooper avoids classifying his account published in *The River*, by terming it a 'journey'.

"John Seale" is referred to by Hooper three times in his index. In one reference, he suggests that Dr. Seale was 'eccentric'. Well, maybe he was. He certainly wasn't a mainstream doctor/researcher. (We discuss his views in chapter seventeen above, section seven.) We certainly didn't get our 'story' from Dr. Seale. We were in to our tenth year of research when Ms. Peg Laurian of Minnesota was kind enough to provide us with a copy of Dr. Seale's report as published by the British House of Commons.

"Might be linked to biowarfare programs." Well, we think that such a linkage is quite reasonable, and we remind Mr. Hooper that, when he was telling the history of David Carr, he states that a Royal Navy doctor had expressed wonder as to what Carr had been vaccinated against. When the doctor skirted a reply, Hooper had suggested to him that "there were germ warfare tests" being conducted around that time. So, apparently Hooper has had thoughts similar to those of Dr. Seale.

However that may be, *The River* is a great history and Mr. Hooper is a great researcher…even if he doesn't examine the foils, he has done a magnificent job in tracking down many of the people, institutions and events in the history of AIDS.

Chapter Twenty-One

ENGAGE THE ENEMY

Donald Gibson

Towards the end of 1995, when we were just beginning our search for answers about chronic fatigue syndrome and beginning to entertain vague doubts that it was a natural epidemic, we received a gift copy of *Battling Wall Street* from the book's author, Prof. Donald Gibson. The book dealt the presidency of John F. Kennedy and the enemies in high places that he had made during his thousand days in office.

The book made a great impression on us for, unlike other books on the subject such as Prof. Peter Dale Scott's *Deep Politics and the Death of JFK* and Harold Weisberg's *Oswald in New Orleans* that were part of our study leading up to Chapter Ten of this work, Professor Gibson did not deal with the mechanics of the assassination…the creation of the Oswald myth as a loner malcontent, or the details of the testimony of Dealey Plaza witnesses…it dealt with a group that Richard Nixon was later to speak about as the 'Establishment', (Ch.15) and whose role in the assassination had not been so specifically addressed in other studies.

We sent our thanks to Prof. Gibson, together with a review of his book written by Paul Lalonde and published in *Ontario Options*. In his review Lalonde had referred to the 'military - industrial complex' that Eisenhower had warned against. Prof. Gibson replied:

> "I did appreciate very much the comments on my book in Paul Lalonde's book review essay. I did wince over the use of the term 'military industrial complex.' I do not think this term accurately represents Kennedy's most powerful enemies. I prefer terms such as the Establishment, East Coast Establishment, Higher Circles, financial establishment, Wall Street, or upper-class elite."   (Letter in our files)

The reference to 'Kennedy's most powerful enemies' was particularly arresting since it moved away from the accepted view that the opposition to Mr. Kennedy was there, but that it was also an intellectual, gentlemanly sort of opposition, expressed politely on paper in journals such as *Life* magazine or the *Wall Street Journal*. One might easily think of the Mafia or of Jimmy Hoffa as dangerous and powerful, but the opposition from the Rockefellers and the Morgan's was polite and civil. Suddenly the reader had to face the fact that the opposition from Wall Street was indeed powerful and by easy extension-dangerous…very dangerous.

Making the opposition from Wall Street even more dangerous was the fact that it was largely hidden from public view. Gibson writes:

> "In one of the supposedly definitive books on President Kennedy, Arthur Schlesinger, Jr., managed to write over a thousand pages which never touched on most of Kennedy's economic initiatives, never mentioned Morgan or David Rockefeller, and barely touched on the attacks on Kennedy. In this was he could wind up portraying the John Birch Society as a prime opponent of President Kennedy."
>
> (Gibson, 1996 Page 76)

We re-read *Battling Wall Street* with new insights, as we continued our research. To our dawning awareness of the truth about the medical and scientific realities of CFS/ME and of AIDS there was added a dawning awareness of just who John F. Kennedy's most powerful and most dangerous enemies were. It had been easy to think of the Mafia as the enemy that could order the murder of the President, but it wasn't easy to picture that murder being covered up at the highest levels of government by that same Mafia ever since! The Mafia was obviously involved at the street level of the murder, but the failure of the justice system of the United States to ever do more than offer the dishonest *Warren Commission Report* with its validation of the myth that Lee Harvey Oswald acting alone was the murderer required that the real murderers have the continuing power to cover-up.

Professor Gibson makes an early and important observation:

> "By the early 1960s the Council on Foreign Relations, Morgan and Rockefeller interests, and the intelligence community

were so extensively inbred as to be virtually a single entity."
(*Ibid*, Page 72)

And one of this cabal's principal points of difference with Mr. Kennedy (and there were many and Gibson deals with most of them in a precise, well-documented way) was the difference over the concept of world population growth rate and its control.

Essentially, Mr. Kennedy believed that a peaceful and reasonable world could sustain a much larger population than it presently supported and could support any increase comfortably and economically. In such an environment of peace, productive employment and sufficiency, the population would regulate itself and smaller families cause the leveling off of the global birth rate.

Mr. Kennedy's Wall Street enemies took the opposite view. Professor Gibson summarizes their position:

> "A committee created in 1958; by President Eisenhower to review military security matters concluded that population growth was a primary cause of instability and backwardness. The 10-man committee included Rockefeller associate John J. McCloy and other notables, such as investment bankers Joseph M. Dodge and William H. Draper, Jr. (the committee was informally called the Draper Committee). Draper, a partner at Dillon, Read, and Co., would organize the Population Crisis Committee in 1965 to act as a lobbying force in Washington, D.C. St. Louis millionaire Hugh Moore assisted Draper in creating the Crisis Committee, and in the 1950s he paid for newspaper ads and pamphlets warning about the danger of a 'population bomb.'" (*Ibid*, Page 93)

It was against this background that Lyndon Johnson assumed the presidency after the murder of Mr. Kennedy, and, as we have already noted (Ch.12) he departed from Mr. Kennedy's position, and gave political expression to the Wall Street position.

And covertly, Johnson was to work to transform the Rockefeller/Dulles MK programs to the VO, SVL and SVC Programs, under which the biological weapons based upon the mycoplasma were tested, developed and deployed into the human population.

The Links to Watergate

The Johnson Shambles and the Presidential Elections of 1968

In November 1963, Lyndon Baines Johnson had succeeded John F. Kennedy as President of the United States.

In the immediate aftermath of Mr. Kennedy's murder, the public was led to believe that the assassination was a random act of a crazed lunatic. This carefully contrived picture was re-enforced by several powerful media such as the *Time-Life* conglomerate of Henry Luce, and the *New York Herald Tribune* under the direction of Jock Whitney. It was also advanced by various government agencies and key personnel including J. Edgar Hoover of the FBI.

In retrospect it is now evident that as part of their pre-assassination planning, the Dulles, Nelson Rockefeller, John J. McCloy, George H. W. Bush conspirators had put a well-planned media program into place. A plan that would assert that: 1. The President had been killed by a lone assassin; and, 2. That the assassin was a communist malcontent named Lee Harvey Oswald. Furthermore, the myth would suggest that, 3. The assassination was in keeping with previous presidential assassinations in this respect (an opinion only held by the grossly mis-informed); and, 4. That the assassination brought no LBJ departure from the policies of JFK. There had not been a *coup d'etat*.

Within hours, this carefully orchestrated media brain washing was in motion, and by and large, the people of the United States bought into it. There was no doubt in the public's mind in the immediate aftermath of the assassination that Lee Harvey Oswald was the killer and when Oswald was in turn murdered by Jack Ruby, cheers went up around the nation.

There is much evidence to show that Lee Harvey Oswald had been carefully selected as one of the potential patsies (you need to know that in case something went wrong and Oswald had failed to turn up at work, there were alternate patsies in place who would only be fingered if required) and had been 'run' by the powers that be to appear as a loner lunatic. Nothing could be further from the truth. Lee Harvey Oswald was a patriot (mis-guided but well-meaning) who is as much a victim as John F. Kennedy.

It was only to be years later that evidence began leaking out which conveyed the truth of the *coup d'etat* that had taken place on November 22, 1963, when the 'shadow government' flexed its hidden and carefully restrained power and removed John F. Kennedy from office by professional assassins and had replaced him with an administration more to its liking.

Despite the powerful and high level support for this warped and dishonest view of the murder, and the continuing official line about the lone assassin myth, the truth is now capable of being stated without equivocation: **John F. Kennedy was murdered in order to change radically the direction in which he was taking the country and which he would undoubtedly have continued after his likely re-election in 1964.**

Author Donald Gibson summarizes this coup well:

> "John Kennedy represented the kind of government activism that they (call them the 'establishment' or 'the secret government' or 'the military-industrial complex' - Ed) found intolerable. They still do. The Morgan's, Rockefeller's, Harriman's, Bushes, and others have never hesitated to use government for their own purposes. In general, however, they view government as a necessary evil. It is to be strictly limited in its functions and powers. President Kennedy was reshaping government policies and using its potential to promote the general welfare of the nation. In his use of credit and loans, in budgetary decisions, in tax reform proposals, in foreign policy, in the promotion of educational opportunities, in the space program and in other areas of science and technology, Kennedy was instituting policies which were increasing the opportunities of people to develop themselves and do something significant with their lives. In the process, he took government policies way beyond what David Rockefeller or Jock Whitney thought was acceptable. These kinds of people, with no significant purpose in their lives beyond the perpetuation of their own power, struck against their enemy: popular, progressive, democratic government. We can't restore to JFK the thirty years of his life that were taken from him. But by recognizing what happened to him and why, it is still possible to return

our government to reasoned, civilized, humane, progress-oriented policies."

Donald Gibson Quoted from *Probe*, Vol.4, No. 1, November-December, 1996 Page 20

Although the basis for the coup of November 22, 1963 was broad and deep, the most immediate change in government policy occurred in the realm of the Vietnam War. Days before the assassination, McGeorge Bundy and Robert McNamara (accompanied for some unknown reason by a large part of the Kennedy cabinet...the reason to emerge later) had met with the Chiefs of Staff in Hawaii, where the war-bound Chiefs were given the decision made by Mr. Kennedy that American military involvement in the Vietnam war was to be wound down, starting immediately with the withdrawal of 1000 American troops and continuing at that rate monthly until all American combat forces were out.

The record of these meetings is still classified, but the evidence is that the Chiefs of Staff were violently opposed to the idea. It was their warped view that the war on the ground in Vietnam could be won if enough American troops were deployed and if the power of American technology...helicopter gun ships, cluster bombs, napalm... was brought to bear on rifle-armed foot soldiers in black pajamas and straw hats. (The same lunatic world-view dominates today in Iraq and Afghanistan.)

This view was also held by Robert McNamara and Vice-President Johnson, but they had been forced for three years to keep their views from Kennedy if they were to keep their jobs.

Just two days before the murder of the president, Bundy and McNamara returned from Hawaii, while the largest part of the Kennedy Cabinet was to proceed west to Japan. *Now the reason for the Cabinet's presence and dispatch to Japan is clear: they were to be safely out of reach when Mr. Kennedy was murdered. If anything went wrong with the assassination plans, anyone who might give leadership against the conspirators had to be put out of the way. Thus, when the President was murdered, his closest Cabinet allies were far out over the Pacific Ocean.*

As a further precaution in case something went wrong with the planned *coup d'etat*, General Lyman Lemnitzer had arranged for several thousand American troops to be flown back from Berlin, just hours before. These thousands of troops, who were being counted upon to obey their field officers if their deployment 'to maintain law and order' was deemed necessary, were in planes over Washington when the President was shot in Dallas that day. Another precaution against any unforeseen resistance, immediately following the murder, was the shutting down of the Washington, D.C. telephone service for several hours.

In the meantime, McGeorge Bundy had prepared a National Security Action Memorandum for President Kennedy which summarized what Bundy and McNamara had told the Chiefs in Hawaii. However, before this Vietnam 'wind-down' Memo could be signed by Kennedy, the President was murdered and one of the first things that the insidious gangster, Lyndon Baines Johnson did, was to pencil in several changes which completely changed the policy direction of the Memo. Rather than a 'wind down' direction, the way was left open for an increased effort by the U.S. Military, following a short period between the November murder and the next year's November elections.

There had been a *coup d'etat* in the United States, and America was on its way to a vastly increased war in Vietnam with the help of the Military, the 'Establishment', the major media…i.e. *New York Times*, the *Time-Life* group, the *Washington Post*, the CIA, FBI and portions of the Secret Service. The 'Deep Politics' crowd was now in charge!

There were probably three hundred key people involved in the assassination, including Allan Dulles, Nelson and David Rockefeller, Tracy Barnes, McGeorge Bundy and army officers such as Lyman Lemnitzer. Most people will scoff at this estimate, using arguments such as 'With that number, someone would be bound to break ranks'. But those who use this argument are not aware of the profound but unspoken depths of the psychological, social, business and professional links the assassin-group had one to the other. This 'awareness' is not limited to a select few…it is right there in the open for all to see if they will only look, (See: Congressional Hearings of June 9, 1969!) and quite frankly, the vast majority prefer not to make that effort of looking. The group which murdered the President was a 'secret society' to which many belonged without ever having consciously joined, but of which with greater or lesser degrees of consciousness they felt themselves a part, and from which none would ever dare exit if he valued his life, his family's lives, and his role or 'place' in the 'establishment'.

An excellent example from history of another unspoken yet very real 'secret' grouping which came together even in a closed and tightly controlled society can be seen in the hundreds of Germans who, in the latter days of World War Two had united to plot the murder of Adolph Hitler. One needs to read about this conspiracy in books such as that by Anton Gill titled, *An Honorable Defeat*. Needless to say, Allan Dulles would know this story intimately.

But, the point of this example is to demonstrate that many people can and will come together in secret to achieve illegal ends if the majority have a common, but very strong, purpose, and if, rightly or wrongly, they feel that they are on the side of the angels; that their purpose is honorable.

Others may join such secret groupings for their own private and selfish ends, but they hide these even from themselves in many cases.

The assassination of Mr. Kennedy was probably initiated by Allan Dulles, motivated most strongly by an urge for private revenge against Mr. Kennedy's firing him following the Bay of Pigs landings.

However, Dulles would advance his plotting by pushing the vulnerable buttons that varied with each participant. When all else failed there was always 'the need to save the nation from a President' and who had crossed the paths of many of the privileged. And they would join, often with deep personal sorrow at the destruction of such an attractive and personable human being, because their 'love of country' made personal sacrifice necessary. As with Brutus in Shakespeare's tragedy: "Not that he loved Caesar less, but that he loved Rome more."

Chapter Twenty-Two

AVIAN FLU…A CAUTIONARY TALE

We began our study of AIDS in 1995 when we were asked for help by a lady with chronic fatigue syndrome. We didn't begin with an axe to grind. In fact, we knew nothing about CFS/ME, and next to nothing about AIDS. Like the vast majority of people what we thought we knew were the myths about a 'gay plague'. However, as we began looking into the facts…not the folk tales and myths…the facts about CFS/ME we quickly learned that it was a real physical disease, not the 'all in the head of the victim' neurotic escape from reality myth widely held by the public and promoted by the public health agencies of the United States and popularized by media assets such as Edward Shorter and Elaine Showalter. We learned of epidemics such as an early outbreak in Iceland and in Punta Gorda, Florida, epidemics that were denied by persons such as Clinton Secretary of Health and Human Services, Donna Shalala. We learned much more, but especially, we learned that there was some kind of link between CFS/ME and AIDS.

Our twelve years of reading and interviewing has confirmed the latter linkage and in this book we have set out some of the evidence that we have found in our search. We have much more evidence that we will continue to develop and report over the time ahead in our quarterly *Journal of Degenerative Diseases*, but in this introduction to our quest we must draw a halt for lack of space.

However, before we do so, we must ask an important series of questions. Is there still the power in the shadows that gave rise to the epidemics of CFS/ME and AIDS? The 'deep politics' of the United States and, as we have seen, their allies in Great Britain, Canada, Australia, Israel and other nations? If there are such…and we are convinced that there are…do they have more plans that are being developed to achieve their world population growth-rate controls?

After all, one of the great lessons of history often repeated in literature but seldom respected in current political practice, is that it allows thinking people to avoid repeating the mistakes of the past.

If there is still the shadowed power and if another AIDS epidemic is being worked upon, what might it be?

We believe that the power is still there and that a strong possibility exists that an 'avian flu' epidemic may be the form that it will take. With such possibilities in mind, we felt that we should take a careful look at what has been and still is going on, and report our findings in this penultimate chapter.

When we began researching and re-reading our files on influenza we were struck by the number of people and institutions that recurred from our study of CFS/ME and AIDS. We wondered: could what has passed be prologue for something yet to come?

It was truly a case of 'that old gang of mine'.

Let us state our concern flat out: many of the same group that brought the world AIDS and CFS/ME are involved in the present avian influenza campaign. Does that mean that the present drumbeat about the hazards of avian flu is bogus, lacking merit in genuine health terms?

No.

It is quite possible that the scientists who are getting so much coverage in *The New York Times* with their worries about just how potentially dangerous an outbreak of avian flu might be are being responsible, informed scientists who have learned from history. The history of the influenza epidemic of 1918 in particular.

However, it might also be that the vaccines currently available or being presently developed are being driven by the money that is to be made from them, *or it may actually be that there is a deeper and more sinister foundation for the 'bird flu' hype.* The same foundation upon which the CIA built the MKULTRA, MKNAOMI, MKDELTA structure to develop and deploy the factors which present as AIDS and CFS/ME, with the collateral damage of other diseases based upon a compromised immune system.

Did the vaccine against hepatitis B offered to gay males in 1976 actually protect the recipients from hepatitis while, at the same time infecting them with the AIDS co-factors? And did those co-factors begin to present in 1980 as AIDS?

In the case of the hepatitis B vaccine program, we have concluded from our research and we have reported in this study, that the latter scenario is what actually happened.

Is the avian flu hype setting humanity up for the next planned pandemic? We must ponder that possibility and examine the people and institutions involved before accepting or rejecting the warning cries.

First, from which institutions are the warnings emanating? The World Health Organization (WHO), the U.S. National Institutes of Health (NIH) and Centers for Disease Control (CDC), plus certain media such as *The New York Times* and writers such as Gina Kolata are the main sources of alarming predictions, and must be examined. Second, the historical record must be searched for possible clues. We begin with a quote from *The Virus Cancer Program* (Ch. 13) that appears relevant:

> "…various live, attenuated adenovirus vaccines were administered to selected human populations as a control measure for debilitating respiratory tract infections. [Emphasis added—Ed] A further complication was introduced when it was discovered that the oncogenic (*i.e.* 'tumor causing'—Ed) papovavirus SV40, acquired from the simian cells used for propagation of the adenoviruses, *was present as a major contaminant* in these vaccine preparations. Since hybrid viruses with a spectrum of biological functions have been isolated from mixed adenovirus-SV40 populations, these adenovirus vaccines undoubtedly contained such recombinant viruses. *Thus, more than one million people were inoculated with representative members of two groups of DNA viruses with known oncogenic properties.*"
>
> (Page 19)

In other words, the United States Government injected a cancer-causing monkey virus into one million U.S. citizens, and then tried to cover up their blunder and silence those who had revealed it.

The record is clear: government agencies are not to be given our unqualified faith. Their claims must be rigorously examined.

But, errors in judgment by authority figures are not the major danger. The evidence derived from our study of the discovery, development and deployment of the AIDS, CFS/ME pathogenic factors shows that powerful forces may be working towards population growth-rate controls through the public health agencies and private and institutional researchers, while employing media assets to mask their real intent. *Money and the power of authority may give those deep political powers the tools to achieve their ends.*

We have seen how, in the 1960s millions of Third World people were rounded up by foreign military occupiers of their countries (authority) and were compelled to take a free vaccination against smallpox. The occupying troops were largely French, British, Belgian and Portuguese and the donor of the free smallpox vaccine was nominally the World Health Organization but in fact was largely the United States Government which had dispatched seventeen teams of people from the Centers for Disease Control in Atlanta to vaccinate millions of innocent people.

The recipients of this American largesse were told that the vaccine would help them escape the risk of smallpox…they would, as it were, give up something old…the disease known as smallpox. However, they would, as the evidence we adduce in this study shows, be getting something new in exchange: AIDS.

We here present what we suggest is another opportunity the world is being given to exchange an ancient disease (a viral influenza) for something new: a 'flu-like illness' caused by a mycoplasmal species. In fact, a large part of the human family have already been contaminated with this deadly new pathogen engineered from its earlier and natural antecedent by the United States Government biowar weapons research, development, testing and deployment agencies and their university and commercial partners.

And, if the support of the media assets is not enough to deliver all citizens over to the vaccine dispensers, other steps can be taken if the citizens let the state have its way.

It appears, from media reports, that shortly the people of the United States and Great Britain are going to be required to accept a vaccination to 'protect' themselves from catching 'influenza'. Just which strain of influenza they are going to be 'protected' against is anyone's guess, but the so-called 'avian flu' species known as H5N1 is being touted in the mass media as the potential culprit. Other gullible 'Coalition' allies such as Poland, the Ukraine, Italy, Spain, and

Australia, going along with the U.S.'s unstated agenda to acquire total control of middle eastern oil by viciously attacking Iraq with the 'shock and awe' bombing followed by a Nazi-style invasion will most likely also go along with their British/American 'Big Brothers' and accept the gift of a vaccination for protection against the flu. Countries, such as Canada, France, Germany, Japan and others will be put under pressure by select media to do the same, but will likely be more resistant.

On this topic it must be emphasized that President George Bush said in September of 2006 that *he may have to call upon the U.S. Military to administer the vaccination program and to confine dissenters to concentration camps until they, too, accept the vaccine offered.* In this, one should recall that Portugal and Belgium used their military power to ensure that the citizens of the occupied colonies in Africa and India (Goa) took the 'free' smallpox vaccines that were pushed upon them in the mid-1960s and early 1970s. (Ch. 7)

Great Britain has also recently announced that **all** citizens may soon be vaccinated 'for their own safety', and that Britain already has a 'plan' in place to achieve just such a goal!

The old 'here's a free vaccine' and the guns of the occupying powers worked with the Third World countries who gave up smallpox in exchange for AIDS. There is reason to believe that it will work again only this time it may be directed at the rest of us when, five years down the line (or even sooner) a new and deadly disease makes its presence known.

Further, it may already well on its way. It will look like influenza and it will kill like influenza and the bacterial sequelae will also be there. But, it won't be influenza!

This doomsday scenario is terrible to contemplate, but who in 1950 would have envisaged the epidemic of AIDS killing 8,000 people a day just fifty years down the line? To help you accept the possibility of this scenario we quote from Dr. Leonard Horowitz' in his 2001 book: *Death in the Air*.

> "…in 1970, immediately after National Security Adviser Henry Kissinger called for drastic Third World depopulation, which sparked secret congressional subsidies into a new generation of bioweapons that Litton Bionetics engineered, *one contract called for the testing of special strains of 'influenza' and 'Para influenza' viruses. As reported by Dr. Horowitz in*

> *Emerging Viruses: AIDS & Ebola- Nature, Accident or Intentional?*
> "these flu viruses were recombined with leukemia viruses for its only rational use - population reduction. Much like the AIDS virus, these new strains could be more rapidly spread to cause slow, non-traceable genocide." [Page 171]

As we stated above, many of the people who turn up in this study of influenza are the same people who have already turned up in our study of AIDS/CFS/ME.

Furthermore, the huge tragedy of 50,000,000 deaths from influenza in the 1918-1919 epidemic *may well have been set loose in the world as a biological war weapon. Period! And its engineered successor could well exceed that mark.*

In case you think that this is an unreasonable possibility, then consider the following quote from a press release distributed by a New York Times science writer, Gina Kolata:

> "Richard H. Ebright, a molecular biologist at Rutgers, said he had serious concerns about the reconstruction of the virus [the 1918 flu virus—Ed] 'There is a risk verging on inevitability, of accidental release of this virus; there is also a risk of *deliberate release of the virus.*'
>
> "And the 1918 flu virus, Dr. Ebright added, 'is perhaps *the most effective bioweapons agent ever known.*'"

We placed a telephone call to Dr. Ebright at 732-932-4636 to talk to him about such a horrible thought, and we left a message with someone who answered our call. Later the same day (Thursday, October 27, 2005) Dr. Ebright returned our call. We asked him if he had been quoted correctly by Ms. Kolata. *He said that he was correctly quoted.* In that case, we asked, does he hold the view that the influenza outbreak of 1918 had been caused by biological weapons research or deployment?

"Oh, no, no. I don't suggest that at all. I just meant that if it were a weapon it would be the most effective ever used..." We let it go at that, but we continue to wonder why he would even talk about bioweapons if, when discussing influenza, it was he who raised the possibility. After all, it was Dr. Ebright who spoke of the possible 'deliberate release of the virus.'

So much for Dr. Ebright! You may have noted that Dr. Ebright was quoted in a press release by Gina Kolata, a science writer for *The New York Times*.

In the search for the truth about influenza we suggest that as with their earlier reporting upon AIDS and CFS/ME, one can trust neither *The New York Times* nor Gina Kolata. We will elaborate.

Gina Kolata published a book in 1999 titled simply, *Flu*. Although it has a lot of valuable information, it is, over all, an unsatisfactory and dishonest book, and has re-enforced our opinion that anyone associated with *The New York Times* should be checked out carefully because of the *Times'* tendency as perceived by certain researchers to employ misinformation or disinformation when reporting upon certain topics.

We'll develop the above claim shortly, but first we want to report upon another book dealing with the 1918 influenza epidemic. The second book we refer to is titled *Hunting the 1918 Flu*, and it is by a Canadian geographer named Kirsty Duncan, Ph.D. In her book Dr. Duncan reports upon an expedition that she organized and led between 1992 and 2002 to a remote Norwegian village on Spitsbergen Island, in the province and archipelago of Svalbard.

There, in the graveyard of Longyearbyen she and her team exhumed the bodies of seven miners who had died of influenza in 1918, hoping to recover viable samples of the deadly virus that had killed them. In the course of her research Dr. Duncan was contacted by Gina Kolata who was covering the story for the Times. The picture of Kolata that emerges from Dr. Duncan's candid account corresponded to the picture that we had developed as we read Kolata's book, Flu. To illustrate what we are referring to, here are some passages from page 233 of Dr. Duncan's *Hunting the 1918 Flu*:

> "While waiting for any PCR results, I (Dr. Kirsty Duncan—Ed) received a call from Gina Kolata…She asked…if I would be willing to be interviewed. I was brutally honest. 'I do not feel comfortable speaking with you, as you have been dishonest with me in the past'…she asked…what I thought (about her latest chapter) 'There are numerous errors and there are outright lies…(I replied)'"

Dr. Duncan had apparently formed the same opinion of Gina Kolata that we had formed as we read and discussed the latter's book!

We say again, as we suggested in Part six above…don't trust the media. If it is *The New York Times* reporting on influenza, AIDS, CFS/ME, or other health issues, double check the report. At this point we will comment upon Kolata's book, *Flu*. We'll limit that look to two paragraphs on pages 268 and 269 where Kolata lists a group of scientists and researchers who participated in a National Institutes of Health (USA) meeting on December 4, 1997, to discuss Dr. Duncan's expedition to Spitsbergen. Here are the paragraphs:

> "Taubenberger was there that day although he had resigned from Duncan's group on September 7, having notified Duncan by fax of his decision. He explained to her that he could not help her with her mission because he had heard from several reporters that she asked them to pay for interviews - a charge Duncan vehemently denies. Once the issue was raised, however, Taubenberger felt he had no choice. Charging the media for access to the Spitsbergen team 'was incompatible with my position as a U.S. government scientist, he said.'
>
> "The meeting room was studded with illustrious scientists - a famous virologist, a famous epidemiologist, a famous expert on respiratory diseases, a famous expert on emerging diseases. In addition to Kirsty Duncan, Robert Webster, and Jeffery Taubenberger, the participants were: Dr. Robert Couch, a microbiologist and influenza expert at Baylor College of Medicine, Dr. Nancy Cox, chief of the influenza branch of the Centers for Disease Control and Prevention, Dr. Donald A. Henderson, a professor at the School of Hygiene and Public Health at Johns Hopkins University, Dr. Peter B. Jahrling, a scientific advisor to the U.S. Army Medical Research Institute of Infectious Diseases in Frederick, Maryland, Dr. William Jordan, an infectious disease expert at the National Institute of Allergy and Infectious Diseases, Dr. Edwin Kilbourne, the influenza expert from New York Medical College, Dr. Brian Mahy, the director of the Division of Viral Diseases at the Centers for Disease Control and Prevention, Dr. John LaMontagne, the director of the Division of Microbiology and Infectious Diseases at

the National Institute of Allergy and Infectious Diseases, Dr. PamelaMcInnes, the chief of the respiratory diseases branch."

Let's start with the second paragraph…then we'll comment upon the first paragraph.

Kolata calls the assembly 'illustrious scientists'? Consider who some of these people are and their particular claims to fame.

The first one worthy of note is Dr. Robert Couch who is, according to Kolata, an 'influenza expert'.

The first time we ran across the name of Dr. R. B. Couch was as a co-author of an article in the *Journal of the American Medical Association* [JAMA] dated February 8, 1964. The title of his article was: 'Infection with Artificially Propagated Eaton Agent (*Mycoplasma pneumoniae*).'

As reported in Chapter 23, Chanock and Couch had been early researchers into the qualities and dangers of the *mycoplasma*.

At this point we feel it necessary to re-state one of our research principles: To the fullest extent possible we use only peer-reviewed scientific articles in well-accepted professional journals and official documents from some government source. We are fully aware of the frequent instances of bias in the journals employed, but at least our sources are on the record and can be readily checked out. And when we identify obvious bias, we point that out to our readers and also identify the source of the challenge so the reader can use his own reason and logic as a basis for his stance. As for the government documents, many of these have been located despite the governments' best efforts to limit public access to them. In either case, it saves us from being accused of forging evidence such as David Baltimore, Robert Gallo and other AIDS researchers have done. (For a thoughtful and careful study of the Baltimore/Gallo and related scholarly dishonesty, see Dr. Serge Lang's book, Challenge 1998; Springer-Verlag, New York, Inc.)

When we noted Kolata's mention of Dr. Couch, we were first struck by the fact that he had been associated as far back as 1964 with Dr. Chanock whose research record demonstrated early involvement with the literature and research of AIDS!

Before we went any further we decided to check it out with Dr. Couch at Baylor College of Medicine. We reached his office and spoke with his secretary, explaining who we were and that we were doing some research into Dr. Couch's early work with mycoplasmas and would appreciate a copy of his full *curriculum vitae*. *The lady informed us that she could only send out such information with the express permission of Dr. Couch and that she would ask him*. She put us on hold, and then returned to say that *Dr. Couch did not want a copy of his full C.V. sent to us, nor did he want to discuss it with us*. We thanked her and went on with our work.

Our next step was to check the index of Kolata's book for any references to Dr. Chanock. There were none, *but we did discover an interesting puzzle*. Although Kolata does not refer to Dr. Chanock in her book in any sense of his work with mycoplasmas or related topics, she does, on an unnumbered page following page 306, write: "I also want to thank…Robert Channock (sic) for providing me with… assistance…"

Well, that 'thank you' note raised all kinds of questions for us. First, was Kolata's 'Channock' simply a misspelling of 'Chanock' or was he a different person? Furthermore, if Channock (?) deserved such a special 'thank you' for his 'assistance', why would Kolata not tell us what that assistance was? Perhaps, we speculated, it was indeed the Chanock who had worked with the 'influenza expert', Dr. Couch, a way back in 1962 when both were pioneering research into the qualities of the mycoplasma and testing them on prisoners in Huntsville Penitentiary in Texas?

If this were the Chanock that would explain why what he helped with…*the role of the mycoplasma in influenza*…*could not be mentioned. Kolata had to leave references to the mycoplasma out of her New York Times reporting because that term is consigned to the memory hole in order to hide significant truth from the masses! Truth, for example, which would shed light on a possible new flu-like pandemic which could hit at any time and be blamed upon an avian flu-virus which had purportedly 'jumped species'?*

There was only one-way to find out: phone Ms. Kolata at *The New York Times* and ask her: 1. Is the Robert Channock she thanks on page 307 actually a misspelling of 'Chanock'? 2. What did Channock (?) assist her with that she never got around to telling her readers in her book? 3. Why does she not have any mention in her book *Flu*, even the faintest whisper, about the role of the mycoplasma in influenza?

We phoned her four times and got her answering machine each time. Each time we left the same message that we were doing some research into her book and there were some brief questions we would like answers to.

Ms. Kolata never returned any of our calls over the period of a week… out reporting, perhaps, on the eminent danger of a flu-like H5N1 pandemic?

The next one of the 'illustrious' gathering that Gina Kolata waxes almost poetic about is Donald Henderson. You may remember him.

Donald A. Henderson was the doctor appointed by the Centers for Disease Control in Atlanta to oversee the main push by the WHO to vaccinate as many people in Third World countries against the scourge of smallpox as they could get their needles into. Henderson was 'ordered' (his word) to take on the job in the mid 1960's. *Millions of Black Africans were given no option by their foreign military occupiers but to allow themselves to be vaccinated with a vaccine grown on monkey kidneys. (MK)!*

Shortly afterwards, as we have reported, the vaccinated innocents of the Third World began to present with the first cases of acquired immune deficiency syndrome.

Kolata then introduces Dr. Brian Mahy who, at one point in his illustrious career had been heavily engaged in research obviously linked to the development of the HIV co-factors. For his efforts, he rose to head the Centers for Disease Control. Along the way, he tried to sabotage Dr. Kirsty Duncan's Norwegian expedition, and then a few years later he 'lost' nearly $4,000,000 given to the CDC by the US Congress to study chronic fatigue syndrome! (Ch. 16)

Four million dollars under Mahy's control simply disappeared, but he was never fired. He knew too much to be fired, so he was given a job with Homeland Security.

And so it goes…Gina Kolata knows an 'illustrious crowd' when she sees one.

The moral of the story: one cannot trust the main stream media when it comes to reporting on hugely important health matters such as AIDS, CFS, and now, the avian FLU.

This principle is frequently recalled when we deal with anything appearing in Time Magazine. After all, it was *Time* which gave AIDS its street name: 'The Gay Plague', and coined the name 'The Yuppie Flu' for chronic fatigue syndrome. However, from time-to-time (no pun intended) we do read selected issues of Luce's legacy. One such exception was the November 7, 2005, Canadian edition of *Time* with its lead article on Global Health. There, under the Letters section was the following letter by a reader:

> **"A Quiet Revenge?"**
> Everyone seems so alarmed by the outbreak of avian flu [Oct.17]. Maybe its time we stopped and looked at the way we raise animals. Seven to nine chickens crammed into a cage the size of a microwave oven is a viral time bomb waiting to explode. Caged chickens stand in their own feces and are never able to flex their wings. Many have been de-beaked, and some have chronic pain and infections. We should ban the inhumane standards of factory farming. I believe that avian flu is the quiet revenge of those millions of chickens, ducks and geese that we torture before they reach our plates. Marcela Donato, Thornhill, ON

Out of the mouths of its readers one gets as close as one is apt to get to the truth in *Time*. However, to return our focus to respiratory diseases, consider the following from Gina Kolata's, *Flu*:

> "On Wednesday, February 4, 1976, eighteen-year-old Private David Lewis felt feverish and achy. His nose was running, his head hurt. And he shivered with cold...He was a new recruit at Fort Dix..." [Page 121]

Question: What is the link between a jam-packed chicken house and a crowded military barracks such as that wherein Private Lewis languished?

Answer: Concentration.

Our research has demonstrated to us the fact that when one concentrates a human or other animal species (including birds) into a relatively confined space, one increases the possibility that respiratory-linked diseases will increase in significance. Consider the following examples. In World War One, thousands of men were packed together in large, often poorly ventilated army barracks. From such cramped barracks, the military recruits were often cramped together even more closely in troop ships, and were forced to re-breathe for hours on end the same air. And what if that air is contaminated by some disease pathogen? Well, in that case the pathogen gets a greater opportunity to concentrate in the respiratory tract and lungs of the victims.

This is especially true of the disease agent *mycoplasma* upon which Drs. Couch and Chanock would later work, and upon which Dr. Robert Huebner (Ch.3), was working for the U.S. Navy, when he discovered that the *mycoplasma* could lead to the 'spontaneous degeneration' of certain human tissues and could lower the body's immune system!

On many factory farms millions of chickens and other fowl are usually placed in wire mesh cages shortly after they are born. The cages are stacked one atop each other for several feet, and bird feces is allowed to drop through the mesh to the ground below where it is salvaged and processed as *a feed protein additive for other farm animals*. Thus, not only is any airborne pathogen concentrated, but any feces-borne pathogen is likewise concentrated.

Consider the following quotation from Dr. Howard Lyman's book, *Mad Cows and Milk Gate*:

> "In April, the Calgary Herald reported the discovery of the first known mad cow case in North America at an elk ranch near Regina, Saskatchewan." [Page 27]

Elk, which normally roamed the wilds with ample free space to graze and breathe...concentrated on factory farms, becoming ill with mad cow disease. Why would that be?

Here we have three examples of concentrating large numbers of men, chickens and elk which had previously existed naturally in spread-out open environments but who were later confined to closely packed barracks, pens, or factory farms, and were subsequently ill with influenza, avian influenza or bovine spongiform encephalomyelitis. What is the connecting link?

It is concentration!

The military recruits stationed in large barracks spent hour after hour in each other's company. As a consequence they breathed and re-breathed each other's air. They did not, as did equivalent young people outside the military barracks, live in separate homes, and have several long hours away from each other. As a result, any pathogenic organisms that might be found in the air of a shared environment would have several extra hours to become concentrated in the lungs of susceptible persons.

The poultry raised on modern factory farms for the production of eggs or for eating are similarly concentrated for their entire lives. They have no daily break for a more individual existence and as with the recruits in military barracks studied by Dr. Huebner, any pathogens in the air are given a greater opportunity to reach dangerous levels of concentration in their lungs. To an extent, the same concentration is achieved on small back yard flocks of poultry in rural areas of Asia where humans, other farm animals (especially swine) and poultry of various kinds share limited space for most of their daily lives. Again the principle is: concentration.

But how about the example of elk farms referred to by the late Dr. Hulse? Are the elk on the farms not just as free and remote from each other as farm-raised animals such as beef steers? Yes, they are, but…they are *concentrated in comparison* to what they were when they roamed the woods and grasslands of their natural habitat. The cattle raised on farms are the descendants of animals raised in similar concentration for hundreds of years and have been able to develop a relative species immunity compared to that which wild elk have been able to develop. Thus, the elk have a lower natural immunity when confined to farms.

In any event, the principle is as we have said, one of concentration.

An Interlude upon the Essential Simplicity of Human Disease

You may recall the acronym often used by language instructors who are working with neophyte writers: 'KISS'…keep it simple, stupid!

That is, if you want your reader or listener to understand what it is that you are talking about, use speech that is as close to the language of the everyday listener as you can achieve.

However, when the National Institutes of Health (NIH) and the Centers for Disease Control and Prevention (CDC) and the pharmaceutical-dominated health industry want to brain wash the public about any topic, they are inclined to employ various techniques to mask their actual intentions while still appearing to be candid and forth-coming. Such 'techniques of obfuscation' have been well summarized by Dr. Serge Lang in his important book *Challenges*. Among such techniques Lang lists -*describing the same thing with multiple names;* leaving out certain documentation; complicating the structures of groups purportedly looking into a matter (*i.e.* 'panel of expert scientific advisors drawn from the extramural research community'); or, putting in unattributed allegations.

Our research has provided us with several examples of the use of such techniques by the NIH, CDC, industry representatives and the media when talking about AIDS and CFS/ME and now when reporting upon influenza and the looming disaster they conjure up of an avian flu pandemic. There is a lot of linguistic sleight-of-hand in many of the public releases and we suggest that the best counter to such drum beating is to put the whole situation into its simple fundamentals (KISS) and we summarize these fundamentals as follows:

- The human body is roughly ninety-seven percent composed of just **FOUR** elements: carbon, hydrogen, nitrogen, and oxygen…or CHNO. The other three percent is made up of traces of other elements such as phosphorus, sulphur, iron, zinc, magnesium etc.
- These four basic elements in varying numbers are then combined into **FIVE** nucleic acids essential to life: adenine, cytosine, guanine, thymine, and uracil.
- The **five** nucleic acids are in turn combined into **TWO** main groups. One **group**, employing adenine, cytosine and guanine together with thymine produce the blueprints of life called deoxyribonucleic acid or **DNA**, which are used in the reproduction of the living organism.
- The other group, employing adenine, cytosine, and guanine together with uracil produce what might be called the 'working drawings' necessary for the translation of the blueprints into actual proteins and hence living organisms, and known as ribonucleic acid or **RNA**.
- The four RNA nucleic acids are then capable of being grouped into trinucleotides or, as the name implies, groups of three, which in turn present as **TWENTY** amino acids. These twenty trinucleotides can then combine to form over sixty-thousand proteins used in the building and operation of the human body.

Against this background we will now take a look at **H5N1** and just what it means and how it is relevant to our present study.

The 'N' in that species label stands for *neuraminidase* and it consists of a string of amino acids which present on the surface of the influenza virus and permit its access to certain human cells. If the sequence of amino acids is altered it presents as a new variant of the virus antigen. It is important to recall that *the mycoplasma, about which Johns Hopkins and Gina Kolata don't seem to have heard (see above) can change certain amino acids in situ and hence alter the neuraminidase code, and thus alter the flu virus cellular access ability. This is one form of viral mutation that you have read so much about.* We will deal further with this matter but at this point, just keep in mind the following fundamentals:

The human body is ninety-seven percent comprised of just four elements: carbon, hydrogen, nitrogen and oxygen.

The elements CHNO combine to form five nucleic acids: adenine, cytosine, guanine, thymine and uracil.

These five acids combine to form a body blueprint (DNA) and working drawings (RNA).

In further groupings of three (trinucleotides) the acids form the twenty amino acids necessary for the creation of the sixty thousand plus proteins of which the human body is composed. We'll return to these fundamentals later. In the meantime, don't be dazzled by all the jargon sleight-of-hand to which you are being subjected in the avian flu hype. The average human body is composed of fifty trillion cells. These cells all start off as a single cell...the egg provided by the female and fertilized by the sperm from the male. Then, immediately after fertilization, the egg begins the process of dividing and differentiating to create the full range of cells which combine in accordance with inherited impulse to create all of the necessary parts of the emerging body.

This is where most people go wrong when thinking about health and disease, including influenza: they start off with the whole body and talk about a single disease at a time. *i.e.*: "I am ill with the flu." Or "My body is wracked by cancer." Wrong on both and any other counts you may cite.

The fundamental thing is to start with individual cells that are attacked by individual pathogens.

Now, the important thing about the so-called influenza pandemics is this: under the rubric of 'influenza', there are a variety of pathogens, which alone or together or one after another, alter the effective working of individual cells at several different sites in the total body. Among the dangerous pathogens are various bacterial, viral, and mycoplasmal species working in the cells of the different body systems. One cannot talk about the 'flu' killing a 'person'. One must think in terms of specific pathogens damaging or destroying specific cells in specific body systems, sometimes to the extent that the whole body ceases to function. So, start your thinking with the cell and go on from there.

Moving on from the fundamental unit of the cell, we must now note the major groupings of those cells into the **TEN** major systems of the functioning human body. Four of these systems work so closely together we group them as pairs rather than as individual systems. The ten systems are: the muscular and skeletal systems; reproductive system; respiratory system; endocrine system; digestive system; urinary system; blood and cardiovascular systems; and the brain and nervous systems.

The disease entity commonly referred to as 'influenza', primarily attacks the respiratory system and the attacking pathogen is a virus.

However, over the years the term influenza has come to cover any of numerous febrile illnesses which reach beyond the respiratory system to affect practically all the other systems of the body! Furthermore, there is now a 'flu-like' illness caused by the *Mycoplasma fermentans* to which we will return in the Summary below.

The viral pathogen primarily focused upon is only **ONE** of **THREE** pathogens which often come into play in attacks of what we broadly call 'the flu'. So, all of this hype about the 'avian flu virus H5N1' has to be responded to with careful thought. What is usually ignored, overlooked or down-played are the roles of certain other pathogens such as bacteria and mycoplasmas. And the latter, especially, is almost totally absent from any reference you will find in print in the literature directed to the average citizen. All the drum beating is about 'avian flu, virus H5N1'…Could it be an intentional misleading emphasis, which will obviate looking for the real danger? We think so.

We are convinced that the ignoring, overlooking and down-playing of the mycoplasma role in influenza is intentional and criminal. You'll see what we mean as we go along.

In summary: influenza is a specific disease entity, but in common parlance the term has come to cover several disease entities such as pneumonia, encephalitis, endocrine dysfunction and more. And, despite the variety of pathogens and the range of body systems that are affected, in each case the beginning point of the illnesses is the individual cell.

At this point we want to elaborate upon the three pathogens that contribute to the symptoms, which collectively are labeled 'influenza.'

It is important to do so because to neglect any one of the three with an undue emphasis upon any one of the others is to expose oneself to danger. The current drum beating about 'H5N1' and 'the flu' and 'get your shot' leads you into a false sense of security if you rush out and roll up your sleeve and let some 'authority' push something into your blood and body.

As we noted above, the poor people of many third world countries were compelled by their gangster occupiers (France, Britain, Belgium, Portugal) working largely on behalf of the American dominated military/industrial/banking/pharmaceutical complex to accept the smallpox vaccines which were laced with the AIDS co-factors.

So, don't accept the simplistic 'an avian flu virus is mutating to become frighteningly dangerous to humans so you better rush out and get a flu shot' line and thus ignore the role of the mycoplasma that Couch & Chanock and others pioneered as disease agents.

We will start with the bacterium, which is essentially a one-celled animal, in contrast with the 50-trillion cells that comprise the human body. Technically this pathogen is summarized as:

> "**bacterium**: any of a group of prokaryotic unicellular round, spiral, or rod-shaped single-celled microorganisms that are aggregated into colonies or motile by means of flagella, that live in soil, water, organic matter, or the bodies of plants and animals, and that are autotrophic, saprophytic, or parasitic in nutrition and important because of their biochemical effects and pathogenicity."   *Webster's Medical Dictionary*; Page 60

As an animal, the bacterium has the capacity to ingest nutrient and process that intake to generate energy necessary if it is to fulfill its inherent functions. However, it also is able to reproduce itself and hence has within itself the necessary DNA genetic code of nucleic acids. We reproduce as Exhibit Three a micrograph of a *Mycoplasma arthriditis* cell at approximately 120,000 magnification. The latter was provided to us by Dr. Harold Clark, Director of the Mycoplasma Institute and Professor Emeritus, George Washington University (Ret'd) who is also the Chairman Emeritus of the Common Cause Medical Research Foundation.

All three variants of microorganisms have a role in the illness that is broadly labeled 'influenza', so allow us to emphasize that there is more to influenza than simply the avian flu virus, species H5N1 which has been touted in the media without let up for some two years to date, while the pathogen known as the mycoplasma has been almost totally ignored. Get that: the role of the mycoplasma has been almost totally ignored, even though scientists like 'influenza expert' Dr. R .B. Couch and 'AIDS expert' Dr. R. M. Chanock began their careers studying the mycoplasma in general and the Mycoplasma pneumoniae specifically. And Gina Kolata, science writer for the media asset *New York Times* managed to discover Dr. Couch and a Dr. Channock (note the spelling) without ever stumbling upon any mention of the mycoplasma? It gets curiouser and curiouser, doesn't it?

In the meantime, back to the bacterium, the virus and the mycoplasma and the role of each in influenza.

First, note that in our drawing we have presented the bacterium and the virus as approximately the same size. This is not the fact in reality. Actually, bacterium (plural: bacteria) range in size from several thousandths of an inch to several hundredths of an inch in length. The average virus, on the other hand, is 10 to 100 times *smaller* than the bacterium.

To make the point more evident, if the bacterium were enlarged to the size of a human body, the virus would be about the size of a human hand, and the mycoplasma would be about the size of the thumbnail on that hand.

Regardless of size, these three microorganisms all play a part in the disease complex known as influenza and *the emphasis upon the virus…especially the avian or bird virus known as H5N1 is misleading… probably intentionally so…as we shall establish. And, the neglect of the mycoplasma is also intentional.*

Although there are exceptions, the bacterium is generally bound by a nonliving cell-wall to protect itself and to contain the fluid interior called the cytoplasm. Floating in the cytoplasm is the ill-defined

blueprint for reproduction called the DNA and throughout the cytoplasm are ribosomal particles which are the **working drawings** called the RNA for the manufacture or assembly of essential proteins and enzymes.

Although the vast majority of bacteria are either innocuous or even helpful in the metabolic processes of life, certain bacteria contain toxins which do great damage to the living cells of other organisms, including humans. To help you appreciate the danger of bacterial toxins we present a paragraph from David S. Goodsell's wonderfully lucid book: *Our Molecular Nature*.

> "A single molecule of the toxin made by diphtheria bacteria can kill an entire cell. Botulism and tetanus toxins are millions of times more toxic than chemical poisons like cyanide. These bacterial toxins are designed for deadliness - they are the most toxic substances known. They combine a specific targeting mechanism, allowing the toxins to seek out and find susceptible cells. With the toxicity only possible with an enzyme. Once inside an unfortunate cell, the toxin jumps from molecule to molecule, destroying one after the next until the cell is killed." (Pp. 113-14)

Here, although we are not concerned with diphtheria, we need to know that bacterial infection often involves *bacterial pneumonia* and it is usually the latter which kills the influenza patient, followed by other blood and nervous system complications, rather than the influenza virus itself.

Before we leave the bacterium there is one more factor we have already reported but must repeat and indeed emphasize. Back in 1946 Dr. Merck, while still director of biological warfare weapons research and development, reported to the Secretary of Defence that the United States researchers had learned how to isolate the *bacterial toxins in crystalline form*. This means that it would no longer be necessary to transport live, toxin-carrying bacteria to an 'enemy' in order to infect him. One need only to take the disease-causing toxin in a crystalline form and convey it to the target by insect vector or by aerosol, or by the food chain.

Thus, one could spread a bacterial illness without leaving any trace of a bacterium!

It is at this point the Government of Canada, the Canadian Military and Queen's University enters the picture. We need to note the details of this entrance because from that point on, human disease contagion was not limited by the forces of nature but were more within the grasp of certain people who could use their new powers to achieve certain social/political/and financial goals such as *population growth control*. At this point we will state a very important fact: When the U.S. learned how to isolate the bacterial toxin in a crystalline form, which could be carried by mosquitoes, they asked the Canadian Government to assist them. The Canadian Government agreed and they started breeding one hundred million mosquitoes a month at the Dominion Parasite Laboratory in Belleville, Canada. Then, they shipped these mosquitoes to Dr. Reid of the Biology Department at Queen's University in Kingston. There, Reid contaminated the mosquitoes with various disease toxins and gave them over to the Canadian Army to share with the American Military for testing upon hundreds of thousands of unsuspecting and innocent citizens of the two countries.

Thus, Queen's University became a vital part of the evil and insidious program of spreading disease among Canadians. Furthermore, the present Queen's administration refuses to co-operate in researching the potential for great harm done to many thousands of Canadians who have developed chronic fatigue, multiple sclerosis, and related diseases from this criminal conspiracy.

Now we can take a look at the microorganism about which the World Health Organization and a number of other governmental and private institutions are generating all the hulla balloo: the virus...with special attention to the bird species labeled H5N1.

> "**virus** n 1: the causative agent of an infectious disease 2: any of a large group of submicroscopic infective agents that are regarded either as extremely simple microorganisms or as extremely complex molecules, that typically contain a protein coat surrounding an RNA or DNA core of genetic material but no semi permeable membrane, that are capable of growth and multiplication only in living cells, and that cause various important diseases."
>
> Webster's *Medical Dictionary*, Page 747

What does all this mean? Well, take another look at the sketch of the bacterium. Notice the meandering line which represents the blueprint for reproduction and which is called the deoxyribonucleic acid [DNA]. For the life of this particular species of bacterium this is an absolutely critical string on nucleic acids if the species is to perpetuate its existence. Now, suppose something were to kill the bacterium, something such as a variant of penicillin that opens a rupture in the bacterial wall. The draining of its cytoplasm will kill this life form, but there is still a will to live in parts of the DNA and RNA. Thus, particles of the DNA or RNA cluster together and quickly assemble a protein protective coat around themselves. Here you have the essential virus: a particle of genetic information with a protein coat.

Take a further look at the bacterium and note the three representative dots labeled ribosomes. In these organelles, and although only three are shown in our sketch, the cytoplasm is full of them, the nucleic acids called ribonucleic acid (RNA) are assembled when it is necessary for the bacterium to manufacture proteins and enzymes for the bacterium to function. As with particles of the DNA, certain bacterial RNA have the capacity to seek to survive when their original life form is threatened by clustering together and self-assembling a protein protective coat.

In a way it is similar to what may happen when a barn burns: the farmer will seek to save the bull and his best cow rather than save twenty or more castrated steers. The latter may supply him with meat for the rest of the year, but the bull and the cow will continue the species line.

Somehow or other, the life force which motivates the bacterium has an inherent sense of which nucleic particles it needs to save when the original life form is threatened. Thus, the various species of virus are select particles of genetic code that have sheltered themselves with a protein coat until they can access another living cell and get on with the business of life.

Unfortunately, in seeking to save their life particles, the viruses often have to destroy other life forms such as human cells. When the latter happens, the destroyed cells present as disease-ravaged remnants of earlier life forms.

At the outset, we noted how the people of many third world countries were compelled by their gangster occupiers to accept a vaccine, which, it was claimed, would protect them from a disease called smallpox.

At this point we want to note in passing, and we will be returning to the subject later, that the virus which is involved with the disease complex called influenza has some close relatives worth mentioning. We'll let Lodish, *et al.* say it for us:

> "Some animal viruses, including influenza virus, rabies virus, and human immunodeficiency virus (HIV), have an outer phospholipid bilayer membrane, or envelope, surrounding the core of the virus particle composed of viral proteins and genetic material." (Molecular Cell Biology; Page 713)

Note: influenza and HIV linked in some mysterious way? Are we getting closer to the links between Dr. Couch, the flu specialist, and Dr. Channock (sic) the AIDS specialist? After all, they worked together a way back in 1964, when the mycoplasma pneumoniae was the center of their interest? More of this later. Let's continue with the three disease pathogens involved.

We have noted two of them, the bacterium and the virus, now on to the third…and most important, albeit the most neglected of the three: the mycoplasma. As we will develop and emphasize, it is the mycoplasma that humanity has to fear, even though the WHO and other 'health' agencies would have you believe that you should fear the avian flu virus, species H5N1.

As we move into this area we again remind you that the world of official medicine apparently doesn't want the average citizen to even know that such an organism exists. To check this out, we refer you again to the *Johns Hopkins Family Health Book*, almost 1,700 pages of information (at least some of which appears to be accurate) and called by its editors 'America's #1 Health Authority'. Or, as we have already mentioned, you can turn to *The New York Times* science writer, Gina Kolata, who has written a book, *Flu*.

Nowhere in her index and apparently nowhere in the book itself does Ms. Kolata get around to mentioning the 'mycoplasma'? Why do you suppose that is? Could it be that neither she nor the Johns Hopkins' 'editors' want you to know about the mycoplasma? We think so…but more of this further along.

And take a look at all of the articles which are and have been appearing in the 'media' about the so-called 'avian flu species H5N1'. Can you find in any one of these articles the word mycoplasma? Probably not.

Note that the bacterium has ribosome's which, as we have seen, are involved in the manufacture of RNA, and note further that sometimes particles of that RNA get loose due to bacterial death and are preserved by being gathered together into groups of eight RNA fragments which are then enclosed in a protective matrix and a cell membrane and voila: there you have the influenza virus!

Now take another look at the bacterium and notice the string of DNA. If the bacterium is killed, not only is there an attempt to preserve its life by the RNA as viruses, but particles of the DNA will also seek to continue as living organisms by creating themselves a membrane and setting off within their environment to find another host cell that will let them inside and give them a refuge. Again this cell wall-less DNA particle becomes a self-replicating but somewhat incomplete life form known as a species of mycoplasma, which we introduced in chapter one of this book! There it was presented as the starting point for AIDS. Here we look at it as a factor in influenza.

Thus, as Dr. Shmuel Razim describes it: the theme underlying the current evolutionary scheme of mycoplasmas is that of *degenerative evolution from walled bacteria.* (Jack Maniloff; 1992 Page 4)

So, one starts with some species of 'walled bacteria' which when it all falls apart (degenerative evolution) for one of a variety of reasons such as the operation of penicillin, gives rise to viral or mycoplasmal life forms (select particles of the bacterial DNA-RNA) and quickly begin a search for some other cell (one of the fifty trillion within the average human body for example) within which it can take up residence.

When, as we have seen, Dr. Robert Huebner (the father of AIDS) was investigating the pathogenic source of atypical pneumonia in U.S. Naval Recruits in the later 1940s and early 1950s, he called the unfamiliar microorganism a 'pleural pneumonia organism', and when he found the same pathogen in the degenerating adenoids of some recruits he called it a 'pleural pneumonia -like organism' [PPLO].

Also about the same time, Monroe Davis Eaton, an American microbiologist had stumbled upon the organism and named it after himself the 'Eaton agent'.

Finally, because the disease onset seemed to be so long in presenting, various researchers, including the above-mentioned Carleton Gajdusek, called the pathogen a 'slow' or 'lenti virus.'

Thus, we are today faced with the original Nocard and Roux microorganism called the 'mycoplasma', but which turns up in the literature as the 'Eaton agent', the' pleural pneumonia-like organism', [PPLO], the 'unconventional virus', the 'lentivirus' and later the 'amyloid' and then the 'prion'.

Some of the name confusion we believe is intentional. When the mycoplasma finds a cell, which will allow it to cross its cellular membrane, the mycoplasma will generally lie peacefully, doing no apparent harm to its new host until it is subjected to some kind of trauma. The body of which the cell is a part, may be subjected to a rear-end automobile accident; or, it may be traumatized by a fall on the ice. Even the news that a dear and valued friend has died can produce a trauma sufficient to rouse the dormant mycoplasma into life.

When so roused into activity, certain species of the DNA mycoplasmal particle will begin to up-take pre-formed sterols from its new host...ultimately killing that host. The totality can be called a 'mycoplasmal infection' and can present as (for example) pneumoniae wherein the cells in the lungs begin to degenerate and release fluid which floods the alveolar or air-containing cells of the lungs.

How do we know that Gina Kolata knows about this important reality about pneumonia but just chooses not to tell the vast rank and file of humanity? Well, she makes four rather laudatory references to Dr. R.B. Couch in her misleading book, Flu. For example, on page 183, she refers to him as: "Robert B. Couch, the flu expert [her term] at Baylor College of Medicine…"

Surely, if she knows that Couch is an 'expert', she knows that back in 1964 he was a co-author of an article in *The Journal of the American Medical Association* [JAMA] (See the chapter below—The Paper Trail to AIDS, 1964: 'Infection With Artificially Propagated Eaton Agent.'

Gina Kolata may also know about Couch's co-author, Dr. R.M. Chanock. However, here we have a problem. On page 307, as we have already mentioned, of her book, Kolata states, "I want to thank… Robert Channock for providing me with articles and letters…"

Now the question is: Is the single 'n' Chanock who wrote the article in Exhibit #3, the same person as the doubled 'nn' Channock in Gina's book? If it is, why does she spell his name wrong? Just an oversight? Alright, but how about her book editor? Did he miss it too, or did Ms. Kolata purposefully spell it *'Channock'* in order to lead one away from Couch's co-author? If the latter is the true explanation, why would Gina Kolata, science writer for *The New York Times* want to do that?

Perhaps the explanation lies in the fact that whereas Dr. Couch went on to become what Kolata calls a 'flu expert', Dr. Chanock, his early co-author, was busily engaged in research which fits into the history of the development of the AIDS co-factors, the mycoplasma and the HIV virus?

[Here we want to repeat our significant research debt to researcher, Robert E. Lee, M.S., M.S.W., who has carefully and meticulously tracked the work of scientists who, *wittingly* or possibly in some cases unwittingly, participated in the hidden agenda of research, development, testing and deployment of the AIDS co-factors.]

At this point, we are entering into what might be called 'The Maze, Mark Two' genre, with Gina Kolata's book, *Flu*, being an example of 'The Maze, Mark One' genre. This latter type of maze is the 'popular' telling of tales about important health issues which subtly leave out critical data, and mis-state other data, to help keep the average citizen in the dark while telling him he is being informed. Another example of *The Maze, Mark One* genre would be Richard Preston's *The Hot Zone*, which purports to tell the story about Ebola.

In *The Maze, Mark One* genre, you will find the names of actual people and descriptions (often rather fanciful, it is true) of some actual events. However, there will be important names and events left out or mis-stated so that by the end of the literary 'masterly recounting of medical history', as Dr. Jerome Groopman of the *Boston Sunday Globe* touts Kolata's book on the back cover thereof, the reader will be essentially a 'well-informed ignoramus.' And who, you may well ask, is Dr. Jerome Groopman. Well, the following brief quote from Bruce Nussbaum's book, *Good Intentions*, will give you some idea:

> "…Dr. Jerome Groopman, a PI from the Harvard Medical School. Groopman was part of an even larger Boston grouping of four institutions doing **AIDS** research headed by Martin Hirsch. Groopman, however, rarely came to the

meetings. Also included…Robert Couch, chairman of the Baylor College of Medicine in Houston, Texas…"   (Page 144)

The 'well-informed ignoramus' that we note, is patterned after some of the characters in Kolata's 'masterly recounting of medical history'.

For example, ignoramus Dr. Peter Jahrling of the United States Army Medical Research of Infectious Diseases [USAMRIID] is depicted up to his armpits in Ebola in Preston's book and is also favorably reported upon by Kolata in her book Flu. However, he emerges as a boor in Dr. Duncan's book (*Hunting the 1918 Flu*). Here is an example:

> "I then looked for team member Peter Jahrling, whom I had never met. He was talking with a friend. I waited patiently for him to finish, but he did not wrap up his conversation. Eventually, I excused myself, 'Dr. Jahrling, I'm Kirsty. I apologize for interrupting your conversation, but I have a plane to catch. I was wondering if you had a minute to talk.'"
>
> He dismissed me, '"I'm speaking, Ms. Duncan."'   (Page 117)

But, before we leave Kolata and her fan club leader, Jerome Groopman, allow us one more quote from Bruce Nussbaum's book:

> "…Kolata [who covered the AIDS beat (! Ed)] said that it was the fault of the new, freer testing system.

It was clearly such blatant nonsense that even the PIs who were quoted in the story said that Kolata had got it wrong."

Thus, *The Maze, Mark One* genre is written by people 'who get it wrong' for people who, as T.S. Eliot has described are:

> "Engaged is devising the perfect refrigerator,
> Engaged in working out a rational morality,
> Engaged in printing as many books as possible…"

Or, they 'come and go, talking of Michelangelo…' or talking about *Flu* or *The Hot Zone*.

The *Maze, Mark Two* genre, on the other hand, is made up of articles reporting upon what purports to be and often is, reproducible scientific evidence, and these often create the picture of a different universe than the universe of Gina Kolata, Richard Preston, or Lewis Carroll. It is in *The Maze, Mark Two* genre that one would place Chanock articles such as:

> Huebner, R. J., Rowe, W.P., and Chanock, R.M. (1958) "Newly recognized respiratory tract viruses." *Ann. Rev. Microbiol.* 12: 49

or

> Huebner, R. J., Chanock, R. M., Rubin, B.A., and Casey, "Induction by adeno-virus type 7 of tumors in hamsters having the antigenic characteristics of SV40 virus." *Proc. Natl. Acad. Sci.* (USA) 52:1333-1340.M. J. (1964)

Both references courtesy of Robert E. Lee (*supra*).

Now, for just a few of *The Maze, Mark Two* features to illustrate what we mean before we wind up this comment upon the mycoplasma.

In the first reference, note that influenza is a 'respiratory tract' disease! Also note that Robert Huebner, the lead author, was an important colleague of none other than Robert Gallo.

Now, look at reference two...notice that Chanock and his friends refer to 'SV40 virus'. That, in case you did not know, stands for the fortieth variant of a simian virus! And how did a simian (*i.e.* a 'monkey') virus get into hamsters? Why Chanock and his friends put it there, just as they put it into humans!

Note especially that Couch and Chanock were using the kidneys of rhesus monkeys upon which to grow their supply of mycoplasma. Then, they were using what they produced on monkey kidneys as an agent to inoculate 'volunteers" with two strains of the agar-grown *M. pneumoniae*.

So, is the mycoplasma important to human health? It is and no amount of obfuscation by Kolata and Couch will hide that fact, if the reader really works at what he is reading. However, if he depends upon *The New York Times* and science writers such as Gina Kolata, the reader will be well-advised to think twice about any action in response to avian flu that he may contemplate based upon what he has 'learned'.

There are some people, few in number we believe, who still believe that Lee Harvey Oswald was the lone shooter in the assassination of President Kennedy. (Ch.9) Much of the growing skepticism about the official Warren Commission fable is attributable to the movie, *JFK*, produced and directed by Oliver Stone.

It is our considered view that the few who do believe the 'lone assassin' theory are simply terribly uninformed; or, are informed strictly on the basis of a diet of articles in *The New York Times*, Time, *Reader's Digest* and similar media assets; or, are just plain gullible.

And so it may well be with influenza…especially H5N1 avian flu. Those who buy into the current drum beating hulla-balloo about 'avian bird flu' mutating to cause a worldwide pandemic and that the noble, courageous workers with the World Health Organization and their assets with *The New York Times*, are doing their level best to save humanity are right in there with the lone assassin crowd and the Flat Earth Society.

Mind you…there may well be a worldwide pandemic and it may well kill thousands of people a day for many days. But, the chances of it being the sole consequence of a mutating H5N1 species of avian flu virus are minuscule or totally unlikely, and the chances of it being a mycoplasmal infection are very high.

If there is such a pandemic, the roots will go much deeper than simply a mutating avian virus. The roots are more likely to be deep in the mysteries of the mycoplasma and its characteristics and its growing prevalence. And more than that, we believe that such a pandemic if it should occur will not be the consequence of chance such as is claimed about the continuing pandemics of AIDS and CFS…An influenza pandemic will be as much a planned event as was the unleashing of AIDS and CFS into the world…all a part of a profound, long range plan to reduce the population of the world.

And the only way to head it off is to urge a significant number of people not to take the easy path of gullibility, but to challenge, challenge, challenge the drum-beating chants of the WHO and its minions.

There is no doubt that the theory of vaccination is a sound, scientific theory. The idea that a little dose of pathogen will stimulate the human immune system to recognize and respond to major pathogenic infections by the same disease agent is sound. However, don't take a flu shot just because the herd is doing so.

The latter philosophy was strengthened back in 1976 when President Gerald Ford was persuaded by the so-called experts to order the mass vaccination of the people of the United States against an anticipated pandemic of swine flu. The same thing is in the works again with President George Bush talking (see above) about using the military to vaccinate all the citizens that he supposedly leads.

Back in 1976 when Ford was being pushed to vaccinate everyone in the U.S., Dr. Russell Alexander said: "My view is that you should be conservative about putting foreign material into the human body." That's always true…especially when you are talking about 200 million bodies. The need should be estimated conservatively. If you don't need to give it, don't.

This is a quote from Gina Kolata's *Flu*, but it is worthy of repeating despite the source.

As far as can be determined, the vaccine used in 1976 killed close to 100 people, while only one known victim of the swine flu died!

In 2004 there was the usual media drumbeat about 'take your shot.'

This was especially true of the local Canadian Broadcasting Corporation's Sudbury station. Then one morning in the spring of 2005 there was their weekly interview with their 'health correspondent', a Dr. Brian Goldman of Toronto. The interview went something like this…(We can't be more precise because we didn't keep notes nor get a transcript):

> **Interviewer**: Well, Dr. Goldman, we haven't seen you for a couple of weeks.
> **Dr. Goldman**: No, I've been off with the flu.
> **Interviewer**: What? Didn't you have your flu shot? You were telling our listeners to get theirs.
> **Dr. Goldman**: Yes, I had my shot just like the others in our office…and I got the worst case of flu I've ever had in my life.

To this point, we have been talking about the public being herded like a bunch of lowing cattle. Now we would like to introduce a related concept…cattle being stampeded rather than being herded. What is the difference between the two? Essentially this, animals are herded only when they participate with a minimum of resistance because some element in the situation engenders their trust and confidence. Usually, their trust is placed in a leader who is willing to betray that trust in order to advance his own well-being. A stampede, on the other hand, is a violent and apparently disorganized movement of the subject animals often leading to their destruction.

An example of this phenomenon was the hunting technique of prairie aboriginal peoples who stampeded herds of buffalo over a cliff in order to kill as many as they deemed necessary to harvest food and hides.

The present governments of many countries, led by the most corrupt government on earth…the United States Government, are presently herding the population into doctors' offices to 'get their shot'. If this fails to achieve their purposes, then those who did not join the lowing, contented herd, will be stampeded by fear to allow some foreign substance to be squirted into them. Even, as President George Bush has said, if the U.S. Military has to be assigned the job of marshaling the stampede.

So, be neither herded nor stampeded into taking a flu shot. Weigh all the facts and arrive at your own personal, reasonable position.

The tough part is getting the facts since, as we have already described and shall develop further the facts are hidden or twisted by the media assets such as *The New York Times* and its science writer, Gina Kolata and others such as Edward Shorter of the University of Toronto who wrote a terrible rant supposedly about chronic fatigue syndrome, but which is really a mess of misinformation titled, *From Paralysis to Fatigue*. Among the important facts about influenza that you need to know are those that we have already alluded to. The three-pronged pathogenic antecedents (bacteria, viruses and mycoplasmas); the tendency of these pathogens to concentrate and hence become more dangerous when potential people or animals are crowded together for extended periods of time; the distinction between the damage done by influenza itself (often, indeed usually innocuous) and that done by the other pathogens to a broad range of human body systems such as the nervous system, the digestive system and the muscoskeletal systems.

Here are some other facts that you should evaluate.

The pattern of disease incidence among a society is shaped broadly like a stretched out W. First, infant and young children are statistically more vulnerable than older children. Then there appears to be a statistical leveling off at a lower incidence until the early twenties at which age influenza rates increase to the age of thirty or so, then decline until age forty. Another leveling off occurs until the late fifties and on into advanced age.

That is, infants whose immune system is not sufficiently developed are potential victims. Now, if you are aware of this fact, you will take additional steps to protect children ten and under. For example, you will not place your youngster in day care, or kindergarten or other group as long as the flu is known to be a possibility. Keep the child at home in a warm, well-aired environment.

Next, for children under ten especially, but for anyone up to fifteen; do not administer aspirin to relieve symptoms. Aspirin has been very well established as a factor in the onset of Reye's syndrome, an encephalitis characterized by high fever and nausea and involving the liver, kidneys and brain.

Third, do not allow family members or others who are just returning from school or work, to pick up an infant or play with a younger child until the returnee has washed their hands and face. This is especially important if there is any flu going around the school or place of work.

Next, never pick up and comfort a young child if you have any hint whatsoever of a cold or the flu. If you must pick up a child in such circumstances, always wear a surgical mask.

For the middle statistical frequency peak of ages 20 to 40, stay home from work if there is any flu circulating at your work place. If you must work, regardless, then carry a handkerchief or package of tissues and cover your mouth and nose if you cough or sneeze.

If you have occasion to touch doorknobs and other public surfaces that someone with the influenza virus or *with a mycoplasma infection* may have touched, keep your hands from your face and wash as frequently as possible.

In particularly risky times, try to avoid long distance travel by plane or train or bus.

As a senior, if you are in your own home, do not join crowds any more than absolutely necessary. Then observe any of the above precautions that you can. If you are in a hospital or nursing home, then observe a high standard of personal hygiene and avoid larger gathering places such as an auditorium, and try to avoid dependence upon an air-conditioning system. Re-circulated air is dangerous. Open windows are probably the healthy source of fresh air.

Also, try to avoid a vaccine. Evidence shows that vaccines often cause other health problems that are as serious as or more serious than the flu. One such study demonstrated that seniors who received flu shots over a four or five year period were several times more likely to develop Alzheimer disease.

In 1976 the vaccines caused several instances of Guillain-Barre syndrome.

Finally, diet and supplements need to be sensible. Our anecdotal evidence shows that anywhere from two to three grams of vitamin C taken with every meal appears to strengthen the body's resistance to any aerosol infectious agent. And, we recommend eating eggs only occasionally…once or twice a week. Most people base their view about the risk of influenza and the need for a vaccination upon the hype of the media.

Other forms of the 'hype' are broadcast in paid advertising, and here too one should be very discriminatory.

These latter sources of information are driven by greed. On occasion, there may be a public-spirited business motivated to do something 'for humanity' or a government that expresses deep-set concern for the welfare of their constituents or of others. But such instances are few and far between.

An example of the latter occurred in the early days of the mad-cow outbreak in Great Britain. When it was realized that there was a likelihood that meat from diseased cattle could plant the seeds of new variant Creutzfeldt-Jakob disease, the British Government was suddenly motivated to send hundreds of tons of questionably safe beef as a 'gift' to the people of the former Soviet Union. The British government and media expressed great indignation when Soviet authorities announced the refusal of a generous gift.

This British Government hypocrisy fades in significance when one considers what happened when the United States Public Health Agencies discovered that large portions of their polio vaccine supplies were contaminated with cancer-causing SV40 (simian virus 40). [See above]

It happened concurrently, that the same Soviet government had asked the United States if the latter could spare any supplies of polio vaccines since many young Soviet children were unprotected. The U.S. Public Health agencies decided to send the SV40 contaminated vaccines and let on that they were motivated by the highest possible human standards.

Fortunately, an audio tape of the discussion happened to be made and has survived and we have a copy, and one public health official can be heard chuckling "We'll be sure to win the Olympics in twenty years time since all the Russians will be carrying forty pound tumors."

However, the final and most tragic 'gift' given to date to any significant group of people was the gift of smallpox vaccines to people in the Third World. They got rid of the smallpox, but as we have noted above, they have inherited AIDS. The mycoplasma which was used to contaminate the smallpox vaccine was also grown on monkey kidneys such as the mycoplasma used by Couch and Chanock.

So, largely ignore the Kolata/Preston reports upon avian flu and the Ebola virus which they publish, and ask why it is that they have not reported upon the mycoplasma?

And then ask why the Johns Hopkins editors of their *Family Health Book* have not seen fit to mention either brucellosis or the mycoplasma.

As we have reported in chapter fourteen, Henry Kissinger wrote a Memorandum titled "National Security Study Memorandum #200" for his pretended boss, President Nixon.

In NSSM 200, Kissinger makes the case for United States Government taking immediate action to reduce the rate at which the world's population was growing. Kissinger pointed out that if the Third World peoples continued to increase in numbers, they would begin to utilize more and more of their own resources which the United States coveted.

Actually, *such population control plans were, as we have reported, well under way* and had been growing as a Rockefeller/Morgan/*nouveau riche* activity for years. The early Rockefeller apparat entrance into 'health' concerns with their 1901 launch of the Rockefeller Medical Institute was as much about killing select populations as it was with keeping other humans alive. There's no cover like that of a doctor treating a patient if the real goal is to kill that patient. We have tracked the activity from the days of Oswald Avery through to the *Special Virus Cancer Program* of Lyndon Johnson and Richard Nixon and our evidence is there: *AIDS was developed in the United States of America as a population control activity. Furthermore, the chronic fatigue syndrome pandemic was a related mycoplasmal-based infectious activity to disable hundreds of thousands of people in the Western Capitalist nations.* After all, in our world of greed-based medicine, one can kill Black people but not White people. The latter can only be disabled, and then be described in the media assets as being 'ill in the head.'

At the Common Cause Medical Research Foundation, we have coined the phrases: Population Control Phase One for AIDS and Population Control Phase Two for CFS. We are now more and more convinced that the WHO and related organizational ballyhoo about H5N1 is to prepare the world for Population Control Phase Three for Flu.

But, will it really be the flu, H5N1 not withstanding?

We doubt it and explain why in the summary below.

As we have reported, we intended to critically evaluate the current WHO, NIH, CDC, George Bush, media asset drum beating about the possibility that the H5N1 strain of the avian influenza virus might jump species and run like wild fire through the human family, as a cautionary tale. The drum beaters protestations that they were dreadfully concerned about the risk to human life *sounded artificial* as we considered the fact that whereas one person a week was dying of the avian flu and *eight thousand persons a day were dying of AIDS* and the WHO, NIH, CDC, George Bush, media asset crowd scarcely seemed to notice the latter.

Why was one person a week so scary and eight thousand a day so passé?

We read Kolata's *Flu* and Duncan's *Hunting the 1918 Flu*. We also read relevant sections of many well-edited scientific texts and sixty or seventy peer-reviewed journal articles (some of which we report in the chapter below.) We detected something that didn't smell right.

The smell was generated by what we already knew about the Rockefeller population control obsession and by the Huebner, Couch, Chanock, Gallo, Koprowski, Baylor College of Medicine, Tulane College of Medicine, Queen's University, the Dominion Parasite Laboratory and the Government of Canada breeding one hundred million mosquitoes a month, Alton Ochsner, monkey kidney, CIA/Military bioweapons research, development, testing and deployment under Projects MK-ULTRA, MK-NAOMI, MK-DELTA, Shyh-Ching Lo, PathogenicMycoplasma Patent, the Uniformed Services

University of the Health Science course unit on the Mycoplasma and other pieces of verifiable evidence, and was accentuated by our careful reading of the current media reporting about avian flu.

Together, all of these factors added up to evil and the WHO, NIH, CDC, media asset drum beating took on a whole new coloration.

Simply stated, we came to realize that it appears that the world is being set up for something and the H5N1 avian flu cover helped not only move the plot forward, but would, after the fact, allow the drum beaters to say…"Well, at least we tried to warn you."

We turned back to Dr. Shyh-Ching Lo's Uniformed Services University of the Health Sciences course unit on the Mycoplasma and read it for the tenth time…and suddenly we realized what one paragraph of that unit was really saying. Here is the paragraph:

> "The most serious presentation of *M(ycoplasma) fermentans* infection is that of a fulminant systemic disease that begins as a **flu-like illness**. Patients rapidly deteriorate developing severe complications including adult respiratory distress syndrome, disseminated intravascular coagulation, and/or multiple organ failure."
> (Page 28, *The Journal of Degenerative Diseases*, Vol. 5; #2)

Now, please note: this is not influenza, but is a 'flu-like illness' which anyone could honestly mistake for the influenza, but it is not the flu and it is not caused by the H5N1 strain of the avian flu virus! It is caused by a pathogen patented by the United States Government!

Thus, if a pandemic of 'influenza' hits and certain doctors try treating what appears to be a bacterial pneumonia with penicillin, the latter will only make the mycoplasmal infection worse!

And the WHO, NIH, CDC, George Bush, media asset claque will be able to say: "We tried to tell you it was coming."

As the prospects of such a scenario developing became more and more intelligible we turned again to our sources…sources written by Huebner and Couch and Chanock and Vernon Castle, and various bioweapons researchers from the U.S. Military and the CIA, and laboratories such as those at the Baylor College of Medicine, the Tulane College of Medicine, the Rockefeller Institute, the Wistar Institute and more.

It was all there!

An Analogy

Suppose that you live on a farm in a wooded area that shelters a vicious breed of wolves. You have learned from experience that the wolves cannot jump higher than six feet, so you have erected an eight-foot fence around your property.

There are two ways by which the wolves can jump the protective fence: either they can evolve (by some genetic mutation) to become longer in the legs and capable of jumping nine feet. Your defense perimeter or 'immunity from wolves' fence will be no good any more.

Or, someone can come stealthily in the night and under the guise of working to protect you and your family, can travel the perimeter of the property, lowering the fence to five feet. The wolves can now overcome your defense system and take a terrible toll of your family.

The population living on your farm will be greatly reduced.

Let's translate this rather simplistic analogy to apply to the subject of this chapter: the chances of an influenza pandemic decimating your family.

The eight-foot fence is your natural immunity acquired over years of living among the wolves but defended from them. The wolves are the pathogenic agents such as the H5N1 avian flu virus that over the centuries has not been able except in very rare instances, to get past the human immune system.

Now, *instead of the pathogen (H5N1) becoming more dangerous, your defense perimeter becomes less of a protective fence.* The fence has been, and is being, lowered. The pathogenic wolves have not really changed size!

It is our considered opinion, based upon as much evidence as we could evaluate to date, that a significant part of the human family has already been contaminated by a mycoplasmal infectious co-agent administered in the myriad of vaccines that have been shoved upon us over the years. There is also a possibility that further vaccines may be similarly contaminated. This leads us to the crux of the situation:

Here we repeat a direct quote from the **Course Curriculum of the Uniformed Services University of the Health Sciences** (Section 6; Ch.1, above):

> "The most serious presentation of the M(ycoplasma) fermentans infection is that of a fulminant systemic disease that begins as a flu-like illness. Patients rapidly deteriorate

> developing severe complications including adult respiratory distress syndrome, disseminated intravascular multiple organ failure." (Reprinted from The JoDD, Vol. 5, #2, Page 28)

What does this mean to the average citizen? Just this: a citizen can present at his medical professional's office with a 'flu-like illness' that **is not the flu at all!** It is a *Mycoplasma fermentans* infection!

The patient will think that he has the flu, and in ninety-nine percent of the cases, his medical professional caregiver will think he has the flu. As a consequence, *the patient will be treated as if he were ill with a viral disease, when actually, he is ill with a mycoplasmal disease!*

And more: if the medical care giver thinks that the 'flu' has led to a bacterial pneumonia and responds by ordering penicillin, the penicillin will only make the mycoplasmal infection worse! And if someone turns to the *Johns Hopkins Family Health Book* and tries to find anything about the *M. fermentans*, he will look in vain, for the information has gone down the Orwellian memory hole.

The quote again:

> "The most serious presentation of *M. fermentans* infection is that of a fulminant systemic disease that begins as a **flu-like illness**. Patients rapidly deteriorate developing severe complications including adult respiratory distress syndrome, disseminated intravascular coagulation, and/or multiple organ failure."

We conclude this cautionary chapter about learning from experience and being alert for the next stage in population growth-rate control by pointing out that the philosophy is still there. The means are still there. Only the truth about the pathogenic agents is still kept from the world at large.

In a September, 1996 appearance at Washington University in St. Louis, Nobel Laureate Edward O. Wilson, an environmental scientist, spoke of the subject of downsizing the earth's population:

> "The mild-mannered Harvard professor of entomology, reported The St. Louis Post-Dispatch (Sept.12th, 1996), explained how the earth's population had to be brought down to 'the hundreds of millions' for a true ecological balance…"

"A single global policy is unfeasible, he said. But efforts are under way in this and other populous nations to achieve zero population growth and even depopulation, he said."

"The March/April, 1996 edition of Foreign Affairs published an article for its elite readership "Why We Need a Smaller U.S. Population and How We Can Achieve It."

"The stuff of fiction? Not any more."

From an article by Paul Likoudis in the January 21, 1999 issue of *The Wanderer*.

PART EIGHT

THE SCIENTIFIC PAPER TRAIL TO AIDS

"He describes the 'fateful meeting' that took place in New York, in January 1952, between Joseph Smadel…Karl Meyer…and himself…"

Edward Hooper, *The River* Page 413

Chapter Twenty-Three

FROM ROSEBURY AND KABAT TO ETERNITY

The Chemical and Research Paper Trail of AIDS

The linkage between bacterial weapons research and the Rockefeller apparat can be seen in an article, 'Bacterial Warfare', written in 1942 but kept secret as a wartime precaution until published in 1947. The authors, Theodor Rosebury and Elvin A. Kabat, were assisted by Martin H. Boldt.

In their overview study they report on page 21:

> "In this connection [aerosol diffusion - authors] it may be noted that a group of investigators supported by *the Rockefeller Foundation* have been conducting epidemiological experiments on tuberculosis in monkeys on a small uninhabited island near Jamaica."

Rosebury and Kabat also cite 306 research articles, including ones by Frank Burnet, Herald Cox, L. D. Fothergill, and Werner Henle, all of whom figure in this study. Their names should be noted.

En passant it can be noted in respect to Burnet and Cox that the causative organism in Q fever (Queensland fever) *Coxiella burnetii* is named for them, and gives just a hint of how bacteriologic warfare research has impacted humanity. Of this, more later; however this brief reference demonstrates the kind of links that will be encountered as we proceed with our study...Rockefeller/Burnet/Cox/Henle...all, and hundreds more, played a role in the discovery, development and deployment of AIDS in the world.

But it starts with wealth seeking to control health

For *the power of wealth to exercise its control of health* requires the obedience of key mass media masters who, through books such as Edward Shorter's *From Paralysis to Fatigue*, and Gina Kolata's, *Flu;*

to newspapers such as *The New York Times* and the *Washington Post*, pass on warped, dishonest and incomplete information about the reality of modern medicine. The Luce media network with *Time-Life* and *Fortune* magazines were in the immediate background of the 1952 election of Eisenhower and much of the misinformation and disinformation about AIDS and CFS ever since.

The same media, which masks the truth about critical health issues, also contribute to the existence of political support for the lies of the Medical Mafia. For example, the elected representatives of the American people dare not take a stand against criminals like the former Director of the Centers for Disease Control, Dr. Brian Mahy; because he participated in the scientific research that led to AIDS (See later in Chapter Five). In brief, he and others know too much to be prosecuted! Furthermore, the media have allowed him to steal millions of dollars of taxpayers' dollars by keeping quiet, and will not take a stand against him in their full reporting and editorials.

In turn, the elected representatives are beholden to the media, and the media are controlled by the wealthy, and the wealthy determine that millions must die to protect sources of raw materials and limit the rate of population growth.

By 1952, and the election of Dwight D. Eisenhower, the *socio-political soil* was ready for the planting of the seeds of AIDS but first, a certain level of scientific, biological and medical research had to have been conducted to find those seeds and to modify them to circumvent humanity's natural defence systems. This latter effort required two things: first, certain zoonotic diseases such as the disease of sheep, now popularly referred to as 'scrapie', but more appropriately called by their Icelandic names *visna, rida* or *maedi*, had to be altered in a way which would enhance their infectious powers in humans. And second, some way had to be found to by-pass the human immune system.

The first condition was achieved with the modification of the visna, maedi, rida (scrapie) retrovirus of sheep to present as the human immunodeficiency virus (HIV) and the second by the discovery and adaptation of the *Brucella*-derived nucleic particle called a mycoplasma.

The Concept of a Paper Trail - Part One

Ms. Shirley Bentley

Sometime around 1998 we received an article and note from Ms. Shirley Bentley of Rochester, N.Y., the President of the Common Cause Medical Research Foundation for the United States. The article that Ms. Bentley sent us was titled "A Study of the Role of Adenoviruses in Acute Respiratory Infections in a Navy Recruit Population" by Wallace P. Rowe, John R. Seal, Robert J. Huebner, James R. Whiteside, Robert L. Woolridge and Horace C. Turner. The article was from the *American Journal of Hygiene*, 1956, Vol. 64: Pages 211-219.

The note from Ms. Bentley, remarking upon the list of authors, read: "Interesting group of names! I wonder if this turned into Eaton Agent? Then evolved to virus-like infectious agent, and then mycoplasma?" Remarking upon several references in the article to "human volunteers", Ms. Bentley then asked, "Are these all experimental studies and observations done on soldiers?"

We began our study of the article with Ms. Bentley's first comment: "Interesting group of names!"

First, we turned to the *Special Virus Cancer Program*, [SVCP] *Progress Report #8* as published by the "Program Staff, Viral Oncology, Etiology Area, National Cancer Institute, July, 1971."

We have already introduced the *Special Virus Cancer Program* in Chapter Twelve.

To recap its history: when the *Program* began in 1964 (just after JFK was murdered) it was labeled by the National Institutes of Health as the *Viral Oncogenic Program* [VO] and then the name was changed to *The Special Virus Leukemia/Lymphoma Program* [SVLP] in 1965. Then it was renamed The *Special Virus Cancer Program* [SVCP] in 1968. In 1974 the Program was again re-titled as *The Virus Cancer Program*. It was finally terminated in 1977.

Thus over the period from circa 1964 to 1977 the *Program* runs from 'VO' to 'SVLP' to 'SVCP', then 'VCP' until terminated on orders from President Jimmy Carter! One program…four different names.

If this sounds confusing it was probably intended to be in order to cloak the work being done in verbiage. *Even Robert Gallo doesn't admit to being a part of the whole thing.* On page 92 of his book '*Virus Hunting*: AIDS, Cancer, & the Human Retrovirus' Gallo writes as follows:

> "…it was around this time [1977 - Ed] that the *Virus Cancer Program,* having begun with such high expectations, came to an inglorious end. Scientifically, the problem was that no one could supply clear evidence of any kind of human *tumor* virus, not even a DNA virus, and most researchers refused to concede that viruses played any important role in human cancers. *Politically,* the Virus Cancer Program was vulnerable because it had attracted a great deal of money and attention and had failed to produce dramatic, visible results. When *the charge was made that the program had been lax in overseeing its contract arrangements,* an independent committee, headed by Norton Zinder of Rockefeller University, was brought in. Following the release of the committee's report, the program was cancelled…The Virus Cancer Program did not come and go without a legacy. Important work in a variety of fields, including the study of oncogenes, was first undertaken and supported *during the seven years of its existence.* Many important methods and reagents were developed by scientists funded under the Virus Cancer Program, methods and reagents that were extremely useful for the future, as we will soon see. Dick Rauscher, *John Moloney* and *Robert Huebner* helped direct money to important yet previously unexplored areas of cancer research."

Now, we will get to the fact that *Robert Huebner* (one of the 'interesting names' referred to by Ms. Bentley) is listed by Gallo, but before we do, we must comment clearly upon Robert Gallo himself and a very important editorial decision we (the authors of this book) have made. We have decided to dispense with certain stylistic niceties and to call a spade a spade. We have determined that Robert Gallo is a liar, and we are going to call him that whenever it is necessary and appropriate to do so. Studies to support our determination are numerous and we have referred to several of these earlier in the book. However, if you would like to check another researcher and see more details, we refer you to two sections of the late Serge Lang's carefully researched book called *Challenges*. The sections are titled "The Gallo Case" (Pages 361 to 600) and "The Case of HIV and AIDS." (Pages 601 to 697)

Here we are stating our editorial determination to call Gallo a liar because, in view of his clearly established dishonesty, he is not entitled to the protection afforded an honest citizen by the 'assumption of innocence' doctrine. With this editorial determination clearly stated, we will return to Gallo's above referenced paragraphs and will evaluate what he says therein about the *Special Virus Cancer Program*.

What difference does one word (cancer) make in the title of the Program? Or the dropping of the word 'Special' from the title? Or, finally, changing from a 'Leukemia/Lymphoma' to a 'cancer' program?

Just this…if, on the basis of Gallo's book, one determines to seek out any reports about a 'Virus Cancer Program' in many of the standard books on the subject, one runs the risk of finding little or nothing about what we are studying. For example, if one turns to the index of Leonard Horowitz' classic study, *Emerging Viruses: AIDS and Ebola*, one will find on page 562 several references to 'virus(es)' but nothing about a *Virus Cancer Program*! However, if one uses the accepted title usage and looks under the index for '*Special Virus Cancer Program*' on page 560, one will find ten (10) references! Gallo is being his usual devious self by failing to clearly identify the program in question.

At this point one should note that Serge Lang (see above) lists several 'techniques of obfuscation' if one wishes to confuse his readers. The first technique reads: "…describing the same thing with multiple names."

Next, Gallo refers to charges about 'lax overseeing of contract arrangements'. Gallo should know of this! As he himself acknowledges on page 38 of *Virus Hunting*: "Although my lab was then officially part of the Cancer Treatment Division of the National Cancer Institute, John Moloney, who was then running the Virus Cancer Program in the Division of Cancer Cause and Prevention, *passed funds from his program to our laboratory*, hoping our work might help his."

In other words, Moloney was siphoning money from a program approved by Congress into certain unspecified efforts of Gallo's laboratory. If the latter efforts were worthy of such money funneling, then they should have been funded legally through proper channels. Why were they not? Why the 'lax overseeing of contract arrangements'? We shall suggest the answer shortly.

Gallo then notes that the chair of a committee appointed by President Carter to assess the work of the (Special) Virus Cancer Program was a member of the Rockefeller apparat. This is the same technique employed by the late Gerald Ford who, as President Richard Nixon's hand-picked successor, appointed none other than Nelson Rockefeller to investigate possible misdeeds by the CIA.

Nelson Rockefeller was, as you will recall, President Eisenhower's 'special assistant' in charge of the CIA when some of those very 'misdeeds' were conceived and carried out. Or the technique employed by Lyndon Johnson when he appointed Allen Dulles to the Warren Commission. The best way to prevent investigators of a crime from revealing the truth about that crime is to appoint the perpetrators to conduct the investigation!

Someone may only be appointed to investigate sensitive (and illegal) activities of government if they can be trusted not to reveal critical truths.

Finally, Gallo alludes to John Moloney and Robert Huebner. The first named had illegally transferred money from an approved budget to a discretionary budget run by Gallo without having to explain to anyone what he was doing. The second named (Robert Huebner) we shall now consider.

We have already introduced Dr. Robert Huebner as the medical scientist who re-discovered the mycoplasma in naval recruits. In the article sent to us by Ms. Bentley, Huebner is one of six authors who link an adenovirus to acute respiratory infections in a Navy recruit population.

Collectively, Ms. Bentley observes that the group of authors' names is 'interesting', and they proved to be that when we referred to the *Special Virus Cancer Program* about which Robert Gallo appeared to be so mixed up. On page 296 of that Program's 'Progress Report, Number Eight', we found that Dr, Huebner is listed as the author or co-author of sixty-two (62) significant articles cited in the Report! So, between the late 1940s and 1970, Huebner shifted from being an 'expert' on epidemiology to being an expert in cancer! Later, as you will see, he emerges as an expert on AIDS.

Is it possible that the *Special Virus Cancer Program* was not really about cancer at all?

And, between 1962 and 1971 when Gallo was researching 'Carcinogenesis with Selected Virus Preparations in the Newborn Monkey' (cited in the SVCP, *Progress Report #8*, pp. 273 to 289) and 1981 when AIDS was first mentioned in the peer-reviewed medical literature, he has shifted from being an 'expert' in cancer to being an expert in AIDS!

Again we must ask: is it possible that the *Special Virus Cancer Program* under which he reported his 'monkey virus' work was not really about cancer at all?

Under the above major question, several further questions arise. First, why should we be concerned about the *Special Virus Cancer Program* in the first place when it is AIDS that we are studying? Second, why is it that Dr. Gallo seems so mixed up about the SVCP when he writes about it? Third, why is there so much confusion about when the Program actually got started and how come it underwent a series of name changes before being terminated?

Let's address each question in order. Why should we be concerned about the *Special Virus Cancer Program?*

We should be concerned because the first 'Progress Report' so-called of that Program that any researchers have been able to find, is numbered as Report Number Eight! Where are Reports One to Seven? The Progress Report #8, in turn, is dated 'July 1971' yet it reports upon activities dating back as far as 1962! For example, on pages 104 to 106 a summary titled 'Investigations of Viral Carcinogenesis in Primates' is presented. And listed in that summary, as one of three Project Officers is none other than Robert Gallo, who as we have seen, didn't remember the name of the Program when he wrote about it in 1991, even though as it turns out, he had been working in that program!

Was Gallo just forgetful, or was he trying to mislead his readers?

It is our considered opinion that Gallo was deliberately misleading his readers because the SVCP was more than its title suggests. We intend to prove, by tracking the work done under that program that *the SVCP was a cover for the determined efforts of the U.S. Government, through its Department of Defense and its Department of Health and Human Services (HHS - formerly Health, Education and Welfare HEW) and its Central Intelligence Agency to develop and deploy the co-factors which present as AIDS in targeted victims.*

We have presented some of that evidence to support this conclusion in previous chapters and we enlarge upon it here.

In the period of the Eisenhower Administration (1953 to 1960) Nelson Rockefeller, first as Eisenhower's Assistant Secretary of Health, Education and Welfare [HEW] introduced a 'war room' into the national Institutes of Health and the Centre for Disease Control whose job it was to tie biological programs for world population control (until then being privately explored and financed by the Rockefeller apparat and its allies) into programs being developed by the Department of Defense and the CIA.

World population growth rate control thus became a part of official U.S. Government policy. Second, when Nelson Rockefeller had completed his agenda with HEW, he asked for and received an assignment from Eisenhower to work with Allen Dulles, the Director of the CIA. In this role, Rockefeller and Dulles set out covertly to integrate certain Rockefeller apparat personnel and research activities into CIA programs.

The first part of the new CIA programs were coded with an 'MK' prefix. The 'MK' standing for 'monkey kidney'. Why monkey kidney? Because Robert Huebner's newly re-discovered mycoplasma (which he had initially called a 'pleural pneumonia-like organism'—PPLO) and certain adenoviruses could best be cultured on monkey kidneys. (See, for example, the discussion below on the "Efficacy of Trivalent Adenovirus (APC) Vaccine in Naval Recruits" (1956) by Joseph A. Bell, et al. (including Robert J. Huebner).

Hence, as reported to the 'Joint Hearing before the Select Committee on Intelligence and the Subcommittee on Health and Scientific Research of the Committee on Human Resources; United States Senate' on August 8, 1977 by CIA Director Stansfield Turner, the title MKULTRA was assigned to the 'umbrella project' under which several subprojects would be hidden (NOTE: This report and others can be purchased from CCMRF. Among these subprojects were MKDELTA and MKNAOMI, with MKDELTA directed towards biological weapons development and MKNAOMI directed towards chemical weapons development.

With a goal of developing a biological weapon which would incorporate the mycoplasma's capacity to damage the immune system, Robert Huebner's 'PPLO' (a species of mycoplasma) was cultured in

Tulane University on the kidneys of Rhesus monkeys at the Delta Primate Farm in Louisiana, and of chimpanzees primarily at Camp Lindi in what was then the Belgium Congo.

Overtly, those parts of the program that had to be referred to in various records (such as NIH- or CDC-funded contracts) were referred to as part of a cancer study titled the Viral Oncogenic Program, begun under Lyndon Johnson in 1964 and re-named the Special Virus Leukemia/Lymphoma Program two years later. When Richard Nixon was elected to the Presidency in 1968, and appointed Henry Kissinger as his National Security adviser, the latter brought the whole program out into the public with the title *Special Virus Cancer Program* as part of Nixon's much touted 'War on Cancer'.

Under the latter politically-appealing title, Kissinger was liberated to move the search for a biological weapon against the world's population growth rate much faster. However, he had a problem: *the essential research and initial deployment had already been done much earlier*, and so great confusion reigned as to what had been done by whom and when, confusing even Gallo who had been a part of it. (Confusing him, that is, when he was not engaged in purposeful obfuscation.) Certainly, by the end of Lyndon Johnson's presidency, the CDC was already in Africa, spreading the AIDS co-factors under the guise of offering Black people a free vaccine against smallpox. And the article under review, sent to us by Ms. Bentley, had dealt with just one part of the scientific activity necessary to reach the point where AIDS could be seeded in Africa.

Thus, the concept of tracking the development of the AIDS co-factors by studying the peer-reviewed literature began to formulate itself in our discussions and initial writings.

The Concept of a Paper Trail - Part Two

Robert E. Lee

Towards the end of September 1999, we received a 300 plus page manuscript from Robert E. Lee, M.S., and M.S.W., of Black Hawk College in Kewanee, Illinois. It was a remarkable typescript document titled *AIDS: The Explosion of the Biological Timebomb?*

Mr. Lee was interested in having the work published. We replied with some suggestions, but received no further communication from him. We subsequently heard that Mr. Lee had found a publisher, but we were unable to learn more, nor to secure a copy of his published book from various bookstores. Our references to his work are therefore based upon the typescript which we acknowledge has been of significant value to us in our research.

The title is Mr. Lee's response to a 1968 article by Gordon Rattray Taylor wherein the author had warned against a possible 'explosion of a biological time bomb' derived from molecular biological research conducted without sufficient moral consideration of possible consequence1s. Mr. Lee suggested in his manuscript that the 'bomb' may already have 'exploded' in the form of the AIDS epidemic which had officially been introduced into the scientific literature by Dr. Michael Gottlieb, et al. in 1981. Mr. Lee traces a scientific paper trail by documenting "…evidence of various experiments of transferring various cancer viruses to various animals including passage of mouse, rat, sheep, cat, dog, primate viruses to humans."(From Mr. Lee's letter) He supports his research by reference to some 1600 research papers dating from the early 1940s and in his introduction he writes: *"…a logical approach to attempt to determine the origin of HIV-1 is the systematic analysis of their (the researchers') and others' historical research."* Mr. Lee does a remarkable job of initiating just such a *systematic analysis*…especially given the fact that he wrote his study in 1988 and copyrighted it in 1989!

Mr. Lee concludes his work by writing: "Such, then, is the purpose of this book – an historical review of *immune deficiency/suppression research* conducted by scientists primarily in the United States, France and England during the last 50 years. An investigation of this type, presented in a systematic and understandable fashion, may help to resolve much of the mystery surrounding the origin of this 'modern plague.'" (Pages 8-9) (To the three countries that Mr. Lee has listed, we would add Israel and Australia, and to a limited degree, Canada.)

Mr. Lee's manuscript supported the position that we had been considering following our receipt of Ms. Bentley's note and the Rowe et al. manuscript described above: *review and analyze the scientific literature dealing with immune suppression* (Dr. Robert Huebner's PPLO) and the introduction of retroviral diseases into humans (Dr.

Sigurdsson's visna viral research). Do such review and analysis in terms of who was doing it and who was paying for it?

The Concept of a Paper Trail - Part Three

Ms. Candace Brown

Near the end of 1999, as we continued our study of CFS and AIDS and the other neuro/systemic degenerative diseases that emerged along the way, we received a remarkable document in the mail. It was a coil-bound manuscript of some 250 pages titled *Huntsville Mystery Illness – Solved; Human Experimentation at the Texas Prisons*. It was dated April 1999, and the author, or perhaps more accurately, the compiler of the document and the writer of a linking narrative was Ms. Candace Brown. As we read through the document it became evident that the remarkable Ms. Brown had been assisted by two other remarkable ladies in the creation of the document: a Ms. Sally Medley, also of Huntsville, Texas, and a Ms. Elizabeth Naugle of College Station, Texas.

From the 16 page annotated 'Table of Contents' it was apparent that Ms. Brown and her associates had actually compiled a scientific paper trail leading from the research of Robert B. Couch, Thomas R. Cate, R. Gordon Douglas, Peter J. Gerone and Vernon Knight as described in an article in *Bacteriological Reviews*, Vol. 50, #3, of September, **1966**, to document item number 46…Which was an extract from the testimony given to a sub-committee of Congress on June 9, **1969**, by Dr. Donald MacArthur, and re-produced in Leonard Horowitz' *Emerging Viruses…AIDS and Ebola*. (See Part Four, ch. 13, above)

The scientific documents from the peer-reviewed literature were interspersed with, linked to, and commented upon by Ms. Brown and a variety of letters to Congressmen, articles from newspapers, and a reproduction of a newsletter of *The Candida and Dysbiosis Foundation* by Ms. Naugle, dated March, 1999 and titled 'Mycoplasmas; Infectious Agents of Chronic Illnesses and Immune Suppression.'

The Huntsville Mystery Illness – Solved is a wonderful document that links the esoteric world of misused science to the consequences for human health of such science, for it traces the work being done in U.S. government-sponsored laboratories through the testing of dangerous pathogens upon ill-informed prisoners in Huntsville Penitentiary to the damage done to citizens of the surrounding community.

It has served us well as the third example of how a scientific paper trail can put the discoveries, testing, development and medical consequences of biological weapons research into perspective for the layperson.

The Concept of a Paper Trail - Part Four

Ms. Sue Oleksyn

Finally, we acknowledge the great help of Ms. Sue Oleksyn of Rochester, N.Y. in our search for the scientific paper trail to AIDS. Near the end of 1999 we received a four inch loose-leaf binder from Ms. Oleksyn which was packed with reproductions of critical documents such as the record of the June 9, 1969 Secret Congressional Hearings wherein Dr. MacArthur had revealed that the Department of Defense was studying the feasibility of developing a 'new microorganism, one which does not naturally exist...and which would be refractory to the human immune system'. The foundation of AIDS!

Also in Ms. Oleksyn's collection was the critical Patent of the Pathogenic Mycoplasma pushed through the Patent Office process by Dr. Shyh-Ching Lo of the American Institute of Pathology wherein it is claimed that "patients with a mycoplasmal infection will be patients diagnosed as having AIDS or ARC, Chronic Fatigue Syndrome, Wegener's Disease, Sarcoidosis, respiratory distress syndrome, Kibuchi's Disease, autoimmune diseases such as Collagen Vascular Disease and Lupus and chronic debilitating diseases such as Alzheimer's disease."

There was also an important chapter from *Field's Virology*, written by Carleton Gajdusek and titled 'Bovine Spongiform Encephalomyelitis' (BSE) and the role of the amyloid in BSE and related diseases.

For our two-person research team, having so many critical documents all in one place and readily available to our work was a valuable aid and saved us many hours of effort.

Thus, this summary of the scientific paper trail to AIDS owes much to Ms. Shirley Bentley (and of course, her husband Don Bentley); to Robert E. Lee; to Ms. Candace Brown, Ms. Sally Medley and Ms. Elizabeth Naugle, and to Ms. Sue Oleksyn.

It is to be noted that all are essentially lay-persons and the most important thing that they have brought to the search for answers about AIDS, CFS and related neuro/systemic diseases has been 'honesty'. The truth has been their starting point, and it is the truth that is still lacking in most of the research and reporting about AIDS and CFS today. Near the end of this short summary of our own research, we quote Dr. Rebecca Culshaw of the University of Texas who has written: "To do the best we can for those affected by AIDS… there urgently needs to be an honest scientific debate." Thank you all.

An Interlude on the Subject of Trails and Evidence and Details

You may have seen on the television news a picture of fifty to one hundred police officers on their hands and knees carefully searching through the grass of a two hundred acre crime scene which has been marked off with rows and columns of tape with each quadrant numbered. Cigarette butts or match book covers or loose buttons or locks of hair caught on a bramble and discovered by the searchers are carefully put into plastic bags and labeled with details about the particular quadrant where they were found.

Each piece of evidence by itself means little or nothing, and it is only when all of the evidence is assembled and viewed in relation to crime suspects or victims, that a picture begins to emerge which has a relevance to the crime. For example, let's say of a hypothetical crime that one of the three crime suspects smoked a particular brand of Philip Morris cigarette. The victim had lost a patch of hair when dragged through a bramble bush. Another crime suspect was known to wear half Wellington boots with high heels that matched several footprints in the soft soil. A large sum of money had been withdrawn from a local bank by the victim just hours before he had failed to return home. Three men, one of whom smoked Philip Morris cigarettes and another of whom wore half Wellington boots, were seen if a local bar with a large amount of money, shortly after the victim had disappeared.

Small, apparently innocent details found in a field near where the body had been located. Details which, when put together against the background of evidence that a crime had been committed, pointed to suspects. But the details if discovered by someone picnicking in a grove just off the crime scene would mean nothing, if indeed they were even noticed.

So it is with a *scientific paper trail* to AIDS that leads from Dr. Robert Huebner's discovery of a 'pleural pneumonia-like organism' to degenerating *lymphoid* tissue adenoids in naval recruits through a 'special virus leukemia/lymphoma program' of the U.S. Government to a *'Special Virus Cancer Program'* of that same Government, and which along the way loses the services of a biological weapons expert, Dr. Rosebury, at Fort Detrick because he is concerned with the role of the Central Intelligence Agency in the research and which suddenly sees the top 'cancer' researcher (Dr. Robert Gallo) transformed into an AIDS expert. An expert who got a boost in his AIDS expertise by the discovery of Dr. Luc Montagnier of France that there was an unusual *'lymphadenopathy* associated virus' (LAV) in the blood of an AIDS victim.

Details, details, details which taken by themselves mean nothing, but which, when put together in chronological order and viewed against the research of Rockefeller protégés such as Bjorn Sigurdsson (retroviral research) and Leonard Hayflick (mycoplasma research) and Hilary Koprowski (vaccine research) lead to reasonable conclusions about AIDS co-factors and vaccination programs against smallpox in Africa among the Black population and against hepatitis in New York, San Francisco and Los Angeles among gay males.

The devil is in the details, and the trail is made harder to find by a conscious effort to obfuscate that evidence.

Note: Although this is a 'scientific' paper trail with the major part made up of peer reviewed articles from the professional medical and scientific journals and a smaller portion of it made up of government documents which have a direct and significant role in the laboratory engineering of the AIDS co-factors, we have inter-leaved certain brief comments to explain apparent anomalies, emphasize significant details and reduce confusion.

Further, some of the articles we list by title and author only, since space prevents us from the full explanation of their special significance, however all contribute to the central purpose of this paper trail…they are part of the effort to comprehend the workings of the immune system, and efforts to find ways to circumvent that immune system.

End of an Interlude

Pre- and Post-1953 Research

Pre-1953 Research

We begin this tracing of a scientific paper trail towards AIDS and other diseases with a paper written in 1942, but not publicly published until 1947: *Bacterial Warfare* by Theodor Rosebury and Elvin A. Kabat, with the assistance of Martin H. Boldt. The authors introduce their article with the following statement:

> "This review was prepared by the writers as private citizens during the months immediately after the entry of this country (the United States—Ed) into the war. (World War Two)—Ed) The authors had no access to confidential information; the paper, therefore, contains only data that were publicly available before 1942. It was treated as confidential during the war emergency and is now published by virtue of the removal of wartime restrictions. Publication of this compilation of data pertaining directly or indirectly to bacterial warfare seems desirable not only for the sake of its value per se, but also as a contribution to an informed discussion of the *portentous moral and political issues involved.*"

> "As the authors became associated with the government's biological warfare project, they are not in a position to

> incorporate into the review data published since 1942. Thus, it cannot be helped that certain portions of the paper are outdated by developments of recent years as, for instance, in the field of virus research. *It will not escape the informed reader, that in a striking number of cases, technical developments discussed as possibilities in this paper have already become realities as evidenced by recent publications."* —Ed

We use this quotation in order to make several points. First, it is evident that as far back as 1942 and even earlier, certain scientists, military personnel, politicians and others were studying the possibility of developing and deploying biological agents as weapons of war. In their bibliography the authors include books and articles such as "The use of biologic agents in warfare" by Major M.C. Fox, of the U.S. Marine Corps dated 1933. Second, although written in 1942, the references cited in the text include persons that we have reported upon in this study such as Frank MacFarlane Burnet who has been associated with Carleton Gajdusek and Henry Kissinger, and Werner Henle. Third, although written before Robert Huebner had rediscovered part of the role of mycoplasmal species (he called them 'PPLO') in human disease, the authors present analyses of brucellosis (a possible genetic antecedent of *Mycoplasma fermentans*) influenza, rift valley fever and other diseases deemed to have potential as agents of bacterial warfare, and all have turned up in our study! Fourth, Rosebury and Kabat make the following statement:

> "(I)t may be noted that a group of investigators supported by the Rockefeller Foundation have been conducting epidemiological experiments on tuberculosis in monkeys on a small uninhabited island near Jamaica." (Page 21)

Thus, this 1942 article by Rosebury and Kabat with its four noted factors and several key researchers, the work of whom has recurred frequently in our study, serves as a good backdrop to our research of AIDS/CFS and the related diseases listed below, and because Dr. Rosebury, in charge of airborne infection research at Fort Detrick, quit his position there in 1943 because of his fear that biological weapons produced there would be used at some point with great hazard for the world. (Lee, Page 25)

Brucellosis

Following comment upon the Rosebury/Kabat paper, we introduce an article about brucellosis. The reason for doing so will become apparent as we proceed. Also, because we are pressed for space, we present just the authors and titles of certain articles, while for the others, we comment upon the significance of the article.

The Scientific Paper Trail

1946
NOTE *Brucellosis; Advances in Diagnosis and Treatment* by Harold J. Harris, M.D. The Journal of the American Medical Association (JAMA), Vol. 131, #18, Pp. 1485-93.

Dr. Harold J. Harris' article of August 1946 provided an excellent overview of brucellosis as we searched the field of scientific literature, looking for clues about the origin of AIDS. Dr. Harris states the challenge of brucellosis as a disease pathogen this way:

> "Brucellosis of animals and man presents an almost unique twofold problem. It is one of the most difficult of all diseases to diagnosis, particularly in the chronic illness. When diagnosis has been arrived at, the problems of treatment are manifold."

We have added emphasis to the final two sentences that are worthy of particular comment. 'Brucellosis'…(as a potential weapon of biological warfare was introduced by Rosebury and Kabat above with this chilling comment)…'*offers the most favorable conditions for military use, whether directly against animals or against man*'. (Page 64)

It is significant to note right off that although brucellosis was early on a prime subject of biological weapons research, it is totally omitted from the June 9, 1969 Pentagon report to Congress (Ch. 13) and *it is also totally absent from the Johns Hopkins Family Health Book (ch. 16). Recall Prof. Scott's 'negative template.'*

Harris refers to a disease 'of animals and man'. That is, the disease is zoonotic and a glance through the literature that we cite demonstrates how important this quality has been in the realm of bioweapons development. Recall Sigurdsson and sheep—Koprowski and chimpanzees—Baltimore and cats…

The twofold problem of 'difficulty in diagnosis and difficulty in treatment' has also loomed large) since these qualities anticipated AIDS, Chronic Fatigue Syndrome and Gulf War Illnesses (Chs. 15 & 19)

Among the signs and symptoms of brucellosis that Harris notes are 'persistent or intermittent high fever, sweating and a palpable *spleen*, with complaints of great fatigue and joint or muscle pains...' all reminiscent of AIDS and CFS (emphasis added).

Harris also introduces the whole idea of 'psychogenic or somatic illness' which were to loom so large later when media asset writers such as Edward Shorter engaged in his efforts on behalf of the NIH to discredit and downplay the suffering of CFS victims. (Ch. 16)

Further along, Harris refers to two important ideas: the idea that *brucella* can co-exist with other disease pathogens and the further possibility that milk of dairy cows (or other domestic cattle such as goats) is an important carrier of the pathogenic microorganism. The idea of pathogenic co-existence or of disease co-factors is critical to our hypothesis about the functioning of AIDS.

Throughout his article Harris makes several references to 'lymphangitis', 'lymphadenitis', 'lymph nodes', and related lymphatic organs which also anticipates the significance of the lymph system in the research of Huebner, Koprowski and others and the fact that the *Special Virus Cancer Program* (SVCP) was, as we noted at the outset, originally called the *Special Virus Leukemia/Lymphoma Program* (SVLP). It is also to be emphasized that when Dr. Luc Montagnier first identified a pathogenic microorganism in the blood of an early AIDS victim, he called it a 'Lymphadenopathy-Associated Virus' (LAV).

There is no doubt that the *lymph-affecting Brucella* bacterium has an apparent linkage to the *lymph-affecting mycoplasma* (PPLO) re-discovered by Robert Huebner. No study of the origins of AIDS and the paper trail of the scientists involved can ignore the role of the lymph system and the latter's effects upon the *immune* system.

1947

Congress on Brucellosis (A Letter from a Special Correspondent) dated November 2, 1946, *Journal of the American Medical Association*; Vol. 133, #11, March 13, 1947

This important letter reports upon the first Inter-American Brucellosis Congress in Mexico City from Oct. 28 to Nov. 2, 1947.

The letter re-states and expands upon many qualities of the brucella bacterium that made it the principal starting point for many biological weapons researchers. The disease signs and symptoms are insidious, hard to identify and harder still to address. And something has happened to brucellosis between the time of the Congress of 1947 and today. In 1947 brucellosis was recognized as a great challenge to the health of both men and animals, and it is still a great challenge… yet somehow, it has disappeared from modern medical practice in North America! It is not even mentioned in the *Johns Hopkins Family Health Book!*

Brucellosis has somehow disappeared down an Orwellian 'memory hole'!

Where has all the brucellosis gone? Our scientific paper trail will lead us to the answer to this question.

The writer of the 1947 letter makes two important initial points: the incidence of brucellosis in both animals and humans is *increasing* and 'pasteurization of milk obviously has not been sufficient to stop brucellosis.' True, pasteurization has apparently stopped brucellosis as far as medical diagnoses of ill people are concerned, but, mysteriously, even though the disease pathogen has apparently been killed by milk pasteurization, the disease symptoms suddenly re-appear in equal or even greater numbers of victims a few years later…and under the name of chronic fatigue syndrome.

The letter then extends the symptom list and the number of focal points associated with brucellosis to include skin manifestations, nasal and bronchial asthma, bone complications, spondylitis, as well as nervous implications, meningomyelitis, meningitis, neuritis, blindness through lesions of the optic nerves and paralysis due to central nervous lesions! Essentially, this protean range of signs and symptoms is that now seen in CFS patients.

The Special Correspondent then reports that presenters Villafore, Di Rienza and Maldonaldo-Allende reported upon their discovery of a link between brucellosis and *spinal disc damage and herniation!* We are reminded by this linkage of a report in our personal files about a middle age couple in Northern Ontario. The wife had a sudden onset of manic-depression (a condition frequently linked to brucellosis) and concurrently the husband had a sudden spinal disc herniation addressed by a spinal fusion. We are now of the view that this couple shared the same pathogenic source of their apparently distinct illnesses. Di Rienza extended this feature protean range nature of brucellosis by also reporting upon the damage in the lungs and the circulatory system!

At this point we want to emphasize that lesions are simply scars. They are the remnants of once healthy cells that have lost their original integrity and no longer function as they once did. The question is: what causes these cells to die? We address this question under **1971 in this chronological trail when we report upon an article by Rottem, Pfendt, and Hayflick. **

The letter makes it very clear why the biowar weapons researchers placed so much emphasis on brucellosis.

1947

Acute Brucellosis among Laboratory Workers by Lieutenant Calderon Howe, (MC) U.S.N.R., Captain Edward S. Miller, M.C., A.U.S., Lieutenant (jg) Emily H. Kelly, H(W) U.S.N.R., Captain Henry L. Bookwalter, M.C., A.U.S., and Major Harold V. Ellingson, M.C., U.S.A. *The New England Journal of Medicine*, Vol. 236, #20, May 15

This article reflects, with its five military authors, that as late as 1947 the World War ll biological weapons research was continuing into peacetime. Furthermore, it demonstrates that brucellosis, noted five years earlier by Rosebury and Kabat, was being studied for its weapons potential.

In an introductory footnote to the article, it is stated that the laboratory work referred to was being conducted at 'The Station Hospital, Camp Detrick, Frederick, Maryland,' which re-enforces the military involvement with brucellosis.

The latter point is significant since brucellosis, like its genome related micro-organism, the *Mycoplasma fermentans*, has been greatly down-played in the official literature by the military and by the public health agencies and co-operating research institutions involved in biological weapons research.

This serves to further illustrate the concept of the 'negative template' suggested by Prof. Peter Dale Scott. As we have already reported, in his important book, *Deep Politics and the Death of JFK*, Professor Scott, noting that several names of key players in the murder of President John F. Kennedy were missing from government-prepared lists wrote:

> "These missing names were recurringly so sensitive that I formed the testable hypothesis that the index itself, or more specifically the residue of names missing from it, provided a negative template or clue for further investigation. In simpler language, for a name to be missing from the Justice Department list was itself a lead, fallible to be sure, that the name might turn out to be that of a significant figure in the political underworld." (Page 60)

Similarly, for the name of an important biological microorganism to be missing from government accounts suggests that that microorganism has significance worth exploring. *In many of the key documents we have studied, the microorganisms brucellosis and mycoplasma are not mentioned even though they play and have played an important role in biological weapons research.* An example of such an omission can be seen in the June 9, 1969 report of Dr. MacArthur already referred to. Dr. MacArthur was asked by Congressman Flood for a list of *incapacitating and lethal biological agents being studied by the Pentagon*. Dr. MacArthur listed these as follows:

Incapacitating:
Rickettsia causing Q-fever
Rift Valley fever virus
Chikungunyu disease virus
Venezuelan equine
    encephalitis virus

Lethal:
Yellow fever virus
Rabbit fever virus
Anthrax bacteria
Psittacosis agent
Rickettsia of Rocky Mountain
Spotted fever
Plague
(Page 121)

**Note that Dr. MacArthur makes no reference to either brucellosis or of any species of mycoplasma, although there is abundant evidence that *both were very much involved in Pentagon research in 1969!* This omission is critical and was undoubtedly intentional. The same two disease agents...brucellosis and the mycoplasma...are also missing (as we shall make later reference)...from *The Johns Hopkins Family Health Book.*

The negative template!

It is also important to note *the symptoms of acute brucellosis* as listed in the article: fever, moderate to marked degree fatigue, aches and pains in the muscles or joints, or both, headaches, shaking chills, mild cough, moderate nausea, vomiting, photophobia and diarrhea.

Finally, it is to be noted that these symptoms of acute brucellosis are essentially the same as the symptoms of chronic fatigue syndrome, and the latter is one of the disease syndromes cited by Dr. Shyh-Ching Lo in the Patent of the Pathogenic Mycoplasma! (Ch. 1) There is evidence that the two diseases, acute brucellosis and chronic fatigue syndrome, are one and the same, and both are linked to AIDS! We will develop this hypothesis later in this article when we review testimony given to a Senate investigating team in the 1970s.

1948

Brucellosis and Multiple sclerosis. Cutaneous reactions to *Brucella* Antigens, By E. R. Kyger, Jr., M.D. and Russell L. Haden, M.D. (From the Cleveland Clinic and the Frank E. Bunts Educational Institute) *The Amer. J. of the Med. Sciences.* 1948

We cite this 1948 article because it is representative of several articles which link brucellosis (and hence, as we have noted, the mycoplasmal species) to *a protean range of diseases,* including multiple sclerosis. We have already cited the diseases associated with the *Mycoplasma fermentans* in the Patent by Dr. Shyh-Ching Lo, and we will be citing diseases associated with the *Brucella melitensis* later under "Colmenero, et al. - **1996**," and we will suggest the likely reason for this shared characteristic of a bacterial disease range and a mycoplasmal disease range.

Kyger and Haden state: "Innumerable case reports attest the ability of acute brucellosis to produce *focal disease of all sorts.* In the central nervous system it may cause meningitis, encephalitis, and encephalomyelitis. [See the article produced by the Rhode Island Department of Health]. It is well known that chronic *Brucella* infection produces lesions in the eye." [See Nussbaum—1990; *Good*

Intentions: pages 192, 203, 211-2 and 279 on AIDS and blindness.] The authors go on to suggest that "multiple sclerosis might be a central nervous system manifestation of chronic brucellosis."

Later the authors cite Dr. L. Foshay (Page 693). This citation is of particular relevance because Foshay was cited five times by Rosebury and Kabat (supra) in their study of bacterial warfare weapons potential (pp. 62-4) and, although the latter references specifically were in respect to *bacterium tularense, (Pasteurella tularensis)* the citations are all part of the web of evidence related to biological warfare weapons research in general. The further relevance of the citations to Dr. Foshay are to be seen in the 1977 U.S. Senate Hearings on "Biological Testing Involving Human Subjects" where, among other tests, one combining Pasteurella tularensis and *Brucella* suis is noted to have taken place at 'Ft. Detrick & DPG' (Dugway Proving Ground) between March and May, 1961. The linkage between tularemia and brucella is further evident when Kyger and Haden state: "Foshay reported limited experience with the several types of *Brucella* antiserum but indicated that the cutaneous reactions were specific for melitensis, suis, or abortus strains." (Page 691)

Although neither Foshay nor Kyger and Haden mention any of the mycoplasma species, the latter authors conclude their article with the following: "Teague...recorded that some of the rabbits inoculated with blood or spinal fluid [of multiple sclerosis victims] died of *wasting infections with an unidentified small gram-negative bacillus* in the blood stream." (Page 692) When one reflects upon the definition of a mycoplasma as "a genus of minute (*i.e.* 'small') pleomorphic (*i.e.* assuming different forms) gram-negative ...microorganisms" it is quite likely that Teague was unwittingly describing a species of mycoplasma about which Kyger and Haden probably had little or no knowledge. The reference to 'wasting infections' is strongly reminiscent of the Icelandic disease of sheep named 'visna' for 'wasting' to which we referred in Chapter 6.

An Interlude about Politics, Power, and Medical Research

The election of Dwight D. Eisenhower opened the door for the eugenics philosophy long advocated by the Rockefeller/Morgan/

Aldrich and other right wing families to become a part, albeit covert at the onset, of official United States Government policy.

The 1950s became a period of hectic activity on several fronts including:

January, 1952 "He (Hilary Koprowski) describes the 'fateful meeting' that took place in New York, in January 1952, between Joseph Smadel (who Koprowski identifies as a later associate director of the U.S. Public Health Service, though he was then a senior scientist at the Walter Reed Army Medical Centre), Karl Meyer (director of the G.W. Hooper Foundation at the University of California), and himself, as follows: 'I was looking for counsel from Nereus and Prometheus. Dr. Smadel was familiar with our work on the immunization of man with living poliomyelitis virus and suggested to Dr. Meyer and myself that we establish a co-operative study. This led to prolonged and fruitful collaboration, when the search for the golden apples of the Hesperides was conducted near the Golden Gate, more precisely, in Jack London's *Valley of the Moon*... Plucking of the golden apples in this eleventh labor of Heracles took several years, but the results...of the investigations were very gratifying." (Hooper, *The River* Page 413)

What was Koprowski talking about? AIDS! But, again a technique in obfuscation, he tells some of what he knows in a lyrical, mythological chant. In effect, he can 'tell' it without revealing it!

Let's take a quick look at those critical years from 1952 until 1959...the period during which Eisenhower golfed on the White House lawn, while deep within the bowels of government Nelson Rockefeller and Allen Dulles put together MKULTRA, MKDELTA and MKNAOMI...and remember the 'MK' is undoubtedly an initialization of 'monkey kidneys' and DELTA refers to the Mississippi delta with Alton Ochsner, Tulane Medical School, the Delta Primate Farm where Rhesus monkeys were raised to provide kidneys for medical research and vaccine manufacture, and the Louisiana State Agriculture facility where researchers were passaging visna virus through cattle to create a 'bovine visna virus'.

March, 1954 Carleton Gajdusek dispatched to New Guinea by Joseph Smadel of Walter Reed Hospital.

1954 Hilary Koprowski dispatched to the Belgium Congo for the establishment of a chimpanzee-stocked research facility at Camp

Lindi where work began 'on a massive scale,' including work on monkey kidneys (chimpanzees) and the creation of a 'polio' vaccine that was forced onto the innocent Black citizens of this Belgian colony.

Mid-1950s Robert Gallo in College is inspired to take courses in cholesterol and the thymus…both of which studies becoming critical in his later work with the N.I.H., with cholesterol being up-taken by an immune suppressing Mycoplasma and the thymus, lymphoid tissue involved in cell-mediated immunity.

1955 Back from Camp Lindi; Koprowski begins 'polio' vaccine experiments upon women prisoners at Clinton Farms. The baby of one of the inmates later presents as an early victim of an AIDS-like illness when she was just 16 years old.

1955 A strange immune deficiency epidemic disease hits the Royal Free Hospital in London, England.

1956 A British Royal Navy seaman is vaccinated with an unknown vaccine against an unstated disease as a 'pre-treatment'…but a pre-treatment for what was not revealed, and the Naval records about the whole affair got 'lost.'

1956 An unusual infestation of Punta Gorda, Florida, by great swarms of mosquitoes is followed by an unusual epidemic of a disease resembling that which had hit Akureyri, Iceland nine years before, and the Royal Free Hospital the year before.

1957 Koprowski moves from Lederle Laboratory to the Wistar Institute, as its Director, where he is able to work with Dr. Leonard Hayflick who is shortly to be put in charge of a new Mycoplasma Laboratory at Stanford University, and with Dr. Fritz Deinhardt who strangely enough also worked with the husband-wife team of doctors (Gertrude and Werner Henle) at the Children's Hospital of Philadelphia (CHOP)…and where CHOP was the name given to one of the vaccines developed by Koprowski at Camp Lindi. Deinhardt had also worked at Camp Lindi on his hepatitis vaccine research, and several years later the hepatitis vaccine was available to be given free of charge to gay men in New York, San Francisco and Los Angeles. (Most of the gays who accepted the free vaccine were later to become the first victims of AIDS in the United States.)

1957 Dr. Alton Ochsner of Tulane Medical School is checked out thoroughly by the FBI in order to clear him for a secret assignment with another unnamed American Agency. Whatever that Agency was or whatever Ochsner's duties were is not known, but it is known that soon Ochsner is making numerous trips to Brazil to work with Portuguese doctors in that country on some unnamed health project. A few years later Brazil had the highest incidence of AIDS in South America...however; it was a different strain of HIV than that in the Congo. (Hooper, Page 159)

1958 Koprowski and the Belgium scientists working with him begin massive trials of their 'polio' vaccine on natives in Ruzizi. A few years later AIDS began to appear in that area in larger numbers than any other place in the world.

1959 David Carr of the Royal Navy, vaccinated three years before as a pretreatment against something (unstated) by the Royal Navy, dies of *Pneumocystis carinii* pneumonia. A major opportunistic disease now largely associated with AIDS.

1959 The United States begins a generous vaccine campaign in 18 West African Nations under the Agency for International Development to eradicate smallpox. The program went into limbo with the unexpected election of John F. Kennedy as President, until 1966 when it was re-started by Lyndon Johnson. Then, in 1969, with Henry Kissinger in charge of the Department of Defence and the CIA, smallpox vaccination programs were started in 'country after country' (Donald A. Henderson, M.D., of Johns Hopkins University, *National Geographic* article, page 804) until by 1971, all Blacks in all countries in Africa were being vaccinated by the Centers for Disease Control in Atlanta, Georgia, with the help of the governments of Belgium and Portugal.

Someone in the United States Government was being very busy in the realm of biological research and disease control.

End of an Interlude

1952

Maedi, a Chronic Progressive Infection of Sheep's Lungs, Bjorn Sigurdsson, et al.. *Journal of Infectious Diseases*, Vol. 90; Pp. 233-241

As we showed earlier, Dr. Bjorn Sigurdsson was from Iceland, but in the early 1940s he turned up in New Jersey, studying plant and animal diseases even though he was a doctor of human medicine, at the Rockefeller Institute. He impressed his Rockefeller patrons, and when he returned to Iceland in 1948 he took with him a large grant to establish an "Institute for Experimental Pathology." Now, you can put that title down to a weak regard for English syntax, but what it really says is 'this is an institute to experiment with various pathogens that cause human disease.' As bad luck would have it (or from the Rockefellers point-of-view it might have been as good luck would have it) a strange disease broke out in schools in Northern Iceland. The disease seemed to be a combination of non-paralytic polio and chronic brucellosis, but there was no laboratory proof that it was either?

However, Sigurdsson was right there to lend his expertise to the disease study, and overnight he went from being an expert on sheep retroviruses, to being an expert in Akureyri Disease, a forerunner of later chronic fatigue epidemics. A unique development in Akureyri was the fact that of the students who became sick, five went on to develop Parkinson's disease!

Sigurdsson went on with further studies and when he died at age forty-six, his Rockefeller funded Institute continued with retroviral study and a daughter and son carried on with the research. Thus, they were already when the first known retrovirus to invade humans (HIV - so called) hit.

(See **1987** - Dr. John Seale below)

1952

Dephosphorylation of Adenosine Triphosphate by Concentrates of the Virus of Avian Erythro-myeloblastosis Leukosis, by Mommaerts, E.B., Eckert, E. A., Beard, D., Sharp, D. G., and Beard, J. Proceedings of the Society of Biological Medicine. Vol. 79; Pp. 450-455

In Professor Robert E. Lee's typescript of *AIDS: An Explosion of the Biological Timebomb?* The author cites the research of Mommaerts, et al. which demonstrates that a Rous sarcoma virus (RSV) - associated avian leukemia, avian erythro-myeloblastosis leukosis (AML) would interfere *in basic metabolic processes*. "Two years later Mommaerts, et al. (1954) contributed to further understanding of the AML-induced metabolic disturbances by isolating specific *particles* (emphasis added—Ed) in the blood that appeared to participate in induction of the too-high-acid metabolic disorder." Then Lee makes the vital observation that Waravdehar, et al. (1955) "...continued investigation by RSV with special focus on hexokinase and aldolase, important metabolic enzymes, both of which, if elevated beyond normal levels, appear related to *immunological deficiency disorders.*" (Emphasis added—Ed)

With this sophisticated observation Lee brings us closer to the nexus of subjects, institutions and people who were engaged in *immune deficiency* research during the period from the early 1950s until AIDS became a household acronym. Among the subjects of such research were cancer, leukemia, lymphoma, poliomyelitis, scrapie, pneumonia etc. Among the institutions were (and many still are) Duke University, Baylor University, University of California, Queen's University of Kingston, Canada, the Children's Hospital of Philadelphia, Wistar Institute, and Sonoma State Home for Children. And finally there were the people such as Cox, Huebner, Mommaerts, Koprowski, Werner and Gertrude Henle, John Enders, Robert Chanock, Bjorn Sigurdsson and others who re-appear in various combinations as the co-factors of AIDS were discovered, altered, tested, combined and deployed.

For example, the cited paper under review (Mommaerts, *et al.* 1952) has much in common with the citation on page 366 of the *Special Virus Cancer Program, Progress Report #8* twenty years later:

Contractor: Duke University
Contract Title: Study and Production of Avian Leukosis Viruses
Principal Investigator: Dr. Joseph W. Beard

How is it that the same subjects, institutions and people come together over a time span of twenty years? Is it a result of a conspiracy or of a coincidence?

If it is by coincidence, then the linkages are becoming more and more fantastic. If they are being brought together and kept together by a conspiracy, then there must be conspirators doing so for a purpose.

Could the purpose be linked to eugenics? Is it just a coincidence that in 1952 when Mommaerts, *et al.* at Duke University were exploring the mechanics of immune deficiency along with hundreds of other researchers in several other universities, Nelson Rockefeller was working with the Department of Health, Education and Welfare in his 'war room' and in 1972 his protégé, Henry Kissinger, was in charge of similar immune deficiency research as Richard Nixon's National

Security advisor, and that a couple of years later Nixon and Agnew would be replaced by Gerald Ford and Nelson Rockefeller?

The scientific paper trail is becoming more coherent!

But, to conclude this study of Mommaerts, *et al.*, note that the subject matter (dephosphorylation of adenosine triphosphate) takes us back to our beginning of this paper trail with Huebner's pleuro-pneumonia studies and Sigurdsson's studies of maedi, a *lung* disease of sheep.

We depart briefly from our chronological ordering of evidence to make note of Andre Voisin's 1959 work wherein he links the evidence of Mommaerts to that of Otto Warburg 'on the respiratory mechanisms of the cancerous cell.'

> "It is enough to say," Voisin writes, "that, according to Warburg's theory, cancer can have thousands of causes: tars, x-rays, radio-activity, carcinogenic substances in foodstuffs, pressure on the organs, etc. But, all of these end up in one final, primary action: the irreversible disturbance of cell respiration." Voisin then concludes: "The cell whose normal respiratory mechanism has broken down beyond repair will try, in order to survive, to create a different method of respiration, 'lactic respiration'. Also called 'lactic fermentation or glycolysis.'" (Voisin, Page 167)

This suggestion opens our trail even wider for, as we shall see, it accounts for the critical work on 'lactic dehydrogenase' by people like de-The and Dr. Brian Mahy.

Now back to our chronological ordering.

1952

Studies on Phagocytosis. Determination of Blood Opsonin for Brucella, Joseph Victor, Abou D., Pollack R., Raymond, and Jeanne R. Valliant. Biological Laboratories, Chemical Corps, Camp Detrick, Frederick, Maryland. 1952

(Note: Phagocytosis refers to the engulfing and destruction of foreign particulate matter such as brucella bacteria that serves as an important part of the body's defence system. Opsonin is an antibody of blood serum that makes such foreign particulate matter more susceptible to the phagocytic action. This article is important because it demonstrates that in 1952 the U.S. biological weapons researchers were still working with brucella as an experimental disease agent. The article also reveals that Dr. Abou D. Pollack, who turns up later in this paper trail to AIDS, was one of several weapons researchers. Dr. Pollack's photograph appears in Norman Covert's book, *Cutting Edge*, a history of Fort Detrick, on page 59. The latter photo is also important because it presents over thirty other researchers including Dr. Herald Cox!

(In 2001 one of the world's leading AIDS researchers, who has requested anonymity, said that he had not located any hard evidence that Cox had been involved with the bioweapons research at Fort Detrick. We were able to settle the question for him by drawing his attention to this photograph.)

The article is highly technical, but like the pieces of evidence uncovered by the careful combing of a crime scene, there are hints of significance in some of the details. Like Polonius, the researcher can "by indirection find direction out."

The major subject of the article is the use of dogs' blood in an effort to make the brucella bacteria more susceptible to the natural immune activity of phagocytes. This suggests rather than states, that the brucella bacteria were posing a problem for the researchers because it was not as subject to phagocytosis as are other bacteria. Apparently dogs' blood put into the blood of a brucella victim, acts as an opsonin. The natural resistance of brucella to such phagocytic action explains in part why brucellosis (and the latter's hypothesized successor the *Mycoplasma fermentans*) is so very hard to clear from the body of the victim, and hence was so attractive to biowar researchers.

However, one of the main clues in this article in our search for the biological origins of AIDS is seen on page 127 in the following sentence: "In other experiments it was found that phagocytosis by dog leucocytes of *Brucella abortus*, **strain 19**, was the same as that of *B. suis*, strain PS111." The key reference is to 'strain B 19' referred to above under 'Mystery Illness at Huntsville, TX.'

'Strain 19' is a mystery factor in so-called canine heart disease and in human juvenile arthritis.

1953

Shepard, Maurice C., Ph.D. The Recovery of Pleuropneumonia-like Organisms (PPLO) from Negro Men with and without Nongonoccal

Urethritis, American Journal of Syphilis, Gonorrhea, and Venereal Diseases, V.38; Pp. 113-124

This long forgotten article from a relatively unknown source is of significance to our scientific paper trail to AIDS for several reasons.

First, it is one of the earliest articles to deal with the PPLO or mycoplasma since Huebner's articles about PPLO in naval recruits six years earlier. However, something new has been added to the research: **an ethnic component has been introduced with a focus upon Negro men.** This element serves to anticipate later research by Robert Gallo in association with Japanese researchers and also the current statistics which reflect a higher incidence of AIDS among Black and aboriginal populations. These features of AIDS are not fortuitous but reflect a eugenics program, as we will show.

Further, it is to be noted that although the article purportedly deals with a respiratory illness, the emphasis is upon genital track infections. And, it is to be noted that Shepard limits his study to patients "…without eye or joint symptoms", both of which symptoms are later associated with AIDS.

It is not until the final page of his article that Shepard presents the crux of his study. This crux is of dramatic significance for our research, for it is in the following two paragraphs that we find data which are vital to our study.

> *"The prevalence of urethral PPLO (a species of mycoplasma - Ed) among Negro men without urethritis indicates that these minute organisms are distributed much more widely among normal Negro men than has heretofore been recognized. This observation emphasizes the need for caution in implicating the pleuropneumonia-like organism as the sole etiologic agent in nongonococcal urethritis in the Negro man."* (Emphasis added—Ed)

> *"The findings among white men college students (controls) are in contrast to the findings among the Negro men clinic controls. Both groups exhibited freedom from urethritis. The respective incidence rates were 2.0 percent and 56 percent. The observed difference is interpreted to suggest a racial factor. The validity of this concept is strengthened by the observation that apparently normal Negro men college students (urethritis*

free) showed an incidence rate for urethral PPLO of 33 percent, in contrast to 2.0 percent for white men students." (Emphasis added—Ed)

This is an absolutely vital finding for it means that if AIDS requires two co-factors, as our growing evidence demonstrates, and one of those factors is a mycoplasma, plus another factor such as the visna retrovirus, and if 33 percent of Negroes already have one of these co-factors in contrast to only 2.0 percent of white men, then the incidence of AIDS will be fifteen times hirer among exposed blacks than among exposed whites when by vaccination or other routes the other of the co-factors is introduced!

This startling ethnic discrimination fits in with current statistics that reveal a hirer per capita incidence of AIDS among the black population of North America than among the white population! It also supports the hypothesis that certain ethnic groups were targeted by their color as potential victims of biological weapons. In this respect it is timely to quote a passage from Robert Lee's document:

> "Clearly, historic investigation of G6PD (which we will explain below—Ed.) which documents interest in racial differences followed by isolation of identical enzymes from rats and mice as well as later appearance of a viral- caused anemia in racially variant G6PD red blood cells and the still later appearance of an immunologically active virus in this type of cell, is a rather interesting chain of developments. That G6PD levels were raised in AIDS patients and that, in the United States, Blacks and minorities are disproportionately infected by HIV-1, given the history of G6PG, appears to suggest that this phenomenon might be due to more than chance. You have, no doubt, heard many reasons for AIDS's disproportionate attack on minorities which have generally specified the 'high occurrence of immoral behavior among these groups.' An alternative hypothesis may rest in *HIV's apparent ability to exploit racial genetic differences governing production of important metabolic enzymes.*"

(Lee: ch.12; Pp. 85-6)

Shepard's article which presents the statistical evidence that fifteen times as many apparently healthy Blacks are infected with a mycoplasmal agent as compared to apparently healthy Whites strongly suggests the latter alternative.

But it wasn't just the racial incidence of a pre-existing mycoplasmal infection that was being studied in the 1950s. Scientists were already aware of and were already studying the fact that there was a genetic difference between Blacks and Whites as to the production of G6PD, and that this difference could affect their susceptibility to *immune disruptive agents*. This difference suggests an explanation for a very unusual sampling of blood from Black residents of the Congo back in 1959. We will quote from Hooper's *The River*:

> "In his very first interview, Gaston Ninane (a Belgian virologist who worked under Ghislain Courtois at Stanleyville in the fifties, and who had helped vaccinate thousands of Blacks in Africa against 'polio' including a 'polio' vaccine campaign in the Ruzizi Valley where, a few years later, the greatest incidence of AIDS anywhere in the world broke out - Ed) mentioned that when he and Motulsky visited Stanleyville… they took blood at the same time, from the same persons. 'When I took a sample of serum for antibodies, he took another ample for testing *Glucose 6* [G6PD deficiency]…'
>
> (Hooper, Page 756)

It is critical to note that one of the above samples of blood was taken from a Black man (known only as L70) who had been vaccinated by Koprowski's CHAT vaccine a few years before. The sample taken a few years after being vaccinated by Koprowski was HIV positive!

Of this, more later. See: **1974** *The Virus Cancer Program*

There are frequent references to the fact that AIDS seems to present more in Black people than in Whites. Dr. Shepard's research suggests how, scientifically, that could be possible. Before leaving this important aspect of the 'ethnic bias' of AIDS, we present the following news account from South Africa. The story is datelined Cape Town-July 28, 1998 and appeared in the *Globe and Mail* on that date:

> "Doctor ordered to testify-
> Wouter Basson, dubbed Dr. Death when he headed the apartheid government's chemical weapons program, was ordered by a judge yesterday to testify before South Africa's Truth and Reconciliation Commission tomorrow.

"His lawyers had argued in the High Court that being forced to give evidence before the commission would prejudice Dr. Basson's criminal trial next month on charges ranging from attempted murder to the manufacture of illegal drugs.

"The lawyers also argued that Dr. Basson's constitutional right to remain silent would be prejudiced if he testified before the TRC.

"Evidence given by military scientists at the start of the TRC hearing last month implicated Dr. Basson in spine-chilling chemical projects, including attempts to sterilize Black women, *to create a bacteria that would kill Blacks only* and to poison Nelson Mandela, now President of South Africa."

Note the italicized portion of the final sentence!

1953

Viral Vaccines and Human Welfare by Herald R. Cox, *The Lancet* July 4, 1953

This article from the July 4, 1953 issue of *The Lancet* is critical in the scientific paper trail to AIDS. The author, Herald Cox, (see entry above) has his name memorialized in the name of a 'pleomorphic rickettsiae bacteria occurring intercellularly in ticks and intracellularly in the cytoplasma of vertebrates and including the causative organism Coxiella-Burnetii of Q (for Queensland) fever. The 'cox' in Coxiella is for Herald Cox and the burnetii is for Frank Burnet of Australia. (Recall that Carleton Gajdusek worked in Australia with Frank Burnet before Gajdusek went on to 'fortuitously' study Kuru among the Fore tribe of New Guinea.

To recap: the year is 1953 - Dwight Eisenhower has just been elected President of the U.S. and Nelson Rockefeller is working in his 'war room' at the Dept. of Health, Education and Welfare (HEW) and Herald Cox is the Director of the Lederle Laboratories Division of American Cyanamid Company at Pearl River, New York.

Notice how certain of the people, places, institutions and research involved with subject's related to immune suppression in this paper trail to AIDS are beginning to recur with increasing frequency!

This article by Herald Cox is, in a way, a lynch pin between the pre-1952 days when the Rockefeller apparat's eugenics efforts were in the private sector and the post-1952 days of the Eisenhower administration when those Rockefeller efforts were largely converted into United States government policies.

The transformation of private Rockefeller goals to U.S. public policy is demonstrated in the title of the subject article: 'Viral Vaccines and Human Welfare'. Vaccines were, as Cox states in the article, of vital importance to Lederle Laboratories. He writes 'The latter vaccine, known as Cox-type or yolk-sac vaccine, was produced on a tremendous scale during World War ll and was administered to several million American, Canadian, and Allied troops as well as to civilian populations in dangerous endemic areas…My laboratory (the Rockefeller-controlled Lederle) contributed significantly to this amount.'

It is reasonable to theorize that this wartime experience with vaccines would plant seeds about the possible dire consequences of contaminated vaccines. Herald Cox was just the kind of person to ponder such possibilities. He was, according to Tom Norton's daughter, Gail, '…a man with problems - a manic-depressive, whose behavior was unpredictable and often bizarre.' (Hooper, Page 445)

Combine the technical and scientific potential of Lederle to produce vaccines, with the Rockefeller interest in vaccines as an immunizing agent against poliomyelitis and with Hilary Koprowski doing the research and neurotic Herald Cox in charge and one has the necessary cover to link the recently re-discovered mycoplasma (PPLO) with other viral agents such as the visna virus of sheep as isolated by Bjorn Sigurdsson! (See entry date above: January, **1952**)

This Cox article foreshadows just such a scenario. Cox alludes to 'This vaccine (yellow fever) is at present used on a very large scale in the French territories in Africa." This anticipates Koprowski's 'polio' vaccine trials in Africa four years later…after he had established his polio bona fides…see entries below for 1955 and 1956 by Koprowski, et al..

Cox then makes a very important statement. He writes: 'It may be possible under certain conditions to adapt or 'train' a virus to become greatly altered from its original properties,,, Dr. Koprowski and Mr. Jack Black have recently succeeded in so modifying the Flury strain of avianised rabies virus…'

Does this anticipate the combination of a mycoplasma/immune suppressor such as that found by Huebner with a retroviral 'lentivirus' such as that found by Sigurdsson to create a 'new microorganism, one which does not naturally exist' and which is refractory to the human immune system? (See entry dated June 9, 1969 of this paper trail to AIDS)

Further along Cox cites the work of John Enders, (who we had noted in earlier issues with his links to Carleton Gajdusek and Joseph L. Melnick) cited eighteen times in Progress Report #8 of the *Special Virus Cancer Program* and who is referred to sixteen times in the index to Hooper's study of AIDS, *The River*.

Now, just because a person is cited in a work about scientific and medical links to AIDS does not mean that they were witting participants in this crime beyond belief. However, it does suggest that their contributions must be scrutinized with rigor and with care.

Finally, and in relation to the year of this article (1953) it is to be noted that the CIA secret MKULTRA program directed by Dr. Sidney Gottlieb, was just being launched, and two of the leading players in this Rockefeller/Dulles crime against humanity were Herald Cox and Hilary Koprowski. Refer especially to the latter's **1955** article below.

1953

The Molecular Biology of Mycoplasma Viruses, Jack Maniloff and Alan Liss. *Annals of New York Academy of Science,* Vol. 225; Pp. 149-158

This short article merits inclusion in our scientific paper trail to AIDS because of its concluding sentence: "…it may be time to examine experimentally the possibility of **mycoplasma lysogenic conversion** and the suggestion of Atanasoff; that **the role of mycoplasmas in disease may be as vectors for viruses.**" Perhaps some of the viruses tested included the retroviruses of sheep?

This possibility echoes the idea expressed by Harris (above) that the *Brucella* bacterium may co-exist with other disease pathogens, hence contributing to the difficulty in diagnosing *Brucella* diseases. It also anticipates the concept of 'co-factors' in the etiology of AIDS.

Post-1953 Research

(In the following three citations note the names in italics)

1954

Adenoidal-Pharyngeal-Conjunctival Agents, Robert J. Huebner, M. D., Wallace P. Rowe, M.D., Thomas G. Ward, M.D., Robert H. Parrott, M.D., and Joseph A. Bell, M.D. *The New England Journal of Medicine*, Vol. 251; #27

This article is important to our tracking of the scientific paper trail because it does a number of things for us. First, it brings us back to Robert Huebner who as we have seen, identified a 'pleural pneumonia-like organism' in the adenoids of naval recruits back in 1946, and who had noted that this PPLO was associated with the 'spontaneous degeneration' of human cells, especially lymph cells essential for the protection of the human body. (Look ahead a few years to the point where Luc Montagnier discovers the foreign particles in an early AIDS victim and notes and calls it a 'Lymphadenopathy Associated Virus!) Furthermore, it is important to note that Huebner and one of his co-authors, Wallace Rowe, turn up seventeen years later, 1971, in the *Special Virus Cancer Program, Progress Report #8*, as experts in cancer! So here he is in 1954 as a researcher in 'undifferentiated respiratory' diseases. What is the link between respiratory diseases and cancer? Could it be a species of mycoplasma?

In 1954 Huebner, *et al.* were apparently but unwittingly tracking the mycoplasma. Obviously, they are puzzled by what their research reveals and in their article they state:" These findings suggest that Type 3 virus represented a kind of 'fellow traveler' (*i.e.*: a co-factor!) producing infection but not illness - the illness probably being due, in this case at least, *"to some other unknown agent or factor."*

It is also to be noted that Huebner's work researching the mycoplasma is concurrent with the work of Koprowski 'researching' polio?

1955

Immunization of Man with Living Poliomyelitis Virus, Hilary Koprowski, *World Health Organization Monograph: Poliomyelitis;* 1955 Pp. 335-357

We will not attempt to précis this speech by Koprowski delivered at Geneva in 1955 under the auspices of the World Health organization. It is what the paper does not say rather than what it does say that is important in our tracking of AIDS. Ed Hooper calls the speech a *tour de force* as far as it goes, but notes that 'certain of the crucial details were missing.' Hooper goes on to suggest that 'The failure to identify which plaque or plaques had been used (to manufacture a certain vaccine- Ed) to make up the actual vaccine pools was therefore surprising and disturbing.' In other words, Koprowski was being his insidious usual self. There was more to the story than he was telling.

As important for our purposes is the fact that Hooper recognizes that Koprowski's move to the Wistar Institute was critical:

> "Free at last of the inhibiting influence of Cox, Koprowski was now his own boss, in charge of a research institute and able both to set the agenda and raise his own funds."

Could it be that Koprowski's move to the Wistar was related to the financial sleight of hand reported by Stansfield Turner in his report to President Carter about MKULTRA some 22 years down the line? We'll take up this possibility later under "1977 Project MKULTRA..."

A Further Background Interlude

From Ed Hooper's, *The River*: "...a total of 25 infants were fed either TN, SM N-90, or both vaccines *between November 1955 and June 1956*. In the next two months, a further seven infants were vaccinated, but only two of these immunizations were recorded in the literature. However, various clues suggest that all seven were fed with variants of SM N-90 as it was transmogrifying into CHAT.

> "After this, *between October 1956 and January 1957* (while Koprowski was still at Lederle), there appears to have been seven feedings of the prototypes of the SM-45, CHAT, and Fox strains, which Koprowski would later announce at the Geneva conference *just after his move to Wistar*..." (Page 694)

"In his Geneva paper, (see immediately above) Koprowski reported on the safety of the excreted viruses of BO, TA, and another vaccinee called GA. The fecal virus from BO ... caused no adverse reactions, but when TA's excreted virus was processed and injected intraspinally into monkeys, *three out of eight became slightly paralyzed...*"   (Pp. 694 and 699)

This background interlude is provided to place these selected articles of our scientific paper trail in the context of what was secretly going ahead. First, it demonstrates that Koprowski's Geneva paper is not candid and completely honest. In other words, like Robert Gallo and others involved in the whole enterprise of AIDS development, testing and deployment, it is necessary to shade the truth because there were things going on behind the scenes that had to be kept from the public.

Further, some of the terms and situations may be confusing to the reader, so we'll explain them.

"Fed" relates to orally administered polio vaccines, some of which were developed at Lederle laboratories in the early 1950s. Notice that the subjects of such vaccine testing were infant children whose mothers were incarcerated in Clinton Farms Women's Prison. Second, Koprowski was initially working for Lederle, which, although a company controlled by the Rockefeller apparat, had professionals whose moral standards in some instances were sufficiently high as to make it difficult to do some of the research and testing necessary to achieve the goals of the eugenics advocates. Thus, although Koprowski could get started towards certain goals at Lederle, he had to move to another venue because it had become apparent that some of those goals might require illicit, immoral or illegal activities. Hence, in the middle of his Lederle work, it is obvious that Koprowski and certain others were secretly planning on making a move to the Wistar Institute where in the beginning; they would be less fettered by morality.

Thus, while appearing in 1955 to be working for Lederle, Koprowski was actually working secretly with some unknown forces to make a move to the Wistar Institute in Philadelphia.

The time frame and the work being done, first at Lederle and then with Koprowski's move, at Wistar, corresponds with the 1952 to 1960 activities of Nelson Rockefeller and MKULTRA of the Eisenhower administration; the January, 1952 Koprowski meeting between Joseph Smadel of the U.S. Military, and Karl Meyer of the

G.W. Hooper Foundation. At the same time Koprowski was involved in meetings with representatives of both Belgium and Portugal. These two countries were engaged in costly wars with black nationalists in their African colonies and the prospects of a biological weapon to employ in these struggles was enough to gain Belgium/Portuguese co-operation.

To develop the latter biological weapon required a cover for Koprowski…a cover that would bear the scrutiny of scientists and medical professionals worldwide. That cover was provided in the form of developing a poliomyelitis vaccine. This effort began with Koprowski's work on polio vaccines…quite legitimate work…but with certain morally questionable aspects at Letchworth Village, a home for mentally retarded children who were said to have 'volunteered for the tests'; and at the Children's Hospital of Philadelphia, where he worked with the Henles and at Clinton Farms Prison for Women.

The polio vaccine cover was then extended into the Belgium Congo Camp Lindi where first chimpanzees were used as test subjects, and then chimpanzee kidneys ('monkey viruses') were used to cultivate vaccines at Wistar and in Belgium and Portugal and deployed throughout Africa.

The hectic of the period accounts for the confusion in reporting Koprowski's movements. This confusion is compounded by the fact that a great deal of obfuscation and outright lies were used by many of those who were involved at the time.

To complicate matters, the 1960 election of anti-eugenicist John F. Kennedy placed the whole program under constraints until Mr. Kennedy was removed from office in the *coup d'etat* of November 22, 1963. However, from 1952 until 1960 the shift from legitimate polio vaccine research to illicit eugenics-motivated research was carried forward, with only the major players knowing what was actually going on. While Koprowski and his confidantes did their work in the shadows, they still had to appear to be working in the full light of day.

End of an Interlude

1956

Efficacy of Trivalent Adenovirus (APC) Vaccine in Naval Recruits, Joseph A. Bell, Bethesda, MD., Captain Matthew J. Hantover (MC),

U.S. Navy, Robert J. Huebner, M.D., Bethesda, Md., and Clayton G. Loosi, M.D., Chicago

This article which can be regarded as a naturally following report on the work cited above under "**1954** Robert J. Huebner, *et al*." is important because of the statement made in its summary: "The opinions expressed herein are those of the authors and cannot be construed as reflecting the views of the Public Health Services at large of the *Department of Health, Education and Welfare*, or of the Naval Service at large of the *Department of Defense*."

Notice that Nelson Rockefeller had been involved in significant roles in both departments italicized.

1956

In the October 6, 1956 issue of *JAMA*, there were two 'Medical Literature Abstracts' which are links in our scientific paper trail:

1. Prevention of *Acute Respiratory Illness in Recruits by Adenovirus (RI-APC-ARD) Vaccine*. M. R. Hilleman, R.A. Stallones, R. L. Gauld, M.S. Warfield and S.A. Anderson, *Proc. Soc. Exper. Biol. & Med.*, V. 92; Pp. 377-383. **and**
2. *Clinical and Laboratory Studies in Patients with Respiratory Disease Caused by Adenoviruses* (RI-APC-ARD Agents), H.E. Dascomb and M. R. Hilleman, *Am. J. Med.* Vol. 21; Pp. 161-174

1956

NOTE *Clinical Findings Six Years After Outbreak of Akureyri Disease*, Bjorn Sigurdsson. Director, Institute for Experimental Pathology, U. of Iceland, Reykjavik, and Kajartan R. Gudmundsson, Clinical Neurologist

1956

Further Outbreak of a Disease Resembling Poliomyelitis, D.W. Sumner; Resident Medical Officer, Manchester Royal Infirmary. *The Lancet* May 26, 1956

1956

Encephalomyelitis Simulating Poliomyelitis, A. Melvin Ramsay and E. O'Sullivan, *The Lancet* May 26, 1956 Pp. 761-762

1956
Present Status of Attenuated Live-Virus Poliomyelitis Vaccine, Albert B. Sabin. *J.A.M.A.* Vol.162; #18 Pp. 1589-1596

1969
Hearings before a Subcommittee of the Committee of Appropriations, House of Representatives; Ninety-First Congress. June 9.

This is one of the top ten documents in our paper trail to AIDS for in it, on page 129, Dr. Donald MacArthur, Deputy Director (Research and Technology), Chemical and Biological Warfare of the Pentagon makes it very clear to a small group of Congressmen who essentially decide upon what activities should be funded in the Defence Budget that the U.S. Government is engaged in the development of biological weapons which could cause a 'worldwide scourge, or a black death type disease that will envelop the world or major geographic areas."(Page 121) However, MacArthur hastens to assure these Congressmen that the Pentagon has imposed restraints upon themselves to ensure that such a disaster does not occur. Then, he undoes all of these assurances by adding: *"We have done a small amount of research on a few agents that do not satisfy this constraint."*

In other words, the work is in progress and that work includes many of the published scientific results that we have summarized this far. These results, taken by themselves and not placed in the context of the whole program of MKULTRA, appear innocent enough by themselves. However, taken as part of the whole they add the necessary details to the crime beyond belief...the creation of the AIDS co-factors.

And just what is it that one of these co-factors possess that makes it so dangerous? As MacArthur puts it:

> "Within 5 to 10 years, it would probably be possible to make a new infective microorganism which could differ in certain important aspects from any known disease-causing organisms. Most important of these is that it might be refractory to the immunological and therapeutic processes upon which we depend to maintain our relative freedom from infectious disease."

That is one of the co-factors of AIDS: an acquired immune deficiency induced by a new microorganism.

If the Congressmen want this new, deadly disease pathogen, then they must budget an extra ten million dollars and chances are good that they will have it within 5 to 10 years. The money is voted and purportedly the crime beyond belief is under way.

However, as we have pointed out in the evidence discussed so far, the new microorganism is probably already developed and deployed.

If this is so, then why does MacArthur make this promise to the Congressmen? Plainly and simply, he wants the Congressmen to retroactively endorse what the CIA and the Defence Department have already done. MacArthur knows that President Johnson had already approved the development and deployment of the AIDS co-factors and that in from five to ten years (*i.e.* by 1980) the AIDS epidemic will already been put in motion, and Congress will be compromised by their vote to proceed.

Essentially, what the researchers will be doing over the next ten years has two parts: first, they will be working to find out how their disease pathogens actually work and second, they will be researching to perfect the disabling component of their two part objective of two biological agents: one agent that is lethal and one that is disabling.

1969 & 1970

Herrera, F., Richard H. Adamson, and Robert C. Gallo, "Uptake of Transfer Ribonucleic Acid by Normal and Leukemic Cells" Proc. of the Nat. Academy of Sciences. Vol. 64, #4; Pp. 1943-1950. This article was presented twice. Once, in 1969 (Cleveland) and later, in 1970, to the NATO International Symposium on Uptake of Informative Molecules by Living Cells, Mol, Belgium.

It is the latter startling fact that merits its inclusion in this paper trail to AIDS, for the North Atlantic Treaty Organization, established in 1949 for the defence of Europe and the North Atlantic against the perceived threat of Soviet aggression. The subject matter in and of itself is interesting and important in that it deals with research demonstrating that transfer ribonucleic acid (in this case from *Escherichia coli*) is uptaken by both normal and leukemia cells and that the uptake is rapid and is not due to altered membrane permeability. Furthermore, 20% of the transferred RNA remains functional and 'apparently intact'. Ordinarily, the normal cell at least could be expected to block that foreign nucleic acid particle from entering as a consequence of its natural immunity. But, as the article demonstrates, the cell's immune defence does not afford the anticipated protection. This leads to the conclusion drawn by the researchers: "The results demonstrate that transfer RNA can enter mammalian cells and suggest that an energy independent, carrier-mediated, mechanism may be operative."(Page 1943) What might that mechanism be? Could it be the mycoplasma acting as a co-factor?

This question is not as important to our research as the question: what does this have to do with a defence alliance between North Atlantic nations?

1970
Murphy, Wm. H., et al.: *Isolation of Mycoplasmas from Leukemic and Non-Leukemic Patients. Journal of National Cancer Institute*, Vol. 45; #2 - August 1970. Pp. 273-251

The critical evidence presented in this article is from the Summary: *"The evidence from this study suggests that mycoplasma, normally inhabiting the mucous membranes, enter the bloodstream and either persist or multiply in patients with leukemia, lymphoma, and other diseases which depress the immune system."*

Consider carefully this sentence and then read the article and weigh what it reveals against the background of our subject: immune depression and the 1964 overt launch of the Special Virus Leukemia/Lymphoma Program under Lyndon B. Johnson.

Also, note the fact that among the sources cited by Murphy *et al.* is one by none other than Hilary Koprowski and Leonard Hayflick! The article is "Direct agar isolation of mycoplasmas from human Leukemic bone marrow." (*Nature*, Vol. 205; Pp. 713-4 1965)

Thus, although Hooper does not make note of the fact anywhere in his book, *The River*, in 1965 Koprowski was obviously sufficiently involved in the study of the role of the mycoplasma in relation to leukemia to write this article.

1970
Werner Henle, Gertrude Henle, et al.: *Anti-body Responses to Epstein-Barr virus and Cytomegaloviruses after Open-Heart Surgery. The N.E.J.M.*, Vol. 282; #19

This article is of interest because of several factors, but the

factor we note here is that the Henle's state: that their research was "Supported by the U.S. Army Research and Development Command"…as well as "the Special Virus Leukemia Program."
1971
Merigan, Thomas C. and David A. Stevens: **Viral infections in man associated with acquired immunological deficiency states**, *Federation Proceedings*; Vol. 30; #6

In the title of this article we see the first reference to an acquired immune deficiency and its links to various viral diseases and this is important since it demonstrates without question that important research on that subject was on-going. It is also important to note that later (as recounted in Johnson's, *Osler's Web*) that Merigan had been an early denier that such an immune deficient syndrome as CFS even existed and he was one of the early advocates of the view that it was 'all in the head' of the sufferers.

1971

In the January 22, 1970 issue of *Nature*, a very interesting letter signed by Lawrence Stone, Edward Scolnick, Kenneth Takemoto and Stuart Aaronson was published. The interest stems from the fact that the writers state: "The demonstration of a visna virus DNA polymerase provides additional evidence of the similarities between visna virus and the avian and murine leukemia viruses previously noted by Thormar." Besides the fact that the letter demonstrates that research was going on which involved the sheep retrovirus 'visna', the linkage to avian leukemia viruses is interesting. This interest is made even greater when one realizes all four of the writers appear in the *SVCP, Progress Report #8!*

1971

Special Virus Cancer Program, Progress Report #8 National Cancer Institute, National Institutes of Health, Public Health Service, U.S. Department of Health, Education and Welfare, Bethesda, MD. Prepared in May 1971, up-dated in July of the same year and presented October 24-27, 1971 to the Annual Joint Working Conference, SVCP at the Hershey Medical Center, Hershey, PA.

This document presents a number of problems, raises a number of concerns, is marked by several anomalies, and possesses some startling details. We have already introduced some of these in chapter eleven and developed those and others in chapter thirteen, so we will simply précis some of that information and repeat other parts for emphasis in our following of the scientific paper trail to AIDS.

First, there is a problem with the title of the 383-page document. It is titled *"Special Virus Cancer Program"*, and it originated with the National Cancer Institute (NCI), one of the institutes within the National Institutes of Health (NIH) in 1971! Yet, according to the former Director of the NCI no such program ever existed. In his fanciful and obfuscating account of the latter agency's work *Virus Hunting: AIDS, Cancer, & the Human Retroviruses* (1991), Robert Gallo makes no mention of SVCP. This is all the more surprising (and confusing) when one considers that Gallo joined the NIH in 1965.

The next problem lies with the numbering of this '*Progress Report #8*'. On the title page we are told that this is "the area's Annual Report", and yet we have been unable to find the seven earlier 'annual reports.' Did such ever exist? Or, is it possible that there were earlier annual reports but these were subsequently destroyed? If the latter we must ask why?

On page two of the document we are told that in 1964 the Congress had provided funds to the NCI for an intensified program in *virus-leukemia/lymphoma research*. The date and subject matter should be noted for 1964 was the year that population growth rate control advocate Lyndon Johnson succeeded population *control opponent* John F. Kennedy as President, and 'leukemia/lymphoma' were consequences of mycoplasmal damage with the latter pathogenic agent having been re-discovered by Robert Huebner back in the late 1940s. We have noted that in 1954 (See above: 'Adenoidal,-Pharyngeal-Conjunctival Agents) Huebner and several other research scientists *were continuing their mycoplasmal research*. Now, in 1971, Huebner-research articles are cited a total sixty-two times!

Very obviously, Huebner was on to something, and that something was the mycoplasmal species later to be implicated publicly by Dr. Shyh-Ching Lo when he patented the *Mycoplasma fermentans* in a protean range of human degenerative diseases. (See chapter one below)

This critical fact is further demonstrated from pages 255 to 256 of *Progress Report #8* where it is revealed that in a June 19, 1969 contract between NIH and Stanford University (Contract: NIH 69-2053) the latter University was to establish 'a Central Mycoplasma Diagnostic Laboratory' under Dr. Leonard Hayflick. It is important to note the following paragraph, which reads:

> "Nine hundred and fifty-five samples were received (Feb. 1-May 30) from SVCP laboratories to be tested for mycoplasma contamination. One hundred thirty-two have been found to be positive. This represents the largest number of mycoplasma samples received in any four month period since the inception of the contract **seven years ago**."

Seven years ago! That means that the degree of interest in mycoplasmas necessary to warrant the establishment of such a laboratory dates back to 1962! Such a display of interest in the mycoplasma lends support to Luc Montagnier's belief that the mycoplasma is a co-factor in the etiology of AIDS and it makes Robert Gallo's dismissal of the mycoplasma as a dangerous microorganism very puzzling. (See Gallo, 1991 Page 286)

There are further problems with *Progress Report #8*. On pages 273 to 289 there is a "Progress Report on Investigation of Carcinogenesis with Selected Virus Preparations in the Newborn Monkey." The Report was submitted by none other than 'Bionetics Research Laboratories, Inc. A Division of Litton Industries'!

Readers will recall that Litton Industries was founded by then Vice-President Nixon's ally, 'whiz-kid' Roy Ash (see chapters eleven and fourteen above.) They will also recall that Gallo had written:

> "Government oversight committees are never comfortable when NIH personnel work too closely with the people with whom they have contract relationships, however, so our move to Pearl Street, to space owned by Litton Bionetics, one of the firms with whom we had a contract relationship, may have raised eyebrows." (Gallo, Page 36)

This is a masterpiece of understatement, but the move demonstrated that the NCI was in a very secret and intimate relationship with Bionetics.

This relationship is further demonstrated in *Progress Report #8* when, on page 300 it is reported that "Ting, R.C." had submitted six research papers to the SVCP! In one of these articles (399) one of his co-authors is Robert Huebner and in another (651), a co-author is Robert Gallo.

Another critical connection between the program to develop the AIDS co-factors and the murder of President John F. Kennedy is to be seen on page 289 where this statement appears:

> "In 1965, twelve rhesus monkeys were transferred from Brooks Air Force Base to Bionetics for continued maintenance and observation. These animals had undergone irradiation treatments from 1957 to 1960."

Consider all of the startling linkages evident in this brief sentence. First notice that it is rhesus monkeys that were the subject of research being done on an Air Force base. Then recall that it was rhesus monkeys, which were later bred in the thousands at the Delta Primate Farm in Louisiana and whose kidneys were used to culture the mycoplasma organisms used by Tulane University Medical School and the Baylor College of Medicine in Huntsville Prison tests. Also note that David Ferrie, friend of Lee Harvey Oswald, had been injecting mice with a 'monkey virus' undoubtedly obtained from Tulane, quite likely through Ferrie's Tulane friend, Mary Sherman, colleague of Alton Ochsner and later murdered. Then consider that Dr. Jose Rivera, who had prior knowledge of Mr. Kennedy's murder, was attached to Brooks Air Force Base. Finally, and taking us back to *Progress Report #8*, note that "Dmochowski, L." is cited on page 294 as having contributed 39 research articles to the Program, and that the 'cancer treatise' found in David Ferrie's apartment after the latter's very suspicious death, cites Dmochowski in its bibliography. Finally note that one of Dmochowski's citations deals with estrogens as an etiological factor in cancer and then refer to *Progress Report #9* of August 1972 and reviewed below.

1971

Takemoto, K. K. and L. B. Stone: *Transformation of Murine Cells by Two 'Slow Viruses,' Visna Virus and Progressive Pneumonia Virus. Journal of Virology*; Vol. 43 #7

Note the nexus of so many factors in this title. First, the visna virus which was the major subject of Bjorn Sigurdsson's research for his Rockefeller patrons, dating from 1942. Then note the 'progressive *pneumonia*", and recall the subject of Robert Huebner's research ten years later: atypical pneumonia in naval recruits. Then note that these two factors obviously play some part in rendering normal murine cells cancerous!

There you have AIDS in a nutshell: an immune suppressant that causes pneumonia, a retrovirus of sheep at work in mouse cells that cause cancer!

1971
Rottem, Pfendt and Hayflick: *Sterol Requirement of T-Strain Mycoplasmas, Journal of Bacteriology*; Vol. 105; #1 January 1971. This article demonstrates that many species of mycoplasma have an absolute growth requirement for sterols, including cholesterol, which they up-take from host cells, largely from the membrane of such cells. Thus, the cell is killed, leaving lesions and the functioning of such cells is impaired or destroyed completely, presenting as a variety of signs and symptoms. For example, if the mycoplasma invades cells of the *substantia nigra*, the latter cells reduce their production of dopamine and Parkinson's disease will present. Or, if the Beta cells of the pancreas are invaded and the production of insulin is reduced, diabetes type one will present. Similarly with several other body systems which can be affected by endocrine imbalance.

It must be emphasized that approximately twenty-five percent of cellular membrane is composed of cholesterol, and the loss of such can severely impede the cellular immune system. (See also below: 1977 Slutzky, *et al.*)

There is also a high degree of endocrine damage since cholesterol is the precursor to many glandular secretions.

1971
Gallo, Sarin, Allen, Newton, Priori, Bowen, and Dmochowski: *Reverse transcriptase in type C virus particles of human origin, Nature New Biology*, Vol. 232, Pp. 140-142

This important article was drawn to our attention by Horowitz (1997) page 70: "Gallo and company, including frequent coauthor Robert Ting (see next citation) from Litton Bionetics, reported modifying simian monkey viruses by infusing them with cat leukemia RNA to make them cause cancers as seen in people with AIDS."

Also of interest is the coauthor, Dmochowski, who was one of the researchers cited in a document found in the apartment of David Ferrie after the latter committed suicide or was murdered. (Haslam, 1995)

It is also important to quote Horowitz' conclusion from the work being done: "I learned that Gallo and his group of researchers created numerous AIDS-like viruses for more than a decade before Luc Montagnier announced the discovery of LAV."(Page 75)

1972
Gallo: Transfer RNA and transfer RNA methylation in growing and 'resting' adult and embryonic tissues and in various oncogenic systems; Cancer Research, Vol. 31; Pp. 621-29

This article advances the research cited above, and fits in with that which follows. Lee (type-script, 1989) demonstrates through several further citations from this period, how the same cast of researchers worked in various combinations to interpret the biological mechanics of reverse transcriptase. And what needs to be emphasized is that all of this work with retroviruses was being done ten years before the entity known as AIDS was officially recognized.

This fits in with one of our major hypotheses, that a species of mycoplasma which lowered the immune defence barriers of infected humans, allowed for a zoonotic disease agent, the visna virus, to invade the victim and so perpetuate the damage. In other words, the mycoplasma species co-factored with the visna virus did the initial damage and then opened the way for other viral illnesses. (See 1971 citation above: Merigan and Stevens)

This hypothesis explains the confluence of the work of Huebner (mycoplasmas), of Sigurdsson (visna) of Koprowski (vaccines) of Gallo (cancer) and of Robert Ting (Litton Bionetics who would provide the production capabilities necessary) and supports the strong likelihood that the AIDS co-factors were first introduced into the human family shortly after Lyndon Johnson succeeded John F. Kennedy. This beginning would be fact-finding in nature and would give Johnson grounds for his January, 1965 State of the Union message where he promised to "seek new ways to use our knowledge to help deal with the explosion of world population." (Johnson, 1971 Pp. 339-40) The first efforts were in African countries where the

Agency for International Development (AID) already had a presence and went full time in 1968 with World Health Organization support under Dr. Donald Henderson, and after Johnson had recruited all of the 'population control' exponents into a "Who's Who of population control", including Wilbur Cohen and John D. Rockefeller lll.(*Ibid*, Page 340)

In other words, the seeds of AIDS were discovered, developed and deployed long before the June 9, 1969 promise to the Congress by Dr. Donald MacArthur. It was only after the epidemic had been launched among humanity that the scientific community went to work to figure out how to control it.

1972
Gallagher, Robert E., Robert Ting, and Robert Gallo. *A Common Change of Aspartyl -tRNA in Polyoma and SV40-Transformed Cells, Biochimica et Biophysica Acta*, Vol. 272; Pp. 568-582

This article brings together a number of the people, elements and subjects of research that entered into the massive and complicated undertaking to develop and deploy disease co-factors which first reduced the normal immunity of the victim and then facilitated various forms of physical damage. Now, with such co-factors deployed and being deployed, it was important for the perpetrators of this crime beyond belief to do several things: first, continue research into the mechanics of immune suppression; second, master the mechanics of transferring zoonotic diseases from animals (in this case primates - SV-40) to humans; third, to mass produce contaminated vaccines for those deploying the co-factors. Signs of all three objectives are seen in this item.

The people to note include, of course, Robert Gallo as one of the authors. But co-author, Robert Ting is critical. Ting is in the employ of Litton Bionetics, and hence, his work and research is beyond the prying eyes of anyone in the Public Health agencies of the U.S. (Even if such an interest as this was decidedly unlikely.) Further, his employer, Litton Bionetics, a major contractor in the U. S. Army biological weapons industry (Horowitz, 1996; Page 78) And you will recall that Litton was founded by 'whiz kid' Roy Ash, friend of Richard Nixon. Also, one must note that at the end of the article the authors acknowledge their 'indebtedness to Dr. K. K. Takemoto.

Takemoto, in turn, provides a link between the immune suppressing mycoplasma and the retrovirus of sheep (visna) having published articles such as that noted above (1971).

Finally, the last sentence of the article reads: "These studies were supported in part by NCI contract NIH-70-2050 and in part by NIH-70-2025, *Special Virus Cancer Program*, NCI."

It must be noted that although funding came in part from the SVCP, and of that funding part would obviously go to co-writer Robert Gallo, the latter in his book *Virus Hunting* seems to have forgotten his role in the Program. This leads us into the next paper trail item: SVCP, Progress Report #9.

In the heading of the article the address of Litton Bionetics is given as '7300 Pearl Street, Bethesda, Md.' now turn to Gallo's highly imaginative account of his research (Gallo, 1991) on page 36 of *Virus Hunting* Gallo writes:

> "Government oversight committees are never comfortable when NIH personnel work too closely with the people with whom they have contract relationships, however, so our move to Pearl Street, to space owned by Litton Bionetics, one of the firms with whom we had a contract relationship, may have raised eyebrows."

The conflict of interest is so dramatically blatant as to boggle the mind of any objective researcher, yet Robert Gallo and his colleagues could get away with it because they obviously had the blessing of powerful people pushing the research along.

1972

Special Virus Cancer Program- Progress Report #9. National Cancer Institute; July 1972

The most important revelation along our scientific paper trail to AIDS in *Progress Report #9* is on page 39 where it is reported:

> "We have for the first time demonstrated that the virogenic markers, group specific antigens (g.s.) and *RNA directed DNA polymerase,* can be activated by alteration of the physiological endocrine balance…The potential for such activation has also been noted by us to be present in certain pesticides…"

With this statement we are beginning to see the scientific linkage between a species of mycoplasma and a co-factor such as the visna virus of sheep, which has been engineered to affect humans. Some species of the mycoplasma as we have noted in the report above (1971: Rottem, Pfend and Hayflick) have an absolute growth requirement for cholesterol. That means that if a mycoplasmal infection uptakes cholesterol from a host, there will be a reduction of hormone generation in the endocrine system. In other words, *there will be an alteration of the endocrine balance!*

When that alteration occurs, then RNA directed DNA polymerase would be activated. The retrovirus can go to work. This is the clue as to why for the first time; a retrovirus has been able to 'affect humans before the advent of AIDS.' (See below 1987: House of Commons Report)

Something else very critical to our hypothesis that AIDS is a mirror-image of CFS is reported on page 110 of SVCP; *Progress Report #9*. There it is revealed that a very large contract was awarded by the *Special Virus Cancer Program* to the *Children's Hospital of Philadelphia*. Readers will recall that this hospital was the base of operations for Werner and Gertrude Henle. (See chapter six above.) They will also recall that Hilary Koprowski and Fritz Deinhardt worked with the Henles. Koprowski's polio vaccine known as CHOP was the initialization of that hospital.

So, does *Progress Report #9* reveal that the Henles were busy with polio vaccine (Koprowski) or with hepatitis vaccine (Deinhardt)? No! When one turns to the summary of the contract on page 168 one finds that they are actually working with Epstein - Barr virus to study whether it is involved with Burkitt's lymphoma (BL) and nasopharyngeal cancer! Now, as you will also recall, BL is a malignant lymphoma that occurs especially among children of central Africa and New Guinea.

This raises the question: how did a disease, primarily of Black children in Africa, come to be a subject of study in Children's Hospital of Philadelphia (CHOP)? And how did it happen that the husband-wife team of Werner and Gertrude Henle who were doing that study also happened to be in charge of research being done in Africa by Dr. Fritz Deinhardt who was studying hepatitis and was using chimpanzees at Camp Lindi in the Congo for his research?

At this point we can refer again to Dr. Carleton Gajdusek who tells us that in the same time frame (1952-3) he had searched the 'swamps and high valleys of Papua New Guinea' on a quest for medical problems in primitive population isolates. (Nobel Lecture; Page 165) Was he looking for biological agents for his boss, Dr. Smadel of Walter Reed Military Hospital?

1973
The Viru -Cancer Program; Progress Report #10
The reader needs to note that the title of the program upon which this document purports to report for the tenth time has been changed from its original form,' The *Special Virus Cancer Program*' by dropping the word 'Special'. This change was purportedly made 'to integrate the Program's research activities into the framework of the new National Cancer Plan.' (Page 2) This may well be, but there are other more logical reasons for the change. First, there is the likelihood that Nixon, at the behest of his National Security Advisor, Henry Kissinger, wanted to distance the program from its antecedents as Viral Oncology Program (in 1964) and then as a Special Virus Leukemia/Lymphoma Program (in 1965 and 1966.) (Page 4) There is also the likelihood that there was a new direction being embarked upon in the research and that was to bring fully on-steam a program to develop the pathogenic basis for a disabling disease…the second part of Dr. MacArthur's report to Congress on June 9, 1969. The seeds of AIDS were already planted; now the evidence suggests that the emphasis will be on developing CFS. We have developed this hypothesis in chapter thirteen.

1973
McBride, Gail: *Clues tantalizing in efforts to link mycoplasmas, infertility.* JAMA, Vol. 226, #3, Pp.263-267
This article links the work of Dr. Shepard (See above: 1953: Dr. Shepard) with both the Mycoplasma and a likely predecessor *Brucella abortus*, and the very significant fact that the mycoplasmal species involved "have the ability to hydroyze urease." (See chapter sixteen) To recapitulate one of the points made there: when the mycoplasma up-takes cholesterol from cell membrane, the neuro-transmitter glutamate may be released. Glutamate, although critical to life in the right place

at the right time and in the right amount may do great damage unless neutralized to glutamine by the up-take of ammonia from urea. This solves one problem but creates another for the loss of ammonia causes the release of cyanide which then captures energy produced by cellular mitochondria, presenting as chronic fatigue syndrome.

1974
The Virus Cancer-Program, Progress Report #11
Continues with the change in emphasis from research into the lethal co-factors in AIDS to the role of the Epstein - Barr virus and CFS.

1977
Project MKULTRA, The CIA's Program in Behavioral Modification.
Joint Hearing Before the Select Committee on Intelligence and the Subcommittee on Health and Scientific Research of the Committee on Human Resources; United States Senate. Ninety-Fifth Congress—August 5, 1977
We have reviewed this document presented by CIA Director, Stansfield Turner on orders from newly elected President Jimmy Carter in chapter two. Here we need only note that the records of the CIA which dealt with the programs MKULTRA, MKDELTA and MKNAOMI were destroyed on orders of the former director of the CIA, William Helms and carried out by Dr. Sidney Gottlieb, Chief of TSD. The very fact that these records were destroyed is in itself sufficient evidence to support the conclusion that the AIDS co-factors were created in U.S. laboratories owned or controlled by the CIA and latterly by a wider spectrum of politicians and officials. The document is also evidence that even though the Carter Administration was an improvement upon those of Eisenhower, Johnson and Nixon/Ford, it is still protected from full disclosure by powerful interests. For example, the title of the document refers to 'Behavioral Modification', and as our research has amply demonstrated, behavioral modification was an infinitely small part of what was actually going on. It was, in fact, a cover for an even more secret effort: the research, discovery, development and deployment of the AIDS/CFS microorganisms with a view to reduce the world population growth rate...*i.e.* genocide on a massive scale.

1977
Hearings before the Subcommittee on Health and Scientific Research of the Committee on Human Resources; U.S. Senate.
A critical discovery is reported on page 70 of this document:

> "In general terms, these are some of the more important accomplishments of the program:
> 4. Production and isolation, for the first time, of a crystalline bacterial toxin…"

This means that the poisons normally caused by various living bacteria can be reduced to a crystalline form and hence be spread by aerosol, food chain or insect vector without leaving any evidence of the bacterial antecedent! If the toxin is related to the bacterial nucleic acid then it could well represent a crystalline form of mycoplasmal species and bacterial diseases could present without any sign of the bacteria.

In the light of this dramatic discovery, consider such statements as the following: "Although there was evidence of inflammation in the fetal membranes of the reproductive 'casualties,' *no bacteria could be found.*" (See above: **1973**: Gail McBride)

Bacterial disease without the bacteria! Chronic brucellosis equals chronic fatigue!

1980
Embree, Joanne E., and Juan A. Embil: *Mycoplasmas in Diseases of Humans, Canadian Medical Association Journal* Vol.123; Pp. 105-113

This article is important for two reasons. First, it is a Canadian article, and it is important to note that many medical jurisdictions differ significantly in several ways from the U.S. Public Health Agencies in their response to many diseases, syndromes and treatment protocols for such conditions as AIDS, CFS and so on. Second, this article does not take the U.S. line of 'mycoplasmas are inconsequential is respect to human health."

Instead of the latter, the authors point out that various mycoplasma species can seriously affect seven human body systems: respiratory; circulatory; musculo-skeletal; cutaneous; gastro-intestinal; genito-urinary; and neurological.

Such a protean range of illnesses is to be expected from a

pathogenic agent which, as we have noted above under **1971**: Rottem, Pfend and Hayflick does its damage by up-taking pre-formed sterols (including cholesterol) from host cells. It also is reminiscent of brucellosis where we started back in the 1940s.

1984

Somewhere around 1980 there was a subtle shift in the subject matter of many journal articles dealing with what is broadly labeled as Chronic Fatigue Syndrome. Prior to this time the articles seemed to be talking about what might be termed a 'non-paralytic' type of poliomyelitis, with additional signs and symptoms Then after 1980 the subject syndromes or diseases seemed to de-emphasize any polio characteristics and to present more as the syndrome we now call CFS.

Let us emphasize: the shift was subtle and most people reading the literature sporadically would not notice it, but as one devotes more time and care to the study of CFS, one can recognize the shift. It is more specifically commented upon in the text edited by Hyde, Goldstein and Levine and published by the Nightingale Research Foundation in 1992:

> "From 1984 until 1992 (the year the book was published-Ed) an endemic period occurred in which an unusually large number of clusters and epidemics of ME/CFS have been recognized in North America. After an apparent initial increase in morbidity in 1983 there seemed to have appeared in late summer of 1984 an unprecedented increase of sporadic and epidemic cases across North America. Although certain geographic hot spots seem to have taken up much of the medical interest, this endemic situation probably represents an unusual and unremitting morbidity in all areas of the United States and Canada. Some of the clusters and epidemics are listed." (Page 185)

Briefly it is this: The initial search of the early eugenist's for a lethal and a disabling biological weapon focused upon several pathogens, principally zoonotic, and included the poliomyelitis virus. However, by the late 1970s the emphasis was gradually shifted to the Huebner mycoplasma, but research and testing involving this pathogen was largely suspended with the election of Jimmy Carter and remained in limbo until 1980 when Ronald Reagan and his new CIA Director, William Casey, resumed power. It took a couple of years until the work was back on track, but then aerosol tests were resumed principally at Tahoe-Truckee High School (1984-85); food chain tests of the pathogenic agent in goats' milk in Lyndonville, New York (1985); and, mosquito vector tests in the St. Lawrence Seaway Cornwall to Montreal area (1984).

1987
Problems Associated with AIDS. Dr. John Seale, Royal Society of Medicine. Published by The House of Commons (Great Britain), Social Services Committee Session 1986-87 Pp. 142-148.

Anyone interested in AIDS should - in fact, must - read these seven critical pages, a copy of which was provided to us by Ms. Peg Laurian. Dr. John Seale is referred to by Leonard Horowitz in his important book: *Emerging Viruses: AIDS and Ebola* where Horowitz discusses the meeting he had with Dr. Robert Strecker. Strecker says:

> "Seale started writing about AIDS in '81 or so…and he was the first guy to say AIDS was not a venereal disease, and that it appeared to be artificial and spreading in an unusual manner, which was really just looking at the fact that the virus appeared in different areas of the world at the same time…How was this virus appearing at different spots in the world at the same time in a sense without any contiguous spread?" (Page 104)

John Seale is also referred to in Hooper's *The River*, pages 153, 165 and 796. Hooper suggests that Seale was a 'brilliant but eccentric British venereologist.' That Seale was brilliant few can argue against, however, he was not eccentric. Hooper apparently thought so because at the time Hooper wrote *The River* he did not accept Seale's belief that AIDS was a biological population growth rate control weapon. It is possible that Hooper will be or is actually re-thinking this assessment of Seale.

Hooper also notes that Seale had written a 7000 word article on AIDS and had submitted it to *The Lancet* in 1990, but that journal had refused to publish it. This emphasizes the bias against reporting such evidence by certain of the major media.

In the House of Commons document, Seale points out several critical facts about AIDS, including: "Half-truths, wishful thinking, flawed scientific hypotheses and deceptions have been perpetrated by scientists, and allowed to flourish as conventional wisdom, aided and abetted by editors of scientific and medical journals." He goes on to note that "AIDS is a contagious, infectious, communicable disease caused by a lentivirus (slow virus), a member of the family of retroviruses. No lentivirus has been known to affect humans before the advent of AIDS."

We cannot précis the entire article, but we can urge everyone to read a copy.

1993

United States Patent #5,242,820 dated September 7, 1993. Subject of patent: **Pathogenic Mycoplasma.** Inventor: Shyh-Ching Lo

This official patent of the pathogenic mycoplasma states that "Some of these patients that are infected with *Mycoplasma fermentans* incognitus will be patients who have been diagnosed as having AIDS or ARC, Cchronic (sic) Fatigue Syndrome, Wegener's Disease, Sarcoidosis, respiratory distress syndrome, Kibuchi's Disease, autoimmune diseases such as Collagen Vascular Disease and Lupus and chronic debilitating diseases such as Alzheimer's Disease." (Page 20)

1993-1994

Department of Microbiology; Uniformed Services University of the Health Sciences (USUHS) 1993-1994 Academic Year, Pages 90-93.

These four pages are critical pages in our scientific paper trail to AIDS. To put them in context before we actually look at what these pages say.

The U.S. Military runs its own University of the Health Sciences for people being trained as medical doctors for the uniformed armed services. As strange as it may seem, this university has subjects in its curriculum, which generally speaking are not included in the curricula of the regular schools of medicine throughout the U.S. One such subject taught to military doctors is the species of microorganism we have seen cropping up all through this study from the work of Dr. Robert Huebner and the coughing recruits (Ch.3) to the preceding item in this paper trail: the Patent of the Pathogenic Mycoplasma by the U.S. Government...the *Mycoplasma*. These four pages are taken from the Curriculum of the USUHS, and they précis the essential details of the mycoplasmal species that the Military thinks that armed services doctors need to know.

This is in sharp contrast to what is taught in the average American university to doctors who will treat ordinary people.

This difference needs to be emphasized. If two 22-year-old males, one a civilian and the other a soldier in the U.S. Army, both six feet tall, both 200 pounds, both in otherwise good health and well-fed, and both presenting with a 'flu-like' illness are examined by their respective doctors, one a military doctor trained at the Uniformed Services University and the other at the School of Medicine, the University of Georgia, the two may well receive different diagnoses of just what is causing their 'flu-like' illness!

Why?

Because the doctor trained at the USUHS may well order tests to determine whether his patient is infected with *M. fermentans*. If the tests are positive, the patient may well be given one of the tetracycline antibiotics and bed rest, with recovery likely to follow.

The doctor trained at Georgia University School of Medicine may diagnose a mild flu and suggest bed rest. Two days later his patient may well check into the emergency ward of the local hospital with adult respiratory distress syndrome, disseminated intravascular coagulation and/or multiple organ failure.

The doctor trained at the USUHS will take the action he did...a rather simple and very effective action if taken in time...because his course of study had taught him that:

> "A. *Mycoplasma fermentans*
> The most serious presentation of *M. fermentans* infection is that of a fulminant systemic disease that begins as a flu-like illness. Patients rapidly deteriorate developing severe complications including adult respiratory distress syndrome, disseminated intravascular coagulation, and /or multiple organ failure." (Page 90)

If one or both doctors suspected that their patient might have AIDS, each could order an HIV test, and both tests could come back positive, at which time the civilian trained doctor could prescribe azidothymidine (AZT) while the USUHS doctor would order a further test for *Mycoplasma genitalium* which is also positive, so the military doctor prescribes a course of Doxycycline to which his patient responds well.

Twelve months later, the military patient is to all appearances fully recovered from his flu-like symptoms, while the civilian patient on AZT endures an onslaught of opportunistic diseases, and finally, with his bone marrow eaten away by the AZT, he dies. (These are hypothetical cases based upon the information in the USUHS course curriculum section dealing with the mycoplasma and drawn partly from information in Nussbaum, 1990, Pp.288-9)

The point is, the U.S. Military which, with the CIA, was instrumental in engineering naturally occurring mycoplasmas to be more infectious and more pathogenic with certain co-factors, is better able to respond to presenting illnesses because they know more of the story than their civilian counterparts.

1993
Katseni, L. Vassiliki, et al.. *Mycoplasma fermentans in individuals seropositive and seronegative for HIV-1*. The Lancet; Vol. 341: Jan.30, 1993

This is another article which advances the possibility that a species of mycoplasma (in this case the *Mycoplasma fermentans*) may act as a co-factor to some other pathogenic agent as etiological factors in AIDS.

> "It has been suggested that mycoplasmas act as a co-factor, enhancing virus replication and accelerating disease progression. This idea was supported by the findings that treatment of HIV- infected cell cultures with tetracycline analogues, active against mycoplasmas, *inhibited cell killing without affecting virus replication, and that certain mycoplasmas enhanced cytopathic changes brought about by HIV-1*…The presence of mycoplasmas in the blood increases the interaction with the immune system. Cytokines [substances secreted by the immune system - Ed] so induced could enhance HIV replication with the increased loss of CD4 cells; in this way the mycoplasma could act as a co-factor."

The findings are somewhat inconclusive, but the fact that mycoplasmas do alter certain cellular metabolic activities make it reasonable to call for more research into the hypothesis that they can indeed act as a co-factor in AIDS. This scientific approach should be contrasted with the position taken by Dr. Mark Wainberg of McGill University who has declared that "HIV deniers should be jailed." See item under **2000** Andre Picard, below.

1995
Shien Tsai, Douglas J. Wear, James Wai-Kuo Shih, and Shyh-Ching Lo. *Mycoplasmas and oncogenesis: Persistent infection and multistage malignant transformation Proceedings National Academy of Sciences*, Vol. 92; Pp. 10197-10201

This is a very significant report since it establishes that certain mycoplasmal species play a role in the initiation and progress of malignant cell proliferation. Especially worthy of notice is the authors' claim that "...all malignant changes were reversible if mycoplasmas were eradicated by antibiotic treatment."

1996
Colmenero, J.D., et al.. *Complications Associated with Brucella melitensis Infection: A Study of 530 Cases. Medicine*, Vol. 75; #4, Pp. 195-211

Despite the fact that *The Johns Hopkins Family Health Book*, which touts itself as 'America's No.1 Medical Authority', makes absolutely no mention of brucellosis in its index (and presumably in the body of the 1800 page text) Drs. Colmenero, *et al.* devote sixteen fact-loaded pages to the disease as they have encountered it in 530 patients they have treated! Where has all the brucellosis gone? The article summarizes the 'signs and symptoms' of patients with brucellosis (Page 200) as follows:

Symptoms	Cases	Signs	Cases
Fever	520	Hepatomegaly	202
Chills	458	Splenomegaly	118
Sweating	450	Adenopathy	48
Constitutional symptoms*	387	Osteoarticular	127
Arthralgias	260	Relative Bradicardia	112
Myalgias	203	Skin lesions	18

Lumbar pain	125	Neurological signs	48
Testicular pain	24		
Epistaxis	12		

*Constitutional symptom = 2 or more of: anorexia, asthenia and malaise.

In addition to this list of generalized symptoms and signs, Colmenero, *et al.* list the following focal forms of brucellosis:

Osteoarticular	Prostatitas	Meningomyeloradiculitis
Spondylitis	**Hepatic**	Spinal arachnoiditis
Monoarthritis	Hepatitis	**Cardiovascular**
Oligoarthritis	Liver abscesses	Endocarditis
Olecranian bursitis	**Neurological**	Pericarditis
Genitourinary	Meningitis	Myocarditis
Orchiepididymitis	Meningoencephalitis	

Given such a protean range of diseases with their signs and symptoms, it is hard to understand how *The Johns Hopkins Family Health Book* editors could omit all references to brucellosis from their text. The only explanation we can offer is that certain of the editors are well aware of the likelihood that various brucella bacteria are phylogenetically antecedent to certain mycoplasmal species and that this relationship must not become generally known and accepted scientifically. In keeping with Dr. Shmuel Razim's expressed hypothesis that…"The theme underlying the current evolutionary scheme of mycoplasmas is that of degenerative evolution from walled bacteria." (Quoted from Maniloff, Page 4), we suggest that a species of brucella bacteria with its capacity to incite the above disease forms with their various signs and symptoms has given rise to a mycoplasma species that carries the same disease potential with it.

Why would the U.S. Government have the audacity to patent such a disease agent? They have one important goal: by having a patent, however frivolous, they essentially erect a barrier, just one of many, to control to a considerable extent, any further research upon the organism. Anyone who wants any funding from the U.S. Public Health Agencies must honor this legal limitation. *Knowledge of and research into the mycoplasmal species is dumbed down.*

1998
Ottenweller, JE, et al.. *"Mouse running activity is lowered by Brucella abortus treatment: A potential Model to study chronic fatigue. Neurobehavioral Unit*, VA Medical Center, East Orange

This important experiment demonstrates the strong likelihood that *Brucella* abortus has an etiological role in the onset of chronic fatigue. This scientific reality is in marked contrast to the nonsense advanced by media assets such as Edward Shorter and Elaine Showalter that CFS/ME is not a real disease. It also supports the concept of a relationship which we have suggested between the nucleic acid of *Brucella* bacteria and the nucleic acid of the *Mycoplasma fermentans* by degenerative evolution has merit.

1999
Huntsville Mystery Illness – Solved, Candace Brown, with the help of Sally Medley and Elizabeth Naugle.

We have reviewed this remarkable document in chapter one. Critical documents found by Ms. Brown and her colleagues and arranged chronologically from 1966 to 1999 trace the testing of mycoplasmal infections on prisoners in the Texas prison system and the consequences of such testing on the community. The document demonstrates what honesty can achieve in exposing the secrecy and evil in high places of the U. S. government. It also ties people like Drs. Chanock, Couch and Castle to the research that went on in the search for biological weapons. Research which ultimately produced AIDS, CFS and much collateral damage, such as the increased incidence of Alzheimer's, Parkinson's, diabetes type one, rheumatoid arthritis and so on.

2000
Andre Picard: **'HIV deniers should be jailed: researcher'**, globeandmail.com Posted 01/05/00

This is a newspaper report and is not peer-reviewed, but we have selected it to demonstrate that the Galileo/Roman Catholic Church dispute about the earth or sun being the center of our galaxy is still alive and well in our world today. The Galileo/Roman Catholic Church dispute was really a case of science (objective observation-based hypotheses) versus authority (claims based upon subjective emotional needs.)

It is unsettling to note that in this case, the accusing 'inquisitorial Cardinal' is Dr. Mark Wainberg, president of the International AIDS Society. Dr. Wainberg, who is also a McGill University researcher (researching what is not specified by Picard) and he is quoted as saying: "If we could succeed and lock a couple of these guys up (the Church locked Galileo up for several months -Ed) I guarantee you the HIV - denier movement would die pretty darn quickly." Just imagine if you are a researcher at McGill looking into the etiology of AIDS and you read some of the careful, peer-reviewed literature that we have been studying and you decide that HIV is not the sole source or even is not a major co-factor in AIDS! Would you dare share your thoughts with Dr. Wainberg?

2005
Garth L. Nicolson, Ph.D., Robert Gan, MB, Ph.D., and Joerg Haier, MD, Ph.D. "Evidence for *Brucella* spp. and *Mycoplasma* spp. Co-Infections in Blood of Chronic Fatigue Syndrome Patients" *Journal of Chronic Fatigue Syndrome*, Vol. 12(2): Pp. 5-17

We started this chapter with a discussion about Brucellosis and we are pleased to include this critical article in our paper trail to AIDS. We will quote from the authors' discussion:

> "In CFS patients we found that multiple co-infections involving *mycoplasma* spp., *C. pneumoniae* and HHV-6 were comm0n, and here we found that some *Mycoplasma* spp. co-infections also involve *Brucella* spp. Thus a common feature of CFS may be the presence of multiple, slow-growing, chronic, intracellular infections. The presence of multiple co-infections in CFS probably play an important role in determining the severity of systemic signs and symptoms found in CF patients. In support of this we found that the severity of signs and symptoms in CFS patients was related to the presence of multiple chronic infections. Since CFS patients that previously tested positive for chronic infections have benefited from therapies directed at their chronic infections, we consider it important that *Brucella* spp. as well as *Mycoplasma* spp. and *C. pneumoniae* infections be carefully considered in the clinical management of CFS."

An Interlude

And 'so it goes…'

And so it goes…if one takes the time and has the interest, one can trace the scientific paper trail from Dr. Robert Huebner and his re-discovery of the mycoplasma and Dr. Bjorn Sigurdsson and his study of retroviruses, to the present, and one can establish clearly that AIDS and CFS and the collateral damage of other neuro/systemic degenerative disease epidemics (ALS; Alzheimer's; Parkinson's; diabetes type one; and so on…) have not emerged from the jungles of Africa, but have emerged from laboratories owned or controlled by the United States Government.

In this brief summary we have noted only three percent of the documents that we have in our files, but space does not permit us to report upon the other 97 percent.

We conclude this review with an article by Celia Farber in *Harper's Magazine* of March 2006, and the Letters to the Editor that were published in the issue of May 2006. Then we present a brief note from the Department of Health, Rhode Island, to the parents of certain school children about…would you believe it…a species of mycoplasma! Finally, we conclude with a warning and a reminder that those who do not learn from history are doomed to re-live it.

End of an Interlude

2006

Celia Farber, *Out of Control; Harper's Magazine*; March, 2006

Ms. Farber's article is not peer-reviewed. If it were peer-reviewed it would never have been published, for the evidence is very clear: if you want to get published or promoted, or even get a job in the first place, in medical science in the U.S. today, then stick with the 'official' paradigm: HIV causes AIDS. Period. Gallo, the liar, says so! Don't say otherwise or you will pay a heavy price. Peer-reviewed articles means that three or so 'authorities' who support the official paradigm, have reviewed what you have written and agree that it is safe to publish it because it does not threaten that paradigm.

Let's take a look at Ms. Farber's article and the letters that it drew.

The article is about a healthy single mother, Joyce Ann Hafford, who became pregnant in 2003. On the basis of one HIV positive test, Ms. Hafford was referred by her doctor to Dr. Edwin Thorpe, a so-called HIV/AIDS specialist who also happened to be an NIH principal investigator.(For a good critique about 'NIH principal investigator's' [P.I.'s] see Nussbaum; 1990) Dr. Thorpe through the University of Tennessee and the St. Jude's Children's Hospital recommended that she enroll in a drug trial sponsored by NIH's Division of AIDS (DAIDS) which Ms. Hafford willingly agreed to do because she wanted to make sure that her baby was protected from any possible health consequences.

We were immediately suspicious because we had, in our tracing of the scientific paper trail to AIDS, run across St. Jude's Children's Research Hospital before. We checked it out and sure enough we learned that *as far back as 1971 St. Jude's had a contract with the Special Virus Cancer Program number NIH- 71 - 2134.* The contract had to do with research into 'Special Animal Leukemia Studies'...And of course, leukemia has figured largely in our research into AIDS.

Then, we were concerned to read that the drugs that this pregnant lady was to be given included nelfinavir and nevirapine. Again red flags went up for we knew from our 2002 edition of *Lippincott's Nursing Drug Guide* that nelfinavir could cause serious adverse effects including anxiety, depression, insomnia, myalgia, dizziness, parethesias, seizures, suicide ideation, diarrhea, nausea, anorexia, vomiting, dyspepsia, liver enzymes elevations, dyspnea, pharyngitis, rhinitis, sinusitis, dermatitis, folliculitis, rash, sweating, urticaria, eye disorders, and sexual dysfunction. As well as put the patient at risk for opportunistic infections. In addition, our very basic Drug Guide told us (under nevirapine) that a rash might be life threatening. Let's repeat that: *a rash might be life threatening.*

Well, within seventy-two hours Ms. Hafford developed a rash... recall from *Lippincott's Drug Guide*, (available to anyone)...a rash can be life threatening...Ms. Hafford called her doctor about the 'life-threatening rash' and she was told to put some hydrocortisone cream on it and to stay in the trial. She did, and she died a month later.

Now, this says an awful lot about AIDS treatment and AIDS research in today's world, even in one of the most scientifically-advanced countries in that world: the United States of America. First off, pregnancy all by itself can produce an HIV positive test result. To treat that one test as final and definitive was a disgrace.Second, no one ever should be put upon such dangerous drugs as nelfinavir and nevirapine without them being fully advised as to the possible dangers. Third, the response of Ms. Hafford's doctor when advised that she had broken out in a terrible rash within seventy-two hours of taking the drug shows a callous lack on interest in the welfare of the patient. We could go on with our review of this terrible tragedy, but, Ms. Hafford's tragic death is only a small blip on the radar screen of AIDS research and treatment and it continues the pattern we have been examining in our research.

The worse is yet to come…and here, according to Ms. Farber, is some of that 'worse'. Ms. Farber writes:

> "By this time, Johns Hopkins AIDS researcher Brooks Jackson had already generated major funding from the NIH to stage a large trial of nevirapine in Kampala, Uganda, where benevolent dictator Yoweri Museveni had opened his country to the lucrative promise of drug research, as well as other kinds of pharmaceutically funded medical research." (Page 42)

Fifteen hundred poor, mostly illiterate, pregnant Ugandan women were to be shot full of the drug that killed Joyce Ann Hafford, with the blessings of a tin pot dictator.

Museveni's actions are in sharp contrast to those of South African President, Thabo Mbeki. Ms. Farber tells us:

> "Because of his concerns about the toxicity of this and other anti-retroviral drugs, President Thabo Mbeki of South Africa was pilloried in the international press as pharmaceutical companies and their well-funded 'activist' ambassadors repeated their mantra about 'life-saving' drugs." (Page 50)

Need we remind you that it was a Centers for Disease Control, later a Johns Hopkins' public health specialist, Donald Henderson who led the American effort to eradicate smallpox from Africa; and, that *Johns Hopkins' Family Health Book* doesn't even mention the mycoplasma…which, as our research demonstrates, is, as an immune suppressor, a the real source of AIDS?

Ms. Farber concludes her article with a brief review of the career of Peter Duesberg, a 'virologist and cancer specialist' at the University of Southern California, who had the courage to challenge the whole

HIV causes AIDS myth. His NIH funding was cut off and he was blackballed in the 'media asset' press...including *Nature*, whose editor Sir John Maddox declared that Duesberg would even be denied the standard scientific 'right of reply' to any articles in the magazine that attacked him! So much for freedom of the press and scientific enquiry.

To conclude with another quotation in Ms. Farber's article:

> "The scientific-medical complex is a $2 trillion industry," says former drug developer Dr. David Rasnick, who now works on nutrition-based AIDS programs in Pretoria, South Africa. "You can buy an awful lot of consensus [that HIV causes AIDS - Ed] for that kind of money." (Page 51)

2006

Letters to the Editor: *Harper's Magazine*, May 2006

Following Ms. Farber's article of March 2006, *Harper's Magazine* published seven letters and added a reply to those letters from Ms. Farber. We will present excerpts of both here and comment upon them against the background of our scientific paper trail to AIDS.

We have already referred to the first letter, which was from Dr. Rebecca Culshaw, who states that "To do the best we can for those affected by AIDS...there urgently needs to be an honest scientific debate." As readers of this book will realize, we have urged for that honest debate...only we would prefer to call it a discussion...for many years. Right from the outset of our studies in 1995, it has been apparent that factions within the U.S. power structure have sought to mask the realities of AIDS, CFS, and certain collateral diseases. We have sought for the truth and we have reported what we have found to date.

Dr. Culshaw also suggests that "...the HIV theory of AIDS begs far more questions than it answers...This debate should have happened long ago (see above: **1987**: Dr. John Seale), before an unproven hypothesis of an immune-destroying retrovirus was thrust upon a vulnerable public, and without being thoroughly critiqued in the scientific literature..."

The next correspondent, Mark A. Bierbaum, PhD, writes: "(my doctor)...agrees with Peter Duesberg regarding the extremely negative, immunosuppressive effects of chronic drug use and malnutrition, and that these are likely important co-factors in AIDS-progression." Again, we agree, but we would add with great emphasis that although both are important, the start has to be where Dr. Robert Huebner started back in the 1940s: with the immune suppressive co-factor of many of the mycoplasma species. Put that defense barrier down and hark, what opportunistic disease agents (including retroviral agents like the visna virus) will follow!

Larry Kramer, an early AIDS victim and activist, has high praise for Dr. Anthony Fauci.

My, oh my. A few years ago Kramer wrote about Fauci as follows: "I called you idiots…now I call you murderers…Yet after three years you have established only a system of waste, chaos, and uselessness… Whose ass are you covering, Tony…? I don't know (though it wouldn't surprise me) if you kept quiet intentionally. I don't know (though it wouldn't surprise me) if you were ordered to keep quiet by higher ups somewhere and you're a good lieutenant, like Adolph Eichmann…"

If Larry Kramer took the time to study the truth about Fauci and the fact that (to quote Bruce Nussbaum, Page 243) "Fauci had spent hundreds of millions of dollars building a drug-testing network that didn't work," he would thank Ms. Farber for the facts she has presented. Facts that our search for the truth compellingly support.

Drs. Richard Marlink and Catherine Wilfert, both of the Elizabeth Glaser Pediatric AIDS Foundation submitted a letter wherein they claim that "Years of careful research have proven beyond a doubt that the HIV virus causes AIDS, that antiretroviral drug treatment saves lives, and that the drug nevirapine is safe and effective in preventing the spread of HIV from mothers to their babies."

The correspondents offer no sources of scientific evidence for these claims, and they ignore much contrary evidence. For example, they ignore the fact that Ms. Farber reported where 561 African women taking **NO** antivirals transmitted HIV at a rate of 12 percent, while the HIV transmission rate for mothers taking nevirapine was 13.1 percent. And is nevirapine safe? The *Lippincott Drug Guide* raises serious doubts about that.

The next letter is the most poignant. It is from Joyce Ann Hafford's sister, Rubbie King who writes: "My sister delivered a baby boy and died three days later from the poison prescribed to her…To the scientists who underreported the deaths in the Uganda Study, the lives of people like my sister meant nothing. She was just another black guinea pig, whose life was reduced to nothing more than an 'oops.'"

Finally, we report that one of the responders to Ms. Farber's article was Dr. Robert Gallo, now Director, Institute of Virology, University of Maryland. Dr. Gallo says many things, but one thing that he said which caught our attention was the following: "That HIV is the single cause of AIDS has been concluded by every single qualified group that has studied the question, including the U.S. National Academy of Sciences; the U.S. Institute of Medicine; the U.S. Institutes of Health; the American Medical Association; the Canadian Centre for Infectious Disease Prevention and Control; the Pasteur Institute; and the World Health Organization."

Any objective and fair-minded reader would have to agree that this is a pretty impressive list. But! Just what is Gallo doing with this list? He is falling back upon 'authority', and he fails to address the objective scientific evidence that suggests that HIV is not the sole cause of AIDS. However, the letter was addressed to Celia Farber, and we'll quote some of her response to it.

Ms. Farber writes: "It is particularly fitting that an article about scientific misconduct should engender a response from Robert Gallo, whose research has been the subject of several devastating investigations, one of which found him guilty of misconduct… Gallo's letter is riddled with assertions of fact that dissolve under careful scrutiny into highly debatable interpretations of ambiguous data…Only carefully designed studies that rigorously test the various hypotheses about AIDS can advance our understanding of this disease. But the suppression and demonization of competing viewpoints, and the refusal to acknowledge mistakes cost lives, will accomplish nothing."

At this point in our study we feel that it is appropriate to quote Robert Gallo when he introduced Peter Duesberg at a scientific gathering back in 1984, before Duesberg released his critique about the possible etiologic origins of AIDS. Gallo said on that occasion: "Peter Duesberg is a man of extraordinary energy and unusual honesty, enormous sense of humour, and a rare critical sense. This critical sense often makes us look twice, then a third time, at a conclusion many of us believed to be foregone."

We will conclude this paper trail to AIDS with a final, important thought. The crux of the AIDS problem is this: Does a much disputed retrovirus 'human immune deficiency virus' (HIV), once called 'lymphadenopathy-associated virus' (LAV) by Dr. Luc Montagnier and 'Human T-cell Leukemia Virus third species' (HTLV-lll) by Dr. Robert Gallo and related to the retrovirus which presents as visna in sheep, act as the sole cause of AIDS in humans or is it (and other pathogenic agents) a co-factor with the mycoplasma?

All the evidence that we have studied in some twelve years of research suggests that the mycoplasma depresses the immune system and allows other pathogens, including the so-called HIV to present as various symptoms, which collectively are diagnosed as AIDS. There are co-factors, period!

However, it is essential for the health powers that be, that the role of the mycoplasma be denied and denigrated in order to cover the tracks of that long period of research which was needed to develop and deploy (to paraphrase Dr. Donald MacArthur of the Pentagon, on June 9, 1969) 'a new microorganism, one which does not naturally exist, and which is refractory to the human immune system upon which we depend to protect us from disease'.

In keeping with this necessary obfuscation of the truth by the U.S. Public Health Agencies and so protect the powers in the shadows who set the tragedy in motion, Dr. Robert Gallo must insist that HIV is the sole cause of AIDS. He does so in his letter to Celia Farber after first quoting some rather garbled and confusing 'facts': "These results alone were sufficient to convince that HIV causes AIDS."

However, back in the late 1980s Gallo had this to say in an article in Discover magazine:

> "...the AIDS retrovirus 'goes into hiding' once it invades the human body. "It remains in the T cell until the cell is kicked into action by another infection. Then the virus comes out of hiding, reproduces and spreads."
>
> (Quoted in Nussbaum, 1990 Page 324)

'Another infection!' That is a co-factor! However, like the politician who finished a speech by saying "And those, ladies and gentlemen, are my principles...and if you don't like them I have others" Robert Gallo is more concerned with enunciating and holding to a political reality rather than a scientific reality.

The truth will not be acknowledged as long as medicine is driven by pharmaceutical company dollars and not by Dr. William Osler's 'facts'.

> "The edifice of medicine reposes entirely upon facts…truth cannot be elicited but from those which have been well and completely observed."
>
> Sir William Osler, *Counsels and Ideals*
> (Quoted in Johnson, 1996)

PART NINE

AS IT MIGHT BE: ON TELLING THE TRUTH

THE ETERNAL STRUGGLE: AUTHORITY VERSUS REASON

Chapter Twenty-Four

THE 9/11 FRAUD

At the conclusion of Chapter 16, Section five above (George W. Bush and the First Gulf War) we stated: "The 'war on terror' all emerges as one colossal lie, beginning with the attacks of September 11 themselves!"

As with most of the world, we were somewhat accepting of the official story that emerged from the September 11, 2001 attacks upon the World Trade Center in New York and the attack upon the Pentagon in Washington. We were also moved by the stories that began to emerge in the days following about a brave band of passengers on United Airlines Flight 93 which had taken off from Newark, New Jersey at 8:42 that morning (just four minutes before the North Tower of the WTC was hit by American Airlines Flight 11 from Boston which, it is claimed, had been hijacked some 45 minutes before.)

There were some things in the news about the attacks that didn't seem to fit, but by-and-large we were too busy with our study of the origins of AIDS to devote the time necessary to track down evidence that would help us to rationalize the conflicting details. Then, we were shocked into a more doubting mode of thinking when we saw the first Canadian showing of The Power Hour's production: '911: In Plane Site.' The occasion was the Sixth Annual Conference of the Common Cause Medical Research Foundation and Joyce Riley, co-host of that radio show with Dave vonKleist, screened the DVD. Several anomalies between the official story and the evidence collected and edited by the DVD's producers were presented in a careful review.

But still we did not devote special time to '9/11' as it had come to be known. We did read all or parts of *The War of Freedom* by Nafeez Ahmed; *Towers of Deception* by Barrie Zwicker; *Debunking 9/11 Myths* by David Dunbar and Brad Reagan; *Flight 93* by Rowland

Morgan; *The 9/11 Commission Report (Authorized Edition)*; and many news stories and magazine articles. But not until July, 2007 did we finally find the time and face the urgent necessity posed by the writing of this book, of trying to re-examine these sources and to plumb the depths of 9/11.

The necessity had arisen from the realization, as we have already stated at various points in this study, which so many of the major tragic events of United States history from 1952 until the First Gulf War seemed to involve the same people and institutions! The record of E. Howard Hunt is one example of a lower echelon participant in many of these criminal events of that era: in Korea he was involved with biological warfare; in Florida he was involved with the Bay of Pigs; in Dallas, he was behind Dealey Plaza on the morning of November 22, 1963. He was a participant in the break-in of the office of Dr. Fielding, the psychiatrist to Daniel Ellsberg; and, finally, he was in charge of the break-in of the Democratic Party offices in the Watergate Hotel. Was E. Howard Hunt present at these scenes of crime while employed by five different employers or were all these events associated with his employer of record: the Central Intelligence Agency? Obviously all of these crimes were linked to the CIA, and that Agency was the secret army of a government in the shadows.

For this study we had to at least consider whether there were such personnel and institutional links between the 9/11 attacks and the operations just cited? We began our review of the evidence but were soon overwhelmed by the volume of unexplained anomalies and the official U.S. Government's resistance to coping with those anomalies. It was obvious that we would have to spend much more time than we had if we were to resolve some of the problems that were evident.

We decided (by necessity) to point out just a few of these anomalies and to leave a further study of these and others to a later time. We would use the bell whether technique that we had employed in our examination of the murder of John F. Kennedy. That is, we would take just one or two of the critical anomalies and see if they could be rationalized in an honest and logical way. If these one or two anomalies could be so rationalized, then we would not feel compelled to look further or to reach any conclusions at this point in time for this study. If, however, the anomalies could not be rationalized we would need to reach and record some reasonable but tentative conclusions as to whether 9/11 was true to the 'official' media asset depiction.

The first major problem that struck us was the fact of Mohamed Atta's movements on September 10, 2001 and September 11, 2001, the day of the attacks. Atta is reputed to be the 'leader' of the hijackers and his movements on the days in question just did not make sense. Therefore, we ask our readers to suspend any memories of Mohamed Atta movements as they may recall them (if they have such memories, for the movements that we focus upon here have been largely ignored by the mainstream media), and to consider carefully and deliberately what those movements were as records show them to have been.

Mohamed Atta's movements on September 10 and September 11

First of all, on September 10, 2001, it is clearly established that Mohamed Atta w as in Boston, Massachusetts.(Keep in mind that on the next day it is purported that he led four other hijackers on to American Airlines Flight 11 at Boston's Logan Airport for a trip to San Francisco, but had seized the plane shortly after take-off at 8:00 am and had flown it southwith pin point accuracy to hit The World Trade Center's (WTC)building number one (The North Tower) at 8:47 a.m.)

That is the official story, yet...on the day in question, September 10, Atta rented a car and (with fellow hi-jackers, Abdulaziz al Omari along) set out to drive north. He drove across the north part of Massachusetts, then across New Hampshire, and finally drove several miles to Portland, Maine. He stayed overnight at Portland, and in the morning he drove his rented car to that city's airport, parked the car and checked his baggage for the flight he was going to take back to Boston's Logan Airport! In other words, he had driven nearly two hundred miles away from his departure point, only to catch a flight back the next morning to Boston. Strange enough in itself, but that is not all there is to puzzle the objective student of the crime.

At the Portland Airport, Atta checked his baggage! And, according to later airport witnesses, he was agitated to learn that he would have to re-check the baggage when he transferred from Flight 5930 (Portland to Boston) to Flight 11 (Boston to San Francisco). Now, keep in mind: he was intending to crash the plane in to the North Tower of the WTC! What possible difference could it make whether he had his luggage routed right through to San Francisco or was re-checked if he and it were to be destroyed with the North Tower of the WTC?

It would make no difference at all!

Or would it? As it turned out, the baggage was to be of critical importance for the framers of the official legend of the crime. (For that …see below!)

However, agitated as he may have been, Atta still caught his flight to Logan Airport in Boston, and is reputed to have then boarded Flight 11 (or did he? Again…see below!) for San Francisco, BUT, his luggage was not transferred, and as a consequence it sat in the baggage handling area until after the Trade Center had been hit and the ever vigilant FBI arrived at Logan to seize and examine the delayed luggage! And what a gold mine of incriminating evidence they found! Even though the baggage, had things gone right, would have been on Flight 11 and would have been lost forever in the subsequent crash and fire, Atta had taken care to pack it with the incriminating evidence! There was a list of 19 hi-jackers! There was a terrorist's manual! It was initially claimed that there was even an airline pilot's uniform, but that claim evaporated when demands to see it were made! Imagine, if you will, that hi-jacker Atta, on his way to blow himself up, was worried that his luggage, packed with incriminating details about his terrorist band would not accompany him.

How was the baggage in question to become so critical? Why, it provided the investigators of '9/11' with a treasure trove of evidence to show that the hi-jacking could be traced back to none other than Osama bin Laden!

And why do we wonder whether Atta actually was aboard Flight 11? Well, there is a rule at Logan Airport in Boston, that transferred luggage is not to be loaded onto a connecting flight, unless the person checking it has first boarded that flight!. If such an individual does not board the flight, neither does his baggage! The evidence demonstrates that Atta did not board Flight 11!

Thus, Atta did not board Flight 11, and so his baggage filled with self-incriminating evidence was available for those who frame the official accounts of such crimes to show to the public through the pliant media!

Now, Atta's strange journey to Portland, Maine can be readily understood in the context of a carefully crafted plot to involve Osama bin Laden and his band of 'terrorists.' The 'official' myth.

There are hundreds more such anomalies, but that doesn't matter. It is not evidence that counts; it is the official media asset version that counts, for it is that version that is broadcast over and over and over until it is part of the accepted wisdom of the race. Don't bother me with the truth; just leave my feel good myths alone. Flight 93 is a prime example.

So, Mohamed Atta and his friends were supposed to have hijacked Flight 11 and flown it into the North Tower of the WTC. How about one of the other hijacked flights of September 11, such as Flight 93 which has had some four or five movies made about it? Movies, which do for 9/11 what *All the President's Men* did for Watergate. It creates a myth that is crap.

Consider: most of the Flight 93 movies end with a group of brave passengers rushing down the aisle of the plane, pushing a trolley or coffee/refreshment dolly to smash in the door to the cockpit and displace the hijackers. You've seen that scene we're sure. Well, consider this excerpt from The 9/11 Commission Report:

> "The hijackers remained at the controls but must have judged that the passengers were only seconds from overcoming them. The airplane headed down; the control wheel was turned hard to the right. The airplane rolled on its back, and one of the hijackers began shouting "Allah is the greatest. Allah is the greatest." With the sounds of the passenger counter-attack continuing, the aircraft plowed into an empty field in Shanksville, Pennsylvania, at 580 miles per hour, about 20 minutes flying time from Washington, D.C.
>
> "Jarrah's objective was to crash his airliner into symbols of the American Republic, the Capitol or the White House. He was defeated by the alerted unarmed passengers of United 93." (Page 14)

Consider, for example, how several films of Flight 93 purport to show that in the final minutes of its flight, a band of brave citizens set out to crash a refreshment dolly into the cockpit door ("Let's roll") and re-take control of the aircraft! Then, consider the fact that the 'black box' data supplied to the 9/11 Commission by the FBI and the Pentagon shows that the plane was upside down when it crashed. Upside down! Picture that…a steel dolly pushed by five or six passengers while flying upside down!

Or, the final point that we will refer to here…the right engine of Flight 93, which supposedly had crashed nose first into the ground near Shanksville, Pa., was found some 1500 yards from the main crash site. The whole plane goes nose-first and upside down into several feet of yielding soil, yet one engine 'bounces' 1,500 yards. How could that be explained? Easily…most likely, Flight 93 was shot down by a heat-seeking missile that struck the right engine, which roared off ahead and to the right of the fuselage and, when the latter plunged upside down into the soft soil, the engine came to earth 1,500 yards away.

Again, consider just what this terrible lie is saying: "The airplane rolled on its back…. with the sounds of the passenger counter-attack continuing…" Remember the dramatic cry of "Let's roll" and the movie shot of the passengers pushing the trolley and running down the aisle? Hold it right there…the plane is on its back! Try pushing a trolley along the ceiling of the plane. And this according to the 'Authorized Edition 'of The 9/11 Commission Report.

The Commission Report is itself a terrible mix of lies with, where they cannot avoid it, some truths. For example, the 'black box' of Flight 93 is extant, and its hard data shows that the plane was on its back. How do you present this fact and then claim that the passengers' counter attack was still in progress? Answer: You don't. You simply present the fact that the plane was upside down, then you tell the lie and back that up with the myth of 'Let's Roll.' Put the latter into a few movies to be broadcast and re-broadcast for years and don't even mention the black box hard data, and it will be the myth that survives.

But how about Atta's September 10 trip to Portland Maine? What does the Commission say about this absolutely nonsensical jaunt? This:

> "No physical, documentary, or analytical evidence provides a convincing explanation of why Atta and Omari drove to Portland Maine, from Boston on the morning of September

10, only to return to Logan on Flight 5930 on the morning of September 11." (Page 451)

The Commission has to say something about Atta's jaunt, after all there is the rental car in Portland, and there are pictures of Atta at the Portland Airport with the date of September 11 on them, and there are receipts of various kinds, and the only reason that he could possibly have had was to make sure that his luggage containing the evidence tracking the whole crime back to Osama bin Laden survived his Flight 11 crash into the North Tower. The only way Atta could achieve that end was to go to Portland, check the luggage, and fly back to Boston. But the Commission says nothing about this likelihood.

So here are just two of the hundreds of anomalies of 9/11. There are many more which we must leave until we have finished this study of the origin of AIDS, and have completed our study of 9/11, but we have seen enough to make it possible to state quite clearly that the whole 9/11 myth is a fraud, committed by President George Bush (who was kept as far away from the actual events of the day as possible because he is too stupid to risk exposing to the public until the 'legend' is well in place) and Vice President Richard Cheney who was actually in charge of the terrible plan and who is devious enough to orchestrate the whole thing while it was unfolding. We will publish our study of 9/11 in about one year's time. In the meanwhile, we must leave it in order to complete our present study of AIDS, with this one thought to keep in mind: where 9/11 caused some 3,000 deaths on that terrible date, AIDS causes some 8,000 deaths per day!

PRESIDENT GEORGE W. BUSH AND $30 BILLION FOR AIDS

To control Health is to control Death…And make Money

On May 31, 2007, President George W. Bush, as reported in the *Globe and Mail* of June 1st, asked the U.S. Congress to double the country's financial commitment to combat AIDS globally, particularly in Africa, to $30-billion over five years.

Paul Zeitz, executive director of the advocacy group Global AIDS Alliance, said Mr. Bush's announcement reaffirms U.S. support to the global fight against AIDS. "We hope that it will leverage other wealthy governments in Europe, like Germany and France, and the U.K. to match the U.S. contribution."

The money, reports Will Dunham of the Reuters News Service, is to provide drugs to treat people infected with the human immunodeficiency virus that causes AIDS and to support prevention efforts as set out in the U.S. President's Emergency Plan for AIDS Relief or PEPFAR Mr. Dunham doesn't say so, but PEPFAR's principal effort is to persuade the people of Africa to abstain from having premarital sex.

The heading to the press story: "Bush seeks $30-billion for AIDS fight in Africa…First lady will travel to stricken regions" creates good public relations for George Bush, but the program is another example of Kurt Vonnegut's space aliens who communicate by farting and tap dancing. Consider the fact that the money to be paid out under PEPFAR is to be directed primarily to the purchase of expensive drugs manufactured in the United States. Literally nothing will be spent helping the people of the affected countries to develop sources of clean water, or to grow nutritious local foods that strengthen the body's immune system. Also consider the fact that the pharmaceutical industry is noted for its price rigging and profiteering, and be aware of the further fact that the Bush family itself along with others in their financial circles are owners of the industry.

The money will be raised in taxes upon the average American taxpayer, and, if Bush *et al.*l have their way, upon the taxpaying citizens of Europe. In other words, PEPFAR will effectively transfer money from low and average American workers to the hugely wealthy and politically powerful few of the American military/industrial (including pharmaceutical) complex.

Michael Culbert has pointed out:

> "Attempts have been made over the decades to pin down the actual costs of producing the synthetic compounds (*i.e.* the expensive drugs that the African recipients will have to import-Ed.) which now dominate Western medicine. It is understood in market economics that the actual cost of producing an item bears little relationship to the cost of the end product to the consumer, so such figures are often misleading- but by any comparison, the drug business (that

is, the 'legal' drug business is a good one to be in.)
(Culbert, 1997 Page 268)

But an even more critical question is: will the drugs do the victims of AIDS in Africa any good? We dealt with that question in the previous chapter, when we looked at Celia Farber's article in *Harpers Magazine*.

Authority's only control is reason. But to exercise reason in the face of authority is to risk one's being…figuratively or often physically.

However, it is unreasonable to believe after studying the history of biological research over the past six decades and learning of the political maneuvering that both responded to such research and advanced certain aspects of it. And considered against the population control worries of many people in powerful positions that AIDS was a zoonotic disease that passed from non-human primates to human primates accidentally.

It is reasonable to conclude from the evidence based upon verifiable facts, that AIDS was purposefully developed then tested and finally deployed against target populations by the powerful people cited above.

The facts are hard to discover because those engaged in the conspiracy took great care to cover their tracks. The starkest example of such track-covering occurred when CIA Director Richard Helms ordered CIA operative Sidney Gottlieb to shred and burn the records of the CIA-Military programs MKULTRA, MKNAOMI and MKDELTA.

Despite the difficulty in finding the evidence, much of it has come to light and it remains only for those who have seen and considered the crime against humanity constituted by the discovery, development, testing and deployment of AIDS to exercise their best efforts to demonstrate the truth to the world. We have tried to do our part by writing this book, and we look for allies.

THERE ARE MANY BATTLES, BUT ONLY ONE WAR

There have been many cruel battles between the forces of light and the forces of darkness over the history of humankind, and although we recognize this fact, we are limited by space to consider only a few of those crimes committed during the late nineteenth and twentieth centuries.

Among those crimes we must include the invasion and occupation of 'colonies' by various nations, principally European, and the abuse, degradation and murder of the original inhabitants. And, although many of the crimes against the displaced peoples have been tempered by a more humane view of the latter's inherent rights, there are still tragic crimes being committed by the occupying peoples against the descendants of the original occupants.

We must also include among the crimes of darkness, the use of superior technical prowess to enslave others for the economic advantage of the enslaver. Among such enslavers are the owners of plantations who compel the labor of the enslaved; the males of patriarchal societies who dominate, degrade and de-humanize the female gender; the owners of property and industries who use their control of police or private armies by virtue of a disproportionate command of generated wealth to deny workers the right of access to and use of a fair share of that wealth.

The crimes against humanity must also include the crime of war. To achieve control of resources, whether such be oil, land, forests, mines or other wealth-generating assets by shooting, bombing, starving, or enslaving others, regardless of how 'glorious' or 'noble' or patriotic it is depicted, is a crime.

But all of these examples of crimes are merely the current battles between factions of mankind. All of the battles are merely incidents in one war: the war between right and wrong; between good and evil; or, as John F. Kennedy said: "between the forces of darkness and the sources of light." *The war between reason and authority.*

In this study we have looked at many battles in that war, by whichever names you ascribe to the protagonists. The battle of scientists who wittingly discover, develop and deploy disease pathogens to disable or kill designated 'enemies.' The battle of political powers to use their positions to enhance their own lives at the expense of those over whom they exercise such powers. The battle between 'believers' and 'non-believers.'

And we have looked at many victims: the vaccinated Blacks of Africa, the Fore tribe of New Guinea, the prisoners in Huntsville penitentiary, the populists of Iran who were denied their reforms and forced to accept the return of the Shah to the Peacock Throne, John F. Kennedy. Lee Harvey Oswald, the people of Vietnam.

Many battles and many victims, but just one war: the war between reason and authority. We have tried to join that struggle by identifying ourselves with the forces we see as the forces of reason. We have looked for facts, facts, and facts. And we have tried to reason out their relationship to each other, and to formulate hypotheses to explain the consequences of their interaction. If we have missed critical facts or if we have not brought sufficient reason to account for their interrelationship, we welcome being told. And, we look for allies.

Such looking for allies has led us to read and consider many documents and books and articles which we have tried to summarize in this study. And, as we have neared the conclusion of this mile in our travel towards what we believe to be the truth, two recent books by influential people dealing with the struggle between authority and reason have provided us with further insights. The books are *god is not great*, by Christopher Hitchens and *The Assault on Reason* by Al Gore.

Both books were promoted as books on the subject of reason versus authority.

AUTHORITY VERSUS REASON

Christopher Hitchins

We have already referred to Hitchens in this work when we commented upon his earlier book, *The Trial of Henry Kissinger*, wherein he meticulously set out the crimes against humanity that Kissinger had committed when he served both Richard Nixon and Gerald Ford during their presidencies. Although we had been impressed by Hitchens' detailed account of those crimes, we had been disappointed by the fact that he never got around to making the point that Kissinger had patrons in high places who had sponsored him and had employed him, hence, giving him the opportunity to do the evil that he did. We wrote to Hitchens about our concerns, but he never answered our letter.

Later, we realized that perhaps Hitchens didn't know about the Hearings of June 9, 1969, or of the Patent of the Pathogenic

Mycoplasma by Dr. Shyh-Ching Lo or even of NSSM 200 by Henry Kissinger, so we wrote him another letter:

June 6, 2001

Dear Mr. Hitchens:

Reference: The Trial of Henry Kissinger
Thank you for an interesting, authoritative and convincing study of Mr. Kissinger, and the crimes done by him on behalf of his sponsors and patrons in the name of the United States National Security.

"I was disappointed to find no reference to what is probably his and America's greatest crime: the development and deployment of the AIDS pathogen as a response to the world population growth rate."

"I communicated this disappointment on page 28 of our current *Journal of Degenerative Diseases;* a copy of which I enclose for your information."

"Since writing the above response I have come to feel that I have perhaps, done you an injustice. Perhaps you are just not aware of NSSM 200 and the Hearings of June 9, 19699 when Dr. Donald MacArthur of the Pentagon shared the American bioweapons plans with twelve Congressmen. At that meeting MacArthur promised to develop for strategic purposes a "new microorganism, one which does not naturally exist and for which no natural immunity could have been acquired!"

"Please try to read the chronology and if you care to respond we will be very pleased to run your reply in our *Journal*. We will also be publishing a more complete review of your book."

Yours sincerely,
Donald W. Scott, M.A., M.Sc. President

Mr. Hitchens did not reply.

Despite this somewhat negative experience, we thought that it might be worthwhile to read Mr. Hitchens' latest call for reason as opposed to misplaced faith in a divine being; however one conceives of such a 'god'. Here is what we found.

On pages 45 to 49 he advances the following:

> "…a group of Islamic religious figures issued a ruling, or fatwa, that declared the polio vaccine to be a conspiracy by the United States, (and amazingly, the United Nations) against the Muslim faith." (Page 45)

Mr. Hitchins' shock that the United Nations *let al.*one the United States, could be suspected of such chicanery suggests that perhaps someone has informed the Muslims of some of the activities of the CIA and the U.S. military in the realm of bioweapons development over the past six decades as we have demonstrated in these pages, but have failed to share such information with him.

> "Would you care to see my video of the advice given by Cardinal Alfonso Lopez de Trujillo, the vatican's (sic) president of the Pontifical Council for the Family, carefully warning his audience that all condoms are secretly made with many microscopic holes through which the AIDS virus can pass?" (Page 45)

No thanks, Mr. Hitchens. We have quite enough to keep us busy without looking at a video of a high church official seeking to frighten his 'flock' in to conforming with rules of sexual abstinence It's up to each member of that congregation, within the limits placed upon them by earlier indoctrination, to weigh the merits of the Cardinal's claims and abstain from sex or otherwise. Our principal hope would be that if any deign to consider what their religious leaders tell them about the possibility of catching AIDS, which they would perhaps happen upon our research. That goes for Mr. Hitchins, too. Have you weighed any of the facts that we have found during our twelve years of research?

> "…science and medicine…have a tendency to break religion's monopoly…" (Page 47)

Our first response to this claim was "Oh?" It's a pretty broad claim. Then, more deliberatively we had a (brief) discussion of our own religious inclinations, and we agreed that the deeper we looked into the science of life, the more awed we became at its mystery and majesty. Then we discussed Mr. Hitchins' reference to 'religion's monopoly'. Again we asked "Oh?" All religions? Monopoly...who claimed such?

Later, when we discussed the following:

> "Fred Hoyle, an ex-agnostic who became infatuated with the idea of "design" was the Cambridge astronomer who coined the term "big bang". (He came up with that silly phrase, incidentally, as an attempt to discredit what is now the accepted theory of the origins of the universe." (Page 65)

Oh? The accepted theory? Who accepts it? On what grounds? Is it the origin (singular) of the universe or origins (plural)) If the latter, how many origins are there?

However, back to pages 45 to 49. On page 48 Mr. Hitchens tells his readers:

> "A condom is, quite simply, a necessary but not sufficient condition for avoiding the transmission of AIDS All qualified authorities, including those who state that abstinence is even better, are agreed on this."

Again...Oh? Is an appeal to 'authorities' the answer to preventing AIDS transmission? This sounds suspiciously like advocating the reference to authority such as was made when Galileo was challenged about his view as to whether the sun or the earth were at the center of things.

> "...the AIDS virus, which was isolated and became treatable, in a great feat of humane scientific research, very soon after it made its lethal appearance."
>
> (Page 49)

When we read this flat out statement several questions came to mind: 'AIDS virus'? Is there such a virus, Mr. Hitchins? If so, why did Gallo initially call it a 'human T-cell *leukemia* virus' (HTLV-III) and why did Montagnier call it a 'lymphadenopathy-associated virus'

(LAV). Or is it none of the above? All of the above? You refer to 'humane scientific research', Mr. Hitchins. Whom do you have in mind? Gallo the thief? Mahy the liar? Baltimore with his fraudulent scientific reports? Dr. Wouter Basson of South Africa? (See below for more on Dr. Basson) Or are you just trying to support a rhetorical fiction?

In summary, we found Mr. Hitchins to be very readable, but very superficial, not just on the subject of AIDS, but in his general intellectual response to challenges of the mind.

Al Gore

As we began Al Gore's book, *The Assault on Reason* we were greatly heartened by the name of the first chapter: 'The Politics of Fear' where we read such lines as "Fear …has always been an enemy of reason" and "Demagogues have always promised security in return for the surrender of freedom." We thought of all the alarmist reports of 'avian flu' and 'Threat to JFK terminal' and 'If we don't stop terror in Iraq, we'll have to stop it here in America'

However, before reading the whole 300 pages, we turned to the Index and looked under 'acquired immune deficiency syndrome- HIV' much to our disappointment, there was nothing, so we returned to the text itself and began to read. On page 163 we read Mr. Gore's new agenda for coping with threats to national and world security. The threats listed were: (1) the global environmental crisis (2) a looming water crisis (3) terrorism (4) drugs and corruption, and (5) new pandemics like HIV/AIDS.

About threat number five Mr. Gore had this to say:

> "We tend to think of threats to security in terms of war and peace. Yet no one can doubt that the havoc wreaked by HIV/AIDS threatens our safety. The heart of the security agenda is protecting lives—and we now know that the number of people who will die of AIDS in the first decade of the twenty-first century will rival the number that died in all the wars of the twentieth century."

> "When hundreds of people in sub-Saharan Africa are infected every hour of every day; when fifteen million

children have already become orphans, and must be raised by other children when a single disease threatens everything from economic strength to peacekeeping- we clearly face a security threat of the greatest magnitude."

"We should follow a policy of 'forward engagement,' as professor Leon Feurth at George Washington University has advocated, and reestablish a robust role for reason in our analysis of and early engagement with the many strategic opportunities and dangers that we must anticipate in building a safer, more secure, and more civilized world for future generations." (Pp. 163-4)

We welcomed Mr. Gore's wisdom, but before we read further, we turned back to the Index and between 'Acid rain' and 'Adams, John' we inked in 'Acquired Immune deficiency syndrome- AIDS, 163-4' and then returned to the thoughtful and thought-provoking text.

The book is the product of a wise, humane person, and sets forth goals for the similarly wise and humane of the American electorate. But there is one cluster of ideas on pages 259 to 270 that we felt were particularly profound. The ideas and observation therein deal with the Internet.

The Internet

"…it is past time for us to examine our role as citizens in allowing and not preventing the dangerous imbalance that has emerged with the executive branch to dominate our constitutional system and reverse the shocking decay and deregulation of our democracy."

"Fortunately, we now have the means available to us by which the people of America can reestablish a robust connection to a vibrant and open exchange of ideas with one another about all the issues most relevant to the course of our democracy.

The Internet has the potential to revitalize the role played by the people in our constitutional framework."

"…In fact the Internet is perhaps the greatest source of hope for reestablishing an open communications environment in which the conversation of democracy can flourish. It has extremely low entry barriers for individuals. The ideas that individuals contribute are dealt with, in the main, according to the rules of meritocracy of ideas. It is the most interactive medium in history and the one with the greatest potential for connecting individuals to one another and to a universe of knowledge." (Al Gore, 2007 Pp. 259-260)

We must admit that, while holding Mr. Gore's views in high regard, we have not availed ourselves of the Internet until just recently. We have been very busy and greatly pressured tracking down evidence which may or may not be somewhere on the Internet. We couldn't take the time to look when we were occupying our time reading research articles in or from the libraries at Laurentian Hospital and Laurentian University, both in Sudbury, Canada. We were trying to find facts and not opinions. We could savor the latter after we had studied such facts as we could locate. And now that we have marshaled the facts summarized in this text, and have drawn conclusions and formulated hypotheses to explain them, we look for our readers' response, and have subscribed to Internet service. Our email address is: wlcscott@yahoo.ca

Using our new medium of communication, we downloaded two items that we deemed useful to the readers of this book. One article is titled "A Mitochondria-K+ Channel Axis is Suppressed in Cancer and its Normalization Promotes Apoptosis and Inhibits Cancer Growth" by Sebastian Bonnet, *et al.*. The article deals with Dichloroacetate as a possible treatment for cancer.

The other article is by Alan Cantwell, M.D., and is titled "More Evidence HIV Was Made at Fort Detrick." We present a précis of the latter and a comment in the penultimate section of this Chapter. In our study of Dr. Cantwell's article, we noted a reference to his book, *Four Women Against Cancer*. We ordered the book and were startled to note a detail on page 70 that Dr. Cantwell presents which suddenly brought all of our twelve years of research full circle and provided us with the nexus of AIDS and cancer...and by natural extension to CFS/ME, and all of the collateral diseases we have encountered over these years. (See Section 10, below)

DICHLOROACETATE - DCA TWO CANCERS; TWO PROTOCOLS; TWO OUTCOMES

In Volume 7, Issue #2 of the Common Cause Medical Research Foundation's *Journal of Degenerative Diseases*, Fall 2006, we published the following short article:

Two Cancers; Two Protocols; Two Outcomes

In August 2005, when we arrived at our Windsor Conference Centre for the Annual Common Cause Medical Research Foundation Conference, I encountered a very dear friend who had been a member and supporter for several years. To protect her identity, I'll call her Helen.

Helen, who was a fifty plus registered nurse, asked to speak with me privately, and she told me that in June she had been diagnosed with cancer in her left breast. In response to the diagnosis, she had undergone a lumpectomy and also had several sentinel lymph nodes removed. Tests by the Oncolal in Boston and MD Labs in New Jersey confirmed cancer in the lymph nodes and also revealed the presence of a *Mycoplasma fermentans* infection. Helen was advised by her doctor to have more surgery, followed by chemotherapy and radiation.

It was at this point in time that we met in Windsor and Helen shared with me the decision that she had reached. She was not going to have any further surgery, nor was she going to take chemotherapy or radiation. I listened to her with respect and sympathy and told her that it was her call, and that should be based upon her studies of objective scientific literature.

Instead of chemotherapy and radiation, Helen began a regimen of minocycline to combat the Mycoplasma, which Dr. Shyh-Ching Lo of the American Institute of Pathology has shown is a key factor in certain cancers. Helen had also had eight treatments of hyperbaric oxygen, and had experienced dramatically rapid wound recovery from the surgery.

After a 'down' period, Helen's health began to improve, but she developed an allergic reaction to the minocycline and switched to colloidal silver.

This latter treatment may seem weird to many, but those who know the affinity free cyanide has for gold, silver or iron, will understand that if there is an excess of cyanide generated by a Mycoplasmal infection, the uptake and voiding of that cyanide is very therapeutic.

In response to a telephone request from me, Helen faxed me a page and a half summary of her current status.

She is still at work and actually missed minimal time. She concludes with this statement:

> "Through this I have learned you must take your health into your own hands and make decisions based upon sound testing. I believe that had I taken more surgery, radiation and chemo, I would not be here now."

Today her health is good, she is working regularly and continues to thrive…all without further (and recommended) surgery, chemotherapy and radiation.

Shortly after I arrived home from Windsor, my wife, Cecile, gave me some unsettling news, a very dear friend and marvelous person, whom I shall call Sue to keep her identity private, had been diagnosed with breast cancer. Like Helen, Sue is a registered nurse in her fifty's. She is a spirited and strong person and Cecile and I were saddened by her diagnosis.

Like Helen, Sue underwent a lumpectomy and was soon advised to have further surgery and to begin a strong regimen of chemo and radiation.

Now, it is my policy never to push my research or studies upon others. They know what I have been studying, and they know that I have developed some alternative considerations for many health problems. If they want to know my take on their situation, I'll share it, but I'll never push it on them.

Sue never asked for my views and she had further surgery, and then began a long and apparently painful series of chemo treatments and radiation that left her badly burned. She has survived this mainstream medical response and we wish her continued improvement. However, unlike Helen, she has not returned to work and I doubt that she will.

Our love and concern go out to both ladies and to all others who face tough choices.

Two cancers; Two protocols; Two outcomes continued

In January of 2007, while visiting in Vancouver, one of the present authors (DWS) received word that Sue had had a further medical check-up and had been told that her cancer was still present and was progressing rapidly. Further chemotherapy and a heavy radiation regimen were recommended by her doctors. At this point DWS decided to depart from his policy noted above, of not promoting the results of the authors' research, but to leave any action to the patients themselves. So, despite not being asked for any opinion, DWS phoned Sue's husband and suggested that he pick up a copy of the above *Journal* and at least read the article and think about Helen's protocol and the results to date. Sue's husband said that he would get a copy of the *Journal* and read the article, but, he never did.

Instead, Sue went ahead with an apparently excruciating regimen of chemicals and radiation. In February we learned that she and her husband had decided to complement her chemotherapy by taking sodium Dichloroacetate (DCA) and they and we hoped for the best. Our hopes were not to be realized and Sue died.

Everyone who knew Sue loved her very much and her death was very hard to accept. It was made even harder by the knowledge that her last few months of life were filled with great pain from the radiation treatments and the chemotherapy.

The authors of this study were especially saddened because Sue, encouraged by those around her, had opted to follow the advice of the traditional cancer treatment specialists, without even considering evidence of other protocols, which might have been helpful. And, if not helpful, such alternative protocols would at least, like the physician who respects the Oath of Hippocrates, 'have done no harm.'

The alternatives that we suggested should be considered were protocols based upon the 1930s research of Dr. Otto Warburg

(Nobel Laureate 1931) wherein he had demonstrated the critical role of oxygen as a response to cancers. We had been heartened by Helen's use of eleven hyperbaric oxygen treatments as a part of her protocol, and, in view of Sue's great suffering our other studies which demonstrated that the oxygen treatments *"...did not produce any discomfort or pain whatsoever."* (Rilling & Viebahn, 1987 Page 103)

Treading a very narrow path between our desire to share what we had learned since 1995 and the right of Sue and her husband to choose whether to look at our evidence and possibly act upon it, or to continue their faith in the edicts of the cancer establishment, we made available what we could and we respected their decision not to look further.

MEDICINE, MONEY AND HEALTH

About three weeks after the death of Sue an article appeared in the June 2, 2007, *Globe and Mail* titled "No money for a miracle" by Anne McIlroy. The gist of the article is that although the drug Dichloroacetate (DCA) had been demonstrated to be effective in dramatically reducing the size of tumors in rats, and although it has been used for years to treat metabolic disorders in patients suffering from various metabolic disorders such as lactic acidosis, researchers at the University of Alberta were finding it very difficult to raise sufficient money to formally and officially test the drug on humans under controlled supervision by qualified medical doctors and other scientists. The reason that such money is so hard to get is that since it is a very simple drug (it is almost table salt in its simplicity and availability) no pharmaceutical company will put up the necessary money to go through all of the regulatory hoops to get it to market.

In other words, the goal is not to save lives of the many but to generate great wealth for the few.

The Cancer Industry

There is a huge and lucrative industry built up around the human misery inflicted upon victims by cancer, and that industry is well critiqued by Dr. Michael Culbert in chapter eleven of his book, *Medical Armageddon*. Dr. Culbert introduces the subject with some thought-provoking quotations:

> "Although it is shielded from the public by high-minded pronouncements and scientific jargon, the cancer establishment is afflicted with a mental and moral malaise. It is more interested in maintaining the status quo than in finding answers to the cancer riddle, and will defend that status quo against all comers. Its struggle to retain credibility and power may well last decades and cost millions of lives, unless the source of its funding…the taxpaying public… requires reform." Gerald B. Dermer, Ph.D.   (Quoted in Culbert: 1997 Page 411)

> "This 'cancer establishment' pushes highly toxic and expensive drugs patented by major pharmaceutical firms which also have close links to cancer centers. Is it any wonder they refuse to investigate innovative approaches developed outside their own institutions? …We clearly need a complete restructuring of the losing war against cancer. Prevention must get the highest priority…Innovative non-toxic therapies must get independent evaluation." Dr. Samuel Epstein.   (Quoted in Culbert: 1997 Page 411)

Despite the billions of dollars that have been and are being raised annually to 'fight cancer', basically the incidence of the disease and the consequent mortality continues to rise.

But what does the cancer industry have to do with AIDS and a crime that is beyond belief?

Just this: the pharmaceutical industry is as much a part of the military /industrial complex that Eisenhower warned against as he left the presidency in 1960 as are the munitions plants, and warship building yards. Just as the manufacturers of the Stealth bomber and the Joint Strike Fighter profit from their multi-million dollar craft fly from the U.S. to inflict 'shock and awe' upon the citizens of Baghdad and fly back, or their Fighter intimidates members of the Taliban the owners of Pfizer, Eli Lilly and Burroughs Wellcome profit from high priced drugs prescribed by doctors to cancer patients.

> "Lockheed and Martin Marietta merged in 1995 to form Lockheed Martin which has become the largest military contractor in the United States and the largest arms exporting company in the world. …In 2001, it was awarded the world's largest weapons contract to date, a $200 billion deal to build the Joint Strike Fighter…"   (Juhasz, 2006 Page 138)

$200 billion for fighters and $30 billion for AIDS to be spent on American made drugs!

However, the same pharmaceutical companies profit from the high cost patented drugs prescribed for AIDS patients. There is an AIDS industry owned and operated by the same financial powers that build the Stealth bombers. And if George W. Bush sells $30 billion of their expensive drugs to be dispensed by 'charitable' agencies in Africa and paid for by American taxpayers (and by European taxpayers too, if they fail to see through the scheme) he has effectively transferred that money from the taxpaying middle class Americans to the members of the American oligarchy. Members who have all manner of 'tax shelters' and front 'foundations' to keep them from really sharing the load.

The AIDS Industry

AIDS and cancer as subjects of U.S. Public Health Agencies and Pentagon research have deep historic and personnel links. As we have learned from the purportedly 'annual reports' of the variously named Special Virus Programs (Ch. 14), it was at the end of 1964 when the CIA 'Monkey Kidney' - MK - programs ended that a 'Viral Oncology' (VO) Program began. The VO ended as abruptly as it began in 1968, but in 1965 a related Program dedicated to research into leukemia and lymphadenopathy had also sprung into being. Like the VO program, the new Special Virus Leukemia/Lymphoma Program (SVLP) ended in 1968 and both it and VO were replaced by a *Special Virus Cancer Program*.

Elsewhere in this study we noted the broad range of programs dealing with research into pathogenic agents which have one thing in common (they depress the human immune system) but the constant switching of program names make it very hard to track just what was going on. The regular change of program names is an effective technique of obfuscation, but such obfuscation should not be allowed to deter honest people from looking for the truth. So, despite all of the name changes for the programs involved, we have formulated the following chronological hypothesis of events:

1952: Nelson Rockefeller and his population control agenda, joins Eisenhower's administration

1953- 1959: Rockefeller and elements of the Rockefeller apparat work with Allen Dulles of the CIA to launch population control programs based upon mycoplasma grown on monkey kidneys and code named **MKULTRA, MKNAOMI** and **MKDELTA**. Trial vaccine programs launched in certain African countries.

1960- 1963: CIA programs go into a period of muffled activity during administration of anti-eugenics/population control President John F. Kennedy. Vice-President Johnson kept secretly up to date on MK programs, just as he was secretly kept up to date on the real situation in Vietnam

November 22, 1963: President Kennedy assassinated and is succeeded by Johnson who quickly (within three days of the murder) reverses Mr. Kennedy's Vietnam withdrawal plans and starts process to bring the CIA biological programs out of the closet as mainstream Public Health Agency Programs.(NIH, including NCI, and CDC)

1964: MKULTRA and sub-projects becomes VO (Viral Oncology) Program 1965: VO extended in personnel and research activities with establishment of **SVLP**. Vaccination programs in Africa extended under the Agency for International Development. (AID or USAID)

1968: Johnson establishes Population Council with John D. Rockefeller lll and William Cohen of HEW as co-chairmen. Directs CDC in Atlanta to go all out with a 'smallpox eradication' program in Africa. Dr. Donald Henderson (later of Johns Hopkins School of Medicine) placed in charge. Full blown AIDS seeding begun.

1968: Nixon elected President, names Henry Kissinger, a Nelson Rockefeller protégé as National Security Advisor. VO and SVLP consolidated as *Special Virus Cancer Program* (**SVCP**)

1969: June 9, 1969. Knowing what is in the pipeline (*i.e.*: that AIDS will begin to present in Africa in astronomic numbers, Dr. Donald MacArthur of the Pentagon tells Congressional sub-committee that they can have an AIDS agent within ten years. (*i.e.* by 1980) Congress votes $10 million for project.

1971: Annual Report number eight of SVCP (where are the first seven reports?) released. Many of the researchers involved in government sponsored research since the 1953-dawn of the MK programs turns up in its pages! These include the Henles, Huebner, Deinhardt, and Dmochowski. All are now suddenly experts in cancer!

1976: NIH and CDC, knowing that an AIDS epidemic will soon be enveloping Africa, offers a 'free' hepatitis vaccine to Gay males in New York, San Francisco and Los Angeles

1980: HIV positive and AIDS victims beginning to appear in African countries, especially those where 'free smallpox' vaccine programs had been most prevalent.

1980: Ronald Reagan elected President. William Casey new CIA Director. 'Mystery' diseases in epidemic proportions occur in a number of American, British Isles, New Zealand and Canadian locales.

1981: First report of AIDS in American medical literature with Dr. Michael Gottlieb article. Labeled the 'Gay Plague' by *Time* magazine. Growing incidence of AIDS in Africa. Research into the disease and help for the victims worldwide hampered by perceived attitude of mainstream America to a 'life-style' disease. Reagan vows: 'No public money will be spent on AIDS.'

1985: Public money finally begins to flow, but 'research' largely controlled and contained by the National *CANCER* Institute- (NCI) and pharmaceutical response although largely paid by Public Agencies, is placed in the hands of the drug companies and the 'Principal Investigators' approved by NIH. Making money is obviously more important than stopping the disease.

As Michael Culbert astutely noted, in a section of his book titled *The Sorry Saga of AZT*, this approach...'Came from the Cancer Inc. apparatus.'(Culbert, 1997 Page 571)

In other words AIDS Inc. is a division of Cancer Inc. and both have as their principal objective, the making of money...which brings us back to Section Seven of this chapter: Dichloroacetate and 'No money for a miracle.'

The Nexus of the Cancer Industry and the AIDS Industry

By 1996 we had moved from our beginning study of chronic fatigue syndrome to include a study of its 'mirror image', AIDS. In the course of that study we learned of the 1964 Lyndon Johnson establishment and funding of a Viral Oncology (VO) program by the National Cancer Institute. *Then, we learned that in the same year the CIA mystery research programs MKULTRA, MKNAOMI, and MKDELTA, which centered upon a huge range of biological research based upon a species of mycoplasma grown upon monkey kidneys had abruptly been terminated.*

We puzzled over questions such as what had happened to the *mycoplasma* research that had been done to date (1964)? What had happened to the researchers such as Dr. Robert Huebner? But we were sufficiently occupied with all of the information we were already working on to give too much thought to these and other questions.

Among the things that we were already at work upon was the linkage between the mycoplasma that Dr. Huebner had found in naval recruits, and the pleuropneumonia like organism (PPLO) in their adenoids and by extension, to the depression of the immune system that accompanied the PPLO. Hence, we focused upon the program launched in 1965 called the *Special Virus Lymphoma/Leukemia Program* (SVLP) and ignored the VO program of the year before.

However, from time-to-time we came upon references to early cancer research by Dr. Peyton Rous and the latter's discovery that one type of sarcoma cancer in chickens was infectious by way of a virus, which was called the 'Rous cancer virus.' Cancer contagious by way of a virus? Very puzzling, but no answers seemed to have made their way into print. We continued our research from mycoplasma to their uptake of pre-formed sterols, to cellular damage to CFS/ME and AIDS as we have presented in this study.

And sometimes we discussed how it had come about that a mycoplasma based infectious disease that caused the 'spontaneous degeneration' of adenoids in sick naval recruits had slowly become part of the work of the National Cancer Institute! After all, one of the accepted 'truths' of the cancer establishment was that cancer was not contagious.

Then, as we were completing the fourth re-write of this book we received and read Dr. Cantwell's book (above) and *there on page 70 was the nexus of AIDS and cancer and the mycoplasma*. We quote:

> "In 1966 Jackson demonstrated in *Growth* that the Rous virus was actually a filterable virus-sized form of the cancer microbe ('Mycoplasma [PPLO] isolated from Rous sarcoma virus'). In 1970 another of her papers was published in the *Annals of the New York Academy of Science* that demonstrated (by use of spectograms [sic] obtained with the ultraviolet spectogramic [sic] microscope) that the RNA Rous sarcoma agent contained traces of DNA - thus indicating the Rous 'virus' was essentially related to bacteria that Eleanor had consistently isolated from cancer." (Page 70)

We re-read the chapter and noted on page 69 that:

> "Rous never named his RNA chicken sarcoma virus 'a virus', but rather 'a filterable transmissible agent.' Like the germ of cancer, the 'agent' passed through a filter designed to hold back bacteria and cells. His original 1911 paper in *JAMA* is titled 'Transmission of a new malignant growth by means of a cell-free filtrate.'"

The sarcoma 'virus' was not a virus after all; it was a mycoplasma! And the mycoplasma is a particle of bacterial DNA.

The information was logical and could sustain rigorous critical analysis. What microbiologist Eleanor Alexander-Jackson, Ph.D. was saying was just this: a one-celled animal (bacterium) contained within its nucleic acids (among other things) the impulse to grow. That impulse as a fragment of the bacterial DNA (*i.e.* a mycoplasma) sought refuge within any vulnerable cell when its original host was killed, and in that host cell's DNA it (under certain prerequisite conditions such as the presence of a growth hormone) gave expression to its unfettered growth-drive. Cancer!

It was only a fragment; or, as Peyton Rous had called it "a filterable transmissible agent." It was not a virus, also a particle of bacterial nucleic acid, because it had no self-assembled protein protective coat that characterizes viruses. It was cell wall-less. It was a mycoplasma or, as Huebner had called it a PPLO. And Dr. Jackson recognized this, and published her proof for other scientists to study and test.

But that is not what happened. Instead of studying and testing the evidence, someone, somewhere along the line in a position of authority sufficient to stop the theory from gaining the attention and further research that it merited, (*i.e.* they controlled the purse strings and the media) dismissed Dr. Jackson's research proof and for whatever reason, the major media buried it. The 'mycoplasma' that Dr. Jackson had identified became a 'virus' to the NIH and NCI and the mycoplasma disappeared from view. *It disappeared to such an extent that it was not until twelve years after we began our study and research into CFS/ME and AIDS that we learned that as far back as 1966 someone with impeccable scientific credentials had tied the mycoplasma to cancer!*

The reason for burying the mycoplasmal theory of a role in cancer was twofold. First, as we have shown, in 1964 the secret 'MK' programs operated by the CIA and the US military and based upon the mycoplasma research of Dr. Huebner were 'officially' terminated, but had to be carried on under some new and public name by the National Institutes of Health. So, Lyndon Johnson authorized the 1964 creation of a Viral Oncology (VO) program. Note that it was a 'viral' program…not a 'mycoplasma' program. Why? Because the mycoplasma was already recognized for its biowar weapons potential and had to be kept from public view as much as possible. The illegal and illicit work was still going on, but it was hidden in the National Cancer Institute.

How do we know that the mycoplasma research was still going on?

We know that the mycoplasma was the subject of active and ongoing research under the *Special Virus Cancer Program*…the successor to the Viral Oncology program…because on page 255 of the SVCP *Progress Report #8* there is a reference to a "Central Mycoplasma Diagnostic Laboratory" run by Stanford University under a renewed NIH contract number (NIH 69- 2053). In the body of the text about this contract it is revealed that the original contract was awarded seven years earlier…or in 1962! It had begun as a CIA project and had been switched to the NCI in 1964.

The powers in the shadows (*i.e.* in the CIA) had to keep their biological weapons research involving the mycoplasma secret, so the term was replaced by the more innocuous 'virus'.

Another reason for burying the research into the mycoplasma was to be found in the fact that if one addressed the bacterial *cum* mycoplasmal roots of cancer, attention would undoubtedly be directed to stopping cancer with relatively low cost antibiotics and oxygen rather than 'treating' it with expensive on-going pharmaceuticals (chemotherapy) and radiation. (See Section 5 above: Two Cancers; Two Protocols; Two Outcomes)

The final piece of our research puzzle had fitted into place.

SOUTH AFRICA

Dr. James Gear was the director of The South African Institute for Medical Research (SAIMR) in the late 1950s and on. During this period he had somehow come into contact and worked closely with Dr. Hilary Koprowski, first of the Lederle Laboratory that had a long association with the bioweapons research being directed by the U.S. Government through Fort Detrick (Covert, 1997 Page 59) and later with the Wistar Institute. (Ch. 5, above) As director of the SAIMR, Gear was heavily involved with vaccination programs in South Africa and other British colonies in Africa. (Hooper, 1999 Pp. 520-1) Gear organized and directed programs to vaccinate millions of Black Africans against measles, mumps, smallpox, hepatitis and other diseases, who had little or no say in the matter. Their British colonial masters mandated their participation in these programs.

However, under great pressure from most Commonwealth nations, especially Canada, and despite American resistance, South Africa was ostracized and placed under heavy economic sanctions. By 1990, the apartheid government began to cave in and in that year they released the African nationalist leader, Nelson Mandela, after 27 years in prison.More reforms followed and in 1994 the first mixed-race elections were held and Nelson Mandela was elected as the first Black President of South Africa. One of his first moves was to apply for re-admission to the Commonwealth. His application was accepted with deep satisfaction by this unique cluster of nations.

Although the re-admission of South Africa had a symbolic value, Mandela did something far more valuable for the advance of humanity and the triumph of truth. In 1969 he authorized the establishment of a Truth and Reconciliation Commission under the Chairmanship of Anglican Archbishop Desmond Tutu. The Rt. Rev. Tutu had won the Nobel Peace Prize in 1984 for his efforts to achieve the peaceful abolition of apartheid in South Africa, and he and Mandela wanted to purge South Africa of the deep rot of the previous political system without the shedding of retributive blood and the perpetuation of racial hatred. Essentially they said to all of the thousands of White South African functionaries who had spent years under the tutelage of the American CIA and Israeli Mossad bullying, torturing, killing, segregating and experimenting upon Black South Africans: "Tell us what you have been doing all of these years and we will forgive you. Refuse to participate and if it subsequently develops that you engaged in any crimes you will be prosecuted to the limits of the law."

AIDS: The Crime Beyond Belief

Although many of the criminals managed to flee to Britain, Canada, the United States and other sanctuaries, thousands more opted to stay in South Africa and tell their stories. And here is where the political events of South Africa are tied to the crime beyond belief… the development and deployment of the AIDS co-factors among the Black population of South Africa and other nations under British colonial rule such as Kenya and Uganda. The Truth and Reconciliation Commission confirmed much of the evidence about the mind set of those who worked with the CIA and Dr. Koprowski from 1952 until the late 1960s.

During its first months of research into the crimes of the apartheid government, the Truth and Reconciliation Commission (TRC) was busy recruiting staff, establishing rules of order, and other housekeeping activities. However, by the middle of 1998 it began to learn some of the terrible activities of medical and biological experimentation that had gone on for several years.

On July 28, 1998, the TRC had its first major showdown with Dr. Wouter Basson who had been in charge of the 'chemical weapons' research during many of the apartheid years. The 'chemical weapons' work included the biological weapons research organization, just as for the first years of its existence, the biological research of the Pentagon had been carried out as part the U.S. Army Chemical Corps. During his tenure Dr. Basson was known to many in the Black Nationalist movement as Dr. Death.

When called before the TRC, Dr. Basson's lawyer's tried to have their client avoid testifying because he had a constitutional right to remain silent. The judge denied the request, and some of the details of Dr. Basson's work came out in testimony over the next few weeks. The papers around the world reported it as the 'Probe reveals horrors of science gone mad.' Actually, it wasn't science gone mad, it was the science delivered to Dr. Basson and his colleagues in the government and military by the United States CIA. The same science that saw over 500,000 American citizens made test guinea pigs in biological and chemical weapons research over the same period.

The news accounts quoted Archbishop Tutu:

> "Here are people of high intelligence, coldly and clinically in white laboratory coats, working on things they know were meant to be instruments of destroying people."

Among such instruments were disease pathogens that would target Black people, but not White people. Here we draw attention to Chapter 22 of this work, and the research done in 1953 by Dr. Maurice Shepard that demonstrated that 33% of healthy Black males carried a species of mycoplasma as compared to 2% of healthy White males. Hence, in any disease with that species of mycoplasma as a co-factor, Blacks would be fifteen times as likely as Whites to become infected.

> "Any researcher who broke ranks because of doubts about the ethics of his work faced possible assassination, scientist Schalk van Rensburg said Wednesday. "We were told in no uncertain terms, if you let the side down you are dead."

Compare this statement with the large number of American microbiologists who have died violent and unexplained deaths over the years, such as that reported by Rampton and Staubb (1997):

> "On May 7, 1996, tragedy struck another scientist, a professor of neurosciences at the University of California-San Diego.

> Tsunao Saitoh and his 13-year-old daughter were gunned down in front of his home by an unknown assailant. At the time of his murder, Saitoh had just published research documenting his discovery of a 'new amyloid component protein,' (NACP) involved in the development of Alzheimer's disease." (Page 195)

It is also important to note that MKULTRA, the American counterpart to the apartheid program, had an 'executive-action-type assassination.' component. (Richelson, 2001 Page 46)

We cite these details to explain why it might be that few have broken CIA ranks to reveal details of the activities they engaged in while working in the programs cited.

> "Run through front companies, the biological and chemical weapons program was controlled by Dr. Wouter Basson..."

This relationship between the government and the private companies is similar to that which was entered into by Robert Gallo when he melded his National Cancer Institute with Litton Bionetics (Gallo, 1991 Page 36) Such shared arrangements limit the amount of oversight that the government can exercise over the joint activities.

It is against this background that the reader should consider the relationship between Hilary Koprowski and James Gear of the South African Institute for Medical Research and the latter's extensive vaccine programs during that period. Whether there is a relationship or not, it is also important to consider that South Africa now has the highest percentage incidence of AIDS of any country in the world.

RE-BIRTH OF DEMOCRACY

The example of Nelson Mandela as president of South Africa and Archbishop Tutu as Chairman of the Truth and Reconciliation set an example of humanity for the world. Either or both could have urged revenge for all of the years that they and their fellow Black citizens endured the de-humanizing oppression of the apartheid years. Instead, these two great leaders and their colleagues in the struggle, both Black and White, created the situation where the truth could be told, and once told, could be forgiven and a new start made for a democratic state.

If there is one regret that we have, it is that the TRC did not know the horrible extent of the CIA eugenics programs and the development and deployment of the AIDS co-factors. As a consequence, although much of the evil was brought to light, much remains in the dark. It is at this point that we would urge Vice-President Al Gore to extend the agenda that he presents in his book, *The Assault on Reason*, by adding on page 164:

> "Finally, we must recognize that the greatest threat to our security, and indeed to the security of all peoples of the world, may lie in the hidden scientific crimes committed over the last half century of biological weapons research, development and deployment. AIDS, CFS/ME and the mycoplasmal- related diseases that have destroyed millions of lives and stand to destroy millions more, can only be contained when the full story of their development and deployment is known and action is taken to compensate the victims and their families and to advance the health of humanity. To this end we need to establish an International Truth and Reconciliation Commission to learn the full scientific details and turn all of our talents to the undoing of the great damage done."

AIDS: THE LIMITS OF BELIEF/DISBELIEF

We accept the anticipated criticism that the facts that we have found in our twelve years of research into AIDS and CFS/ME will sound beyond belief to the average reader. We also accept the fact that where there were great blanks in the discovered evidence (often because the powers that held the evidence had destroyed huge parts of it) our suggested hypotheses to fill those gaps will be equally beyond belief. We do not ask you to believe what we have come to believe, but rather, that you seek out ours and any other sources you can find, and submit our facts and hypotheses to rigorous examination. Then share those with us so that if we are in error, we may correct those errors and if we are right, then we can unite with you as a new ally in the crusade for truth.

EPILOGUE

On the title page of this book we stated 'One cannot study any major aspect of North American Medicine of this age without concurrently studying economics and politics.'

Over the intervening pages we have attempted to establish our basis for that claim, especially as it applies to that area of North American medicine from 1952 to the present that was involved with the discovery, development and deployment of acquired immune deficiency diseases.

Today, we conclude our study of *AIDS: The Crime Beyond Belief* by quoting in full an editorial from The Toronto *Globe and Mail*, dated July 12, 2007:

> **United States Surgeon-general in fetters:**
>
> A surgeon-general who is not allowed to write or talk about stem cells, secondhand smoke, sex education, prison, mental health, emergency contraception or global issues is not worth much. Richard Carmona, who spent four years as U.S. surgeon-general—"the nation's doctor"—under President George W. Bush, told a congressional committee seeking ways to improve the office that he was muzzled on major issues for political reasons. It's a shame he didn't come forward earlier to say so. But most shameful of all is the White House's apparent willingness to put public health at risk.
>
> Trust and credibility are essential to the role of the surgeon-general- to communicate the best available science on issues affecting the nation's health. (The position has no national counterpart in Canada.) That is no less crucial today than when the job was created in 1873 to oversee the response ti such health threats as yellow fever and tuberculosis. But in practice, the surgeon-general lacks independence. As C. Edward Koop, a previous surgeon-general told the congressional committee, the office holder needs the permission and support of others to issue a

report, hold a news conference or attend a meeting out of town. He said he was discouraged during the Reagan years, from talking about the emerging AIDS crisis; he did so anyway. David Satcher, another surgeon-general, told how, in the Clinton years, he was asked not to release a report on sexual behavior because of Bill Clinton's dalliance with intern Monica Lewinsky.

But these stories paled next to the pressure on Dr. Carmona, a war hero who described himself as "politically naive" when he took the job. He was to mention Mr. Bush's name three times on each page of his speeches. He was discouraged from attending Special Olympics because the event is supported by the Democratic Kennedy family. His report on the dangers of second-hand tobacco smoke was held up for years.

The politics of faith and family values have often trumped science during the Bush years. Forty-eight Nobel laureates and former presidential science advisers signed a petition three years ago calling for scientific integrity to be restored to government policymaking. The nation's doctor needs the freedom to speak fearlessly."

In closing this study, we welcome the support for scientific integrity as expressed editorially by The *Globe and Mail*; however, we ask their editorial decision makers to at least read Chapter Eighteen, Section Four (B) of this book: A brief burst of reality almost spoils 'feel good' parade.'

The *Globe and Mail* is probably the most important daily newspaper in Canada. This newspaper and its 'Public Health Reporter', Mr. Andre Picard, have an obligation to report with scientific integrity to their readers.

Neither is doing their job. They should stop telling the government of the United States what its duties are in respect to their Surgeon-General and start telling the world the truth about AIDS and the mycoplasma.

"And, although devoted philanthropists in appearance to the outside world, the vehicle for Rockefeller political expression throughout the years has been the Republican Party, which was always adamantly opposed to having the government carry on analogous benign activity even with taxpayer consent. All government 'intervention' in the fields of science, medicine, higher education, social uplift, art, individual amelioration has been fought openly or indirectly impeded by the Republican Party. For government to do it on a large and effective scale is bad; for the Rockefellers and other Republicans to do it on a restricted tax-saving scale is good—so they say. For the latter is private—that is, sacred."

"If one looks at the Rockefellers as philanthropists, how does one account for this seeming contradiction? How can tough politics be squared with philanthropic benignity? The point is: it isn't philanthropy and it is tax avoidance and power building." Lundberg (1975), Page 359

The Complete Paradigm of Life:

OIL > WEALTH > ROCKEFELLERS > ESTABLISHMENT > MEDIA CONTROL > POLITICAL POWER > CIA > RESOURCE CONTROL > HIDDEN WARS > AIDS > HOT WARS > TRUTH > RECONCILIATION > MAN AND MAN > MAN AND GOD.

For the fact is that if one enters the complete paradigm of life at any point in the honest search for the reality of anything he will be led to the truth about everything.

APPENDICES

EXHIBIT ONE
Mycoplasma pneumoniae Clinical Manifestation of Infection
Laboratory Test Handbook, Page 488

Respiratory	Pneumonia Pharyngitis Otitis media Bullous myringitis Sinusitis Laryngotracheobronchitis Bronchiolitis Nonspecific upper respiratory symptoms
Neurologic	Meningoencephalitis Encephalitis Transverse myelitis Cranial neuropathy Poliomyelitis-like syndrome Psychosis Cerebral infarction Guillian-Barre syndrome
Cardiac	Pericarditis Myocarditis Complete heart block Congestive heart failure Myocardial infarction
Gastrointestinal	Hepatic dysfunction Pancreatitis
Hematological	Autoimmune hemolytic anemia Bone marrow suppression Thrombocytopenia Disseminated intravascular coagulation
Musculoskeletal	Myalgias Arthralgias Arthritis
Genitourinary	Glomerulonephritis Tubolointerstitial nephritis Tubo-ovarian abscess
Immunologic	Depressed cellular immunity and neutrophils chemo taxis

EXHIBIT TWO

Author's Adenoid Drawing

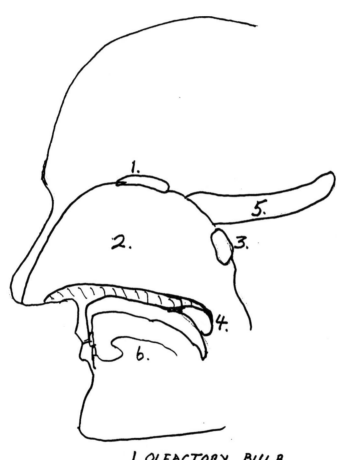

1. OLFACTORY BULB
2. NASAL CAVITY
3. ADENOIDS
4. TONSILS
5. HIPPOCAMPUS
6. TONGUE

EXHIBIT THREE

Micrograph of a *Mycoplasma arthriditis* cell at approximately 120,000 magnification

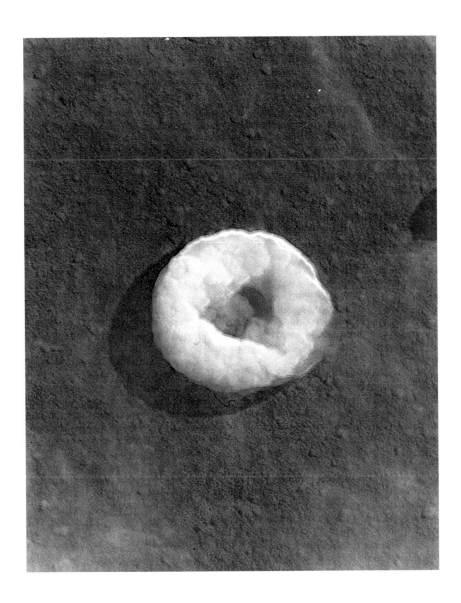

EXHIBIT FOUR

LIFE'S LIES
Exert from article entitled
'Ends to Nagging Rumors: The Six Critical Seconds'
printed in *Life* magazine, December 06, 1963, page 52F

wasn't satisfied and, accordingly, it was a week of breathless rumors: that Oswald had been a hired killer; that Oswald had used an accomplice; that Oswald had not killed the President at all; that Oswald had been framed and then shot to silence him. The rumors grew because the best evidence which could dissolve them, the contents of Oswald's mind, was now irretrievable. But even though the investigations were just under way, there was already enough other evidence on hand to answer some of the hard questions.

Was it really Oswald who shot the President?

Yes. The evidence against him is circumstantial and it received an incredibly bush-league battering around by the Dallas police, but it appears to be positive.

Three shots were fired. Two struck the President, one Governor Connally. All three bullets have been recovered—one, deformed, from the floor of the limousine; one from the stretcher that carried the President; one that entered the President's body. All were fired from the 6.5mm Carcano carbine which Lee Oswald bought by mail last March.

The murder weapon, although subsequently manhandled for the benefit of TV, still showed Oswald's palm print. His own carbine was missing from its usual place. A witness had seen him bring a long, gun-sized package to work. And threads from Oswald's clothing were found in the warehouse sniper's nest.

from an adjoining building. He had put another box off in a corner so he could sit on it and look out the window—again so as not to be seen. Finally, in front of the window he had stacked three boxes as a rest for his carbine. Two big pipes ran vertically along a wall near his window, natural braces for a shoulder. His position while shooting at a car going away to his right would have been comfortable and rock-steady, and Oswald had both the time and the ability to zero in three times.

The description of the President's two wounds by a Dallas doctor who tried to save him have added to the rumors. The doctor said one bullet passed from back to front on the right side of the President's head. But the other, the doctor reported, entered the President's throat from the front and then lodged in his body.

Since by this time the limousine was 50 yards past Oswald and the President's back was turned almost directly to the sniper, it has been hard to understand how the bullet could enter the front of his throat. Hence the recurring guess that there was a second sniper somewhere else. But the 8mm film shows the President turning his body far around to the right as he waves to someone in the crowd. His throat is exposed—toward the sniper's nest—just before he clutches it.

Had authorities been watching Oswald?

They had—but not when it mattered. Oswald first came to the FBI's atten-

EXHIBIT FIVE

Man claims he cured AIDS

Convicted in three countries, 'doctor' to speak in Sudbury

BY DENIS ST. PIERRE
The Sudbury Star

A convicted criminal who has spent several years in prison and who has promoted alleged cures for AIDS, cancer and other diseases, will be a guest speaker at an alternative medical research conference in Sudbury.

Basil Earle Wainwright is scheduled to deliver a lecture at the Conference on Human and Social Health Crises, to be held Nov. 17-19 at a downtown hotel. The conference is sponsored by the Common Cause Medical Research Foundation.

The Common Cause foundation, created by retired Sudbury teacher Donald Scott, promotes research that is distinctly outside and often attacked by mainstream scientific circles.

The foundation suggests there is a common cause behind many diseases and that governments and the scientific establishment dismiss and even cover up such evidence.

In an interview, Scott said he was not aware of Wainwright's criminal past, which includes jail terms in Great Britain and the United States. Scott suggested Wainwright, 72, is among the "world leaders" in AIDS research and treatment, but he has been unfairly attacked by critics.

"There has been a really conscious effort to blacken his name," he said.

Wainwright has had dramatic success in treating AIDS and other diseases, Scott said.

"He has had a great deal of success with an ozone apheresis machine," he said. "It takes blood out of an arm, for six seconds total and exposes it to ozone, which kills the micro-organisms immediately and puts it back into the blood."

Wainwright has demonstrated that, "people with AIDS, who tested positive for HIV/AIDS, after a few weeks of his treatment ... they had no symptoms and no measure of HIV," Scott said.

Those results have been verified by the Common Cause Foundation, which has reviewed "vast amounts" of documents provided by Wainwright to validate his claims, Scott said.

___

> "There has been a really conscious effort to blacken his name."
>
> **Don Scott**

___

"He sent us about 30 pounds of records," he said. "I know his science is credible. It's very solid science."

However, government authorities on at least three continents have had significantly different views of Wainwright and his various endeavours for more than three decades.

News reports indicate Wainwright's legal troubles date back at least to the early 1980s in his native Great Britain, where he was convicted and jailed for numerous counts of theft, fraud and forgery.

Stated the judge in that case: "I am satisfied — and so is the jury — that you are thoroughly dishonest."

In 1985, after being released from jail, Wainwright pleaded guilty to another fraud charge in Britain.

In 1990, by which time he was living in the United States, Wainwright was imprisoned for four years on charges of fraudulently holding himself out as a doctor, reported The Independent newspaper of London, as well as other media.

While in custody on those offences, Wainwright formed a new scheme for treating blood with ozone to kill AIDS and hepatitis viruses, the U.S. Food and Drug Administration reported.

Wainwright pleaded no contest to the charges related to that scheme and was sentenced to five years in prison, the FDA said. He served 18 months and was released in the spring of 1992.

The FDA investigation found Wainwright had been selling unapproved ozone generators "as a cure for serious illnesses such as cancer and AIDS."

The scheme "swindled investors and desperate patients out of hundreds of thousands of dollars," the FDA said.

Victims of the scheme were found in several states and "at least three patients who bought the so-called 'cure' died," the agency said.

An FDA officer described Wainwright as a "career criminal, who has spent almost his entire adult life perpetrating frauds and left a trail of human misery in his wake."

Among other things, Wainwright encouraged individuals to use his ozone machines to "self-administer ozone through the rectum or vagina," using tubes and needles, the FDA said.

Wainwright has operated a number of companies over the years. The websites of some of his companies have suggested he is a three-time nominee for the Nobel Prize for Medicine and that his apheresis treatment reverses HIV and cures diseases such as cancer, tumours, hepatitis, tuberculosis, multiple sclerosis and pneumonia.

dstpierre@thesudburystar.com

BIBLIOGRAPHY

SECONDARY SOURCES

Agee, Philip: *CIA Diary*, Middlesex, England: Penguin Books (1975)
Agee, Philip and Louis Wolf: *Dirty Work*, Secaucus, NJ (1978)
Ahmed, Nafeez Mossaddeq: *The War on Freedom*, Joshua Tree, CA; Tree of Life Publications (2002)
Albright, Madeleine: *Madam Secretary—A Memoir*, New York; Hyperion Press (2003)
Ambrose, Stephen E.: *Eisenhower (Volume Two) The President*, New York; Simon and Schuster (1984)
Anderson, Jack (with James Boyd): *Fiasco*, New York; The New York Times Book Co., (1983)
Apple, R. W.: *The Watergate Hearings*, New York; New York Times / Bantam Books (1973)
Avirgan, Tony and Martha Honey: *La Penca: on Trial in Costa Rica*, Costa Rica; Editorial Porvenir (1987)
Barnes-Svarney, Patricia: *Science Desk Book*, New York; A Stonesong Press Book Macmillan (1995)
Bellett, Gerald: *Age of Secrets*, Maitland, Ontario; Voyageur North America (1995)
Bird, Kai: *The Chairman*, New York; Simon & Schuster (1992)
Blitzer, Wolf: *Territory of Lies*, New York; Harper Paperbacks (1989)
Blum, Deborah: *The Monkey Wars*, New York; Oxford University Press (1994)
Blum, William: *Killing Hope: U.S. Military and C.I.A. Interventions since World War II*, Monroe, Maine Common Courage Press (2004)
Blum, William: *Rogue State*, 3rd. Ed. Monroe, ME; Common Courage Press (2005)
Bowart, W. H.: *Operation Mind Control*, New York; A Dell Book (1978)
Brendon, Piers: *Ike: His Life and Times*, New York; Harper & Row Publishers (1986)
Bryden, John: *Best - Kept Secret*, Toronto; Lester Publishing (1993)
Brodie, Fawn M.: *Richard Nixon: The Shaping of His Character*, New York; W. W.Norton & Company (1981)

Bundy, McGeorge: *Danger and Survival*, New York; Vintage Books/A Division of Random House, Inc. (1990)
Campbell, Rodney: *The Luciano Project*, New York; McGraw-Hill Book Company (1977)
Cantwell Jr., Alan: *Queer Blood: The Secret AIDS Genocide Plot*, Los Angeles; Aries Rising Press (1993)
Cantwell Jr., Alan: *AIDS and the Doctors of Death: An Inquiry into the Origin of the AIDS Epidemic*, Los Angeles; Aries Rising Press (1988)
Carroll, Michael C.: *Lab 257*, New York; HarperCollins (2004)
Caute, David: *The Great Fear*, New York; Simon & Schuster (1978)
Chernow, Ron: *The Warburgs*, New York; Random House (1993)
Chester, Lewis, et al: *Watergate*, New York; Ballantine Books (1973)
Clark, Harold W.: *Why Arthritis? Searching for the Cause and the Cure of Rheumatoid Disease*, Tampa, FL; Axelrod Publishing (1997)
Collier, Peter and David Horowitz: *The Rockefellers*, New Jersey; New American Library (1977)
Colodny, Len & Gettlin, Robert: *Silent Coup: The Removal of a President*, New York; St. Martin's Press (1991)
Conn, Rex B.: *Current Diagnosis 8*, Philadelphia; W.B. Saunders Company (1991)
Cook, Fred J.: *The Warfare State*, New York; The Macmillan Company (1962)
Covert, Norman M.: *Cutting Edge*, Frederick, MD; Public Affairs Office U.S. Army (1997)
Cuddy, Dennis Laurence: *September 11 Prior Knowledge: Waiting for the Next Shoe to Drop*, Oklahoma City; Hearthstone Publishing, Ltd. (2002)
Culbert, Michael: *Medical Armageddon*, San Diego, CA; C and C Communications (1997)
D'Adesky, Anne-Christine: *Moving Mountains: The Race to Treat Global AIDS*; London, New York; Verso (2004)
Dean, John W.: *Blind Ambition: The Whitehouse Years*, New York; Simon & Schuster (1976)
Dean, John W.: *Lost Honor*, New York; Stratford Press (1982)
Di Eugenio, James: *Destiny Betrayed: JFK, Cuba and the Garrison Case*, New York; Sheridan Square Press (1992)

Duffy, James R.: *Conspiracy: Who Killed JFK?* New York; Shaposky Publishers, Inc. (1992)
Duncan, Kirsty: Hunting the 1918 *Flu*, Toronto; University of Toronto Press (2003)
Ehrlichman, John: *Witness to Power, The Nixon Years*, New York; Simon & Schuster (1982)
Ellsberg, Daniel: *Papers on the War*, New York; Pocket Books (1972)
Emery, Fred: *Watergate: The Corruption of American Politics and the Fall of Richard Nixon*, New York; Simon & Schuster (1994)
Endicott, Stephen and Edward Hagerman: *The United States and Biological Warfare*, Bloomington and Indianapolis, IN; Indiana University Press (1998)
Epstein, Edward Jay: *Legend: The Secret World of Lee Harvey Oswald*, Reader's Digest Press (1978)
Ehrlichman, John: *Witness to Power: The Nixon Years*, New York; Simon and Schuster (1982)
Ewing, Michael and Bernard Fensterwald, Jr.: *Assassination of JFK*, New York; Zebra Books (1977)
Fox, Michael J.: *Lucky Man A Memoir*, New York; Hyperion (2002)
Friedman, Alan: *Spider's Web: The secret history of how the White House illegally armed Iraq*, New York; Bantam Books (1993)
Geballe, Shelley, Gruendel, Janice and Andiman, Warren: *Forgotten Children of the AIDS Epidemic*, New Haven; Yale University Press (1995)
Galbraith, John Kenneth: *Annals of an Abiding Liberal*, Boston; Houghton Mifflin Company (1979)
Galbraith, John Kenneth: *A Life in our Times*, Boston; Houghton Mifflin Company (1981)
Gallo, Robert: *Virus Hunting*, A New Republic Book / Basic Books (1991)
Garrison, Jim: *On the Trail of the Assassins*, New York; Warner Books (1988)
Gibson, Donald: *Battling Wall Street*, New York; Sheridan Square Press. (1994)
Gill, Anton: *An Honourable Defeat*, New York; Henry Holt and Company (1994)
Greig, Charlotte: *Conspiracy: History's Greatest Plots, Collusions and Cover-Ups*, London; Arcturius Publishing Limited (2007)

Groden, Robert J.: *The Killing of a President*, New York; Viking Studio Books (1993)

Groden, Robert J.: *The Search for Lee Harvey Oswald*, New York; Penguin Studio Books (1995)

Grose, Peter: *Gentleman Spy*, Boston New York; Houghton Mifflin (1994)

Goulden, Joseph C.: *Fit to Print*, New Jersey; Lyle Stuart Inc (1988)

Guthman, Edwin O. and Shulman, Jeffrey (Eds.): *Robert Kennedy In His Own Words*, New York; Bantam Books (1988)

Haig, Jr., Alexander M.: *Caveat: Realism, Reagan, and Foreign Policy*, New York; Macmillan Publishing Co. (1984)

Halberstam, David: *The Powers That Be*, New York; Alfred A. Knopf (1979)

Haldeman, H. R.: *The Haldeman Diaries: Inside the Nixon Whitehouse*, New York; G. P. Putnam's Sons (1994)

Haslam, Edward T.: *Mary, Ferrie & the Monkey Virus*, Albuquerque, New Mexico; Wordsworth Communications (1995)

Hepburn, James: *Farewell America*, Frontiers Publishing (1968)

Hitchens, Christopher: *The Trial of Henry Kissinger*, London / New York; Verso (2001)

Ho, Mae-Wan and Burcher, Sam and Veljkovic, Veljko: *Unraveling AIDS: The Independent Science and Promising Alternative Therapies*, Ridgefield, CT; Vital Health Publishing (2005)

Hoffman, Paul: *Spiro!* New York; Tower Publications (1971)

Hooper, Edward: *The River*, New York; Little, Brown and Company (1999)

Hoopes, Townsend and Brinkley, Douglas: *Driven Patriot*, New York; Alfred A. Knopf (1992)

Horowitz, Leonard: *Emerging Viruses: AIDS and Ebola*, Rockport, MA; Tetrahedron Press (1997)

Horowitz, Leonard: *Death in the Air*, Sandpoint, Idaho; Tetrahedron Press (2001)

Hougan, Jim: *Secret Agenda: Watergate, Deep Throat and the CIA*, New York; Random House (1984)

Hougan, Jim: *Spooks*, New York; William Morrow and Company, Inc. (1978)

Hulse, Virgil: *Mad Cows and Milk Gate*, Phoenix, OR; Marble Mountain Publishing (1996)

Humphrey, George: *Uncommon Sense, Your Choice: The Blue pill or the Red Pill?* (2002)

Humphreys, Margaret: *Yellow Fever and the South*, Baltimore and London; The Johns Hopkins University Press (1992)

Hung, Nguyen Tien and Jerrold L. Schecter: *The Palace File*, New York; Harper & Row (1986)

Hurt, Henry: *Reasonable Doubt: An Investigation into the Assassination of John F. Kennedy*, New York; Holt, Rinehart and Winston (1985)

Hyde, Byron Marshall: *The Clinical and Scientific Basis of Myalgic Encephalomyelitis Chronic Fatigue Syndrome*, Ottawa, ON; The Nightingale Research Foundation (1992)

Irvine, Reed and Kincaid, Cliff: *Profiles of Deception: How The News Media Are Deceiving The American People*, Smithtown, NY; Book Distributors, Inc. (1990)

Isaacson, Walter: *Kissinger*, New York; Simon & Schuster (1992)

Jacobs, David S.; Kasten, Jr., Bernard L.; DeMott, Wayne R.; Wolfson, William L.: *Laboratory Test Handbook*, Cleveland, OH; Lexi-Comp Inc. (1988)

Johnson, Hillary: *Osler's Web*, New York; Random House (1996)

Johnson, Lady Bird: *A White House Diary*, New York; Dell Publishing Co., Inc. (1970)

Johnson, Lyndon Baines: *The Vantage Point*, New York; Popular Library (1971)

Juhasz, Antonia: *The Bush Agenda: Invading the World One Economy at a Time*, New York; HarperCollins (2006)

Kalb, Marvin and Bernard Kalb: *Kissinger*, Boston - Toronto; Little, Brown and Company (1974)

Kantor, Seth: *The Ruby Cover-up*, New York; Zebra Books (1978)

Karnow, Stanley: *Vietnam... A History*, New York; Vietnam (1983)

Kolata, Gina: *Flu*, New York; Simon & Schuster (1999)

Kutler, Stanley I.: *Abuse of Power: The New Nixon Tapes*, New York; The Free Press (1997)

Land, Serge: *Challenges*, New York; Springer-Verlag (1998)

Leigh, David: *The Wilson Plot*, New York; Pantheon Books (1988)

Leonard, Jerry: *AIDS: The "Perfect" Disease*, 1st Books Library (2002)

Leonard, Jerry: *The Perfect Assassin: Lee Harvey Oswald, The CIA and Mind Control*, Harrisburg, NC; Winston Smith Publishing (2002)

Livingstone, Harrison Edward: *Killing Kennedy and the Hoax of the Century*, New York; Carroll & Graf Publishers, Inc. (1995)

Lundberg, Ferdinand: *The Rich and the Super-Rich*, New York; Bantam Books (1968)

Lundberg, Ferdinand: *The Rockefeller Syndrome*, New Jersey; Lyle Stuart Inc. (1975)

Magruder, Jeb Stuart: *An American Life*, New York; Pocket Books (1975)

Mangold, Tom: *Cold Warrior: James Jesus Angleton: The CIA's Master Spy Hunter*, New York; Simon & Schuster (1991)

Maniloff, Jack: *Mycoplasmas*, Washington, D.C.; American Society for Microbiology (1992)

Mankiewicz, Frank: *U.S. vs. Richard M. Nixon*, New York; Ballantine Books (1975)

Martin, Al: *The Conspirators, Secrets of an Iran-Contra Insider*, Pray, Montana; National Liberty Press (2002)

Martin, Ralph G.: *Henry and Clare: An Intimate Portrait of the Luces*, New York; G. P. Putnam's Sons (1991)

Marsa, Linda: *Prescription for Profits*, New York; Scribner (1997)

McMillan, Priscilla J.: *The Ruin of J. Oppenheimer and the Birth of the Modern Arms Race*, New York; Penguin Books Ltd. (2005)

Melanson, Philip H.: *The Martin Luther King Assassination*, New York; Shapolsky Publishers, Inc. (1991)

Miller, Judith and Engelberg, Stephen and Broad, William: *Germs: Biological Weapons and America's Secret War*, New York; Simon & Schuster (2002)

Miller, Merle: *Plain Speaking*, New York; Berkley Books (1974)

Monteith, Stanley: *The Unnecessary Epidemic: America Under Siege*, Sevierville, TN; Covenant House Books (1991)

Morgan, Rowland: *Flight 93 Revealed: What really happened on the 9/11 "Let's Roll" flight?* New York; Carroll & Graf Publishers (2006)

Morris, Roger: *Haig: The General's Progress*, Playboy Press (1982)

Morrow, Robert D.: *Betrayal*, New York; Warner Books (1976)

Neustadt, Richard E.: *Presidential Power: The Politics of Leadership*, New York; John Wiley & Sons, Inc. (1960)

Newman, John: *Oswald and the CIA*, New York; Carroll & Graf Publishers, Inc. (1995)

Newman, John M.: *JFK and Vietnam*, New York; Warner Books (1992)

Nicolson, Garth and Nancy: *Project Day Lily: An American Biological Warfare Tragedy*, Xlibris (2005)

North, Mark: *Act of Treason: The Role of J. Edgar Hoover in the Assassination of President Kennedy*, New York; Carroll & Graf Publishers, Inc. (1991)

North - Broome, Nicholas: *The Nixon - Hughes "Loan"*, New York; APAI Books (1972)

Nussbaum, Bruce: *Good Intentions*, New York; The Atlantic Monthly Press (1990)

Nusslein-Volhard, Christianne: *Coming to Life - How Genes Drive Development*, Kales Press (2006)

Panno, Joseph: *Stem Cell Research*, New York; Facts on File, Inc. (2005)

Panno, Joseph: *Gene Therapy*, New York; Facts on File, Inc. (2005)

Parson, Ann B.: *The Proteus Effect*, Washington, D.C.; Joseph Henry Press (2004)

Penrose, Barrie and Roger Courtiour: *The Pencourt File*, New York; Harper & Row, Publishers (1978)

Pinchot, Roy (Editor): *The Human Body - Blood: The River of Life*, New York; Torstar Books, Inc. (1985)

Piper, Michael Collins: *Final Judgment*, Washington, D.C.; The Wolfe Press (1993)

Prouty, L. Fletcher: *JFK*, New York; Carol Publishing Group (1992)

Quirk, John Patrick: *The Central Intelligence Agency*, Guilford, Connecticut; Foreign Intelligence Press (1986)

Reed, Terry and John Cummings: *Compromised: Clinton, Bush and the CIA*, New York; S.P.I. / Shapolsky Publishers, Inc. (1994)

Reeves, Richard: *President Kennedy Profile of Power*, New York; Simon & Schuster (1993)

Richelson, Jeffery T.: *The Wizards of Langley*, Boulder, CO; Westview Press (2001)

Risen, James: *State of War: The Secret History of the CIA and the Bush Administration*, New York; Free Press (2006)

Roberts, Paul William: *A War Against Truth*, Vancouver, B.C.; Raincoast Books (2004)

Rosenberg, Steven A.: *The Transformed Cell - Unlocking the Mysteries of Cancer*, New York; G. P. Putnam's Sons (1992)
Russell, Dick: *The Man Who Knew Too Much*, New York; Carroll & Graf Publishers/ Richard Gallen (1992)
Safire, William: *Before the Fall*, New York; Ballantyne Books (1977)
Sampson, Anthony: *The Seven Sisters*, New York; Bantam Books (1976)
Sayer, Ian and Douglas Botting: *Nazi Gold*, London; Granada Publishing Ltd. (1985)
Schlafly, Phyllis and Chester Ward: *Kissinger on the Couch*, New Rochelle, N.Y. (1975)
Schlesinger, Arthur M. Jr.: *A Thousand Days*, Boston; Houghton Mifflin Company (1965)
Schoenebaum, Eleanora W.: *Profiles of an Era*, New York and London; Harcourt Brace Jovanovich (1979)
Schorr, Daniel: *Clearing the Air*, Boston; Houghton Mifflin Company (1977)
Schrodinger, Erwin: *What is Life? The Physical Aspect of the Living Cell*, London; Cambridge University Press (2001)
Scott, Donald W. and William L.C. Scott: *Life: From Plants to Animals to Us*, Sudbury, Canada; The Chelmsford Publishers (2005)
Scott, Peter Dale: *Deep Politics and the Death of JFK*, Berkeley; University of California Press (1993)
Scott, Peter Dale: *Crime and Cover-up*, Santa Barbara, CA; Open Archive Press (1977)
Shar, Erik & Novak, Viveca: *Inside the Wire*, New York; The Penguin Press (2005)
Sheehan, Neil: *A Bright and Shining Lie*, New York; Random House (1988)
Shilts, Randy: *And the Band Played On: Politics, People and the AIDS Epidemic*, New York; St. Martin's Press (1987)
Shorter, Edward: *From Paralysis to Fatigue*, New York; The Free Press (1992)
Shorter, Edward: *The Health Century*, New York; Doubleday (1987)
Simpson, Christopher: *Blowback*, New York; Weidenfeld and Nicolson (1988)
Sirica, John J.: *To Set the Record Straight*, New York; W.W. Norton & Company (1979)

Sklar, Holly (Ed): *Trilateralism: The Trilateral Commission and Elite Planning for World Management*, Boston; South End Press (1980)
Sloan, Bill with Hill, Jean: *JFK The Last Dissenting Witness*, Gretna, LA; Pelican Publishing Company (1992)
Snead, Eva Lee: *Some call it "AIDS" I call it murder!*, San Antonio, TX; AUM Publications (1992)
Stratton, Allan: *Chanda's Secrets*, Toronto + New York + Vancouver; Annick Press (2004)
Summers, Anthony: *Conspiracy*, New York; McGraw-Hill Book Company (1980)
Swanberg, W. A.: *Luce and His Empire*, New York; Charles Scribner's Sons (1972)
Tanaka, Yuki: *Hidden Horrors*, Boulder, Colorado; Westview Press (1998)
Taylor, L. B. and C.L. Taylor: *Chemical and Biological Warfare*, New York; Franklin Watts; An Impact Book (1985)
Teicher, Howard & Teicher Gayle Radley: *Twin Pillars to Desert Storm*, New York; William Morrow & Company, Inc. (1993)
Thomas, William: *Bringing the War Home*, Anchorage, Alaska; Earthpulse Press (1998)
Thornley, Kerry: *The Dreadlock Recollections*, Manuscript (c. 1988-1989)
Timmerman, Kenneth R.: *The Death Lobby: How the West Armed Iraq*, Boston; Houghton Mifflin Company (1991)
Turner, Stansfield: *Secrecy and Democracy; The CIA in Transition*, Boston; Houghton Mifflin Company (1985)
Vestal, Bud: *Jerry Ford, Up Close: An Investigative Biography*, New York; Coward, McCann and Geoghegan (1974)
Weberman, Alan J. & Canfield, Michael: *Coup D'etat in America: The CIA and the Assassination of John F. Kennedy*, San Francisco; Quick American Archives (1992)
Weinberg, Robert A.: *One Renegade Cell - How Cancer Begins*, New York; Basic Books (1998)
Weinberg, Robert A.: *Racing to the Beginning of the Road*, New York; Harmony Books (1996)
Weisberg, Harold: *Frame-up; The Martin Luther King / James Earl Ray Case*, New York; Outerbridge & Dienstfrey (1971)

Weisberg, Harold: *Selections from Whitewash*, New York; Carroll & Graf Publishers / Richard Gallen (1994)
White, Theodore H.: *Breach of Faith*, New York; A Dell Book (1976)
Wills, Garry: *The Kennedy Imprisonment, A Meditation on Power*, Boston/ Toronto; Little, Brown and Company (1981)
Wright, Lawrence: *The Looming Tower - Al-Qaeda and the Road to 9/11*, New York; Alfred A. Knopf (2006)
Zwicker, Barrie: *Towers of Deception - The Media Cover-up of 9/11*, Gabriola Island, BC; New Society Publishers (2006)

PRIMARY SOURCES A

Articles reporting critical research

We are indebted to the compilation in a single loose-leaf volume of several of these articles by Ms. Sue Oleksyn of Rochester, New York, and to Ms. Shirley Bentley, also of Rochester, for several of the most critical of these articles. We also acknowledge our debt to John Scott, for drawing our attention to the extremely valuable article by Burroughs and Edelson: "*Medical Care of the HIV-Infected Child*"

Ben-Menachem, Gil; Rottem, Shlomo; Tarshis, Mark; Barash, Varda; Brenner, Talma: *Mycoplasma fermentans Glycolipid Triggers Inflammatory Response in Rat Astrocytes*, Elsevier Science (1998) Pp. 34-38

Burroughs, Margaret H., MD, and Paul J. Edelson, MD: *Medical Care of the HIV-Infected Child*, Pediatric Clinics of North America - Vol. 38, No. 1, Feb. 1991. Pp. 45-67

Colmenero, J. D.; Reguera, J. M.; Martos, F.; Sanchez-de-Mora, D.; Delgado, M.; Causse, M.; Martin-Farfan, A.; Juarez, C.: *Complications Associated with Brucella melitensis Infection: A Study of 530 Cases*, Medicine 1996 Vol. 75, No. 4 Pp. 195-211

Crewdson, John: *In Gallo case, truth termed a casualty*: Report: Science Subverted in AIDS Dispute; Chicago Tribune, January 1, 1995

Fu, Michael; Wong, K. S.; Lam, Wynnie W. M.; Wong, Gary W.K.: *Middle cerebral artery occlusion after recent Mycoplasma pneumoniae infection*, Journal of Neurological Sciences 157 (1998) Pp. 113-115

Hayflick, L. et al: *Mycoplasma pneumoniae: Proposed Nomenclature for Atypical Pneumonia Organism (Eaton Agent)*, Science Volume 140, Page 662

Hayflick, L.; Koprowski, H.: *Direct Agar Isolation of Mycoplasmas from Human Leukaemic Bone Marrow*, Nature February 13, 1965 Pp. 713-714

Levine, P.H., Ablashi, D.V., Berard, C.W., Carbone, P.P., Waggoner, D.E., and Malan, L.: *Cancer* 27: 416 - 421, 1971

Memorandum by Dr. John Seale, Royal Society of Medicine: Third Report from the Social Services Committee (Session 1986-87), *Problems Associated with AIDS*, London, Her Majesty's Stationery Office, May 13, 1987

Nasralla, M.; Haier, J.; Nicolson, G. L.: *Multiple Mycoplasmal Infections Detected in Blood of Patients with Chronic Fatigue Syndrome and/or Fibromyalgia Syndrome*, Eur J. Clinical Infectious Disease; Vol. 18: Pp. 859-856, Spring (1999)

Nishimura, M.; Saida, T.; Kuroki, S.; Kawabata, T.; Obayashi, H.; Saida, K.; Uchiyama, T.: *Post-infectious encephalitis with anti-galactocerebroside antibody subsequent to Mycoplasma pneumoniae infection*, Journal of Neurological Sciences 140 (1996) Pp. 91-95

Paton, G. R.; Jacobs, J. P.; Perkins, Dr. F. T.: *Chromosome changes in Human Diploid-cell Cultures Infected with Mycoplasma*, Nature July 3, 1965 Pp. 43-45

Pearce, Jane L.; Luke, Richard K. J.; Bettleheim, Karl A.: *Sudden Infant Death Syndrome: What Questions Should we Ask?* FEMS Immunology and Medical Microbiology, Vol. 25 (1999) Pp. 7-10

Rottem, S; Pfendt, E.A.; Hayflick, L.: *Sterol Requirements of T-Strain Mycoplasmas*, Journal of Bacteriology, January 1971 Pp. 323-330

Rowe, Wallace P.; Seal, Captain MC USN John R.; Huebner, Robert J.; Whiteside, Comdr. MC USN, Woolridge, Robert L.; Turner, Horace C.: *A Study of the Role of Adenoviruses in Acute Respiratory Infections in a Navy Recruit Population*, Am. Journal of Hygiene 1956, Volume 64 Pp. 211-219

The RT Hon The Lord of Berwick - Chairman, *Independent Public Inquiry on Gulf War Illnesses*; Published by The Lloyd Inquiry, United Kingdom, November 17, 2004

Vernon, Suzanne D.; Unger, Elizabeth R.; Dimulescu, Irina M.; Mangalathu, Rajeevan; Reeves, William C.: *Utility of the blood for gene expression profiling and biomarker discovery in chronic fatigue syndrome*, Disease Markers 18 (2002) Pp. 193-199

Vojdani, A.; Choppa, P. C.; Tagle, C.; Andrin, R.; Samimi, B.; Lapp, C.W.: *Detection of Mycoplasma genus and Mycoplasma fermentans by PCR in Patients with Chronic Fatigue Syndrome*, FEMS Immunology and Medical Microbiology, Vol. 22 (1998) Pp. 355-365

Williamson, M. E.: *"Lethal reticuloproliferative disease induced in Cebus albifrons monkeys by Herpes virus saimiri."* Int. J. Cancer 06-431 (1970)

Yirmiya, Raz; Weidenfeld, Joseph; Barak, Ohr; Avitsur, Ronit; Pollak, Yehuda; Gallily, Ruth; Wohlman, Avital; Ovadia, Haim; Ben-hur, Tamir: *The Role of Brain Cytokines in Mediating the Behavioral and Neuroendocrine Effects of Intracerebal Mycoplasma fermentans*, Brain Research 829 (1999) Pp. 28-28

PRIMARY SOURCES B

United States Government Documents

Special Virus Cancer Program, Progress Report # 8; U. S. Department of Health, Education, and Welfare, National Institutes of Health, July 1971

Special Virus Cancer Program, Progress Report # 9; U.S. Department of Health, Education, and Welfare, National Institutes of Health, August 1972

The Virus Cancer Program, Progress report # 10; U.S. Department of Health, Education, and Welfare, National Institutes of Health, July 1973

The Virus Cancer Program, Progress Report # 13, U.S. Department of Health, Education, and Welfare, National Institutes of Health, August 1976

The Virus Cancer Program, Progress Report # 14, U.S. Department of Health, Education, and Welfare, National Institutes of Health, June 1977

Project MKULTRA, the CIA's Program of Research in Behavioral Modification, Joint Hearing before the Select Committee on Intelligence and the Subcommittee on Health and Scientific Research of the Committee on Human Resources, United States Senate, Ninety-Fifth Congress, August 3, 1977

United States Patent # 5,242,820; *Pathogenic Mycoplasma*, Inventor, Dr. Shyh-Ching Lo, American Registry of Pathology, Washington, D.C.; September 7, 1993

Staff Report to U.S. Senator Donald W. Riegle, Jr.; *Gulf War Syndrome: The Case For Multiple Origin Mixed Chemical/Biotoxin Warfare Related Disorders*, September 9, 1993

United States Dual-Use Exports to Iraq and Their Impact on the Health of the Persian Gulf War Veterans, *Hearing before the Committee on Banking, Housing, and Urban Affairs*; United States Senate, One Hundred Third Congress, U.S. Government Printing Office, Washington, D.C.; May 25, 1994

Department of Defense Appropriations for 1970, *Hearings before a Subcommittee of the Committee on Appropriations*; House of Representatives Ninety-First Congress, June 9, 1969

National Security Study Memorandum 200 (NSSM 200): *Implications of Worldwide Population Growth for U.S. Security and Oversea Interests*, Henry A. Kissinger, December 10, 1974

Investigation of the Institutional Response to the HIV Blood Test Patent Dispute and Related Matters, Subcommittee on Oversight and Investigations, Committee on Energy and Commerce, U.S. House of Representatives

Isaiah 40

28 Hast thou not known? Hast thou not heard, that the everlasting God, the Lord, the Creator of the ends of the earth, fainteth not, neither is weary? There is no searching of his understanding.

29 He giveth power to the faint; and to them that have no might he increaseth strength.

30 Even the youths shall faint and be weary, and the young men shall utterly fall.

31 But they that wait upon the Lord shall renew their strength; they shall mount up with wings as eagles; they shall run, and not be weary; and they shall walk, and not faint.

1 Timothy 6
10 For the love of money is the root of all evil; which while some coveted after, they have erred from the faith, and pierced themselves through with many sorrows.
11 But thou, O man of God, flee these things; and follow after righteousness, godliness, faith, love, patience, meekness.
12 Fight the good fight of faith, and lay hold on eternal life, whereunto thou art called, and hath professed a good profession before many witnesses.

INDEX

A

Ablashi, Dharam 109, 239, 241, 449
A Bright and Shining Lie 69, 642
Acquired Immunodeficiency Syndrome 4, 271
Adenoids 393
AIDS i, ii, v, vi, ix–xiv, xviii–xxi, xxiii–xxvii, xxix, xxx, 3–15, 18–28, 34, 35, 37–39, 41–43, 45, 46, 48–52, 56, 61, 66, 67, 71, 74, 76, 78, 79, 81, 82, 87, 88, 90–92, 94, 96, 97, 99, 103, 105, 108–111, 113, 117–119, 124–128, 132, 133, 141–143, 198, 207, 209–212, 215, 217, 220, 228, 229, 231, 234, 235, 237, 239–243, 246, 253, 255, 259, 260–278, 286, 290, 302–304, 306–308, 310, 313, 322, 323, 337, 338, 343, 344, 346, 347, 349, 350, 354, 372, 377–379, 382–384, 386, 388, 392, 393, 399, 402, 407–409, 411–432, 434, 435, 439–441, 443, 444, 455–458, 460, 467–475, 477, 481, 484, 485, 489–493, 495, 500, 501, 507, 509, 510, 512–526, 530–536, 538–547, 550, 551, 554–564, 566, 567, 569, 570, 572–580, 585, 591–593, 596–600, 602, 606–612, 614, 616, 617, 621–623, 636–639, 642–645
Akureyri 95, 447, 533, 535, 549
Albright, Madeleine 340, 342
Aldrich, Senator Nelson W. 55
Aldrich, Winthrop 63
Alzheimer's disease 10, 42, 83, 307, 322, 348, 349, 392, 393, 395, 520, 616
American Caesar 35, 284
American Cyanamid 76, 102, 243, 542
American Institute of Pathology xxvi, 424, 428, 431, 520, 602
Amyloid 398
An Honourable Defeat 139, 637
Ash, Roy L. 76–78, 242, 243, 261–263, 555, 559
avian flu 56, 430, 468–470, 476, 478, 481–485, 489, 490, 494, 495, 500–503, 599
AZT 569, 609

B

bacterium 8, 43, 54, 83, 93, 394, 451, 484–490, 526, 527, 531, 544, 611

Baghdad 196, 218, 308, 311, 313, 326, 327, 332, 606
Baker, Marion 139, 140, 151, 166, 171, 172, 176, 179, 181, 189, 199, 204, 217
Baltimore, David 25, 475
Barnes, Tracy xi, 61, 136, 207, 212–214, 287, 465
Bawden, Jim 196
Baylor College of Medicine ix, 53, 66, 474, 476, 491, 493, 501, 502, 556
Bay of Pigs 47, 60, 61, 73, 135, 141, 185, 212, 214, 219, 262, 280, 281, 286, 288, 291, 360, 466, 586
Belgium Congo 14, 34, 58, 71, 517, 533, 548
Belin, David 194, 199
Bell, Karen xiii, 446, 450, 451
Belleville 80, 228, 392, 487
Ben-Gurion 136, 137
Bentley, Shirley xiv, 511, 521, 644
Bethesda Naval Hospital 191, 195
Bissell, Richard 72, 73, 135, 213, 214, 282
Blackwell Corporation 58
Blum, William 66, 67, 271, 433, 435
Boggs, Hale 202, 219
Brooks Air Force Base 242, 556
Brucellosis iii, 337, 446, 451, 525, 526– 528, 530, 573
Bundy, McGeorge 134, 138, 214, 464, 465
Burnet, Frank 34, 108, 118, 125, 441, 509, 542
Burroughs, Dr. Margaret 56
Bush, George W. xiv, 258, 311, 340, 341, 343, 423, 585, 591, 607, 621

C

Caldwell, Dr. Harvey 22, 417
Camp Lindi 71, 72, 104, 108, 109, 112, 117, 118, 126, 517, 533, 548, 562
Canada ii, xi, xvii, xxix, 64, 80, 81, 123, 207, 214, 215, 223, 228, 229, 259, 275, 308, 314, 319, 321, 331, 332–334, 336–339, 345, 347, 348, 350, 352, 353, 355, 356, 359, 370, 388, 408, 420, 430, 432, 435, 467, 471, 487, 501, 518, 536, 565, 601, 613, 614, 621, 622, 642
Canada Packers Limited xvii
Canadian Broadcasting Corporation 196, 353, 496

Cancer xi, xiii, xiv, 31, 41, 53, 76, 87, 88, 91, 97, 100, 108, 126, 142, 209, 210, 233–238, 240, 243–245, 247, 263, 273, 349, 381, 387, 388, 407, 413, 419, 433, 439, 449, 469, 500, 511–515, 517, 522, 526, 536, 541, 544, 545, 552–554, 558, 560–563, 575, 601, 605, 607–612, 616, 642, 643, 645, 646

Carr, David 79, 81, 111, 116, 230, 458, 534

Carter, Jimmy xii, 25, 64, 299, 300, 301, 304, 511, 563, 566

Castro, Fidel 73, 140, 199, 281, 359, 360

C.D.C xxv

Centers for Disease Control xxv, 4, 116, 119, 227, 240, 242, 267, 273, 384, 385, 388, 469, 470, 474, 477, 480, 510, 534, 576

Central Intelligence Agency ii, ix, x, xi, 8, 46, 47, 48, 49, 58, 60, 64, 66, 101, 128, 135, 254, 263, 279, 287, 291, 297, 303, 313, 516, 522, 586, 641

CFS ix, xiii, xix, xxiv, xxv, xxvi, xxvii, 9, 11, 18, 21, 22, 23, 24, 26, 41, 43, 49, 90, 96, 97, 105, 108, 109, 110, 113, 128, 212, 215, 229, 231, 235, 237, 239, 241, 242, 253, 261, 307, 323, 330, 331, 337, 343, 348, 349, 350, 351, 377–379, 384, 385, 386, 388, 393–395, 407, 408, 416, 430, 431, 434, 435, 439, 440, 443, 444, 446, 449–453, 457, 460, 467, 468, 470, 472–474, 477, 481, 495, 501, 510, 519, 521, 524, 526, 527, 553, 561–565, 572–574, 577, 602, 610, 612, 617

Challenges 24, 244, 481, 513, 639

Chambers, Whittaker 61, 69

Chase Bank 62

Cheney, Paul xiii, 446, 448

China 30, 48, 61, 115, 116, 135, 212, 260, 303, 413

Chrétien, Rt. Hon. Jean 81

Churchill, Winston 45, 361

CIA ii, ix, xii, xxvi, xxvii, 25, 26, 47, 48, 49, 57–61, 64–69, 72–76, 78, 79, 82, 101, 103, 115–117, 120, 127, 128, 134–136, 138–140, 143, 146, 147, 177–179, 187, 199, 202, 203, 209, 212, 219, 221, 222, 230, 233, 236, 243, 245–247, 251, 252, 254, 259–263, 267, 275, 276, 279–282, 285, 286, 288, 291–294, 297–310, 313, 314, 344, 346, 354–357, 359, 360–363, 365, 366, 368, 371, 372, 378, 413, 445, 455, 457, 465, 468, 501, 502,
514, 516, 534, 544, 551, 563, 566, 569, 586, 593, 597, 607–610, 612–617, 623, 635, 638–641, 643, 647

Clark, Ramsey 195, 196, 218

Clinton, William (Bill) Jefferson 124, 154, 340, 341, 342, 368, 421–425, 622

Common Cause Medical Research Foundation 24, 337, 345, 418, 421, 430, 435, 448, 450, 485, 501, 511, 585, 602

Connally, John 154, 171, 194

Conn's Current Diagnosis #8 4

Cook, Major Timothy xii, 82, 319

Council on Foreign Relations 48, 63, 68, 116, 461

Courtois, Ghislain 72, 117, 118, 127, 541

Coxiella burnetii 509

Creutzfeldt-Jakob disease 38, 39, 499

Crohn's-colitis 83

Cuba x, 47, 49, 72, 73, 75, 196, 212, 258, 280, 281, 302, 339, 359, 360, 636

Cytometrics Laboratory of San Diego 23

D

Dallas x, 19, 36, 60, 131, 134, 138–140, 145, 148, 150, 151, 153, 154, 162–164, 166–169, 171–173, 175, 177, 179, 181, 183–190, 192, 193, 195–197, 208, 212, 214, 217, 282, 288, 308, 361, 465, 586

Dealey Plaza 36, 60, 145, 146, 148, 149, 151, 162, 163, 166, 168, 171–179, 185, 186, 190, 192, 193, 198, 199, 212, 214, 217, 280, 282, 288, 459, 586

DeFreitas, Elaine xiii, 239, 242, 450, 451

deoxyribonucleic acid 24, 43, 481, 488

de The, Guy 387

diabetes type one xix, xx, xxvi, 83, 274, 557, 572, 574

Dillon, C. Douglas 63

Dinkin, Eugene 137

DNA 24, 27, 43, 54, 90, 92, 100, 126, 382, 383, 387, 401, 469, 481, 482, 485–488, 490, 491, 512, 553, 560, 561, 611

Dominion Parasite Laboratory 80, 228, 487, 501

Duesberg, Peter 51, 576, 577, 579

Dulles, Allen 47, 53, 60, 61, 64, 66, 67, 69, 72, 73, 75, 76, 135–139, 202, 213, 214, 219, 222, 233, 278, 281, 282, 355, 514, 516, 532, 608

E

Eaton, Monroe Davis 9, 490
Einosuke, Hirano 30
Eisenhower, Dwight D. xxix, 20, 24, 45, 82, 262, 268, 510, 532
Ellsberg, Daniel 60, 212, 586
Emerging Viruses...AIDS and Ebola 25, 31, 244, 246, 407, 417, 440, 472, 513, 519, 566
Enders, John 35, 37, 536, 544
England , xxvi, 79, 215, 306, 336, 418–420, 426, 518, 528, 533, 545, 635

F

Fauci, Anthony 578
FBI xi, 135, 138, 140, 146, 177–180, 183, 187, 192, 193, 208, 243, 250, 286, 297, 354, 462, 465, 534, 588, 590
Federal Bureau of Investigation 135, 249, 262
Federal Reserve 55
Flexner, Simon 56
Flu xiii, 467, 473, 474, 477, 478, 489, 491–493, 496, 501, 510, 637, 639
Ford, Gerald xii, 161, 170, 194, 202, 203, 219, 255, 259, 286, 294, 295, 297, 299, 304, 356, 360, 362, 496, 514, 537, 595
Fore Tribe 29
Forrestal, James 63, 355
Fort Detrick 3, 40, 74, 102, 142, 143, 235, 305, 455, 522, 524, 538, 601, 613
Fortune 510
France 6, 12, 69, 70, 115, 137, 215, 270, 275, 290, 291, 293, 310, 355, 471, 484, 518, 522, 592
Friedland, G. H 4, 6
From Paralysis to Fatigue 22, 385, 497, 510, 642

G

Gajdusek, Dr. D. Carleton ix, 24, 31, 33–35, 37–39, 42, 46, 108, 238, 322, 349, 377, 391, 395, 398, 400, 447, 491, 520, 524, 532, 542, 544, 562
Galbraith, Kenneth 61, 69, 288
Gallo, Robert xiii, xxv, 12, 25, 28, 34, 38, 43, 49, 52, 76, 79, 87, 88, 94, 95, 97, 99, 105, 142, 209, 238, 239, 241–244, 261, 263, 269, 270, 273, 276–380, 383, 388, 422, 475, 494, 512, 514, 515, 522, 533, 539, 547, 554–556, 559, 560, 579, 580, 616
Garrison, Jim 195, 199, 207, 214
Gibbs, C. Joseph 238
Gill, Anton 139, 466
Gonda, Mathew 12
Goodsell, David 44
Gottlieb, Dr. Michael xxvi, 518, 609
Gottlieb, Dr. Sidney 25, 300, 301, 544, 563
Great Britain xxix, 64, 115, 116, 215, 259, 275, 308, 439, 467, 470, 471, 499, 566
Griffin, G. Edward 243
Guatemala x, 47, 68, 73, 74, 75, 141, 280

H

Harper's Magazine 5, 259, 373, 574, 577
Hayflick, Leonard xxvi, 65, 103, 382, 522, 533, 552, 555
Health, Education and Welfare 39, 57, 236, 515, 516, 536, 542, 549, 553
Helms, CIA Director Richard 25, 64, 233, 300, 301, 303, 304, 593
Henderson, Donald 228, 237, 267, 277, 381, 477, 559, 576, 608
Henle, Gertrude 104, 107, 109, 110, 112, 536, 552, 561
Henle, Werner 108, 509, 524, 533, 552
Hidden Horrors 238, 643
Hilleman, Maurice 97
HIV xix, 5–8, 12–14, 24, 27, 28, 30, 50–52, 56, 79, 81, 87, 109, 117, 119, 120, 121, 126, 129, 241, 270, 346–349, 352, 377, 408–412, 414–420, 422, 424–426, 441, 455, 477, 489, 492, 510, 513, 518, 534, 535, 540, 541, 568–570, 572–575, 577–580, 599, 601, 609
Ho, David 408, 409
Hoffa, Jimmy 135, 140, 460

Hooper, Edward xiii, xxv, 24, 52, 79, 104, 108–111, 455, 507
Hoover, J. Edgar xi, 138, 140, 158, 159, 169, 178, 201, 218, 219, 262, 297, 462, 641
Hopkins, Johns 56, 74, 195, 474, 482, 489, 500, 504, 525, 527, 530, 534, 570, 571, 576, 608, 639
Horowitz, Dr. Leonard 25, 31, 242, 272, 471
Houston 53, 66, 152, 166, 171, 173–178, 493
Huebner, Robert x, xxv, xxx, 3, 8, 9, 19, 38, 43, 65, 75, 76, 81, 87, 92, 95, 99, 109, 240, 241, 244, 262–264, 273, 379, 381, 393, 479, 490, 494, 512, 514, 516, 517, 519, 522, 524, 526, 545, 554, 556–568, 574, 578, 610
Hughes, Howard 77, 161, 262
human immunodeficiency virus 12, 13, 27, 28, 79, 489, 510, 592
Hunt, E. Howard xi, xii, 36, 60, 61, 72, 136, 138, 177, 179, 207, 212–214, 278–283, 285–289, 586
Huntsville Mystery Illness 519, 520, 572
Hussein, Saddam 196, 218, 308, 310–312, 314, 316, 318, 341, 342
Hyams, Captain 'Craig' 334

I

I Came to Kill 61
Iceland 65, 94, 95, 96, 98, 126, 143, 230, 447, 467, 533–535, 549
Institute of Experimental Pathology xxx, 65, 94, 97
Iraq 49, 82, 196, 212, 308, 310, 311, 313–318, 326, 332, 335, 341–343, 464, 471, 599, 637, 643, 647
Israel xi, xxix, 136, 137, 139, 215, 259, 292, 310, 467, 518

J

Japan 29, 30, 31, 33, 45, 115, 396, 464, 471
Jenkins, Walter 158, 201, 218
JFK and Vietnam 69, 641
Johns Hopkins Family Health Book 56, 489, 504, 525, 527, 530, 570, 571
Johnson, Hillary xiii, xxiv, xxv, 21, 22, 107, 108, 110, 234, 240, 268, 407, 440, 443, 446, 447, 451, 453
Johnson, Lyndon B. xxx, 38, 55, 74, 88, 158, 199, 230, 234, 236, 237, 552
Joint Chiefs xi, 10, 34, 136, 139, 283, 286, 307, 378

K

Kaposi's sarcoma xix, 6, 19, 23, 65, 91, 95, 269, 270
Karnow, Stanley 69
Kennedy, John F. xi, xxx, 19, 20, 34–36, 55, 61, 73–75, 82, 117, 127, 131, 134, 136, 137, 145, 147, 150, 151, 171, 180, 182, 186, 190, 199, 207, 210–212, 221, 222, 230, 234, 236, 242, 260–262, 273, 276, 281, 282, 284–288, 293, 300, 301, 307, 308, 340, 344, 359, 360, 373, 439, 440, 459, 460, 462, 463, 529, 534, 548, 554, 556, 558, 586, 594, 595, 608, 639, 643
Kenya 72, 115, 434, 614
Khomeini, Ayatollah 68, 310
Kibuchi's Disease 432, 520, 567
Kingston xiii, 80, 392, 453, 487, 536
Kissinger, Henry xii, xxvii, 34, 79, 108, 125, 128, 231, 242, 250, 251, 253–263, 267, 273, 276, 285, 293, 346, 355, 356, 358, 362, 363, 366, 367, 372, 373, 400, 417, 441, 471, 500, 517, 524, 534, 537, 562, 595, 596, 608, 638
Koch, Robert 13
Kolata, Gina 66, 211, 430, 469, 472, 473, 474, 477, 478, 482, 485, 489, 491, 492, 494, 496, 497, 510
Koprowski, Hilary x, xxv, 34, 37, 38, 71, 97, 99, 102, 105, 108–111, 117, 118, 125, 126, 241, 264, 304, 377, 451, 522, 532, 533, 543, 544, 546, 552, 561, 613, 616
KS 65
Kuru 31, 34, 39, 41, 238, 395, 401, 402, 542

L

Laden, Osama Bin 67
Landon, Dr. John 244
Lang, Serge 23, 51, 244, 475, 481, 513
Lansky, Meyer 'Little Man' 135, 137, 139, 140, 178
Laurentian Hospital 23, 601
Laurentian University 23, 419, 432, 601
LAV 11–14, 269, 270, 377, 383, 522, 526, 558, 580, 599

Lederle Laboratories 66, 102, 125, 542, 543
Lemnitzer, Lyman 136, 299, 464, 465
Lennette, Edward H. 102, 125
Lennette, Evelyne 107, 109, 110
Lentivirus
Levine, Paul 239, 240, 241, 449, 565
Lewinski, Monica 340, 342
Litton Industries xi, 76–78, 209, 238, 242–244, 262, 263, 383, 555
Lo, Dr. Shyh-Ching xxvi, 9, 10, 26, 42, 90, 391–393, 428, 431, 457, 502, 520, 530, 554, 596, 602, 647
Lovett, Robert A. 63
Lumumba, Patrice 58, 71, 116
Lundberg, Ferdinand 62
Lupus 10, 42, 83, 322, 393, 396, 397, 432, 520, 567
Lyme disease xx, 83, 124, 143, 326
lymphadenopathy virus 12
lymphoid interstitial pneumonitis 19

M

MacArthur, Douglas 31–33, 284, 285, 396
MacArthur, Dr. Donald M. 271
Maedi 96, 230, 323, 534
Mahy, Brian xiii, 25, 97, 242, 377, 384–387, 389, 452, 474, 477, 510, 537
Manchester 79, 111, 166, 181, 230, 284, 549
Mannlicher-Carcano 6.5 mm 197
Marcello, Carlos 135, 140, 208, 211, 214
Marleau, Hon. Diane 81
McLean, J. S. xvii, xviii
McCloy, John J. 63, 177, 194, 202, 219, 254, 278, 286, 292, 294, 461, 462
MF ix, xiii, xxv, 10, 18, 24, 26, 43, 49, 97, 105, 108–110, 113, 128, 212, 215, 253, 261, 343, 348–351, 377–379, 384–386, 388, 394, 395, 407, 408, 416, 443, 446, 449–451, 453, 457, 460, 467, 468, 470, 472–474, 481, 565, 572, 602, 610, 612, 617, 635
Merigan, Thomas C. xxiii
Michigan State University 195
Miller, Merle 64

Minow, Nell 77
Mitchell, William 57
Mitochondria 601
MKDELTA ix, xxix, 25, 53, 57, 72, 74, 76, 78, 102, 116, 120, 128, 209, 211, 233, 236, 237, 246, 247, 277, 300, 301, 304, 306, 354, 468, 516, 532, 563, 593, 608, 610
MKNAOMI ix, xxix, 25, 57, 76, 102, 116, 128, 209, 233, 236, 246, 247, 277, 300–302, 468, 516, 532, 563, 593, 608, 610
MKULTRA ix, x, xii, xxix, 25, 53, 57, 64–66, 72, 74–76, 78, 101–103, 116, 117, 128, 136, 209, 233, 236, 237, 246, 247, 252, 277, 300–306, 354, 468, 516, 532, 544, 546, 548, 550, 563, 593, 608, 610, 616, 647
MMWR 4
Moloney, John 388, 512–514
Monks, Robert 77
Montagnier, Luc ix, 12, 49, 50, 52, 87, 269, 270, 377, 383, 522, 526, 545, 555, 558, 580
Montreal 138, 337, 354, 453, 566
Morbidity and Mortality Weekly Report 4
Mossadegh, Mohammad 67, 309
Mossad, Israeli 134, 135, 137, 614
Muguga 72
multiple sclerosis xx, 42, 44, 49, 83, 274, 349, 434, 487, 530, 531
Munich 197
Myalgic Encephalomyelitis 443, 639
mycoplasma xiii, xix, xxvi, xxx, 3, 8–10, 12, 14–19, 24, 26–28, 31, 41, 42, 44, 50–56, 65, 66, 75, 76, 81, 83, 89–92, 95–97, 99, 100, 102, 104, 108, 109, 111, 112, 143, 211, 229, 230, 233, 235, 238, 244, 245, 247, 261–263, 266, 273–275, 302, 319, 321–323, 327, 329, 332–334, 336, 349–351, 354, 379–383, 387, 389–391, 393–396, 398–401, 403, 423, 424, 428, 431, 434, 461, 475–477, 479, 482, 484, 485, 489–492, 494, 495, 498, 500, 510, 511, 514–517, 522, 526, 529–531, 539, 540, 543–545, 552, 555–558, 560–562, 564, 565, 567, 569, 571, 573, 574, 576, 578, 580, 608, 610–613, 615, 622

Mycoplasma ix, xx, xxvi, xxx, 8–12, 14, 17–19, 26, 27, 42, 54, 82, 103, 274, 321, 322, 326, 327, 332, 333, 335, 336, 382, 392, 398, 400, 424, 428, 431, 475, 483, 485, 502, 504, 520, 524, 528, 530, 533, 538, 544, 554, 555, 562, 567–569, 572, 573, 596, 602, 611, 612, 627, 629, 644–647

N

Nagell, Richard Case xi, 140
Nasser, Gamel Abdel 136
National Institute of Allergy and Infectious Diseases xxiv, 52, 474, 475
National Institutes of Health xxv, 21, 40, 46, 58, 59, 76, 88, 116, 244, 330, 380, 443, 469, 474, 480, 511, 553, 554, 612, 646
National Security Action Memorandum 136, 233, 465, 136, 233, 465
National Security Archive 21
National Security Council 70, 213, 252
New England Journal of Medicine xxvi, 306, 336, 419, 420, 528, 545
New Guinea 29–31, 33–35, 3–43, 143, 238, 360, 361, 395, 447, 532, 542, 561, 562, 594
Newman, John 69
New Orleans 66, 120, 127, 135, 140, 147, 153, 178, 190, 195, 207, 208, 210, 211, 214, 215, 338, 359, 459
New York xiii, xxix, 35, 43, 51, 56, 63, 66, 67, 71, 104, 119, 123, 124, 127, 128, 141, 149, 153, 182, 183, 185, 211, 212, 235, 243, 249, 254, 259, 262, 265, 279, 289, 293, 308, 340, 343, 366, 367, 388, 401, 417, 430, 443, 444, 446, 450, 462, 465, 468, 469, 472–476, 485, 489, 492, 494, 495, 497, 507, 510, 522, 532, 533, 542, 544, 566, 585, 609, 611, 635, 636–641, 642–644
Nicolson, Dr. Garth 328, 329, 335, 337, 349, 433, 450
N.I.H xxv, 533
Ninane, Gaston 72, 541
Nixon, Richard xii, 35, 38, 49, 55, 61, 69, 72, 73, 76, 78, 82, 117, 128, 133, 136, 139, 212, 219, 231, 234, 235, 242, 249, 251, 252, 257, 259, 261–264, 276, 280, 285, 288, 290, 297, 299, 300, 301, 354, 362, 459, 500, 514, 517, 537, 560, 595, 635, 637
Nocard, Dr. Edmond-Isidore 50
North Korea 61
Nucker, Christine M. 10
Nussbaum, Bruce 28, 492, 493, 578

O

Ochsner, Alton 38, 66, 120, 209, 211, 501, 532, 533, 556
Oleksyn, Sue xiv, 520, 521, 644
Oliver Stone 204, 288, 495
Olson, Dr. Frank 65
Osler's Web xxiv, xxv, 21, 22, 24, 107, 108, 110, 239, 241, 268, 407, 443, 444, 446, 447, 553, 639
Osler, William 22, 581
Osterrieth, Paul 72
Oswald, Lee Harvey 131, 139, 140, 145–148, 150–154, 156, 159, 160, 165, 167–169, 171, 172, 179–182, 184–187, 189, 193, 194, 196, 197, 199, 203, 204, 208, 210–212, 214, 217–219, 242, 286, 452, 460, 462, 463, 495, 556, 595, 637, 638, 639
Oswald, Marina 197, 199
Ottawa 80, 320, 329, 337, 639

P

Pahlavi, Shah Mohammad Reza 67
Paris 8, 19, 137, 383
Parkinson's disease xix, xxvi, 42, 44, 83, 95, 126, 348, 349, 390, 392, 396, 402, 535, 557
Parkland Hospital 19, 148, 162, 181, 186, 191, 194
Pasteur Institute xxx, 8, 19, 65, 89, 383, 420, 579
Patent Number 5, 242, 820
Patterson, Robert 63
PCP xix, 65, 111
Pentagon xxiii, xxiv, xxvi, 11, 34, 49, 74, 88, 93, 118, 123–126, 137, 138, 212, 229, 231, 252, 253, 261, 265, 271, 272, 275, 285, 289, 308, 315, 316, 325, 326, 343, 344, 347, 378, 408, 412, 413, 416, 417, 419, 451, 456, 457, 525, 529, 530, 550, 580, 585, 590, 596, 607, 609, 615
Peterson, Daniel xiii, 63, 446, 447

Philadelphia 71, 102, 104, 108, 109, 111, 533, 536, 547, 548, 561, 636
Plain Speaking 64, 640
pleural pneumonia-like organism 9, 19, 65, 89, 92, 491, 516, 522, 545
Pneumocystis carinii pneumonia xix, 6, 23, 65, 111, 269, 534
Power and Accountability 77
PPLO 9, 19, 65, 66, 81, 89, 91, 99, 109, 121, 211, 229, 233, 240, 244, 273, 387, 393, 400, 490, 491, 516, 517, 519, 524, 526, 539, 540, 543, 545, 610–612
Preston, D.R. 10
Prion 398
Prouty, Fletcher 59, 69, 283
Prusiner, Stanley 24, 399, 401

Q
Queensland fever 125, 509
Queen's University 80, 81, 338, 392, 487, 501, 536

R
Rauscher, Frank 31, 512
Ray, James Earl xi, 207, 214–216, 643
Reagan, Ronald xii, 270, 293, 299, 300, 306, 307, 316, 566, 609
Reed, Dr. Guilford B. 80, 229
Republican Party 63, 252, 339, 623
respiratory distress syndrome 10, 27, 42, 83, 241, 322, 393, 397, 428, 431, 502, 504, 520, 567, 568
retroviral x, xix, xxx, 3, 8, 38, 93, 97, 100, 108, 109, 242, 263, 519, 522, 535, 544, 576, 578
Rheumatoid Arthritis vi, 83
Rhode Island 55, 530, 574
ribonucleic acid 24, 43, 481, 488, 551
Riegle, Donald W. 317
Rivera, Dr. Jose 242, 452, 556
RNA 24, 27, 43, 54, 90, 92, 100, 126, 383, 387, 400, 401, 481, 482, 486–488, 490, 551, 552, 558, 560, 561, 611
Rockefeller, David 55, 213, 252, 254, 380, 460, 463, 465

Rockefeller Institute for Medical Research 59
Rockefeller, Nelson Aldrich 38, 45, 47, 55–60, 63, 65–69, 74, 76, 101, 116, 125, 127, 136, 209, 212, 229, 231, 233, 234, 242, 249–252, 254, 259, 277, 285, 286, 292, 295, 298, 343, 462, 514, 516, 532, 536, 537, 542, 547, 548, 608
Rockefellers' Medical Research Institute 56
Rockefeller Syndrome 62, 640
Rockefeller University 56, 409, 512
Rogue State 66, 67, 271, 433, 635
Rous, Peyton 610, 611
Roux, Dr. Pierre xxx, 8, 9, 19, 24, 50, 65, 89, 491
Ruby, Jack 134, 139, 140, 146, 186, 187, 189, 190, 195, 217, 218, 462
Russell, Dick 138, 140, 197, 284
Russell, Richard 219

S
Sabin, Albert 99, 550
Samuels, J. C.
San Francisco xxix, 68, 71, 104, 119, 124, 235, 239, 240, 416, 444, 522, 533, 587, 588, 609, 643
Sarcoidosis 10, 42, 83, 322, 392, 397, 431, 520, 567
Schlesinger, Arthur M. 63, 221
Scott, Donald W. i–iii, vii, xxv, 336, 351, 353, 448, 596
Scott, Peter Dale v, 133, 139, 146, 178, 197, 208, 260, 284, 287, 289, 291, 354, 384, 440, 459, 529
Scott, William L.C. i, iii, xxv, 337, 351, 353, 432
Shalala, Donna 340, 467
Shaw, Clay 147, 195, 208, 211, 214
Shea Jr., Quinlan J. 21
Sheehan, Neil 69
Shepard, Dr. Maurice C. 4
Sherman, John 202, 219
Shiro, Dr. Ishii ix, 29
Shorter, Dr. Edward 22, 385
Sigurdsson, Bjorn x, xxx, 3, 24, 38, 65, 93–95, 97, 105, 126, 230, 263, 267, 302, 382, 447, 522, 534, 536, 543, 549, 557, 574
Simpson, Leslie O. 331, 335, 450
Singer, S. Jonathon 44

Sirhan, Sirhan 223
SKMCC 243
Sloan-Kettering Memorial Cancer Center 243
Smadel, Dr. Joseph E. 34–37, 43, 46, 102, 105, 304, 507, 532, 547, 562
smallpox vaccination program 227, 261
Snead, Dr. Eva Lee 239
Some call it "AIDS" – I call it murder! 239
Speakes, Larry 234
Special Virus Cancer Program xi, 31, 53, 87, 91, 100, 108, 126, 233, 235, 238, 243, 245, 381, 419, 449, 500, 511, 513–515, 517, 522, 526, 536, 544, 545, 553, 554, 560–562, 575, 607, 608, 612, 646
Special Virus Leukemia/Lymphoma Program xxx, 230, 233, 235, 247, 252, 380, 381, 511, 517, 526, 552, 562, 607
Specter, Arlen 150, 194, 219
Standard Oil 62, 139, 143, 360
Stanleyville 71, 72, 117, 541
Starr, Ken 340, 342
Stevens, David A. xxiii, 553
Stone, Oliver 204, 288, 495
Straus, Stephen xxv
Sudbury ii, iii, 23, 81, 337, 345, 353, 402, 403, 408, 422, 425, 428, 429, 432–436, 448, 496, 601, 642
SVCP xi, 14, 31, 87, 91, 103, 126, 209, 231, 233–236, 238, 240, 242, 244, 246, 247, 274, 354, 380–382, 388, 419, 420, 511, 515, 526, 553–556, 560, 561, 608, 609, 612
SVLP xi, 14, 87, 88, 102, 116, 230, 231, 233, 235, 237, 244, 247, 252, 303, 354, 380–382, 387, 388, 511, 526, 607, 608, 610

T

Tanaka, Yuki 29, 238
The Health Century 58, 59, 642
The Journal of Degenerative Diseases 24, 421, 502
The Man Who Knew Too Much 140, 197, 642
The Passionate Eye 196
The Riegle Report 143, 318
The River xxv, 4, 24, 37, 72, 79, 108, 110, 241, 412, 441, 455, 457, 458, 507, 532, 541, 544, 546, 552, 566, 638, 641
The Vantage Point 220, 234, 236, 639
Thousand Days, A 63, 221, 222, 642
Time-Life 462, 465, 510
Ting, Dr. Robert 76, 243
Tripp, Linda 340, 342
Truly, Roy 140, 152, 154, 155, 157, 161, 163, 166, 171, 176, 179, 180, 200, 204, 205, 217
Truman, Harry 46, 47, 48, 64
Tulane University 66, 120, 127, 207, 209–211, 517, 556
Turner, Stansfield 64, 74, 75, 300, 301, 304, 516, 546, 563

U

United States ii, v, xii, xv, xvii, xx, xxiii, xxiv, xxv, xxvi, xxvii, xxix, 5, 7–11, 13, 20, 24, 35, 45, 47, 48, 49, 55, 56, 61, 62, 64, 66–72, 78, 79–83, 87, 90, 93, 95, 101, 102, 107, 110, 112, 115, 117, 119, 123, 127, 135, 137–139, 141, 150, 153, 158, 178, 182, 195, 196, 198, 203, 210, 212–215, 218–220, 222, 227, 236, 249, 250, 252–257, 259–265, 268, 269, 272, 273, 27–277, 280, 282, 286, 287, 289, 291, 292, 295, 297, 298, 308, 309, 310, 312, 313, 315, 317–320, 322, 325–328, 330, 331–335, 338–344, 350, 355, 359–362, 365, 383, 388, 393, 417, 419, 420, 422, 428, 431–433, 439, 441, 443, 444, 448, 453, 460, 462, 465, 467, 469, 470, 486, 493, 496, 497, 499, 500, 502, 511, 516, 518, 523, 532–534, 540, 543, 563, 565, 567, 574, 575, 586, 592, 596, 597, 607, 614, 615, 621, 622, 637, 646, 647
United States Armed Forces Institute of Pathology 9
United States Army 110, 137, 493
United States Government xv, xxv, xxvii, 7, 8, 24, 55, 64, 66, 69, 78, 83, 123, 263, 265, 272, 286, 383, 388, 393, 428, 469, 470, 497, 500, 502, 532, 534, 574, 646
United States of America v, xii, xvii, xxix, 254, 260, 312, 318, 500, 575
University of Guelph 22

V

Valerio, David 244
Vietnam x, 47–49, 66, 69, 70, 73–75, 115, 125, 128, 136, 137, 141, 212, 223, 224, 254, 258, 279, 280, 291, 293, 301, 308, 309, 343, 361, 365, 378, 380, 464, 465, 595, 608, 639, 641
virus xxix, xxx, 5–8, 12, 13, 15, 18, 19, 27–31, 33, 37, 38, 41, 42, 50, 54, 65, 79, 81, 91, 95, 96, 99, 107, 125, 132, 141, 209, 211, 234, 239–241, 245, 246, 267, 269, 322, 323, 352, 380, 382, 383, 387, 398–401, 409–411, 414, 416, 417, 424, 469, 472, 473, 476, 482–492, 494, 495, 498–503, 510–513, 515, 522, 524, 529, 532, 535, 540, 543–545, 547, 552–554, 556–558, 561, 563, 565–567, 569, 578, 580, 592, 597, 598, 610–613, 646
Virus Hunting 142, 209, 243, 378, 380, 382, 383, 512, 513, 554, 560, 637
Visna 96, 97, 230, 322, 323, 395, 556

W

Walker, Edwin 196, 197
Walter Reed Army Institute of Research 38
Warburg, Paul M. 55
Warren, Chief Justice Earl 202, 219
Warren Commission 138, 139, 148–151, 154, 158–160, 167–169, 171, 199, 200, 202–204, 211, 220, 222, 254, 288, 297, 299, 460, 495, 514
Warren Report 145, 147, 151–155, 159–161, 166, 170–174, 177, 180, 190, 194, 195, 199, 200, 203, 204, 222, 288
Washington, D.C. 9, 21, 36, 38, 138, 209, 219, 282, 288, 289, 317, 343, 433, 435, 461, 465, 589, 640, 641, 647
Washington Post 251, 265, 282, 283, 286, 378, 417, 465, 510
Watergate xii, xiii, 25, 36, 53, 60, 64, 103, 140, 177, 212, 214, 233, 249, 251, 254, 263, 264, 280, 282, 283, 285–289, 294, 298, 299, 301, 304, 370, 378, 445, 462, 586, 589, 635–638
Wegener's Disease 10, 42, 83, 392, 397, 431, 520, 567
Weisberg, Harold 146, 147, 153, 167, 181, 197, 199, 440, 459
Welch, Dr. William 56
West Germany 41, 137, 197
WHO xi, xxvi, 72, 227, 228, 229, 237, 253, 261, 378, 381, 383, 469, 477, 489, 495, 501, 502
Wiktor, Dr. T. J. 72
Wistar Institute 71, 102, 105, 109, 110, 118, 126, 127, 382, 451, 502, 533, 536, 546, 547, 613
World Health Organization xxvi, 55, 56, 227, 267, 277, 469, 470, 487, 495, 546, 559, 579
World Without Cancer 243
Wormsley, Susan xxv, 23

Z

Zaire 70, 71

Printed in the United States
111040LV00003B/95/P